Dedication

To our life's greatest works: Jessica "God's Grace" and our source of riches, Jared our one true "descendant from angels," and Eric and Alex our double miracle, strength, and inspiration. You are all our most precious treasures in life. It is through you that our values and accomplishments will be measured. Never forget that our love is for always and forever, Mom and Dad.

RJC
JBC

W9-CIO-262

Foreword

Among the pleasures which accrue from having been around a long time is that occasionally people ask you to do things that turn out to be both important *and* fun. One of the things I like to do is to review manuscripts of new text books. I know this does not sound like fun, but consider that if you stick with the process you get to see something that started as an idea progress from the concept stage through the various development phases until it develops and matures into a valuable addition to the literature. It is, in a sense, like watching a child or student grow in body and mind.

Usually the authors and reviewers don't know each others' identities at first—this makes for a level playing field. Occasionally, one or more of the reviewer–author combinations "click," and there begins a synergy where the ideas and applications of the authors and the critiques of the reviewer build upon each other to produce a work that is truly special. Among the best honor or award that a reviewer can receive is a request to write a foreword or introduction to a book that he or she has reviewed. So it is with a sense of honor that I respond to the authors' request to introduce their excellent laboratory manual.

While text books are difficult and time consuming to write, laboratory manuals may have more inherent problems of authorship and relevancy. This is especially so in the fast-changing field of respiratory care. Each program, each hospital, or alternate care site have their own particular mix of technology and technique—each assume that, in one fashion or another, their way is either superior or of a better "fit" than the next institution's methods. Attempting to develop and write a laboratory manual that will provide a comprehensive yet flexible guide through the intricacies of respiratory care equipment and procedures is in itself challenging. But to do so in a manner that is both student- and teacher-friendly is another matter entirely. Butler, Close, and Close have met these four challenges admirably.

From clearly stated objectives, a glossary, well thought out laboratory exercises and activities to valuable and usable appendices, this lab manual is an unusually thoughtful and well-conceived work. The use of plentiful illustrations and the detailed chapter introductory summaries of relevant theory set the stage for the various laboratory exercises. The manual should provide both students and instructors with tools that will ease the sometimes daunting path to mastery of respiratory care equipment, techniques, and procedures.

To the student: Good luck in your studies; to the instructors: Thanks for helping to insure and secure our futures; and to the authors: Congratulations on a job well done—and thank you for the privilege of both reviewing this fine work and allowing me to write this foreword.

Breathe Easy,
Paul J Mathews EdS, RRT, FCCM
Associate Professor
Respiratory Care Education
School of Allied Health
The University of Kansas Medical Center
Kansas City, Kansas

Preface

One of the most challenging tasks for any teacher is to invent, design, concoct, or manipulate learning activities that enhance critical thinking skills. Cookbook methodologies that simply have students assemble equipment and follow prescribed steps do not achieve any goal except slavish adherence to a procedure that has no variability. Additionally, when is the student permitted to explore and experiment with various pieces of equipment? Certainly not in the clinical setting!

This text had its conception in trying to achieve those goals. We wanted students to challenge themselves by exploring all possibilities. "What happens if I turn this up all the way?" "What if I connect this end instead?" Many of the exercises contained in this manual were inspired by actual events from our respiratory care laboratory. Over the years we have watched students try these things when we were not looking. Eventually we realized that we should not be stifling intellectual curiosity, but maximizing it to the benefit of the student and the profession. The exercises were then revised to be flexible while not being brand specific and the procedural competency evaluations (PCEs) adapted for laboratory or clinical evaluation. We hope that you join us in this philosophy and obtain the maximum benefit from this text.

Thomas J. Butler
Janice Blaer Close
Robert J. Close

Acknowledgments

A major project of this magnitude can never be accomplished single-handedly. The quality of the work is always enhanced through the contributions of others. We would like to thank several people who have assisted us over the long haul and without whose assistance this book would not have been completed.

First and foremost, a special thanks to Susan Gilbert, medical illustrator, whose dedication and perseverance was indispensable. Her vision and tremendous talent enabled her to take our vague and unclear instructions and turn them into fabulous illustrations.

We would like to thank the following reviewers, whose excellent input and insight helped broaden our perspective and expand the creativity of the exercises:

Lawrence A. Dahl, EdD, RRT
Instructor/Coordinator
Respiratory Therapy Technology Program
Hawkeye Community College
Waterloo, IA

Linda Dickson, BA, RRT
Clinical Director
Department of Respiratory Therapy
Sandhills Community College
Pinehurst, NC

Paul J. Mathews, EdS, RRT, FCCM
Associate Professor
Respiratory Care Education Department
University of Kansas Medical Center
School of Allied Health
Kansas City, KS

Yvonne Jo Robbins, MEd, RRT
Director, Respiratory Care
Main Line Health Hospitals
Bryn Mawr, PA

Their collective experiences helped improve the content and scope of all the chapters. We would especially like to thank Paul Mathews for staying with us from the beginning to the end of this long and sometimes arduous endeavor, and for his always thorough and valuable critiques. It was both a pleasure and an honor to have worked with such a distinguished professional.

We would also like to thank the following people, who reviewed the manuscript proposal:

William A. Byrtus, MEd, RRT
Program Director
Respiratory Care Department
Sandhills Community College
Pinehurst, NC

Bob DeLorme, EdS, RRT, RCP
Division Chair, Health Sciences
Program Director, Respiratory Therapy
Gwinnett Tech
Lawrenceville, GA

Martha DeSilva, MEd, BS, RRT
Program Director
Respiratory Therapy Department
Massasoit Community College
Brockton, MA

Ken D. McCarty, MS, RRT, RCP
Former Assistant Professor/Director of Clinical Education
Cardiopulmonary Department
Loma Linda University
Loma Linda, CA

Thank you alone can never fully express our gratitude to Mary Leighton, the world's best laboratory assistant, without whom the labs at Rockland Community College would never run.

Lastly, we would like to thank the students and graduates of Rockland Community College over the last years, who served as our experimental subjects to test the clarity of the text and the feasibility of the exercises included in the book. Often their curiosity, questions, and mistakes were the inspiration for our ideas.

Thomas J. Butler
Janice Blaer Close
Robert J. Close

Procedural Competency Evaluations

Contents

Introduction

Purpose and Scope of This Book

Over the last several decades, respiratory care has evolved from a limited technical support service to a sophisticated profession requiring complex skills and behaviors. Enrollment in a respiratory care program may represent a student's first exposure to professional education. As in other modes of education, a body of specialized knowledge must be mastered. Professional education is unique, however, in that it requires the student to skillfully apply this knowledge in practical settings, often with the patient's life in the balance. In addition, specific interpersonal skills and behavioral attributes must be developed for effective professional competence.[1]

Laboratory exercises are an essential and integral part of health professions education. Any laboratory text must include practice of the basic cognitive, psychomotor, and affective principles related to respiratory practice. This text is designed to provide the hands-on and communication skills necessary to integrate theory and clinical practice. This book is *not* intended to be an all-inclusive compendium of respiratory equipment or tasks or a replacement for the theoretical content found in other respiratory care texts; it is a complementary tool to be used in conjunction with other resources. It can, however, be used by students and instructors as a teaching, study, and evaluation tool in the preclinical or clinical setting.

The laboratory should be used as a risk-free environment for formative development of respiratory care skills. Students will be asked to assess their "patients," perform procedures, manipulate equipment, and determine settings to observe and experience the resulting consequences. The exercises are designed to promote critical thinking rather than solely to practice psychomotor skills. Some of the exercises are designed for students to *purposely* set up or use equipment incorrectly in order for them to differentiate the right way from the wrong way. It is better to explore these situations in a controlled laboratory setting than in a patient care environment. The text is flexible and general enough to cover these principles without being too specific as to particular brand name products, which may not always be available.

The manual is formatted so that most chapters can be completed in one or more formally scheduled 2-hour laboratory periods. The longer chapters may be divided into sections. The sequence of chapters is not intended to be rigid and may be assigned to suit curricular needs. The text is, however, detailed enough so that students could perform the exercises with minimal supervision in an independent practice setting as a supplement or replacement for a scheduled laboratory period.

Each chapter includes the following:

- An introduction
- Objectives
- Key terms
- A list of required equipment
- Exercises appropriate to content
- Tables summarizing normal, abnormal, and critical values where appropriate
- References
- Related readings
- A laboratory report form
- Procedural competency evaluations (PCEs) for each skill assessment
- Performance rating scale forms for each PCE

The key terms are not limited to vocabulary found in the text of the chapter. Terms that may be necessary to communicate effectively, understand concepts, or answer chapter questions are also included. All are defined in the glossary. Objectives are not limited to manipulation of equipment, but are geared toward both basic and higher-level cognitive, psychomotor, and affective skills. Troubleshooting exercises and verbal and written communication exercises are included where appropriate. Charting of procedures performed is extensively practiced.

Evaluation is a vital link in the teaching-learning process. A procedural competency evaluation (PCE) involves a demonstration of a specific respiratory care skill in conjunction with an assessment of the student's understanding and ability to apply the related theory. A copy of the PCE for each skill is available in each chapter for laboratory or clinical application. A complete list of all PCEs is included at the beginning of the text for easy reference. The skills included represent the most common entry-level and advanced procedures required of the respiratory care practitioner. The PCEs are intended to be used as study tools as well as evaluation tools. All procedures are in compliance with the AARC Clinical Practice Guidelines (CPGs).

The laboratory report form documents data collection during the exercises. Questions and clinically relevant scenarios are included in the report to enhance critical thinking skills, integrate theory with practice, and focus on the affective domain. The placement of this report allows for easy removal so that it may be submitted to the instructor, leaving the remainder of the manual intact for study, review, and additional practice.

References and recommended related readings are also included in each chapter. Relevant journal articles are included to encourage skills needed for lifelong learning. A glossary and appendices summarizing clinical formulas and common "rules of thumb" are found at the end of the main text.

Procedural Competency Evaluations

The task to be evaluated is identified on each PCE form. The evaluator may be a peer or an instructor. The PCE form may be used for student review or peer evaluation, preclinical evaluation in the laboratory setting, and for clinical competency evaluation. Multiple copies should be made for these purposes. Each competency evaluation consists of a list of steps in the task or procedure, definitions of acceptable performance, a scoring scheme, and a performance rating form.

When both the student and evaluator believe that a skill has been mastered, an evaluation session may be scheduled. It therefore follows that students should be fully prepared to demonstrate mastery *without assistance of any kind.* If it becomes necessary for the evaluator to intervene either to safeguard the patient's welfare or to expedite completion of the procedure, additional practice, laboratory or clinical, will be required and a repeat evaluation session will be necessary.

The student should fill out his or her complete name and the date of the evaluation, including the year. The conditions should be described, such as the level of patient cooperation; whether the procedure was performed on an infant, child, or adult; unexpected emergencies; if the procedure was simulated on a peer; or any other applicable variables. The equipment used (e.g., a particular brand of ventilator or spirometer) should be identified.

Detailed steps are included for each procedure. The sequence may occasionally vary, but there is usually a critical order for many steps. Certain common elements are required as part of every procedural competency to meet national practice standards and provide quality patient care. Three main categories of behaviors are Equipment and Patient Preparation, Assessment and Implementation, and Follow-up. Legal issues, such as verifying orders or respiratory protocols, patient identification, compliance with OSHA regulations or CDC guidelines for infection control, and documentation, are addressed. The procedures are not brand specific regarding equipment, but are intended to verify that the student can select, obtain, assemble, verify function, and correct malfunctions of the required equipment for the procedure. Students should always clean up after the procedure, adhering to infection control guidelines. The manner in which the student interacts with patients or other health care professionals should also be assessed. Students should be able to react appropriately to adverse reactions, notify appropriate personnel, and make recommendations to modify the patient care plan according to patient needs.

The scoring criteria reflect what the student knows, does, and says. Students should demonstrate knowledge of essential concepts as part of the procedural evaluation. The ability to apply, analyze, and synthesize didactic information in the clinical setting is needed for higher ratings. The procedures must be completed in a reasonable time frame consistent with patient safety and national time frame standards. Performance is rated as satisfactory or unsatisfactory. To obtain a satisfactory rating, the step must have been performed without critical error, without errors of omission or commission, and without significant prompting by the instructor. The instructor also has the option of choosing "not observed" or "not applicable" for any step. The "not observed" rating would be an addition to a satisfactory or unsatisfactory, where it is obvious that the step was done, but the instructor did not directly observe the activity. An example would be if a patient already had a blood pressure cuff on when the instructor entered the room to evaluate the PCE for blood pressure measurement. This may have been done correctly or incorrectly. "Not observed" may also indicate errors of omission, in conjunction with an unsatisfactory rating. If the student can correct noncritical errors without endangering patient safety or the validity of data, without prompting from the evaluator, a satisfactory rating should result.

Satisfactory completion of a given PCE requires more than a rigid adherence to the listed steps. The performance criteria include behaviors to be evaluated in addition to the procedural steps. Students are graded on these criteria using a scale of 1 to 5, with Level 1 being unacceptable performance and Level 5 being excellent, outstanding, or independent performance. Each item should be rated individually and independently, avoiding "middle-of-the-road" ratings.

Student performance should be rated using Level 3 as the starting point. Level 3 represents average or minimal competency. This level indicates that the student's performance is safe and effective without critical errors. The student is able to self-correct errors, reports information accurately, and demonstrates awareness of his or her own limitations. No directive cues or prompting is needed, but the student may require supportive cues. Some unnecessary energy may be used to complete the activity, and the student may occasionally be anxious and distracted as skills become more complex.

Performance at Level 1 indicates critical errors and unsafe practice, inability to demonstrate the behavior, or potentially harmful behaviors are noted frequently. The student demonstrates a lack of understanding of the basic concepts, inability to apply concepts or adapt to changing situations and is unaware of his or her limitations. The student lacks organization, appears frozen or is nonproductive, and requires continuous directive cues.

A rating at Level 2 is below minimal competency. Performance is marginal or below average, and although the student may perform safely under direct supervision, performance is not always accurate, and some critical errors are noted. Improvement is needed and significant problem areas still exist.

Level 4, above average or supervised performance, indicates that the student requires no directive prompting or correction, is able to self-correct errors, and is aware of his or her own limitations. Minimal supportive cues may be needed and some unnecessary energy may be used to complete activities.

A Level 5 performance rating is reserved for flawless performance, far exceeding expected level of performance. This is intended for the student who has superior knowledge, judgment, independence, and initiative. The student contributes to his or her own and the group's learning, spends minimal time on tasks, applies theory and rationale accurately each time, and uses subtle cues to modify his or her own behaviors.

The summary performance evaluation and recommendations section has two general ratings: satisfactory or unsatisfactory. Satisfactory performance in the preclinical setting allows the student to first apply the skill in the clinical setting. Satisfactory performance in the clinical setting verifies the student's terminal competency to perform the skill with minimal supervision and is achieved only when the student is capable of independent function. Unsatisfactory performance may include minor deficiencies requiring additional supervised clinical practice. More severe omissions or commissions result in additional required laboratory practice.

The evaluator should review the completed PCE evaluation with the student, emphasizing positive performance elements as well as areas needing improvement. Both evaluator and student should sign the completed PCE.

Laboratory Report

Efficient use of laboratory time depends on adequate preparation by the student. The assigned chapter should be read before the scheduled laboratory session, and related didactic information should be reviewed. Students are encouraged to practice all skills as frequently as necessary in order to master the art of communication and the performance of psychomotor tasks. This will require additional independent laboratory time outside of scheduled sessions. Students should not realistically expect to be competent after performing a skill once or twice in a laboratory setting or watching someone else perform the task.

Data collection and observations performed during the laboratory exercises should be documented completely and neatly on the laboratory report form. Each section of exercises and subsets that require documentation of data or observations is correlated with the corresponding number in the chapter. Exercises that do not require any documentation are excluded.

The laboratory session is intended for hands-on practice. Questions and calculations that do not involve direct contact with equipment or performance of procedures should be completed outside of laboratory time. Answers to the Critical Thinking Questions should be written out neatly or word processed and attached to the laboratory report. The question and corresponding number should be included in the attachment to facilitate ease of grading for the instructor.

The questions at the end of each laboratory report are not designed to be answered solely from performing the laboratory exercises and procedures, nor from a single reference source. Students are expected to research a variety of supplemental readings. Keeping current with the literature is an important part of professional development.

Students are expected to complete the laboratory report and all questions. The report should be submitted to the instructor by the assigned date. Deductions for late reports, according to individual programs' policies, are to be expected. The remainder of the laboratory chapter should be kept intact. Students may wish to keep returned graded laboratory reports for further review and study.

Laboratory Rules and Safety

In both the educational setting and clinical workplace, respiratory care students and practitioners will be working with equipment and materials and performing procedures that may result in injury or illness.

According to the Occupational Safety and Health Administration (OSHA) Hazard Communication Standard[2] and regulations in many states, employees have the right to know what they work with or could be exposed to that may be hazardous. They must be informed regarding what can be done to avoid injury or illness when working with these materials.

Students should be aware that in all health care facilities, respiratory care departments are required to maintain current policy and procedure manuals. These manuals include infection control and blood-borne pathogen plans, chemical hygiene plans, and other "right to know" information that may be required by state or federal regulations. The details of these policies and plans are beyond the scope of this book. However, students and instructors are strongly encouraged to review these materials during their clinical rotations.

Before performing any exercises from this book, the student should be oriented to the laboratory setting. The orientation should include the location of all equipment; waste and sharps disposal policies and procedures; and the mechanism for reporting defective equipment, needle sticks, and other injuries. Location of Material Safety Data Sheets (MSDSs) should be indicated. Orientation to these sheets is crucial and will also be beneficial in the clinical area.

There are some basic rules that must be followed in order to make the laboratory a safe and meaningful experience.

1. Students must read the assignments *before* the start of each laboratory session. It is important that there be a familiarity with terminology, equipment, and the types of exercises before beginning any practice.

2. For any independent practice, students must sign in and out according to laboratory policies.

3. Smoking, eating, and drinking should not be allowed in the laboratory area. Food should not be stored in the laboratory area. "No Smoking" signs should be posted even though most educational and health care institutions are "smoke free."

4. Applying cosmetics or contact lenses should not be permitted in the laboratory area.

5. All equipment must be handled with care. Compressed gas cylinders must never be left freestanding. Oil, grease, and any other flammable materials should not be used near oxygen equipment. Equipment should not be handled before instruction in its use is given by the instructor. Any defective or broken equipment must be reported immediately to the laboratory instructor or supervisor. This includes any equipment with frayed wires or loose connections. Immediately report any electrical equipment that is sparking or that causes a shock.

6. Personal protective equipment (PPE) should be used as required in the exercises.

7. Handle all chemicals and disinfecting solutions as instructed. MSDSs should be available for all substances kept in the laboratory. As an example, the MSDS for Clorox bleach is shown in Figure 1. The location and identification of the health risk, flammability, reactivity, personal protective equipment recommendations, and first aid procedures to be followed for this substance should be familiar to the student. The explanations of the codes used on an MSDS are given in Table 1.

8. Needles should *not* be recapped. All sharps should be disposed of in the puncture-proof containers provided.

9. Any injury or accidental needle stick should be reported immediately to the instructor or laboratory supervisor.

10. All students are responsible for cleaning up after each laboratory session. The laboratory personnel are not substitutes for housekeeping or mothers. Discard any papers or disposable equipment and supplies properly before leaving the laboratory.

11. Make sure all equipment is turned off and returned to its proper place before leaving.

12. Any disposable equipment that is assigned to students for repeated use (such as oxygen devices, noseclips, or mouthpieces) should be stored in a designated container and labeled with the student's name. It is the student's responsibility to maintain this equipment and have it available for the laboratory exercises.

13. Never remove equipment from the laboratory unless instructed to do so.

Where Does the Laboratory Fit In?

The laboratory experience is an invaluable part of respiratory care education. There is no substitute for hands-on investigation of the application of principles learned in the didactic portion of the educational program.

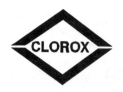

The Clorox Company
7200 Johnson Drive
Pleasanton, California 94588
Tel. (510) 847-6100

Material Safety Data Sheet

I Product:	CLOROX BLEACH - FOR INSTITUTIONAL USE
Description:	CLEAR, LIGHT YELLOW LIQUID WITH CHLORINE ODOR

Other Designations	Manufacturer	Emergency Telephone No.
EPA Reg. No. 5813-1 Sodium hypochlorite soultion Liquid chlorine bleach Clorox Liquid Bleach Clorox Germicidal Bleach	The Clorox Company 1221 Broadway Oakland, CA 94612	For Medical Emergencies, call Rocky Mountain Poison Center: 1-800-446-1014 For Transportation Emergencies, call: Chemtrec: 1-800-424-9300

II Health Hazard Data

*Causes substantial but temporary eye injury. May cause nausea and vomiting if ingested. Exposure to vapor or mist may irritate nose, throat and lungs. The following medical conditions may be aggravated by exposure to high concentrations of vapor or mist; heart conditions or chronic respiratory problems such as asthma, chronic bronchitis or obstructive lung disease. Under normal consumer use conditions the likelihood of any adverse health effects are low.

FIRST AID: EYE CONTACT: Immediately flush eyes with plenty of water. If irritation persists, see a doctor. SKIN CONTACT: Remove contaminated clothing. Wash area with water. INGESTION: Drink a glassful of water and call a physician. INHALATION: If breathing problems develop remove to fresh air.

III Hazardous Ingredients

Ingredients	Concentration	Worker Exposure Limit
Sodium hypochlorite CAS # 7681-52-9	5.25%	not established

None of the ingredients in this product are on the IARC, NTP or OSHA carcinogen list. Occasional clinical reports suggest a low potential for sensitization upon exaggerated exposure to sodium hypochlorite if skin damage (e.g. irritation) occurs during exposure. Routine clinical tests conducted on intact skin with Clorox Liquid Bleach found no sensitization in the test subjects.

IV Special Protection and Precautions

Hygienic Practices: Wear safety glasses. With repeated or prolonged use, wear gloves.

Engineering Controls: Use general ventilation to minimize exposure to vapor or mist.

Work Practices: Avoid eye and skin contact and inhalation of vapor or mist.

Keep out of the reach of children.

V Transportation and Regulatory Data

U.S. DOT Hazard Class: Not restricted

U.S. DOT Proper Shipping Name: Hypochlorite solution with not more than 7% available chlorine. Not Restricted per 49CFR172.101(c)(12)(iv).

EPA CERCLA/SARA TITLE III Superfund Amendment and Reauthorization Act:

	CERLA/304		
	RQ (lbs)	311/312	313
Sodium hypochlorite	100	----	---
Sodium hydroxide	1000	Yes	---

VI Spill or Leak Procedures

Small Spills (<5 gallons)
1) Absorb, containerize, and landfill in accordance with local regulations.
(2) Wash down residual to sanitary sewer.*

Large Spills (>5 gallons)
1) Absorb, containerize, and landfill in accordance with local regulations; wash down residual to sanitary sewer.* - OR - (2) Pump material to waste drum(s) and dispose in accordance with local regulations; wash down residual to sanitary sewer.*

VII Reactivity Data

Stable under normal use and storage conditions. Strong oxidizing agent. Reacts with other household chemicals such as toilet bowl cleaners, rust removers, vinegar, acids or ammonia containing products to produce hazardous gases, such as chlorine and other chlorinated species. Prolonged contact with metal may cause pitting or discoloration.

VIII Fire and Explosion Data

Not flammable or explosive. In a fire, cool containers to prevent rupture and release of sodium chlorate.

IX Physical Data

Boiling point . . . . 212°F/100°C decomposes)
Specific Gravity (H₂O=1) 1.085
Solubility in Water . . . . complete
pH 11.4

FIGURE 1   Material safety data sheet (MSDS) for Clorox. (Courtesy of the Clorox Co., Oakland, CA.)

HAZARDOUS MATERIAL IDENTIFICATION GUIDE

TYPE HAZARD

- ⬤ **HEALTH**
- ⬤ **FLAMMABILITY**
- ⬤ **REACTIVITY**
- ◯ **PROTECTIVE EQUIPMENT**

- 4 - Extreme
- 3 - Serious
- 2 - Moderate
- 1 - Slight
- 0 - Minimal

HAZARD RATING

Health

4—Extreme: Highly toxic— May be fatal on short-term exposure. Special protective equipment required.

3—Serious: Toxic—Avoid inhalation or skin contact.

2—Moderate: Moderately Toxic— May be harmful if inhaled or absorbed.

1—Slight: Slightly Toxic— May cause slight irritation.

0—Minimal: All chemicals have some degree of toxicity.

Flammability

4—Extreme: Extremely flammable gas or liquid—Flash Point below 73°F.

3—Serious: Flammable—Flash Point 73°F to 100°F.

2—Moderate: Combustible— Requires moderate heating to ignite. Flash Point 100°F to 200°F.

1—Slight: Slightly Combustible— requires strong heating to ignite.

0—Minimal: Will not burn under normal conditions.

Reactivity

4—Extreme: Explosive at room temperature.

3—Serious: May explode if shocked, heated under confinement or mixed with water.

2—Moderate: Unstable—may react with water.

1—Slight: May react if heated or mixed with water.

0—Minimal: Normally stable—does not react with water.

PROTECTIVE EQUIP.

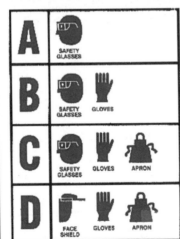

A — SAFETY GLASSES
B — SAFETY GLASSES, GLOVES
C — SAFETY GLASSES, GLOVES, APRON
D — FACE SHIELD, GLOVES, APRON

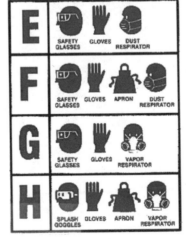

E — SAFETY GLASSES, GLOVES, DUST RESPIRATOR
F — SAFETY GLASSES, GLOVES, APRON, DUST RESPIRATOR
G — SAFETY GLASSES, GLOVES, VAPOR RESPIRATOR
H — SPLASH GOGGLES, GLOVES, APRON, VAPOR RESPIRATOR

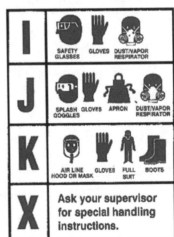

I — SAFETY GLASSES, GLOVES, DUST/VAPOR RESPIRATOR
J — SPLASH GOGGLES, GLOVES, APRON, DUST/VAPOR RESPIRATOR
K — AIR LINE HOOD OR MASK, GLOVES, FULL SUIT, BOOTS
X — Ask your supervisor for special handling instructions.

Lab Safety Supply Inc.

Reorder No. 20548R

TABLE 1 Hazardous material identification guide. (Sign courtesy of Lab Safety Supply Inc., Janesville, WI.)

Equipment and technology are constantly changing. It would be impossible for any text to address the extensive variety of equipment available or regional differences in procedures and techniques. National standards have been employed wherever possible. It is more important for students to integrate the basic principles and develop the critical thinking skills that can then be applied to any future circumstance.

Cognitive and psychomotor competency is only part of the total skills needed to be an effective respiratory care practitioner. Mastering affective behaviors such as verbal, written, and communication skills, self-direction, and responsibility; exhibiting sound judgment; establishing priorities; demonstrating thoroughness to detail and safety, and dependability are crucial to success during the educational process and in the job market.

Most important, health care workers are in a helping profession. Consideration of the patient's medical, physical, social, and psychological needs should be the primary concern. Competent respiratory care practitioners do more than turn dials, press buttons, and compile data. The human being at the other end of the machine is easily lost in the modern health care facility. Issues of patient confidentiality and emotional needs, as well as the practitioner's ability to interact effectively with other members of the health care team, are an integral part of respiratory care education.

The goal of the educational program should be to prepare respiratory care practitioners who can not only evaluate patients and situations, but adjust to changing conditions and make recommendations and modifications in the respiratory care plan in order to provide optimal but cost-effective patient care. Respiratory care practitioners must function as part of the health care team and develop multiple skills to succeed in the future.

It is the authors' fervent hope that this laboratory manual will help contribute to the education of well-rounded, competent respiratory care practitioners who can lead us in the next century.

References

1. Scanlan, C et al: Respiratory Therapy Competency Evaluation Manual. Blackwell Scientific, Boston, 1984, p vii.
2. Centers for Disease Control (CDC): NIOSH Recommendations for Occupational Safety and Health: Compendium of Policy Documents and Statements. U.S. Department of Health and Human Services, Public Health Service, DHHS (NIOSH) publication no. 92-100, 1992.

Related Readings

Selected Journal Articles

American Association for Respiratory Care: AARC Clinical Practice Guideline: Training the health-care professional for the role of patient and caregiver educator. Respir Care 41:654–657, 1996.
American Association for Respiratory Care: AARC Clinical Practice Guideline: Providing patient and caregiver training. Respir Care 41:658–663, 1996.

Infection Control

For centuries, infectious diseases have been the major cause of death in humans. Until recently, the scientific community believed that advances in the development of vaccines and antibiotic therapy would eliminate many infectious diseases by the 21st century. However, misuse and overuse of antibiotics, lax attitudes regarding the application of these advances, and the remarkable ability of microorganisms to adapt are threatening much of the progress made in the fight against infection.

As a result, we now find ourselves faced with a resurgence of diseases that were thought to be no longer a problem, including tuberculosis, measles, cholera, and typhoid.

Resistant strains of microorganisms and the discovery of previously unheard-of infectious diseases such as human immunodeficiency virus (HIV) are appearing in **epidemic** proportions. All are challenging our medical technology and altering the way health care is delivered.

The combination of a susceptible host, invasive procedures providing a route of transmission, and the presence of **virulent** and antibiotic-resistant strains of microbial organisms makes health care settings the perfect location for the transmission of infectious disease.

Recent concerns center around the protection of health care workers from blood-borne pathogens, which include but are not limited to hepatitis B virus, HIV, and related transmissible illnesses such as tuberculosis.[1]

Infection control in the health care setting has two primary goals. The first is to protect health care workers from transmissible diseases. The second is to reduce the incidence of **nosocomial** infections in susceptible patients. All health care personnel must maintain an up-to-date knowledge and compliance with most current guidelines.

We can reduce the risks to health care workers and patients by four methods[2]:

1. *Providing barriers to transmission.* This includes understanding the routes of transmission and applying standard (formerly universal) precautions and transmission-based isolation procedures to prevent transmission.

2. *Eliminating sources of infectious agents.* This includes decontamination, disinfection, and sterilization of equipment; proper disposal of infectious waste; and, most important, handwashing before and after patient contact, attending to any personal hygiene activities, and proper handling of dirty and clean equipment.

3. *Reducing host susceptibility.* This includes factors related to the patient's immune status, reducing exposure to sources of infection, appropriate use of antimicrobial agents, and limiting invasive procedures to only those that are essential.

4. *Monitoring and evaluating the effectiveness of infection control procedures.* This includes epidemiologic surveillance and quality management procedures.

Respiratory care practitioners, as part of the health care team, should be intimately familiar with issues concerning the **etiology** and **epidemiology** of infectious disorders. Each practitioner must adhere to established guidelines. Knowledgeable respiratory care practitioners can serve as positive role models and educators to reinforce the importance of every health care provider's responsibility in preventing and controlling infection.

1. Demonstrate effective handwashing technique.

2. Apply standard precautions and transmission-based isolation procedures according to Centers for Disease Control and Prevention (CDC) guidelines.

3. Distinguish between various types of isolation procedures and apply applicable precautions for each.

4. Practice procedures mandated by the Occupational Safety and Health Administration (OSHA) for the handling and disposal of infectious waste or equipment.

5. Differentiate between the methods for **decontamination, disinfection,** and **sterilization.**

6. Prepare equipment for the most commonly used methods of decontamination, disinfection, and sterilization.

7. Practice monitoring techniques for evaluating the effectiveness of infection control procedures.

8. Practice communication skills needed to explain infection control procedures to patients.
9. Practice documentation of infection control procedures.

KEY TERMS

aerobe
anaerobe
antiseptic
asepsis
aseptic
bacteremia
bactericidal
bacteriostatic
cell-mediated
colonization
commensalism
condensate
debilitated
decontamination
desiccation

disinfectant
disinfection
endemic
endocytosis
endotoxin
enteric
epidemic
epidemiology
etiology
eukaryotic
exotoxin
facilitate
facultative
fastidious
fomite
hemolytic

homogeneous
humoral
immunology
immunosuppression
infection
inhibition
morphology
mutualism
mycology
necrosis
nosocomial
obligate
opportunistic
optimum
parasitism
pathogen

phagocytosis
prokaryotic
proliferation
prophylactic
prophylaxis
pus
sepsis
septicemia
sterilization
symbiosis
synergism
vector
virology
virulence
virulent

EQUIPMENT REQUIRED

- Sink with running water
- Antimicrobial liquid soap in dispenser
- Bar soap
- Paper towels
- Stopwatch
- Disposable latex and vinyl gloves in various sizes
- Sterile gloves in various sizes
- Surgical masks
- Isolation head and foot coverings
- Disposable isolation gowns
- Protective eyewear
- Disposable high efficiency particulate aerosol (HEPA) filter masks
- Sample isolation signs
- Sharps containers
- Sample syringes, "contaminated" equipment and waste
- Infectious waste bags with biohazard labels
- Agar plates
- Culture swabs
- Various size equipment brushes
- Detergent solution
- **Aseptic** area/field for drying equipment
- Various bags and wraps for equipment packaging
- Chemical indicator tape
- Biological indicator vials

● EXERCISES

EXERCISE 1.1 Handwashing

Proper handwashing before and after any patient contact is one of the single most important infection control procedures.

1. Remove jewelry and watch.
2. Adjust water flow and temperature using foot pedals, if available, as shown in Figure 1.1, or hand faucet controls.
3. Wet forearms and hands.
4. Apply disinfectant liquid soap liberally.

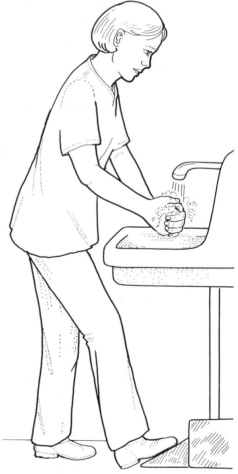

FIGURE 1.1   Adjusting water flow using foot pedals.

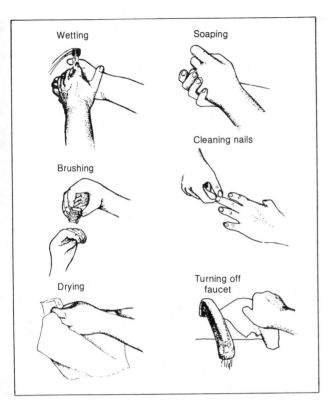

FIGURE 1.2 Handwashing technique. (From McLaughlin, AJ Jr: Manual of Infection Control in Respiratory Care. Little, Brown & Co., Boston, 1983, p. 85, with permission.)

5. Wash with strong friction for as long as you feel appropriate. Have your partner use a stopwatch to time how long you wash. *Record the initial time on your laboratory report.* You should scrub the following as shown in Figure 1.2:
   a. Palms
   b. Between digits
   c. Under fingernails and around cuticles with a brush
   d. Wrists and forearms
   NOTE: Make sure you do not touch the sink with your hands or body.
6. Handwashing should be done for a minimum of 15 seconds.[3] If you did not achieve this time initially, repeat step 5.
7. Rinse from the forearm to the fingertips, ensuring that all soap solution has been removed.
8. Obtain paper towels aseptically.
9. Dry hands individually, using separate towels.
10. Turn off water faucets using a dry, clean towel if foot pedals are not available.
11. Discard paper towels in an appropriate waste container.

EXERCISE 1.2 Barrier Precautions/ Personal Protective Equipment

EXERCISE 1.2.1 Standard Precautions/ Transmission-Based Isolation Procedures

Protecting our patients and ourselves against infection requires strict adherence to current infection control procedures.[1,4] To create barriers to transmission, one must be aware of the routes of transmission of infectious disease (Fig. 1.3).

1. Review all signs and posters for standard precautions and transmission-based isolation procedures.
2. Review all category-specific isolation precautions[4] as in Table 1.1. The CDC classifies four categories for isolation procedures: standard, airborne, droplet, and contact precautions. Standard precautions synthesized the major features of universal (blood and body fluid precautions) and body substance isolation.[5] Transmission-based precautions are designed for patients documented or suspected to be infected with highly transmissible or epidemiologically important pathogens for which additional precautions are needed to interrupt transmission.[5] Airborne precautions are designed to reduce the risk of transmission of infectious agents by droplet nuclei or dust particles. Droplet precautions reduce the transmission of infectious agents through large droplet contact (greater than 5 μ) such as occurs with coughing, sneezing, or talking. Immunocompromised patients, such as those with cancer, leukemia, severe burns, or organ transplants, are generally at increased risk for bacterial, fungal, parasitic, and viral infections from both endogenous and exogenous sources.[6] The use of standard precautions for all patients and transmission-based precautions for specified patient should reduce the acquisition by these patients of nosocomial infections.
3. Obtain all personal protective equipment (PPE) required for standard transmission-based isolation procedures. Hands should be washed before this procedure. Apply the equipment in the following order[3] (Fig. 1.4):
   a. Hair and foot coverings. Make sure all of your hair is covered.
   b. Gown.
      (1) Open gown fully.
      (2) With the opening in the back, insert your arms into the sleeves.
      (3) Fasten ties at the neck and waist.
   c. Mask. Make sure that both your nose and mouth are completely covered and the mask is tied to the back of the head. A surgical mask should be changed frequently because it is ineffective once it becomes wet.
   d. Goggles or face shield. Although not part of required strict isolation equipment, goggles or face shield may be necessary if splashing of blood or body fluids is anticipated.
   e. Gloves. Gloves should fit well. Examine for any tears or holes and replace if necessary. Vinyl gloves may be substituted if latex sensitivity is a problem.

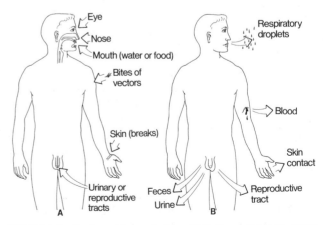

FIGURE 1.3 Routes of transmission of infectious diseases. (From Scanlon, VC and Sanders, T: Essentials of Anatomy and Physiology, ed 2. FA Davis, Philadelphia, 1991, p. 510, with permission.)

Know this table.

TABLE 1.1 **Isolation Precautions**

Category*	Requirements	Selected Indications
Standard (Universal)	Handwashing with nonantimicrobial soap	Routine; before and after all patient contact
	Handwashing with antimicrobial soap	For specific outbreaks as defined by infection control program
	Gloves	When touching blood, body fluids, secretions, mucous membranes, nonintact skin
	Mask, eye protection, face shield	For procedures likely to generate splashes or sprays of blood, body fluids, secretions, and excretions
	Gown	For procedures and activities that are likely to generate sprays or splashes or cause soiling
	Patient-care equipment	To prevent skin and mucous membrane exposures and contamination of clothing; clean and reprocess reusable equipment between patients; discard single-use items
	Environmental control	Routine care: cleaning and disinfection of environmental surfaces, beds, bedrails, bedside equipment; blood spills should be cleaned up promptly with 5.25% solution sodium hypochlorite diluted 1:10 with water
	Linen	Handle, transport, and process used linen soiled with blood, body fluids, secretions, and excretions to prevent skin and mucous membrane exposures, contamination of clothing and avoid transfer of microorganisms to other patients and environments
	Occupational health and blood-borne pathogens	Prevent injuries when using, cleaning, or disposing of needles, scalpels, and other sharps; do not bend, break, or otherwise manipulate by hand; never recap using any technique involving point of sharp toward any part of the body
	Private room	For patient who contaminates the environment or who cannot assist in maintaining hygiene or environmental control
Airborne	_In addition to standard precautions:_ Private room with door closed and monitored negative air pressure; 6 to 12 air changes per hour; discharge of air outdoors or monitored HEPA filtration of room air Respiratory protection Limit patient transport, mask patient	Patients known or suspected by organisms transmitted by airborne droplet nuclei; measles (rubeola); chicken pox varicella; tuberculosis
Droplet	_In addition to standard precautions:_ Private room Mask when working within 3 feet of patient Limit patient transport, mask patient	Known or suspected to be infected with microorganisms transmitted by large particle droplet (>5µ) that can be generated during coughing; sneezing, talking, or performance of procedures
		Invasive _Hemophilus influenzae_ type disease including meningitis, pneumonia, epiglottitis and sepsis; invasive Neisseria meningitidis disease including meningitis, pneumonia and sepsis; diphtheria, _Mycoplasma_ pneumonia, pertussis, pneumonic plague, streptococcal, pharyngitis, pneumonia or scarlet fever in infants and young children; adenovirus, influenza, mumps rubella
Contact	_In addition to standard precautions:_ Private room Masks Gloves when entering room; change when soiled and before leaving room Gowns when entering room if soiling likely change after contact with infective material	Gastrointestinal, respiratory, skin and wound or colonization by multidrug-resistant bacterial infections such as methacillin resistant _Staphylococcus aureus_ (MRSA) Enteric infections with low infectious dose including _Clostridium difficile_; infectious diarrhea from _Escherichia coli, Shigella,_ hepatitis A or rotovirus Respiratory syncytial virus, parainfluenza virus or enteroviral infections in infants and young children Skin infections that are highly contagious including diphtheria (cutaneous), herpes simplex virus, impetigo, major abscesses, cellulitis or decubiti, pediculosis, scabies; zoster; viral hemorrhagic conjunctivitis; viral hemorrhagic infections including Ebola, Lassa, and Marburg virus

(handwritten annotations: "AFB MRSA acid fast Bacilli unicreant" / "TB" near Airborne row; "Vancomizin antibiotic" near MRSA)

*NOTE: Hands must be washed after touching patient or potentially contaminated articles for all categories. Contaminated articles should be discarded or bagged and labeled.

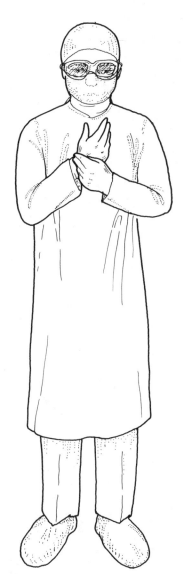

FIGURE 1.4 Personal protective equipment (PPE).

4. Remove all PPE in the following sequence:
   a. Head and foot coverings.
   b. Mask and goggles.
   c. Gloves. Gloves should be removed by pulling down from the wrist and turning them inside out.
   d. Gown. After untying neck and waist, remove gown inside out.
5. Discard disposable items in infectious waste container. (For purposes of laboratory practice, PPE may be saved to reuse in later exercises.)
6. Wash hands.

EXERCISE 1.2.2 Application of Sterile Gloves

When applying sterile gloves it is important to follow the proper sequence of steps to prevent contamination, as shown in Figure 1.5.

During this exercise, you will be placing a glove on your dominant hand first, using the opposite (nondominant) hand to handle the glove. If you are right-handed, your right hand is your dominant hand and your left hand is your nondominant hand. If you are left-handed, the opposite is true.

1. Obtain proper size package of sterile gloves.
2. Wash hands.
3. Open package aseptically and unfold it completely, making sure both gloves are accessible. Do not touch the inside of the package (Fig. 1.5 A).
4. Using your nondominant hand, insert two or three fingers into the cuffed (folded) portion of the glove that will be pulled onto your dominant hand. Make sure not to touch any part of the glove other than the outside of the folded portion of the cuff (Fig. 1.5 B).
5. Slide your dominant hand into the glove as far as possible. Now raise your hand and apply the glove completely. Use your nondominant hand to pull the glove on while touching only the *inside* of the glove (Fig. 1.5 C).
6. Using your gloved dominant hand, pick up the other glove, again using two or three fingers inserted into the cuffed portion (Fig. 1.5 D).
7. Slide your ungloved nondominant hand into the glove as far as possible. Now raise your hand and apply the glove completely. Do not touch your skin with the sterile gloved hand. Pull the glove on by the cuff while touching only the *outside* of the glove (Fig. 1.5 E).
8. Remove gloves. Gloves should be removed by pulling them down from the wrist and turning them inside out.
9. Discard gloves in infectious waste container.

EXERCISE 1.2.3 Airborne/Droplet Precautions

OSHA regulations for tuberculosis precautions now require the use of a high efficiency particulate aerosol (HEPA) mask as part of personal protective equipment or other similar devices recommended by the National Institute for Occupational Safety and Health (NIOSH).[5,6] NIOSH certifies three types of masks as acceptable: HEPA 100, with a 99.97 percent efficiency rate; HEPA 99, with a 99 percent efficiency rate; and HEPA 95, with a 95 percent efficiency rate. OSHA relies on NIOSH certification for its recommendations. Review the current CDC recommendations for respiratory/tuberculosis isolation precautions.

1. Obtain disposable HEPA filter mask. Read the directions on the manufacturer's label.
2. Apply the mask according to the manufacturer's directions, as shown in Figure 1.6. Make sure the mask fits well.

   NOTE: Facial hair may interfere with the effective functioning of this mask. Also, health care providers may need medical clearance to wear these types of masks for any length of time. Preexisting pulmonary disease or reduced flow rates may cause difficulty in breathing through these masks. Your medical director should be consulted regarding guidelines.
3. Leave the mask on for 5 minutes, as tolerated. *Record your observations on your laboratory report.*

EXERCISE 1.3 Handling and Disposal of Infectious Equipment and Waste

In this exercise, you are simulating entering the room of a patient in contact isolation to discard disposable infectious waste and safely remove a piece of reusable respiratory equipment for transport to the disinfection area. The instructor will have the "room" prepared with equipment to be discarded and to be transported.

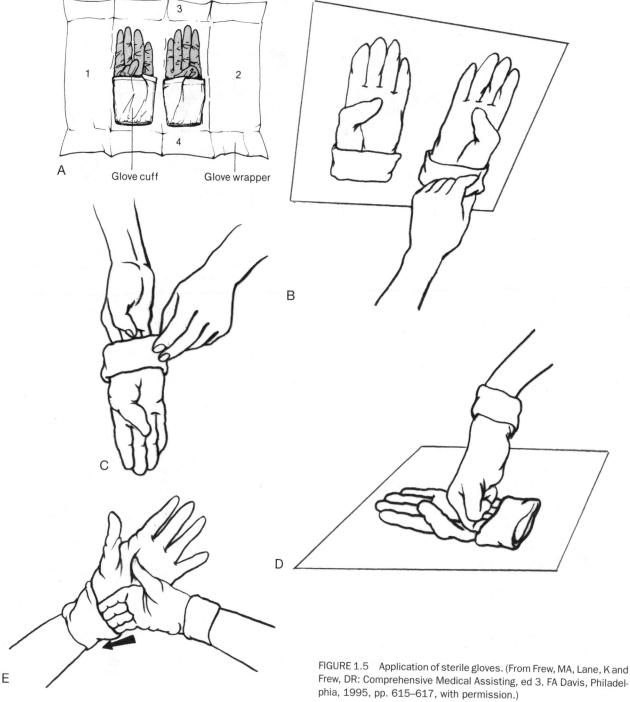

Glove cuff   Glove wrapper

A

B

C

D

E

FIGURE 1.5   Application of sterile gloves. (From Frew, MA, Lane, K and Frew, DR: Comprehensive Medical Assisting, ed 3. FA Davis, Philadelphia, 1995, pp. 615–617, with permission.)

1. Wash your hands as previously instructed.
2. Apply the required PPE for contact isolation.
3. Enter the "patient's room."
4. Carefully dispose of any sharps (needles, syringes, lancets) into the puncture-proof sharps container (Fig. 1.7). If the container is full, replace it with a new one.
5. Obtain infectious waste bags labeled with a biohazard indicator.
6. Place the reusable equipment into the infectious waste bag, secure it, and label it as in Figure 1.8. Be careful not to contaminate the outside of the bag.

7. Leave the "room." Remove your PPE in the sequence previously described, and discard it in an infectious waste container.

EXERCISE 1.4 Preparation of Equipment for Disinfection/Sterilization

The instructor will provide nondisposable equipment for this exercise. Although specific requirements vary with the method of disinfection or sterilization to be used, there are steps in equipment preparation common to all modalities.

• Fitting instructions to be followed each time respirator is worn

1 Prestretch top and bottom straps before placing respirator on the face.

2 Cup the respirator in your hand, with the nosepiece at your fingertips, allowing the headbands to hang freely below your hand.

3 Position the respirator under your chin with the nosepiece up. Pull the top strap over your head resting it high at the top back of your head. Pull the bottom strap over your head and position it around the neck below the ears.

4 Place your fingertips from both hands at the top of the metal nosepiece. Using two hands, mold the nose area to the shape of your nose by pushing inward while moving your fingertips down both sides of the nosepiece. Pinching the nosepiece using one hand may cause a bad fit and result in less effective respirator performance. Use two hands.

5 The seal of the respirator on the face should be fit checked prior to each wearing. To check fit, place both hands completely over the respirator and exhale. Be careful not to disturb the position of the respirator. If air leaks around nose, readjust the nosepiece as described in step 4.

If air leaks at the respirator edges, work the straps back along the sides of your head.

FIGURE 1.6   Application of high efficiency particulate aerosol (HEPA) filter mask. (Courtesy of 3M Occupational Health and Environmental Safety Division, St. Paul, Minnesota.)

Not all schools have the facilities to conduct all parts of this exercise. If access to disinfection/sterilization equipment and areas is available, students should perform all elements. If not, students should perform steps 1 through 8 and then examine the materials necessary for the remaining steps.

1. Put on PPE, including gloves and gown.
2. Completely disassemble the equipment into its smallest parts.
3. Examine the equipment for any tears, cracks, or pitting. Equipment should be discarded if defective because these defects can provide a safe hiding place for microorganisms.
4. Soak the equipment for at least 10 minutes in a warm solution of disinfecting detergent agent.
5. Scrub the equipment parts thoroughly, making sure to get into any crevices (Fig. 1.9).
6. Rinse the equipment thoroughly with tap water.
7. Set the equipment out to dry on aseptic absorbent disposable towels provided for this purpose.
8. Reassemble the equipment. Loosely secure any parts so that the disinfection/sterilization method can penetrate.
9. Once the equipment is reassembled, it is ready for the appropriate sterilization method:
   a. For autoclave or "gas sterilization" with ethylene oxide, the equipment is first packaged in the appropriate materials; sealed; labeled with time, date, load, and technician signature; and marked with chemical indicator tape (Fig. 1.10). The equipment is then sterilized and aerated, if necessary. Any required paperwork should be completed according to institution policy.
   b. For "cold sterilization" with glutaraldehyde, protective eyewear should be worn. The equipment is next soaked in the disinfecting solution for 10 minutes to 10 hours,

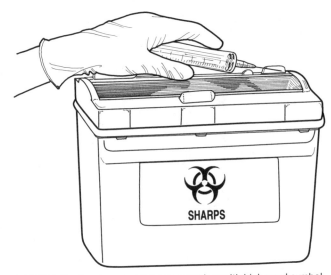

FIGURE 1.7   Puncture-proof sharps container with biohazard symbol.

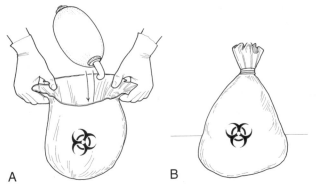

FIGURE 1.8   Bagging of contaminated equipment.

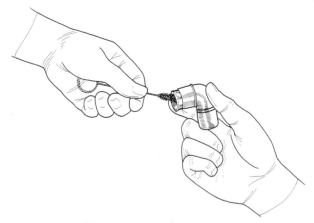

FIGURE 1.9 Scrubbing equipment.

depending on whether disinfection or sterilization is to be achieved. The technician then puts on sterile gloves and prepares a sterile field. The equipment is then aseptically rinsed with sterile water, dried on the sterile field, and packaged for storage. The package should be labeled with the date, time, and technician signature. Any required paperwork should be completed according to institution policy.

c. For pasteurization, the equipment is loaded into the machine and run through the cycle. The equipment is then dried and packaged for storage. The package should be labeled with the date, time, and technician signature. Any required paperwork should be completed according to institution policy.

EXERCISE 1.5 Monitoring Infection Control Procedures

Monitoring of infection control techniques is essential in evaluating their effectiveness. This can be accomplished by a variety of microbial culture techniques, depending on the item to be cultured.

Not all schools have the facilities to conduct all parts of this exercise. If access to a microbiology laboratory is available, students should perform all elements.

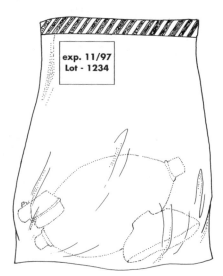

exp. 11/97
Lot - 1234

FIGURE 1.10 Packaging of equipment for sterilization.

EXERCISE 1.5.1 Biological Monitors

Examine the biological monitor vials or strips used for autoclave and ethylene oxide sterilization (Fig. 1.11).

EXERCISE 1.5.2 Swab Culturing

Swab culturing may be used to take spot cultures of various surfaces, such as tracheostomy stoma sites (Fig. 1.12).

1. Wash your hands thoroughly.
2. Obtain the sterile swabs and culture medium tubes.
3. Using separate culture swabs and tubes, culture each of the following:
   a. The palms of your hands
   b. The drain area of the sink
   c. Bar soap
4. Rub the swab back and forth over the area to be cultured. Aseptically replace the swab in the culture tube.
5. Seal the culture tube. Label it with the date, time, and area cultured.
6. Send the culture tube to the microbiology laboratory for culturing and identification.
7. When results are available, *record them on your laboratory report.*

EXERCISE 1.5.3 Culturing Aerosol and Gas Sources

For this exercise, the instructor will have a large-volume aerosol delivery system available.

1. Wash your hands thoroughly and put on gloves.
2. Obtain an agar plate.
3. Expose the surface of the plate to the aerosol directly, as shown in Figure 1.13, without allowing the tube to touch the surface of the agar. A commercially available funnel device may be used to minimize contamination of the sample.

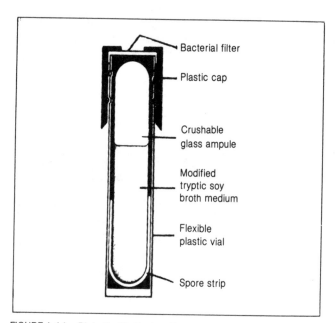

FIGURE 1.11 Biological indicator. (From McLaughlin, AJ Jr: Manual of Infection Control in Respiratory Care. Little, Brown & Co., Boston, 1983, p. 72, with permission.)

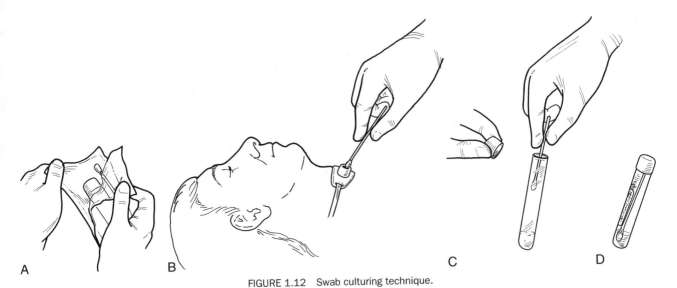

FIGURE 1.12   Swab culturing technique.

4. Seal the agar plate. Label with the date, time, source of sample, and technician signature.

5. Send the sample for culturing.

6. When results are available, *record them on your laboratory report.*

References

1. Occupational Safety and Health Administration: Regulations for bloodborne pathogens. Federal Register, 29 CFR Section 1910.103, January 29, 1992, pp 41–47.

2. Scanlan, C et al (eds): Egan's Fundamentals of Respiratory Care, ed 6. Mosby, St Louis, 1995, p 52.

3. Centers for Disease Control: Guideline for handwashing and hospital environmental control, 1985. US Department of Health and Human Services, Atlanta, 1985.

4. Centers for Disease Control and Prevention: Guideline for isolation precautions in hospitals. Part II: Recommendations for isolation precautions in hospitals. AJIC 24:32–52, 1996.

5. Centers for Disease Control and Prevention: Guideline for isolation precautions in hospitals. Part II: Recommendations for isolation precautions in hospitals. AJIC 24:36–37, 1996.

6. Centers for Disease Control and Prevention: Guidelines for preventing the transmission of *Mycobacterium tuberculosis* in health-care facilities, 1994. US Department of Health and Human Services, Atlanta, 1994, 43:1–32.

Related Readings

Eubanks, DH and Bone, RC: Principles and Applications of Cardiorespiratory Care Equipment. Mosby, St Louis, 1994.

Hopp, J and Rogers, E: AIDS and the Allied Health Professions. FA Davis, Philadelphia, 1989.

McLaughlin, AJ and Palermo, R: Manual of Infection Control in Respiratory Care, ed 2. Aspen, Gaithersburg, MD, 1996.

McPherson, S: Respiratory Care Equipment, ed 5. Mosby, St Louis, 1995.

NYU Regional AIDS Education Center: HIV/AIDS Education: A Curriculum Guide, Part I, III. AIDS Education Center, New York, 1989.

Rau, J: Respiratory Care Pharmacology, ed 4. Mosby, St Louis, 1994.

Rukeyser, J: HIV/AIDS Education: A Curriculum Guide for Respiratory Therapists and Cardiovascular Technologists. State University of New York at Stony Brook, Stony Brook, NY, 1993.

Scanlan, C et al (eds): Egan's Fundamentals of Respiratory Care, ed 6. Mosby, St Louis, 1995.

Selected Journal Articles

AHA questions cost, scope of CDC draft TB guidelines. TB Monitor, 1:41–42, 1994.

Boyce, J: Increasing prevalence of methicillin-resistant *Staphylococcus aureus* in the United States. Infect Control Hosp Epidemiol 11:639–642, 1990.

Boyce, JM: Methicillin resistant *Staphylococcus aureus* in hospitals and long-term care facilities: Microbiology, epidemiology and pre-

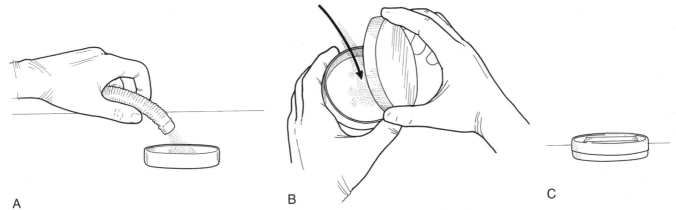

FIGURE 1.13   Technique for aerosol or gas source culturing.

ventive measures. Infect Control Hosp Epidemiol 13:725–737, 1992.

Brudney, K and Dobkin, J: Resurgent tuberculosis in New York City. Am Rev Respir Dis 144:745–749, 1991.

Centers for Disease Control and Prevention: Essential components of a tuberculosis prevention and control program: Screening for tuberculosis and tuberculosis infection in high risk populations. MMWR 8:RR-11, 1995.

Centers for Disease Control: Guideline for handwashing and hospital environmental control, 1985. US Department of Health and Human Services, Atlanta, 1985.

Centers for Disease Control and Prevention: Guidelines for preventing the transmission of *Mycobacterium tuberculosis* in health-care facilities, 1994. US Department of Health and Human Services, Atlanta, 43:RR-13, pp 33–34.

Centers for Disease Control and Prevention: Guideline for prevention of nosocomial pneumonia. Respir Care 39:1191–1236, 1994.

Centers for Disease Control and Prevention: Recommendations for preventing the spread of vancomycin resistance. MMWR 44:RR-12, 1995.

Centers for Disease Control: Update: Universal precautions for prevention of transmission of human immunodeficiency virus, hepatitis B virus, and other blood-borne pathogens in the health care setting. MMWR 37:377–399, 1988.

Chatburn, R: Decontamination of respiratory care equipment: What should be done, what can be done. Respir Care 34:98–110, 1989.

Chatburn, R et al: A comparison of acetic acid with a quaternary ammonium compound for disinfection of hand held nebulizers. Respir Care 33:179–187, 1988.

Craven, D and Steger, K: Pathogenesis and prevention of nosocomial pneumonia in the mechanically ventilated patient. Respir Care 34:85–97, 1989.

Culver, DH et al: Surveillance of HIV infection and zidovudine use among health care workers after occupational exposure to HIV-infected blood. Ann Intern Med 118:913–919, 1993.

Hess, D: Guideline for prevention of nosocomial pneumonia and ventilator circuits: Time for change? Respir Care 39:1149–1153, 1994.

Hierholzer, WJ: Guideline for prevention of nosocomial pneumonia. Respir Care 39:1191–1237, 1994.

Hooton, T: Protecting ourselves and our patients from nosocomial infections. Respir Care 34:111–115, 1989.

Horan, TC et al: Nosocomial infections in surgical patients in the United States. Infect Control Hosp Epidemiol 14:73–80, 1993.

McQueen, MJ: Conflicting rights of patients and health care workers exposed to blood-borne infection. Can Med Assoc J 147:299–302, 1992.

New CDC TB guidelines: Risk assessments trigger move to formal TB programs. Hospital Infection Control 20:149–154, 1993.

Occupational Safety and Health Administration: Regulations for blood-borne pathogens. Federal Register, January, 1992, pp 41–47.

Panlilio, AL et al: Methicillin-resistant *Staphylococcus aureus* in US hospitals. Infect Control Hosp Epidemiol 13:582–586, 1992.

Schaberg, DR: Enterococcal infections: An increasing problem in hospitalized patients. Infect Control Hosp Epidemiol 9:457–461, 1988.

Schaberg, DR: How infections spread in the hospital. Respir Care 34:81–84, 1989.

Schaberg, D and Culver, D: Major trends in the microbial etiology of nosocomial infections. Am J Med 91(suppl 3B):72S–75S, 1991.

Steinberg, KP: Nosocomial pneumonia: From prophylaxis to management. RT 7:74–76, 1994.

LABORATORY REPORT

CHAPTER 1: INFECTION CONTROL

Name _____   Date _____

Course/Section _____   Instructor _____

Data Collection

EXERCISE 1.1   Handwashing

Time of initial handwashing in seconds: _____

EXERCISE 1.2.3   Airborne/Droplet Precautions

Observations wearing HEPA filter mask: _____

_____

_____

EXERCISE 1.5.2   Swab Culturing

Date	Time	Source	Results
_____	_____	_____	_____
_____	_____	_____	_____
_____	_____	_____	_____
_____	_____	_____	_____

EXERCISE 1.5.3   Culturing Aerosol and Gas Sources

Date	Time	Source	Results
_____	_____	_____	_____
_____	_____	_____	_____

CRITICAL THINKING QUESTIONS

Mr. Abraham is a 40-year-old man being mechanically ventilated with an oral endotracheal tube in place. You note on his chart that a methicillin-resistant form of *Staphylococcus aureus* (MRSA) has been cultured from his sputum.

1. What types of transmission-based isolation precautions should be taken before entering the room? List the PPE required.

2. What type of antimicrobial therapy would be recommended to treat this patient's infection?

3. Describe how intensive care and mechanical ventilation may have contributed to the development of this nosocomial infection.

Ms. Holland is a 27-year-old woman who is HIV positive. She was admitted for respiratory difficulty. Sputum analysis has proved positive for acid-fast bacillus.

4. What type of transmission-based isolation precautions are indicated in this patient?

5. Describe what infection control precautions (relating to the equipment, the patient, and yourself) should be taken when performing an arterial blood gas on this patient.

6. You inadvertently spill some blood on the floor while performing the arterial blood gas on this patient. What action or actions should be taken to clean up the spill?

7. After an unsuccessful resuscitation, you are requested to remove the manual resuscitator bag from the patient's room. The bag is made of a silicone material. Describe how this equipment should be transported and disinfected.

Memorize this at home.

PROCEDURAL COMPETENCY EVALUATION

Name _Celia Ayala_   Date _6/9/00_

Standard Precautions/Transmission-Based Isolation Techniques

Setting: ☑ Lab ☐ Clinical   Evaluator: ☐ Peer ☑ Instructor

Conditions (describe): _____

_____

Equipment Used

_____

_____

	S A T I S F A C T O R Y	U N S A T I S F A C T O R Y	N O T O B S E R V E D	N O T A P P L I C A B L E

Assessment and Implementation

1. Removes jewelry and watch — ☑ ☐ ☐ ☐
2. Adjusts water flow and temperature — ☑ ☐ ☐ ☐
3. Wets forearms and hands — ☑ ☐ ☐ ☐
4. Applies disinfectant soap liberally — ☑ ☐ ☐ ☐
5. Washes the following for a minimum of 15 seconds with strong friction:
   a. Palms — ☑ ☐ ☐ ☐
   b. Between digits — ☑ ☐ ☐ ☐
   c. Under fingernails and around cuticles — ☑ ☐ ☐ ☐   *is critical if you don't do it you may fail your test*
6. Never touches sink with hands or body — ☑ ☐ ☐ ☐
7. Rinses from the forearm to the fingertips — ☑ ☐ ☐ ☐
8. Obtains towels aseptically — ☑ ☐ ☐ ☐
9. Dries hands individually using separate towels — ☑ ☐ ☐ ☐
10. Turns off water using dry, clean towel (if no foot pedals) — ☑ ☐ ☐ ☐
11. Reviews patient chart and surveys patient room for any transmission-based isolation precautions posted — ☑ ☐ ☐ ☐
12. Obtains and applies PPE as appropriate in the following sequence:
    a. Hair and foot coverings: for isolation — ☑ ☐ ☐ ☐
    b. Gown: for potential soiling — ☑ ☐ ☐ ☐
    c. Mask — ☑ ☐ ☐ ☐
    d. Goggles or face shield: for potential splattering — ☑ ☐ ☐ ☐
    e. Gloves: for any direct contact with body fluids; examines for any tears or holes and replaces if necessary — ☑ ☐ ☐ ☐
13. Performs procedure — ☑ ☐ ☐ ☐

Follow-up

14. Maintains/processes equipment — ☑ ☐ ☐ ☐
    a. Bags, seals, labels, and transfers contaminated equipment — ☑ ☐ ☐ ☐
15. Removes PPE in the following sequence:
    a. Head and foot coverings — ☑ ☐ ☐ ☐
    b. Mask and goggles — ☑ ☐ ☐ ☐

(Memorize it)

	SATISFACTORY	UNSATISFACTORY	NOT OBSERVED	NOT APPLICABLE
c. Gloves: removed by pulling gloves down from wrist and turning them inside out	☑	☐	☐	☐
d. Gown: removed from inside out	☑	☐	☐	☐
16. Disposes of infectious waste	☑	☐	☐	☐
17. Washes hands	☑	☐	☐	☐
18. Transports contaminated equipment in low-traffic areas	☑	☐	☐	☐

_____
Signature of Evaluator

_____
Signature of Student

6/9/00 : Needs to review
Dsd. Table.

PERFORMANCE RATING SCALE

5 EXCELLENT—FAR EXCEEDS EXPECTED LEVEL, FLAWLESS PERFORMANCE
4 ABOVE AVERAGE—NO PROMPTING REQUIRED, ABLE TO SELF-CORRECT
3 AVERAGE—THE MINIMUM COMPETENCY LEVEL, NO CRITICAL ERRORS
2 IMPROVEMENT NEEDED—PROBLEM AREAS EXIST; CRITICAL ERRORS, CORRECTIONS NEEDED
1 POOR AND UNACCEPTABLE PERFORMANCE—GROSS INACCURACIES, POTENTIALLY HARMFUL

PERFORMANCE CRITERIA		SCALE			
1. DISPLAYS KNOWLEDGE OF ESSENTIAL CONCEPTS	5	4	3	2	1
2. DEMONSTRATES THE RELATIONSHIP BETWEEN THEORY AND CLINICAL PRACTICE	5	4	3	2	1
3. FOLLOWS DIRECTIONS, EXHIBITS SOUND JUDGMENT, AND DEMONSTRATES ATTENTION TO SAFETY AND DETAIL	5	4	3	2	1
4. EXHIBITS THE REQUIRED MANUAL DEXTERITY	5	4	3	2	1
5. PERFORMS PROCEDURE IN A REASONABLE TIME FRAME	5	4	3	2	1
6. MAINTAINS STERILE OR ASEPTIC TECHNIQUE	5	4	3	2	1
7. INITIATES UNAMBIGUOUS GOAL-DIRECTED COMMUNICATION	5	4	3	2	1
8. PROVIDES FOR ADEQUATE CARE AND MAINTENANCE OF EQUIPMENT AND SUPPLIES	5	4	3	2	1
9. EXHIBITS COURTEOUS AND PLEASANT DEMEANOR	5	4	3	2	1
10. MAINTAINS CONCISE AND ACCURATE RECORDS	5	4	3	2	1

ADDITIONAL COMMENTS: INCLUDE ERRORS OF OMISSION OR COMMISSION, COMMUNICATIVE SKILLS, AND EFFECTIVENESS OF PATIENT INTERACTION:

SUMMARY PERFORMANCE EVALUATION AND RECOMMENDATIONS

SATISFACTORY PERFORMANCE—Performed without error or prompting, or able to self-correct, no critical errors.

_____ LABORATORY EVALUATION. SKILLS MAY BE APPLIED/OBSERVED IN THE CLINICAL SETTING.

_____ CLINICAL EVALUATION. STUDENT READY FOR MINIMALLY SUPERVISED APPLICATION AND REFINEMENT.

UNSATISFACTORY PERFORMANCE—Prompting required; performed with critical errors, potentially harmful.

_____ STUDENT REQUIRES ADDITIONAL LABORATORY PRACTICE.

_____ STUDENT REQUIRES ADDITIONAL SUPERVISED CLINICAL PRACTICE.

SIGNATURES

STUDENT: _____   EVALUATOR: _____

DATE: _____   DATE: _____

PROCEDURAL COMPETENCY EVALUATION

Name _____ Date _____

Sterilization/Disinfection

Setting: ☐ Lab ☐ Clinical   Evaluator: ☐ Peer ☐ Instructor

Conditions (describe): _____

_____

Equipment Used

_____

_____

	S A T I S F A C T O R Y	U N S A T I S F A C T O R Y	N O T O B S E R V E D	N O T A P P L I C A B L E
Equipment and Patient Preparation				
1. Isolates, gathers, and transports equipment to processing site	☐	☐	☐	☐
2. Applies PPE, including gloves and gown	☐	☐	☐	☐
3. Disinfects sink (washer)	☐	☐	☐	☐
4. Fills sink, adds detergent	☐	☐	☐	☐
5. Sorts, disassembles equipment into smallest parts	☐	☐	☐	☐
6. Examines equipment for any tears, cracks, or pitting; discards defective equipment	☐	☐	☐	☐
7. Immerses equipment in solution and soaks for 20 minutes (institutes wash cycle)	☐	☐	☐	☐
8. Scrubs parts thoroughly, including any crevices	☐	☐	☐	☐
9. Rinses equipment thoroughly with tap water or sterile water as appropriate (institutes rinse cycle)	☐	☐	☐	☐
10. Removes equipment and drains sink	☐	☐	☐	☐
11. Sets equipment out to dry on aseptic absorbent surface	☐	☐	☐	☐
12. Reassembles equipment; loosely secures any parts so disinfection/sterilization method can penetrate	☐	☐	☐	☐
13. Prepares for appropriate sterilization method:				
a. Autoclave or gas sterilization: packages item in the appropriate materials and marks with chemical indicator tape	☐	☐	☐	☐
b. "Cold sterilization" with glutaraldehyde: checks solution expiration date; immerses equipment in solution; soaks in disinfecting solution for 10 minutes to 10 hours, as specified; puts on sterile gloves and prepares sterile field; aseptically rinses equipment with sterile water, dries on sterile field, and packages for storage	☐	☐	☐	☐
c. Pasteurization: loads equipment into machine and runs through cycle; dries and packages for storage; seals package	☐	☐	☐	☐
d. All methods: labels with time, date, load, and signature	☐	☐	☐	☐
Follow-up				
14. Maintains/processes equipment:				
a. Disinfects sink	☐	☐	☐	☐
b. Cultures equipment samples	☐	☐	☐	☐
c. Stores equipment, rotates stock	☐	☐	☐	☐
15. Disposes of infectious waste	☐	☐	☐	☐
16. Washes hands	☐	☐	☐	☐
17. Completes any required paperwork according to institution policy	☐	☐	☐	☐

_____   _____
Signature of Evaluator   Signature of Student

PERFORMANCE RATING SCALE

5 EXCELLENT—FAR EXCEEDS EXPECTED LEVEL, FLAWLESS PERFORMANCE
4 ABOVE AVERAGE—NO PROMPTING REQUIRED, ABLE TO SELF-CORRECT
3 AVERAGE—THE MINIMUM COMPETENCY LEVEL, NO CRITICAL ERRORS
2 IMPROVEMENT NEEDED—PROBLEM AREAS EXIST; CRITICAL ERRORS, CORRECTIONS NEEDED
1 POOR AND UNACCEPTABLE PERFORMANCE—GROSS INACCURACIES, POTENTIALLY HARMFUL

PERFORMANCE CRITERIA		SCALE			
1. DISPLAYS KNOWLEDGE OF ESSENTIAL CONCEPTS	5	4	3	2	1
2. DEMONSTRATES THE RELATIONSHIP BETWEEN THEORY AND CLINICAL PRACTICE	5	4	3	2	1
3. FOLLOWS DIRECTIONS, EXHIBITS SOUND JUDGMENT, AND DEMONSTRATES ATTENTION TO SAFETY AND DETAIL	5	4	3	2	1
4. EXHIBITS THE REQUIRED MANUAL DEXTERITY	5	4	3	2	1
5. PERFORMS PROCEDURE IN A REASONABLE TIME FRAME	5	4	3	2	1
6. MAINTAINS STERILE OR ASEPTIC TECHNIQUE	5	4	3	2	1
7. INITIATES UNAMBIGUOUS GOAL-DIRECTED COMMUNICATION	5	4	3	2	1
8. PROVIDES FOR ADEQUATE CARE AND MAINTENANCE OF EQUIPMENT AND SUPPLIES	5	4	3	2	1
9. EXHIBITS COURTEOUS AND PLEASANT DEMEANOR	5	4	3	2	1
10. MAINTAINS CONCISE AND ACCURATE RECORDS	5	4	3	2	1

ADDITIONAL COMMENTS: INCLUDE ERRORS OF OMISSION OR COMMISSION, COMMUNICATIVE SKILLS, AND EFFECTIVENESS OF PATIENT INTERACTION:

SUMMARY PERFORMANCE EVALUATION AND RECOMMENDATIONS

SATISFACTORY PERFORMANCE—Performed without error or prompting, or able to self-correct, no critical errors.

_____ LABORATORY EVALUATION. SKILLS MAY BE APPLIED/OBSERVED IN THE CLINICAL SETTING.

_____ CLINICAL EVALUATION. STUDENT READY FOR MINIMALLY SUPERVISED APPLICATION AND REFINEMENT.

UNSATISFACTORY PERFORMANCE—Prompting required; performed with critical errors, potentially harmful.

_____ STUDENT REQUIRES ADDITIONAL LABORATORY PRACTICE.

_____ STUDENT REQUIRES ADDITIONAL SUPERVISED CLINICAL PRACTICE.

SIGNATURES

STUDENT: _____   EVALUATOR: _____

DATE: _____   DATE: _____

Patient Assessment

Effective patient assessment is the single most important component in providing competent respiratory care. Initiation, modification, and discontinuance of all respiratory care skills and procedures depend on adequately assessing the patient's changing condition.[1] To effectively participate in the decision-making process or successfully implement respiratory care, therapist-driven protocols (TDPs), the respiratory care practitioner must be proficient in patient assessment techniques.

The basic elements of patient assessment include the following:

1. Scene survey
2. Primary survey
3. Patient history and interview
4. Vital signs
5. Secondary survey
6. Physical assessment of the chest
   a. Observation
   b. **Palpation**
   c. Diagnostic chest **percussion**
   d. **Auscultation**

OBJECTIVES
Upon completion of this chapter, the student will be able to:

1. Critically observe the environment as part of a scene survey.
2. Conduct a primary survey.
3. Use therapeutic communication skills to establish patient rapport and elicit information during a patient interview.
4. Practice the techniques of simple vital sign measurements.
5. Perform the elements of a secondary survey.
6. Practice the techniques of observation, palpation, percussion, and auscultation for physical examination of the chest.
7. Explain how cultural or ethnic differences may affect the performance of patient assessment techniques.
8. Practice medical charting for the documentation of performance of patient assessment procedures.
9. Apply infection control guidelines and standards associated with equipment and procedures, according to OSHA regulations and CDC guidelines.

KEY TERMS

acute
adventitious
alleviating
ambulatory
aneroid
antecubital
anterior
apical
apnea
aspiration
asterixis
asymmetrical
ataxia
atelectasis
atrophy

auscultation
basilar
bifurcation
bilateral
binaural
Biot's respiration
blanching
bradycardia
bronchoconstriction
bronchodilation
bronchorrhea
bronchospasm
cachectic
caudad
cephalad
Cheyne-Stokes respiration

chronic
clubbing
collateral
consolidation
contraindication
contralateral
copious
crepitation
cyanosis
debilitated
decubitus
demographics
density
diagnosis
diaphoresis
distal

dyspnea
ecchymosis
edema
egophony
electrolyte
empyema
epistaxis
epithelium
erythema
eupnea
febrile
fetid
flail
flaring
Fowler's position
fremitus

25

hematocrit	lordosis	pleural friction rub	surrogate
hemoptysis	malaise	pleuritic (pain)	symmetrical
homeostasis	medial	pneumoconiosis	syncope
hyperinflation	mucoid	pneumothorax	systemic
hyperpnea	mucopurulent	polycythemia	systolic pressure
hyperresonant	nodules	posterior	tachycardia
hypertension	obtunded	prone	tachypnea
hyperthermia	orthopnea	proximal	tenacious
hypertrophy	orthostatic	purulent	tetany
hypervolemia	pallor	rales	torr
hypopnea	palpation	resonance	Trendelenburg position
hypotension	paradoxical	retractions	turbulent
hypothermia	paresthesia	rhonchi	turgor
hypovolemia	paroxysmal (cough)	scoliosis	tympanitic
inferior	patency	sensorium	unilateral
inspissated	pectoriloquy	serous	vascular
ischemia	pectus carinatum	somnolent	vasoconstriction
jaundice	pectus excavatum	sphygmomanometer	vasodilation
Kussmaul's respiration	percussion	stoma	ventilation
kyphosis	perfusion	stridor	wheezing
lateral	phalanges	subcutaneous emphysema	
lesions	phonation	superior	
lethargic	pleural effusion	supine	

EQUIPMENT REQUIRED

- Patient mannequin (or student)
- Hospital bed or equivalent
- **Sphygmomanometer** (mercury and **aneroid**)
- Various size blood pressure cuffs
- **Binaural** stethoscopes (teaching models, if available)
- Watch with second hand
- Stopwatch
- Electronic oral or ear thermometer and sheaths (optional)
- Cassette player
- Recording of breath sounds
- Video of physical assessment of the chest
- Video player and monitor
- Disposable gloves, various sizes
- Alcohol prep pads

● EXERCISES

EXERCISE 2.1 Scene Survey

Before performing any procedure, the practitioner must assess the surrounding environment to ensure his or her own safety,

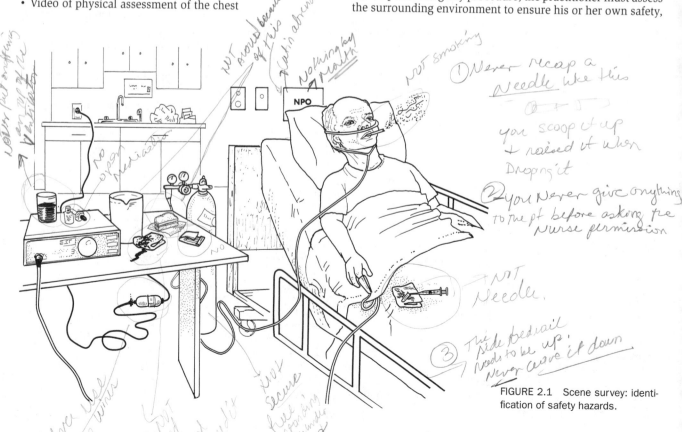

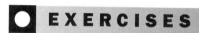

FIGURE 2.1 Scene survey: identification of safety hazards.

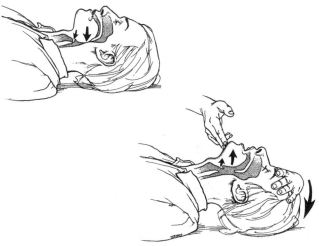

FIGURE 2.2 Opening the airway. (Reproduced with permission. © *Textbook of Basic Life Support for Healthcare Providers*, 1994. Copyright American Heart Association.)

the safety of the patient, and the safety of other healthcare workers. Wash your hands and apply standard precautions or transmission-based isolation procedures as appropriate.

EXERCISE 2.1.1 Identification of Safety Hazards—Diagram

Identify at least 10 safety hazards in Figure 2.1. *Record your list on the laboratory report.*

EXERCISE 2.1.2 Identification of Safety Hazards—Scenario

In this exercise, the instructor uses a mannequin or student to act as a **surrogate** patient. With the "patient" in bed, the instructor prepares the scene to include possible safety hazards. The student then performs the following:

1. When entering the "patient" area, quickly observe your surroundings. Look up, down, and all around. Take a maximum of 45 seconds.
2. Turn away from the scene and *record on your laboratory report* all your recollections about the scene for the following factors:
   a. Was the scene safe? List any hazardous conditions.
   b. What equipment did you see in the immediate area?
   c. Were the conditions conducive to patient comfort?
      (1) What were the environmental conditions like? Describe the temperature, humidity, lighting, and cleanliness.
      (2) Were the patient's material needs within easy reach?

EXERCISE 2.2 Primary Survey

The primary survey includes the initial impression of the patient, observing for any immediate life-threatening conditions only. The primary survey consists of checking airway, breathing, and circulation (the ABCs): **A**irway—is the airway open? **B**reathing—is breathing present? **C**irculation—is pulse present? Is there any severe bleeding? Immediate action must be taken for any life-threatening condition before proceeding to the next step.

It is expected that the student will have already had instruction in basic life support for health providers before this laboratory exercise.

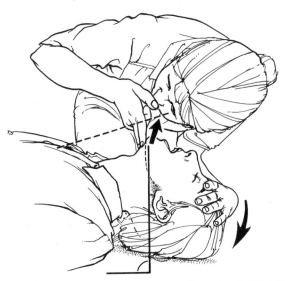

FIGURE 2.3 Determining breathlessness. (Reproduced with permission. © *Textbook of Basic Life Support for Healthcare Providers*, 1994. Copyright American Heart Association.)

In this exercise the instructor will set up one or more of the following scenarios. Refer to current American Heart Association (AHA) or American Red Cross (ARC) cardiopulmonary resuscitation (CPR) guidelines for specific details.

Students should apply standard precautions and transmission-based isolation procedures as appropriate. Approach the patient and assess the ABCs. Perform any necessary steps as determined by your findings.

1. A conscious and alert patient who is breathing and has a pulse
   a. Determine responsiveness.
   b. Quickly observe the patient for chest rise and fall.
   c. Ask the patient a question that requires a response to determine that the subject has a patent airway and is able to move air.
   d. Quickly observe for any severe bleeding by scanning the patient from head to toe.
2. An unconscious patient who is breathing and has a pulse
   a. Determine unresponsiveness.
   b. Activate the emergency medical services (EMS) system.
   c. Use the head-tilt/chin-lift maneuver (Fig. 2.2) to open the airway. Look, listen, and feel for breathing (Fig. 2.3). If spinal injury is suspected, use a modified jaw thrust (Fig. 2.4) to open the airway.

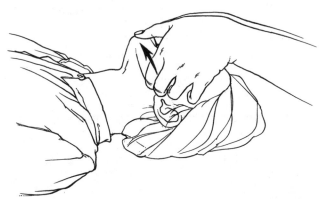

FIGURE 2.4 Jaw-thrust maneuver. (Reproduced with permission. © *Textbook of Basic Life Support for Healthcare Providers*, 1994. Copyright American Heart Association.)

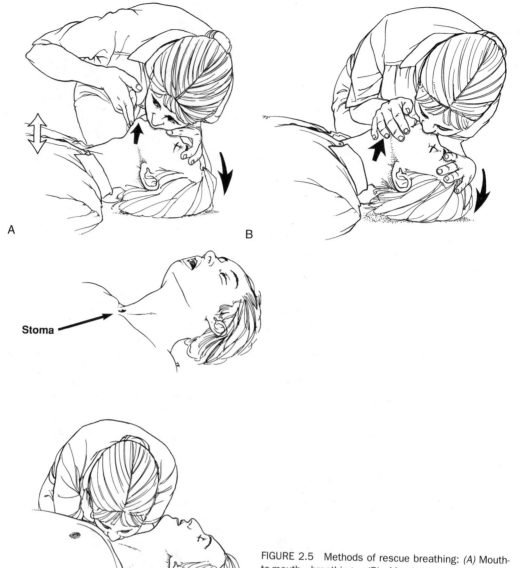

A

B

Stoma →

C

FIGURE 2.5   Methods of rescue breathing: *(A)* Mouth-to-mouth breathing, *(B)* Mouth-to-nose breathing, *(C)* Mouth-to-stoma breathing. (Reproduced with permission. © *Textbook of Basic Life Support for Healthcare Providers*, 1994. Copyright American Heart Association.)

d. If the patient is breathing, maintain head-tilt/chin-lift position with one hand. Continue to monitor for breathing and carotid pulse.

3. An unconscious patient who is not breathing but who has a pulse
   a. Determine unresponsiveness.
   b. Activate the EMS system.
   c. Use the head-tilt/chin-lift maneuver to open the airway, and maintain it with one hand. Look, listen, and feel for breathing.
   d. If breathing is absent, begin rescue breathing. Various methods of **ventilation** are shown in Figure 2.5.
   e. Practice mouth-to-mask ventilation as shown in Figure 2.6.

NOTE: Ventilations should be simulated if student is acting as surrogate patient.

   f. Check the carotid pulse for 5 to 10 sec (Fig. 2.7). If the pulse is present, continue rescue breathing. Monitor the pulse periodically.

4. An unconscious patient who is not breathing and has no pulse
   a. Determine unresponsiveness.
   b. Activate the EMS system.
   c. Position the patient.
   d. Use the head-tilt/chin-lift maneuver to open the airway, and maintain it with one hand. Look, listen, and feel for breathing.
   e. If breathing is absent, give ventilations.
   f. Check the carotid pulse for 5 to 10 sec.
   g. If pulse is absent, begin chest compressions (Fig. 2.8) and continue CPR according to current AHA or ARC guidelines.

NOTE: Compressions should be simulated if student is acting as surrogate patient.

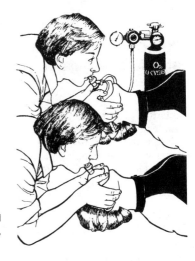

FIGURE 2.6 Mouth-to-mask ventilation with a one-way valve and supplemental oxygen. (Courtesy of Laerdal Medical Corporation, Wappingers Falls, NY.)

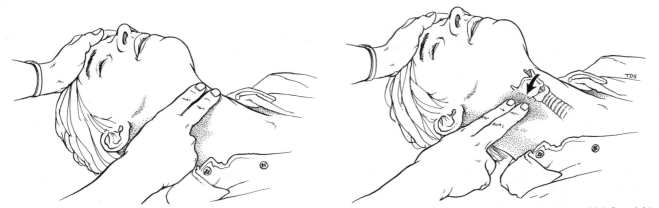

FIGURE 2.7 Checking the carotid pulse. (Reproduced with permission. © *Textbook of Basic Life Support for Healthcare Providers*, 1994. Copyright American Heart Association.)

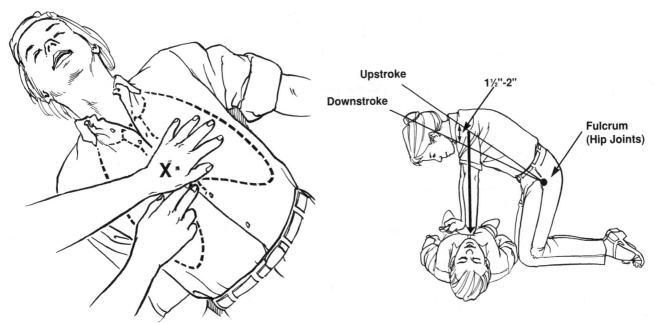

FIGURE 2.8 Proper positioning for chest compressions. (Reproduced with permission. © *Textbook of Basic Life Support for Healthcare Providers*, 1994. Copyright American Heart Association.)

EXERCISE 2.3 Chart Review, Patient Interview, and History

Effective communication skills are necessary to establish a rapport with the patient and to elicit useful information to supplement the physical examination (Fig. 2.9). It also provides the patient's perspective on the problem at hand.[1] In this exercise, the student will practice communication and questioning techniques, with a fellow student acting as the patient surrogate.

EXERCISE 2.3.1 Review of the Medical Record

Before entering the "patient's room," check the "chart" for all pertinent information. Your review of the chart should include the following priority areas:

1. Patient **demographics**
2. Chief complaint/**diagnosis**
3. History of present illness, including smoking history
4. Past medical history—major surgeries, **hypertension,** tuberculosis, diabetes, cardiac or pulmonary disease, and any other *major* illness
5. Social history—living arrangements, drinking, sexual activity
6. Occupational history
7. Allergies
8. Current medications
9. Results of recent diagnostic procedures (x-ray, laboratory, pulmonary function tests, electrocardiogram, etc.)
10. Recent progress notes
11. Physician orders

    NOTE: This activity may be performed with actual patient charts, if they are available in the lab, or by describing the information to your lab partner. It may also be performed in the clinical setting.

12. *Record your findings on your laboratory report.*

EXERCISE 2.3.2 Patient Interview and History

Students should wash hands and apply standard precautions and transmission-based isolation procedures as appropriate. The exercise requires using a laboratory partner as a surrogate. Approach your "patient" and perform the following:

1. Introduce yourself to the patient and explain why you are there.
2. Verify your patient's identification by checking the name band.
3. The interview should be used to assess the following general information:
   a. Level of consciousness and **sensorium**—orientation to person, place, and time
   b. Ability to follow directions
   c. Emotional status
   d. Level of **dyspnea**
   e. Nutritional status
   f. Tolerance of activities of daily living (ADLs)
4. Ask the patient questions in order to verify the information obtained from the chart regarding the following:
   a. Demographics
   b. Chief complaint: onset, duration, frequency, severity (quantity), character (quality), location, radiation, aggravating factors, **alleviating** factors, associated manifestations
   c. History of present illness, including smoking history
   d. Past medical history
   e. Psychosocial assessment:
      (1) Birthplace
      (2) Race
      (3) Religion
      (4) Culture

Interviewer	SENSORY/EMOTIONAL FACTORS	Patient
INTERNAL FACTORS	Fear	INTERNAL FACTORS
Previous experiences	Stress, anxiety	Previous experiences
Attitudes, values	Pain	Attitudes, values
Cultural heritage	Mental acuity, brain damage, hypoxia	Cultural heritage
Religious beliefs	Sight, hearing, speech impairment	Religious beliefs
Self concept		Self-concept
Listening habits	ENVIRONMENTAL FACTORS	Listening habits
Preoccupations, feelings	Lighting	Preoccupations, feelings
	Noise	Illness
	Privacy	
	Distance	
	Temperature	

VERBAL EXPRESSION — Language barrier, Jargon, Choice of words/questions, Feedback, voice tone

NONVERBAL EXPRESSION — Body movement, Facial expression, Dress, professionalism, Warmth, interest

FIGURE 2.9 Factors influencing communication. (From Wilkins, RL, Sheldon, RL and Krider, SJ: Clinical Assessment in Respiratory Care, ed 2. Mosby-Year Book, St. Louis, 1990, with permission.)

TABLE 2.1 **Some Characteristics of an Effective Listener**

1. Seek to understand the person who is speaking, not simply to respond to his or her statements.
2. Listen to a person's tone and inflection as well as his or her choice of words.
3. Look at the person speaking and pay attention to body language. Does the person's body give you the same message as his or her words?
4. Don't rush in with opinions and judgments. Give the person the freedom to express himself or herself.
5. When you speak, make it clear that you have understood what the person has said. You can even restate the person's point more clearly than he or she might have made it originally.

From Soreff, SM and Cadigan, RT: EMS Street Strategies. FA Davis, Philadelphia, 1992, p. 45, with permission.

    (5) Language(s) spoken
    (6) Highest education level
    (7) Sexual activity
    (8) Living arrangements (e.g., live alone?)
    (9) Alcohol intake
    (10) Drug use
  f. Occupational history
  g. Allergies
  h. Current medications

5. Ask the patient questions to ascertain specific pulmonary symptoms:
  a. Dyspnea—on exertion or rest; **orthopnea**
  b. Cough
  c. Sputum production—amount, color, consistency, presence of blood
  d. Chest pain—quality, location, radiation, aggravating factors, alleviating factors, associated manifestations
6. Ask the patient questions to determine current comfort level or needs.
7. *Record your interview findings on your laboratory report.*

EXERCISE 2.3.3 Communication Exercise

Discuss with your laboratory partner any experiences each of you may have had as patients in a hospital or other setting. Describe your feelings in this situation. Include in your discussion attitudes toward health care that are culturally based. Do you feel that the quality of your care was affected by cultural, ethnic, or racial issues? If you and your partner have never had these experiences, describe what concerns would be most important in the event one of you were hospitalized. *Record your laboratory partner's responses on your laboratory report* (Table 2.1).

TABLE 2.2 **Causes of Hypothermia and Hyperthermia**

Causes of Hypothermia	Causes of Hyperthermia
Cold exposure	Fever
Shock, blood loss	Heat exposure
Drugs	Drugs
Brain injuries	Dehydration
	Anesthesia
	Atelectasis
	Surgery
	Brain injuries

[handwritten annotations: "Infections or Septis" pointing to Fever/Heat exposure; "collapsed the alviou" next to Atelectasis]

EXERCISE 2.4 Vital Signs

EXERCISE 2.4.1 Taking Oral/Ear Temperatures (Optional Exercise)

Each student will measure the oral or ear temperature of a laboratory partner (Table 2.2, Fig. 2.10). Wash your hands and apply standard precautions and transmission-based isolation procedures as appropriate.

Thermometer
Several types of thermometers measure body temperature: glass-mercury, chemical dot, digital, and electronic digital. Each type provides accurate readings when used properly.

Glass-mercury thermometer

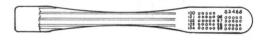

Oral thermometer

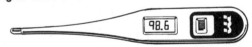

Rectal thermometer

Chemical dot thermometer

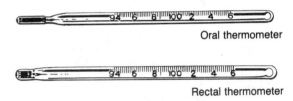

Digital thermometer

Electronic digital thermometer

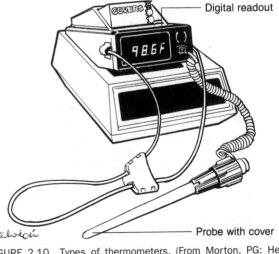

FIGURE 2.10   Types of thermometers. (From Morton, PG: Health Assessment in Nursing, ed 2. FA Davis, Philadelphia, 1993, p. 74, with permission.)

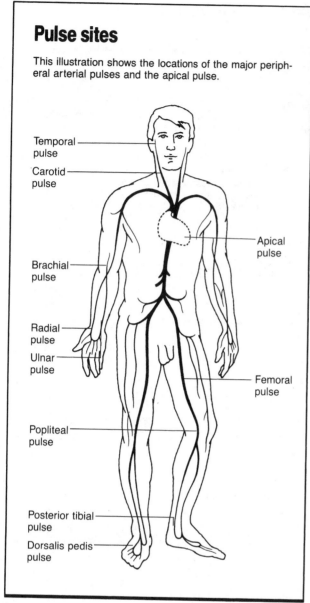

Pulse sites

This illustration shows the locations of the major peripheral arterial pulses and the apical pulse.

Temporal pulse

Carotid pulse

Apical pulse

Brachial pulse

Radial pulse

Ulnar pulse

Femoral pulse

Popliteal pulse

Posterior tibial pulse

Dorsalis pedis pulse

FIGURE 2.11   Location of pulses. (From Morton, PG: Health Assessment in Nursing, ed 2. FA Davis, Philadelphia, 1993, p. 96, with permission.)

1. Place the thermometer probe in a disposable sheath.
2. Press the "Start" button, or shake down the mercury column if using a glass thermometer.
3. Place the probe of the thermometer under your lab partner's tongue (or in ear if using an ear thermometer). Leave it in place until the thermometer indicates a final reading (about 30 sec). If you are using an oral glass thermometer, leave it in place for 3 to 5 min.
4. Remove the thermometer, discard the sheath, and *record the temperature on your laboratory report.*

EXERCISE 2.4.2 Location and Measurement of Pulse

A. Location of Common Pulse Points

Wash your hands and apply standard precautions and transmission-based isolation procedures as appropriate. Iden-

tify the following pulse points as shown in Figure 2.11 on your laboratory partner or yourself:

1. Radial
2. Ulnar
3. Brachial
4. Carotid
5. Femoral
6. Temporal
7. Popliteal
8. Dorsalis pedis
9. **Posterior** tibial

NOTE: To properly palpate pulses, use the index and middle fingers as shown in Figure 2.12. Press firmly but gently. *The thumb should not be used.* Excessive pressure can obliterate the pulse. Ideally the pulse should be measured for a full minute, particularly in subjects with an irregular heart rate or rhythm.

B. Measurement of Pulse Rate

Wash your hands and apply standard precautions and transmission-based isolation procedures as appropriate.

1. Using a watch with a second hand, measure your partner's radial pulse for ~~15~~ 30 and 60 sec. *Record the results on your laboratory report.*
2. Describe the quality of the pulses you felt. Include assessment of pulse strength and regularity. *Record this on your laboratory report.*
3. Have your partner run in place for 1 min. Remeasure the radial pulse. *Record the result on your laboratory report.*

C. Measurement of Apical-Radial Pulse

The apex of the heart is located on the left side of the chest. You can hear the heart beating with a stethoscope (Table 2.3).

1. Measure the **apical** pulse rate on your laboratory partner and compare it with the result from B.1.
2. *Record the pulse rate on your laboratory report.*

D. Capillary Refill

Capillary refill helps one to assess local **perfusion.**

1. Gently squeeze the tip of each finger (one at a time) until a **blanching** is noticed (nailbed turns white), as shown in Figure 2.13.
2. Using a stopwatch, *record the time it takes for the fingertip to turn pink.* A slow refill greater than 3 sec indicates poor perfusion.

TABLE 2.3   **Causes of Bradycardia and Tachycardia**

Causes of Bradycardia	Causes of Tachycardia
Heart block	Hypoxia or (Hypoxemia
Athletic conditioning	Fever
Hypothermia	Anxiety/stress
Severe trauma	Pain Most C
Adrenergic blocking agents	Drugs
Vagal stimulation	Hyperthyroidism
Increased intracranial pressure	Shock
Drugs	Hypercapnia ↑ CO_2
	Heart dysrhythmias

HR → Contraction
Pulse → diff. of systolic + Diastolic

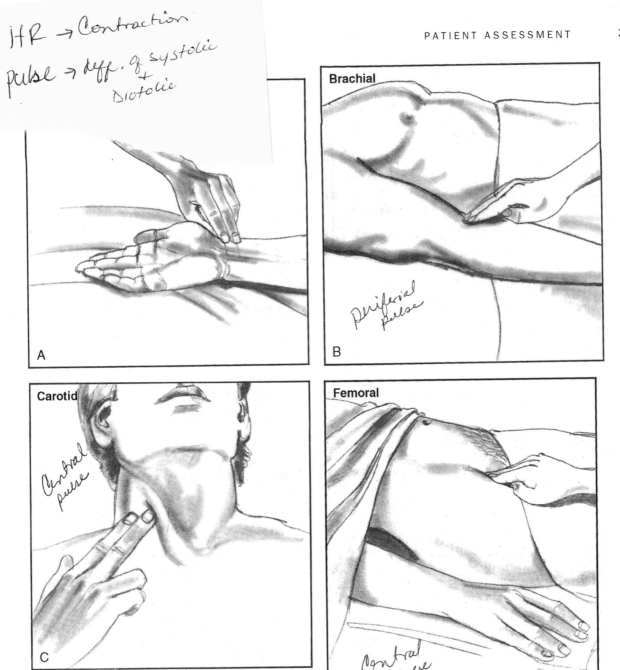

FIGURE 2.12   Palpation of pulses: *(A)* radial pulse, *(B)* brachial pulse, *(C)* carotid pulse, *(D)* femoral pulse.   *Continued*

EXERCISE 2.4.3 Assessment of Breathing (Respiration)

A. Measuring Respiratory Frequency

Wash your hands and apply standard precautions and transmission-based isolation procedures as appropriate.

1. Observe your partner's chest for movement. The chest rises during inspiration. Count *one* full respiration as a cycle from the beginning of one inspiration to the beginning of the next.

   NOTE: Many patients unintentionally alter their respiratory rate or pattern if they become aware that you are counting their respirations. This can be avoided if you appear to be taking the pulse while you are actually counting the respiratory rate.

2. Using a watch with a second hand, count your partner's respirations *(f)* for 15 and 60 sec. *Record the results on your laboratory report.*

3. Describe the quality of the respirations you observed. Assessment should include evaluation of the rate and depth, whether there is labored breathing, and the pattern of respiration.

B. Inspiration : Expiration Ratio (I : E)

Expiration is normally twice as long as inspiration. The ratio of inspiratory time (I) to expiratory time (E) should be approximately 1 : 2. It is extremely difficult to manually measure the I : E ratio. In a clinical setting (e.g., a patient on mechanical ventilation) the I : E ratio is measured by computerized technology. However, it is clinically important to be able to assess and compare the length of inspiratory and expiratory cycles with "normal."

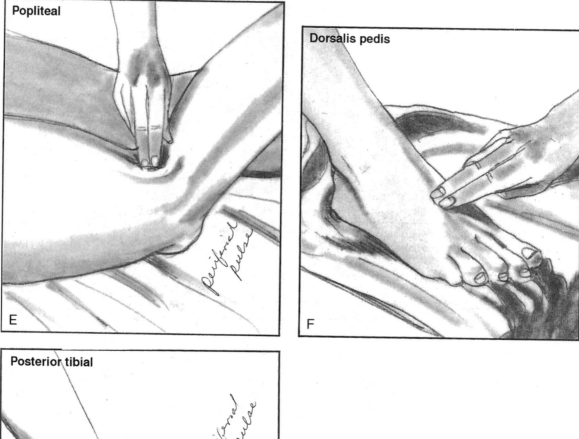

FIGURE 2.12 *Continued*   *(E)* popliteal pulse, *(F)* dorsalis pedis, *(G)* posterior tibial. (From Morton, PG: Health Assessment in Nursing, ed 2. FA Davis, Philadelphia, 1993, pp. 312–313, with permission.)

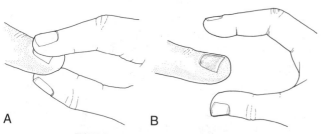

FIGURE 2.13   Assessing capillary refill.

Formulas:
f = respiratory rate
T (total time) = $60/f$
$E = T - I$
$I = T - E$
$I:E = 1:E/I$
$$I = \frac{T}{I + E}$$

1. Using a watch with a second hand, measure the time it takes for one full respiration from the beginning of inspiration to the beginning of the next inspiration.

2. Watch your laboratory partner closely. Measure your partner's inspiratory time (from beginning of inspiration to beginning of expiration) in seconds. _Record the results on your laboratory report._

3. Measure your partner's expiratory time (from beginning of expiration to beginning of inspiration) in seconds. _Record the results on your laboratory report._

NOTE: The inspiratory time and expiratory time should equal the total time. Because of the difficulty of manual measurement, times may not be exact.

EXERCISE 2.4.4 Arterial Blood Pressure

Most health care facilities have sphygmomanometers with a mercury manometer mounted on a wheeled cart or on the wall. An aneroid manometer with a needle gauge that shows the pressure may also be used (Fig. 2.14).

To measure blood pressure with an aneroid (optional) and mercury sphygmomanometer, take your laboratory partner's blood pressure while sitting, using both an aneroid manometer and a mercury manometer. _Record the results on your laboratory report._

1. Wash your hands and apply standard precautions and transmission-based isolation procedures as appropriate.

2. Wrap the sphygmomanometer cuff snugly around your partner's arm approximately 1 inch above the inner aspect of the elbow (the **antecubital** area) as shown in Figure 2.15. Proper cuff size is essential. The cuff should be about 1.5 times the size of the limb. Ensure that the cuff bladder is centered over the brachial artery. Most cuffs have arrows to indicate artery and cuff alignment. The mercury manometer should be kept at eye level. If using an aneroid gauge, the gauge should be kept at the level of your partner's arm. Your partner's arm should be kept at heart level. The arm must remain relaxed. Any muscle tension used to keep the arm straight will alter the reading.

3. Palpate the brachial pulse, and then rapidly inflate the cuff to approximately 30 mm Hg above the level at which the pulse disappears.

4. Deflate the cuff _slowly_ until the pulse reappears. Make a mental note of that number. Deflate the cuff completely.

5. Place the stethoscope in your ears and place the bell of the stethoscope over the brachial pulse, slightly distal to or partially under the cuff, as shown in Figure 2.16.

6. Watching the manometer, pump up the cuff until the level is about 30 mm Hg above the point at which the pulse disappeared (from step 4).

7. Slowly open the air valve to deflate the cuff, and watch carefully as the column of mercury (or needle) drops. The speed should be approximately 2 to 4 mm Hg per second.

8. Listen for the sound of blood pulsating through the brachial artery while watching the manometer. The point at which this occurs is the systolic pressure. Make a mental note of this number. This is the **systolic pressure.**

9. Continue to deflate the cuff at the same rate until all sound disappears. Note this number. This is the **diastolic pressure.**

10. Remove the cuff and _record the blood pressure on your laboratory report_ as systolic/diastolic.

Sphygmomanometer
Most hospitals have sphygmomanometers with a mercury manometer mounted on a wheeled cart or on the wall; others may have an aneroid manometer with a needle gauge that shows the pressure.

Mercury manometer

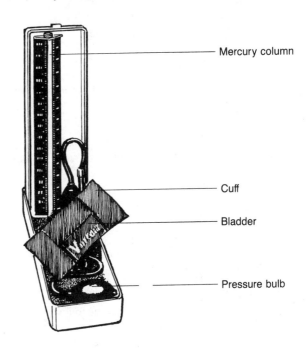

Mercury column

Cuff

Bladder

Pressure bulb

Aneroid manometer

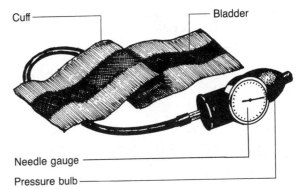

Cuff

Bladder

Needle gauge

Pressure bulb

FIGURE 2.14 Mercury and aneroid sphygmomanometers. (From Morton, PG: Health Assessment in Nursing, ed 2. FA Davis, Philadelphia, 1993, p. 75, with permission.)

11. Repeat the blood pressure measurement while your partner is standing and then lying down. _Record these measurements on your laboratory report._

12. Have your partner run in place for 1 min, and then repeat the standing blood pressure measurement. _Record the measurement on your laboratory report._

EXERCISE 2.5 Secondary Survey

The secondary survey is a brief head-to-toe observation of your patient to ascertain any injuries or problems other than the chief complaint that may require attention.

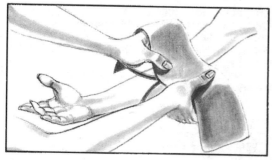

FIGURE 2.15 Blood pressure cuff application. (From Morton, PG: Health Assessment in Nursing, ed 2. FA Davis, Philadelphia, 1993, p. 99, with permission.)

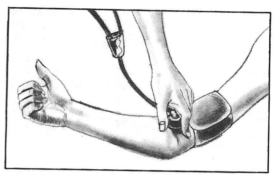

FIGURE 2.16 Measuring blood pressure. (From Morton, PG: Health Assessment in Nursing, ed 2. FA Davis, Philadelphia, 1993, p. 99, with permission.)

Perform a brief head-to-toe survey of your lab partner, as shown in Figure 2.17. Wash your hands and apply standard precautions and transmission-based isolation procedures as appropriate.

1. Head. Examine the head as follows:
   a. Observe and palpate for the presence of any cuts or bruises.
   b. Inspect the nose and ears for fluid or blood.
   c. Inspect the mouth for blood, broken teeth, or loose teeth.
   d. Check the breath odor.
   e. Check skin temperature and texture.
   f. Check mucous membranes for color.

2. Neck. Inspect and palpate the neck for the following:
   a. Jugular vein distention
   b. Tracheal deviation _The trachea Has To be in The MidLine position_
   c. Presence of **stoma** → _whole that is left on the tracheostomy surgery_
   d. Any **masses**
   e. Medic Alert pendant
   f. **Subcutaneous emphysema** → _when you have a leak from lungs_
   g. Use of accessory muscles
   h. Transtracheal oxygen catheter _2 types percoual cuthstor_
   i. Any other **invasive catheters** _Pice Line (control circulation) Control cathet_

3. Chest. This area will be covered in the next exercise.

4. Abdomen. Palpate the four quadrants and observe for the following: _acute abdomen due to_
   a. Pain
   b. Distention
   c. Rigidity
   d. Bruising

5. Extremities. Observe and palpate for the following:
   a. Deformities
   b. **Edema** (Fig. 2.18)
   c. Peripheral pulses
   d. Temperature and color
   e. Capillary refill → _enlargement 'distal Fibrosis, COPD cause by cystic Fibrosis_ _of the fingers_
   f. **Clubbing** of the distal phalanges (Fig. 2.19)
   g. Tobacco stains on the fingers
   h. Medic Alert bracelet

6. *Record your findings on the laboratory report.*

EXERCISE 2.6 Physical Assessment of the Chest

For a practitioner to perform a complete physical assessment, the room should be well lit, and the patient should ideally be naked to the waist. However, for female patients, the patient's modesty must be considered and safeguarded. The patient should be in the **Fowler's position,** and the practitioner should explain the process and reassure the patient before performing the assessment.

This section is best completed using a male volunteer with shirt removed. A video demonstration may be substituted. Wash your hands and apply standard precautions and transmission-based isolation procedures as appropriate. Have the subject sit upright.

A. Observation _Assessment_

1. Observe the patient for overall appearance, age, sex, and weight.

2. Stand directly in front of the patient and observe the chest for the following:
   a. General shape and appearance (Fig. 2.20):
      (1) **Anterior** to posterior diameter
      (2) Sternal deformities
   b. Surgical or other scars.
   c. **Symmetrical** expansion (Fig. 2.21)—observe for any **paradoxical** or unequal expansion.
   d. Presence of chest tubes.

3. From the back of the patient, observe spinal curvature.

4. Observe skin for **cyanosis, pallor,** mottling, **diaphoresis,** swelling, bruises, and **erythema.**

5. Observe skin for any obvious masses, **lesions,** or **nodules.**

6. Assess the respiratory pattern. Look for regularity, accessory muscle use, rate and depth, and patient positioning for breathing (Fig. 2.22). _pulling of skin_

7. Observe for **retractions,** pursed-lip breathing, and nasal flaring. _absorp pareciendo los labios junto para respirar._

B. Palpation

1. Palpate the position of the trachea by inserting two fingers from the same hand on either side of the trachea and moving your fingers downward (Fig. 2.23).

2. Palpate the skin for the presence of subcutaneous emphysema, which may be felt as **crepitation** or crackling under the skin ("rice-krispies").

3. Place your hands in the "butterfly" position with your thumbs on the spine and your hands on the posterior rib margins. Palpate for equal **bilateral** expansion using the steps in Figure 2.24.

4. Tactile **fremitus.** Palpate the chest wall over each of the lung lobes as shown in Figure 2.25 while the patient says "ninety-nine." Feel for any vibrations with the palms of your hands. Avoid bony prominences.

5. Palpate for spinal curvature. Place two fingers from the same hand along either side of the spine and move them

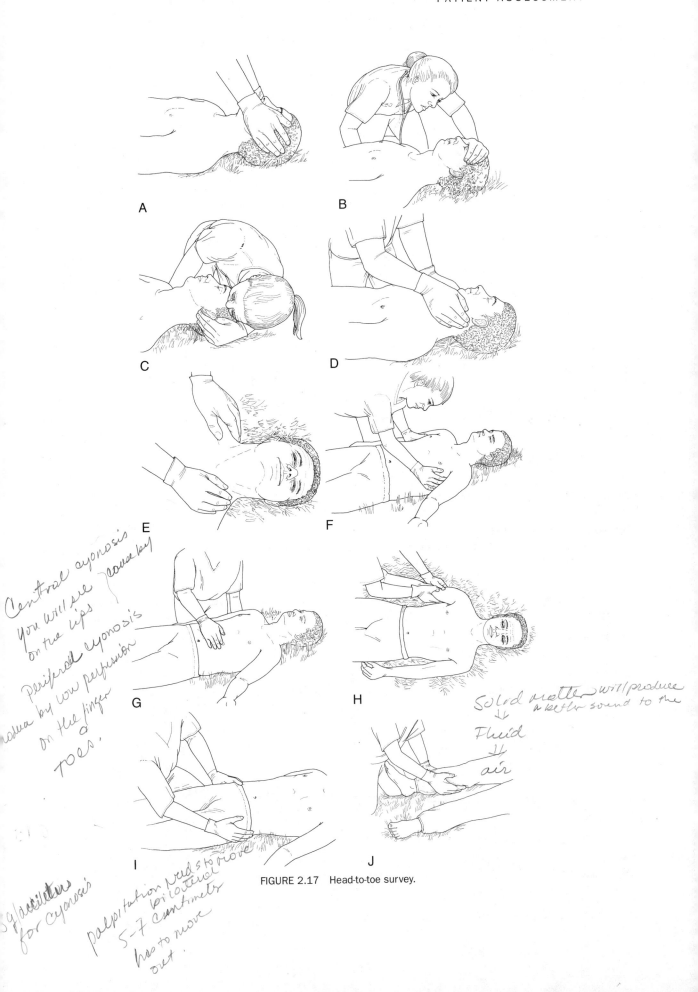

A

B

C

D

E

F

G

H

I

J

FIGURE 2.17   Head-to-toe survey.

Handwritten notes:

Central cyanosis you will see probably on the lips

Peripheral cyanosis produce by low perfusion on the finger a toes.

vasodilators for cyanosis

palpitation need to move bilateral move 5-7 centimeter has to move out.

Solid matter will produce a dull sound to the
↓
Fluid
↓
air

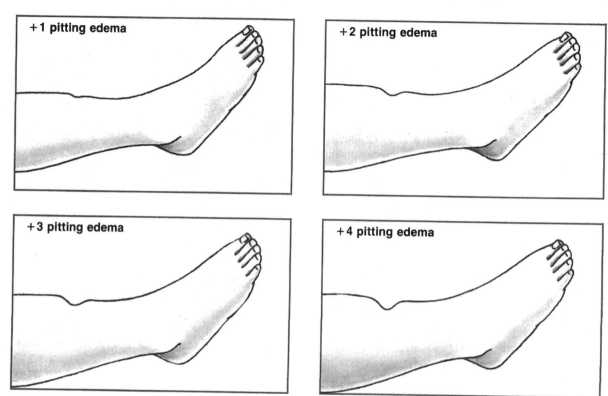

FIGURE 2.18   Evaluating pitting edema. (From Morton, PG: Health Assessment in Nursing, ed 2. FA Davis, Philadelphia, 1993, p. 399, with permission.)

downward, using sufficient pressure to cause skin blanching. Note any deviations.

6. Assess peripheral perfusion by palpating pulses and capillary refill.

C. Diagnostic Chest Percussion

Diagnostic chest percussion may be performed by directly striking the chest wall with a finger between the ribs. It may be performed indirectly by placing one hand on the chest wall and striking the middle or index finger with your other hand, as shown in Figure 2.26. Comparison of bilateral percussion notes for quality and intensity should be made. Table 2.4 shows the important percussion notes, location, and common causes. Diaphragmatic excursion can also be estimated by percussion of the posterior chest wall.[2]

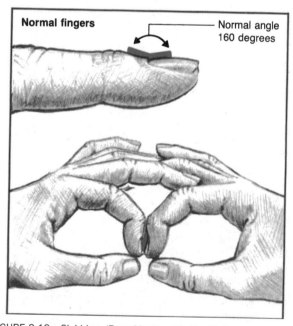
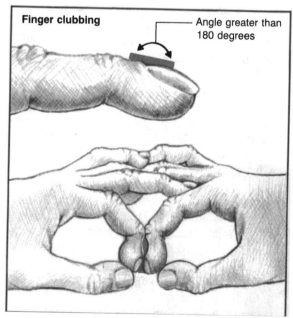

FIGURE 2.19   Clubbing. (From Morton, PG: Health Assessment in Nursing, ed 2. FA Davis, Philadelphia, 1993, p. 261, with permission.)

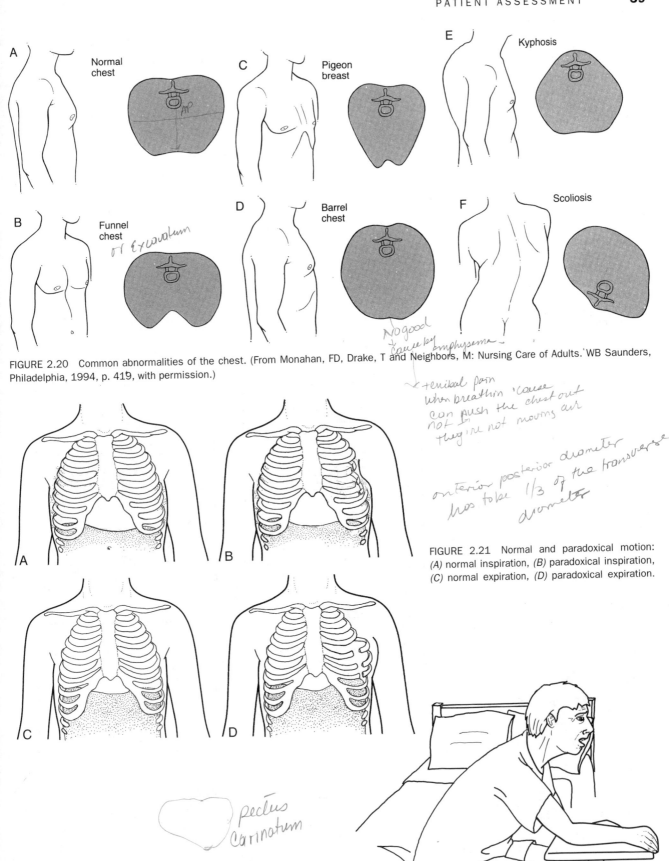

FIGURE 2.20 Common abnormalities of the chest. (From Monahan, FD, Drake, T and Neighbors, M: Nursing Care of Adults. WB Saunders, Philadelphia, 1994, p. 419, with permission.)

(handwritten annotations on Figure 2.20)

A — Normal chest — *AP*
B — Funnel chest — *or Excavatum*
C — Pigeon breast
D — Barrel chest — *No good — cause by emphysema*
E — Kyphosis
F — Scoliosis

terrical pain when breathin 'cause can push the chest out not — they're not moving air

anterior posterior diameter has to be 1/3 of the transverse diameter

FIGURE 2.21 Normal and paradoxical motion: (A) normal inspiration, (B) paradoxical inspiration, (C) normal expiration, (D) paradoxical expiration.

(handwritten) pectus carinatum

(handwritten) Look at the bilateral movement on the trachea. ex

FIGURE 2.22 The tripod position.

(handwritten) If the tube goes in the R side the L side will collapse

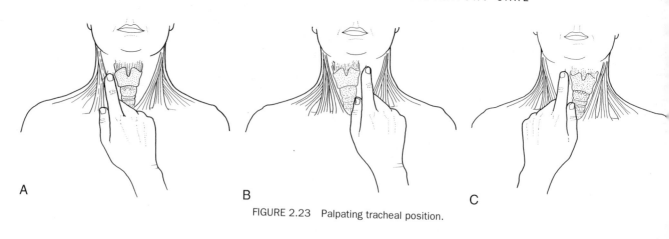

FIGURE 2.23 Palpating tracheal position.

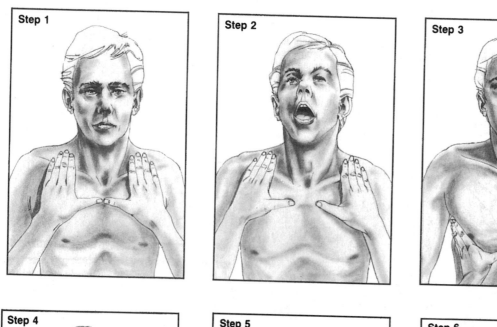

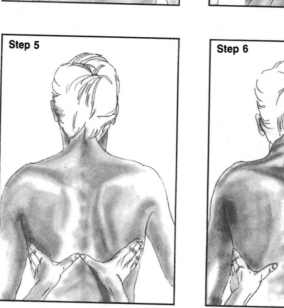

FIGURE 2.24 Palpating for chest excursion. (From Morton, PG: Health Assessment in Nursing, ed 2. FA Davis, Philadelphia, 1993, pp. 266–267, with permission.)

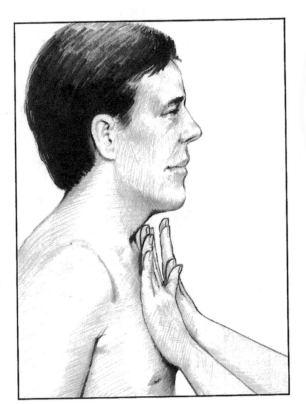

FIGURE 2.25 Palpating for tactile fremitus. (From Morton, PG: Health Assessment in Nursing, ed 2. FA Davis, Philadelphia, 1993, p. 275, with permission.)

TABLE 2.4 **Percussion Sounds** *ONly.*

Sound	Quality	Source
Resonant *(Normal lungs)*	Hollow	Normal lung
Dull *(solid)*	Thudlike	Liver, consolidated lung, pleural effusion
Hyperresonant/ tympanitic *- Sound*	Drumlike	Hyperinflated lung (as in emphysema), gastric air bubble, pneumothorax
Flat	Flat	Muscle, bone

Percussion assessment diaphragmatic Excursion. 3-5 centimeter up+ Down.

Stethoscope

All stethoscopes have earpieces, binaurals, tubing, and a chestpiece (head). However, some have several removable chestpieces suitable for adult and pediatric clients. Others, designed specifically for use on an adult or a child, have only one chestpiece.

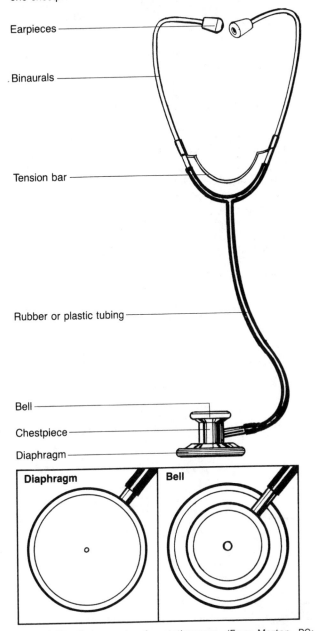

Earpieces

Binaurals

Tension bar

Rubber or plastic tubing

Bell

Chestpiece

Diaphragm

Diaphragm   Bell

FIGURE 2.27 Components of a stethoscope. (From Morton, PG: Health Assessment in Nursing, ed 2. FA Davis, Philadelphia, 1993, p. 99, with permission.)

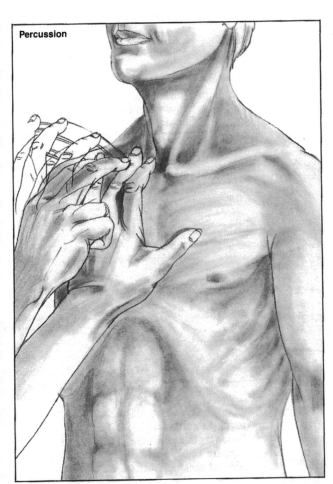

Percussion

FIGURE 2.26 Diagnostic chest percussion. (From Morton, PG: Health Assessment in Nursing, ed 2. FA Davis, Philadelphia, 1993, p. 268, with permission.)

Anterior chest

Posterior chest

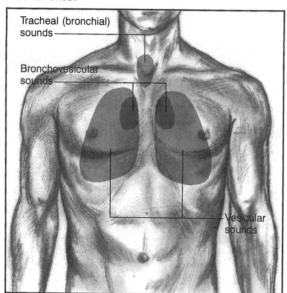
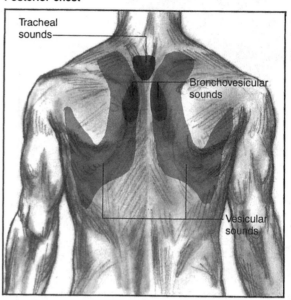

FIGURE 2.28   Location of normal breath sounds. (From Morton, PG: Health Assessment in Nursing, ed 2. FA Davis, Philadelphia, 1993, p. 270, with permission.)

1. Percuss over a solid structure such as the liver, thigh, or heart to create a dull percussion note.

2. Percuss over normal lung tissue to hear a resonant percussion note. Compare the sounds bilaterally.

3. Percuss over the stomach to hear a **hyperresonant** or **tympanitic** percussion note.

4. Estimate diaphragmatic excursion by first instructing the patient to take a full, deep breath. Determine the lowest margin of **resonance** by percussing over the lower lung field and moving downward in small increments until a definite change in the percussion note is detected. Then instruct the patient to exhale maximally and hold this position while percussion is repeated.

D. Auscultation

The stethoscope (Fig. 2.27) is a valuable and essential assessment tool for the respiratory care practitioner. It consists of four basic parts: (1) a bell for low-frequency sounds, such as heart sounds; (2) a diaphragm for higher-pitched lung sounds; (3) tubing, which is ideally 11 to 16 inches in length and thick enough to exclude external noise; and (4) binaural earpieces, which should be pointed in toward the ear canals.[3]

1. Listen to the breath sound tape (if available).

2. Auscultate your laboratory partner.
   a. Check your stethoscope for function. Wipe the earpieces and diaphragm with an alcohol swab. Place the earpieces securely in your ears. Turn the head of the stethoscope to

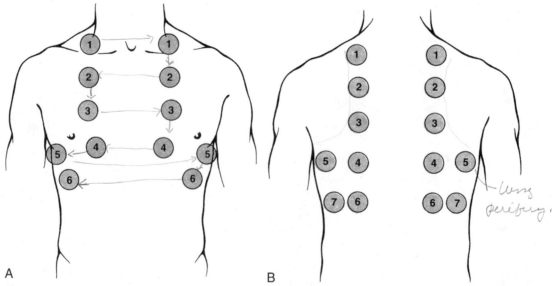

A   B

FIGURE 2.29   Sequence for chest auscultation. (From Hogstel, MO and Keen-Payne, R: Practical Guide to Health Assessment Through the Lifespan. FA Davis, Philadelphia, 1993, pp. 94–95, with permission.)

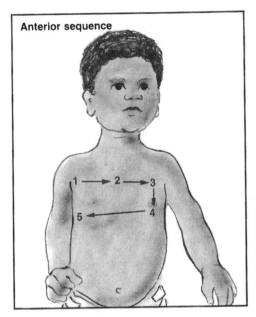

Anterior sequence

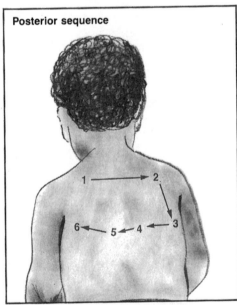

Posterior sequence

FIGURE 2.30 Auscultation positions in children. (From Morton, PG: Health Assessment in Nursing, ed 2. FA Davis, Philadelphia, 1993, p. 274, with permission.)

the diaphragm side and gently tap on it. If you do not hear anything, turn the chestpiece 180 degrees and repeat. Examine the chestpiece and tubing regularly for cracks and other defects. Clean the earpieces of wax and dirt.

b. Warm the diaphragm piece with your hands.

c. Instruct your "patient" to sit up, lean forward, and breath through the mouth with the head turned away from you. Place the diaphragm firmly against the chest wall.

d. Identify the location of normal breath sounds, as shown in Figure 2.28.

e. Auscultate the posterior chest wall in at least six places, comparing sounds bilaterally, as shown in Figure 2.29. You may proceed from **apexes** to bases or from bases to

apexes as long as you make bilateral comparisons. Figure 2.30 demonstrates the auscultation positions in children.

f. Auscultate the anterior chest wall, with the patient leaning slightly back, in at least six places. Compare sounds bilaterally.

References

1. Scanlan, C et al (eds): Egan's Fundamentals of Respiratory Care, ed 6. Mosby, St Louis, 1995, p 361.
2. Wilkins, RL, Krider, SJ and Sheldon, RL: Clinical Assessment in Respiratory Care, ed 3. Mosby, St Louis, 1990, p 61.
3. Wilkins, RL, Krider, SJ and Sheldon, RL: Clinical assessment in Respiratory Care, ed 3. Mosby, St Louis, 1990, p 62.

Related Readings

American Red Cross: Standard First Aid. American National Red Cross, New York, 1991.

Eubanks, DH and Bone, RC: Principles and Applications of Cardiorespiratory Care Equipment. Mosby, St Louis, 1994.

Freedberg, PD, Hoffman, LA and Cagno, JA: Physical Examination of the Chest (video). WB Saunders, Philadelphia, 1989.

McPherson, S: Respiratory Care Equipment, ed 5. Mosby, St Louis, 1995.

Morton, P: Health Assessment in Nursing. FA Davis, Philadelphia, 1993.

Scanlan, C et al (eds): Egan's Fundamentals of Respiratory Care, ed 6. Mosby, St Louis, 1995.

Wilkins, T, Hodgkin, J and Lopez, B: Lung Sounds: A Practical Guide, ed 2. Mosby, St Louis, 1996.

Wilkins, R, Sheldon, R and Krider, S: Clinical Assessment in Respiratory Care, ed 3. Mosby, St Louis, 1995.

Selected Journal Articles

American Association for Respiratory Care: AARC clinical practice guidelines, providing patient and caregiver training. Respir Care 41(7):658–663, 1996.

American Heart Association: Guidelines for cardiopulmonary resuscitation and emergency cardiac care: Recommendations of the 1992 National Conference. JAMA 268:16, 1992.

Appenheimer, L: The thoracic patient: Physical assessment of the chest. ADRN J 40:732–737, 1984.

Blumsohn, D: Clubbing of the fingers, with special reference to Schamroth's diagnostic method. Heart Lung 10:1069–1072, 1981.

Carrieri-Kohlman, V: Dyspnea in the weaning patient: Assessment and intervention. AACN Clin Issues Crit Care Nurs 2:462–473, 1991.

Carrieri, VK et al: The sensation of dyspnea: A review. Heart Lung 13:436–437, 1984.

Clinical maneuvers to assess dyspnea. Emerg Med 22:103, 106, 1990.

Gift, AG and Cahill, CA: Psychophysiologic aspects of dyspnea in chronic obstructive pulmonary disease: A pilot study. Heart Lung 19:252–257, 1990.

Halperin, HR et al: Compression techniques and blood flow during cardiopulmonary resuscitation. Respir Care 40:380–392, 1995.

Halpern, JS: Mnemonics used for patient assessment. J Emerg Nurs 20:219–221, 1994.

Kanematsu, T et al: Clubbing of the fingers and smooth muscle proliferation in patients with idiopathic pulmonary fibrosis. Chest 105:339–342, 1994.

King, DE: Assessment and evaluation of the paradoxical pulse. DCCN 1:266–274, 1982.

Luce, JM and Culver, BH: Respiratory muscle function in health and disease. Chest 81:82–90, 1982.

Luer, MJ: Sedation and chemical relaxation in critical pulmonary illness: suggestions for patient assessment and drug monitoring. AACN Clin Issues Adv Pract Acute Crit Care 6:333–343, 1995.

Mahler, DA and Horowitz, MB: Clinical evaluation of exertional dyspnea. Clin Chest Med 15:259–269, 1994.

LABORATORY REPORT

CHAPTER 2: PATIENT ASSESSMENT

Name _____   Date _____

Course/Section _____   Instructor _____

Data Collection

EXERCISE 2.1   Scene Survey

EXERCISE 2.1.1   Identification of Safety Hazards—Diagram

List 10 safety hazards:

_____   _____

_____   _____

_____   _____

_____   _____

_____   _____

EXERCISE 2.1.2   Identification of Safety Hazards—Scenario

1. Was the scene safe? List any hazardous conditions.

_____   _____

_____   _____

_____   _____

_____   _____

_____   _____

2. What equipment did you see in the immediate area?

3. Were the conditions conducive to patient comfort?
   a. What were the environmental conditions like? Describe the temperature, humidity, lighting, and cleanliness.
   b. Were the patient's material needs within easy reach?

CRITICAL THINKING QUESTION

Scenario: You are asked to enter a patient's room to perform morning vital signs. When you approach the patient, you put the side rail of the bed down to allow better access to the patient. There is an intravenous (IV) pump on the same side on which you are standing. As you grab the IV pump to move it out of the way, you feel a mild tingling sensation in your hand.

1. What would your next actions be? Why?

EXERCISE 2.2   Primary Survey

Scenario: You have entered the patient's room to administer a respiratory treatment. You find the patient lying face down on the bathroom floor.

1. What are the first *three* steps you would take under these circumstances?

2. You have determined that the victim is not breathing. You attempt manual ventilation and do not see the chest rise and fall or feel air entering the victim. What are the first *three* steps you would take under these circumstances?

EXERCISE 2.3   Chart Review, Patient Interview, and History
EXERCISE 2.3.1   Review of the Medical Record
If an actual patient chart was used, *record your findings on a separate piece of paper.*

EXERCISE 2.3.2   Patient Interview and History
DEMOGRAPHICS

Name: _____ Date of birth: _____ Sex: **M** ☐ **F** ☐

Weight: _____ Height: _____

CHIEF COMPLAINT: _____

_____

HISTORY OF PRESENT ILLNESS: _____

_____

Smoking History: _____

☐ Never smoked

☐ Smoker

☐ Former smoker

Age started _____ Age when quit _____ Current age _____ Packs/day _____

PAST MEDICAL HISTORY
Head:

☐ Neurological problem _____

☐ Seizure history _____

☐ Mental status _____

Eyes: _____ Ears, nose, throat: _____

Teeth: ☐ Dentures _____

Lungs:

☐ Asthma _____

☐ Emphysema _____

☐ Bronchitus _____

☐ Pneumonia _____

☐ Tuberculosis _____

☐ Other _____

☐ Dyspnea _____

　　☐ On exertion _____

　　☐ At rest _____

☐ Cough _____

☐ Sputum production _____

☐ Chest pain _____

Heart:

☐ Chest pain _____

☐ Pacemaker _____

☐ Hypertension _____

☐ Heart attack _____

☐ Other _____

Gastrointestinal:

☐ Ulcers _____

☐ Liver disease _____

☐ Hepatitis _____

☐ Bowel problems _____

☐ Other _____

Nutritional status: _____

Genitourinary: _____

Endocrine:

☐ Diabetes _____

☐ Thyroid _____

☐ Other _____

Bone/muscle: _____

Skin: _____

Gynecological: _____

Surgical procedures: _____

_____

ALLERGIES: _____

CURRENT MEDICATIONS: _____

_____

PSYCHOSOCIAL ASSESSMENT:

Birthplace: _____   Race: _____

Religion: _____   Language(s) spoken: _____

Culture: _____   Highest educational level: _____

Sexual activity: _____

Alcohol intake: _____

Drug use: _____

Assessment of ADL: _____

_____

OCCUPATIONAL HISTORY: _____

EXERCISE 2.3.3   Communications Exercise

_____

_____

_____

_____

_____

_____

CRITICAL THINKING QUESTION

1. How might differences in cultural or ethnic background between the practitioner and the patient affect the practitioner's ability to perform a patient assessment?

EXERCISE 2.4   Vital Signs
EXERCISE 2.4.1   Temperature

Temperature = _____ °F
Convert temperature to centigrade. Show your work!

$$°C = \frac{5(°F - 32)}{9}$$ Temperature = _____ °C

Temperature = 35°C
Convert temperature to Fahrenheit. Show your work!

$$°F = \frac{°C \times 9}{5} + 32$$ Temperature = _____ °F

CRITICAL THINKING QUESTIONS

1. Name two respiratory care procedures or modalities that can interfere with the accurate measurement of an oral temperature.

2. Convert the following Fahrenheit temperatures to centigrade. Show your work!

   95°F = _____ °C   105°F = _____ °C

EXERCISE 2.4.2   Pulse

15 sec   Pulse = _____ × 4

                = _____ /min

60 sec   Pulse = _____ /min

Quality of pulse: _____

Compare the two measurement methods: _____

_____

Pulse after exercise = _____ /min

Apical pulse rate (resting) = _____ /min

Pulse deficit = Apical − Radial = _____

Capillary refill time = _____ sec

CRITICAL THINKING QUESTIONS

1. When would it be recommended to count the pulse for 30 to 60 sec rather than 15 sec?

2. What conditions or circumstances may cause the apical and radial pulse to be different from each other?

3. A patient is noted to be tachycardic with a pulse rate of 140/min. What other signs and symptoms would you expect to find on physical examination if the tachycardia is caused by hypoxia?

EXERCISE 2.4.3   Assessment of Breathing (Respiration)

1. Measuring respiratory frequency

   a. f: 15 sec = _____ × 4

      = _____ /min

   b. f: 30 sec = _____ /min

   c. Quality of respirations: _____

2. Inspiration : Expiration ratio

   a. Measured respiratory total time = _____ sec

   b. Measured inspiratory time: = _____ sec

   Calculating expiratory time. Using steps 2.a and 2.b, calculate the following. Show your work!

   Expiratory time $T - I = E$ _____ (sec)

   I : E ratio = 1 : _____

   c. Measured expiratory time = _____ sec

   Calculating inspiratory time. (Do not use your measured value of I time for this calculation!) Using steps 2.a and 2.c, calculate the following. Show your work!

   $T - E$ (measured) = I _____ sec

   I : E ratio = 1 : _____

CRITICAL THINKING QUESTIONS

1. If the patient's total respiratory time and respiratory rate stayed the same, but expiratory time was increased, would inspiratory time increase or decrease?

2. If the patient's total respiratory time was 6 sec, what would this person's respiratory rate per minute be? Show your work!

3. If a patient's I : E ratio was 1 : 2 and expiration was 4 sec long, what would the inspiratory time be? Show your work!

4. If a patient's I : E ratio was 1 : 3 and respiratory rate was 30/min, calculate the following. Show your work!

   $T =$ _____

   Inspiratory time = _____

   Expiratory time = _____

EXERCISE 2.4.4   Arterial Blood Pressure

1. Blood pressure (BP) sitting = _____ mm Hg (mercury)

   Pulse pressure = Systolic − Diastolic = _____

   BP sitting = _____ mm Hg (aneroid)

Pulse pressure = _____

2. BP standing = _____ mm Hg

   BP supine = _____ mm Hg

3. BP after exercise = _____ mm Hg

CRITICAL THINKING QUESTIONS

1. Explain how and why pulsus paradoxus occurs.

2. How will the blood pressure measurement be affected if excessive pressure is used in cuff inflation or if pressure is held in the cuff too long?

3. What happens if a blood pressure cuff is too small?

EXERCISE 2.5   Secondary Survey

1. Head

   _____

2. Neck

   _____

3. Chest

   _____

4. Abdomen

   _____

5. Extremities

   _____

CRITICAL THINKING QUESTIONS

Scenario 1: A patient with diabetes enters the emergency room in a coma. You perform a secondary survey on this patient.

1. What would you expect to find when assessing the patient's breath?

2. The patient's capillary refill time is noted to be 10 sec. What would this indicate? Why?

3. What type of respiratory rate and pattern would you expect to find?

Scenario 2: You are called to the emergency room to evaluate Mr. C. O. Tu. Mr. Tu has a long-standing history of chronic obstructive pulmonary disease (COPD). He has been brought to the emergency room (ER) by ambulance. He complains of increasing shortness of breath and productive cough with thick, green sputum.

1. Identify five clinical findings you could detect by direct observation that would indicate to you that Mr. Tu has an increased work of breathing.

2. What values would you expect to find when measuring vital signs (pulse, respirations, blood pressure, temperature)?

During physical examination of the chest, you notice a hyperresonant percussion note with decreased fremitus over most of the lung fields except for the right lower lobe (RLL), which has a dull percussion note and increased fremitus.

3. Identify a possible explanation for these differences in your findings.

4. Based on your findings, describe what you would expect to hear on auscultation over the RLL.

PROCEDURAL COMPETEN̶C̶... ...LUATION

Name _Celia Ayala_   Date ____ ...00

Medical Records

Setting: ☐ Lab ☑ Clinical   Evaluator: ☐ Peer ☑ Instructor

Conditions (describe): _____

_____

Equipment Used

_____

_____

	S A T I S F A C T O R Y	U N S A T I S F A C T O R Y	N O T O B S E R V E D	N O T A P P L I C A B L E

Equipment and Patient Preparation

1. Obtains and verifies the correct chart — ☑ ☐ ☐ ☐

2. Informs the nurse or unit secretary if removing the chart from the nurse's station — ☑ ☐ ☐ ☐
or Somebody incharged

Assessment and Implementation

3. Locates and evaluates the following:
   - Patient demographics → Age, sex, hight + Weight — ☑ ☐ ☐ ☐
   - Chief complaint/diagnosis → c/c /Dx The pts complaint Don't always look at THER. — ☑ ☐ ☐ ☐
   - History of present illness → When did you Vomiting, vomiting, caughing — ☑ ☐ ☐ ☐
   - Smoking history (packs/yrs.) → have you ever smoke always round of gathen — ☑ ☐ ☐ ☐
   - Past medical history — ☑ ☐ ☐ ☐
   - Social history: drinking, sexual activity, home situation — ☑ ☐ ☐ ☐
   - Occupational history → disease that are related w/ the patient symptom — ☑ ☐ ☐ ☐
   - Allergies → — ☑ ☐ ☐ ☐
   - Current medications — ☑ ☐ ☐ ☐
   - Results of recent diagnostic procedures — ☑ ☐ ☐ ☐

4. Reads and evaluates the recent progress notes — ☑ ☐ ☐ ☐

5. Locates and evaluates the physician's orders or protocols — ☑ ☐ ☐ ☐

6. Charts procedures performed, or shift note, including, as applicable:
   a. Date — ☑ ☐ ☐ ☐
   b. Time — ☑ ☐ ☐ ☐
   c. Modality, method, procedure — ☑ ☐ ☐ ☐
   d. Medication, dosage, dilution DO NOT TAKE A Medication that does not have dosage. — ☑ ☐ ☐ ☐
   e. Duration eg treatment — ☑ ☐ ☐ ☐
   pre   ROS assessment
   f. Subjective, objective assessment before and after therapy — ☑ ☐ ☐ ☐
   → always record patients reaction
   g. Adverse reactions, other comments — ☑ ☐ ☐ ☐
   h. Plan → ex continue w/ the assessment — ☑ ☐ ☐ ☐
   i. Signature, credentials — ☑ ☐ ☐ ☐

Follow-up

7. Returns the chart to its proper location — ☐ ☐ ☐ ☐

_____   _____
Signature of Evaluator   Signature of Student

To get information history (hx) of smoking you do this
The Amount of packs X Amount of year   ex   3ppd x 20y
(ppd)   60 Pack Per Year
                                                 (PPY)

PERFORMANCE RATING SCALE

5 EXCELLENT—FAR EXCEEDS EXPECTED LEVEL, FLAWLESS PERFORMANCE
4 ABOVE AVERAGE—NO PROMPTING REQUIRED, ABLE TO SELF-CORRECT
3 AVERAGE—THE MINIMUM COMPETENCY LEVEL, NO CRITICAL ERRORS
2 IMPROVEMENT NEEDED—PROBLEM AREAS EXIST; CRITICAL ERRORS, CORRECTIONS NEEDED
1 POOR AND UNACCEPTABLE PERFORMANCE—GROSS INACCURACIES, POTENTIALLY HARMFUL

PERFORMANCE CRITERIA		SCALE			
1. DISPLAYS KNOWLEDGE OF ESSENTIAL CONCEPTS	5	4	3	2	1
2. DEMONSTRATES THE RELATIONSHIP BETWEEN THEORY AND CLINICAL PRACTICE	5	4	3	2	1
3. FOLLOWS DIRECTIONS, EXHIBITS SOUND JUDGMENT, AND DEMONSTRATES ATTENTION TO SAFETY AND DETAIL	5	4	3	2	1
4. EXHIBITS THE REQUIRED MANUAL DEXTERITY	5	4	3	2	1
5. PERFORMS PROCEDURE IN A REASONABLE TIME FRAME	5	4	3	2	1
6. MAINTAINS STERILE OR ASEPTIC TECHNIQUE	5	4	3	2	1
7. INITIATES UNAMBIGUOUS GOAL-DIRECTED COMMUNICATION	5	4	3	2	1
8. PROVIDES FOR ADEQUATE CARE AND MAINTENANCE OF EQUIPMENT AND SUPPLIES	5	4	3	2	1
9. EXHIBITS COURTEOUS AND PLEASANT DEMEANOR	5	4	3	2	1
10. MAINTAINS CONCISE AND ACCURATE RECORDS	5	4	3	2	1

ADDITIONAL COMMENTS: INCLUDE ERRORS OF OMISSION OR COMMISSION, COMMUNICATIVE SKILLS, AND EFFECTIVENESS OF PATIENT INTERACTION:

SUMMARY PERFORMANCE EVALUATION AND RECOMMENDATIONS

SATISFACTORY PERFORMANCE—Performed without error or prompting, or able to self-correct, no critical errors.

——— LABORATORY EVALUATION. SKILLS MAY BE APPLIED/OBSERVED IN THE CLINICAL SETTING.

——— CLINICAL EVALUATION. STUDENT READY FOR MINIMALLY SUPERVISED APPLICATION AND REFINEMENT.

UNSATISFACTORY PERFORMANCE—Prompting required; performed with critical errors, potentially harmful.

——— STUDENT REQUIRES ADDITIONAL LABORATORY PRACTICE.

——— STUDENT REQUIRES ADDITIONAL SUPERVISED CLINICAL PRACTICE.

SIGNATURES

STUDENT: _____ EVALUATOR: _____

DATE: _____ DATE: _____

PROCEDURAL COMPETENCY EVALUATION

Name _Celia Ayala_   Date _6/13/00_

Patient Interview and History

Setting: ☐ Lab ☑ Clinical   Evaluator: ☐ Peer ☑ Instructor

Conditions (describe): _____

_____

Equipment Used

_____

_____

	SATISFACTORY	UNSATISFACTORY	NOT OBSERVED	NOT APPLICABLE
Equipment and Patient Preparation				
1. Washes hands and applies standard precautions and transmission-based isolation procedures as appropriate	☑	☐	☐	☐
2. Identifies patient, introduces self and department	☑	☐	☐	☐
3. Explains purpose of the procedure and confirms patient understanding	☑	☐	☐	☐

Assessment and Implementation

4. Uses therapeutic communication skills to determine the following: *→ perfect pt / Oriented x2 = ok pt / Oriented x1 = NOT good / disoriented*

Sense clock + TV → Oriented x 3

	SATISFACTORY	UNSATISFACTORY	NOT OBSERVED	NOT APPLICABLE
a. Level of consciousness and sensorium—orientation to person, place, and time 0x1	☑	☐	☐	☐
b. Ability to follow directions and level of cooperation → *by asking pt to squeeze your hands + you wiggle your toes, can you open your eyes*	☑	☐	☐	☐
c. Emotional status → *do not ask the pt (you need to asses it) Then you write it down*	☑	☐	☐	☐
d. Level of dyspnea *diff in breathing (you need to ask the pt.)*	☑	☐	☐	☐
e. Nutritional status → *apply to children + home care*	☑	☐	☐	☐
f. Tolerance of ADL *(Activity of daily life) how to asses Ex Can you cook, clean, walk.*	☑	☐	☐	☐

5. Asks the patient questions in order to verify the information obtained from the chart regarding the following:

	SATISFACTORY	UNSATISFACTORY	NOT OBSERVED	NOT APPLICABLE
a. Demographics *Age sex, hight + weight*	☑	☐	☐	☐
b. Chief complaint: onset, duration, frequency, severity (quantity), character (quality), location, radiation, aggravating factors, alleviating factors, associated manifestations *Color*	☑	☐	☐	☐
c. History of present illness:				
(1) Smoking history	☑	●	☐	☐
(2) Sexual activity → *consider*	☑	☐	☐	☐
d. Past medical history	☑	☐	☐	☐
e. Psychosocial assessment:				
(1) Birthplace	☑	☐	☐	☐
(2) Race	☑	☐	☐	☐
(3) Religion → *do not disrespect*	☑	☐	☐	☐
(4) Culture →	☑	☐	☐	☐
(5) Language(s) spoken → *Ask the pt to repeat back to you what you have say*	☑	☐	☐	☐
(6) Highest education level	☑	☐	☐	☐
(7) Alcohol intake →	☑	☐	☐	☐
(8) Drug use	☑	☐	☐	☐

IVDA — (Internal Drugs Avuser)

	SATISFACTORY	UNSATISFACTORY	NOT OBSERVED	NOT APPLICABLE
f. Occupational history	☑	☐	☐	☐
g. Allergies	☑	☐	☐	☐
h. Current medications	☑	☐	☐	☐

SOB shortness of breath

6. Asks the patient questions to ascertain specific pulmonary symptoms:

a. Dyspnea—on exertion or rest; orthopnea *difficulty breathing when you lay flat*	☑	☐	☐	☐
b. Cough	☑	☐	☐	☐
c. Sputum production—amount, color, *& smell color, consistency* consistency, presence of blood *(hemoptasis)*	☑	☐	☐	☐
d. Chest pain—quality, location, radiation, aggravating factors, alleviating factors, associated manifestations	☑	☐	☐	☐

| 7. Asks the patient questions to determine current comfort level or needs | ☑ | ☐ | ☐ | ☐ |

Follow-up

8. Disposes of infectious waste and washes hands	☑	☐	☐	☐
9. Records pertinent data in chart and departmental records	☑	☐	☐	☐
10. Notifies appropriate personnel and makes any necessary recommendations or modifications to the patient care plan	☑	☐	☐	☐

_____
Signature of Evaluator

_____
Signature of Student

Air Entrainment 24-50%
FIO₂ - is up to 50

• *RSV — Respiratory*

COPD these people Need
↓
Low FIO₂
< 3-4   *Stable Pt | Nasal conmule*

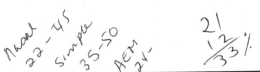

PERFORMANCE RATING SCALE

5 EXCELLENT—FAR EXCEEDS EXPECTED LEVEL, FLAWLESS PERFORMANCE
4 ABOVE AVERAGE—NO PROMPTING REQUIRED, ABLE TO SELF-CORRECT
3 AVERAGE—THE MINIMUM COMPETENCY LEVEL, NO CRITICAL ERRORS
2 IMPROVEMENT NEEDED—PROBLEM AREAS EXIST; CRITICAL ERRORS, CORRECTIONS NEEDED
1 POOR AND UNACCEPTABLE PERFORMANCE—GROSS INACCURACIES, POTENTIALLY HARMFUL

PERFORMANCE CRITERIA		SCALE			
1. DISPLAYS KNOWLEDGE OF ESSENTIAL CONCEPTS	5	4	3	2	1
2. DEMONSTRATES THE RELATIONSHIP BETWEEN THEORY AND CLINICAL PRACTICE	5	4	3	2	1
3. FOLLOWS DIRECTIONS, EXHIBITS SOUND JUDGMENT, AND DEMONSTRATES ATTENTION TO SAFETY AND DETAIL	5	4	3	2	1
4. EXHIBITS THE REQUIRED MANUAL DEXTERITY	5	4	3	2	1
5. PERFORMS PROCEDURE IN A REASONABLE TIME FRAME	5	4	3	2	1
6. MAINTAINS STERILE OR ASEPTIC TECHNIQUE	5	4	3	2	1
7. INITIATES UNAMBIGUOUS GOAL-DIRECTED COMMUNICATION	5	4	3	2	1
8. PROVIDES FOR ADEQUATE CARE AND MAINTENANCE OF EQUIPMENT AND SUPPLIES	5	4	3	2	1
9. EXHIBITS COURTEOUS AND PLEASANT DEMEANOR	5	4	3	2	1
10. MAINTAINS CONCISE AND ACCURATE RECORDS	5	4	3	2	1

ADDITIONAL COMMENTS: INCLUDE ERRORS OF OMISSION OR COMMISSION, COMMUNICATIVE SKILLS, AND EFFECTIVENESS OF PATIENT INTERACTION:

SUMMARY PERFORMANCE EVALUATION AND RECOMMENDATIONS

SATISFACTORY PERFORMANCE—Performed without error or prompting, or able to self-correct, no critical errors.

_____ LABORATORY EVALUATION. SKILLS MAY BE APPLIED/OBSERVED IN THE CLINICAL SETTING.

_____ CLINICAL EVALUATION. STUDENT READY FOR MINIMALLY SUPERVISED APPLICATION AND REFINEMENT.

UNSATISFACTORY PERFORMANCE—Prompting required; performed with critical errors, potentially harmful.

_____ STUDENT REQUIRES ADDITIONAL LABORATORY PRACTICE.

_____ STUDENT REQUIRES ADDITIONAL SUPERVISED CLINICAL PRACTICE.

SIGNATURES

STUDENT: _____   EVALUATOR: _____

DATE: _____   DATE: _____

PROCEDURAL COMPETENCY EVALUATION

Name _Cerlis Ayals_   Date _6/13/00_

Vital Signs: Pulse and Respiration

Setting: ☐ Lab ☑ Clinical   Evaluator: ☐ Peer ☑ Instructor

Conditions (describe): _____

_____

Equipment Used

_____

_____

	S A T I S F A C T O R Y	U N S A T I S F A C T O R Y	N O T O B S E R V E D	N O T A P P L I C A B L E
Equipment and Patient Preparation				
1. Washes hands and applies standard precautions and transmission-based isolation procedures as appropriate	☑	☐	☐	☐
2. Identifies patient, introduces self and department	☑	☐	☐	☐
3. Explains purpose of the procedure and confirms patient understanding	☑	☐	☐	☐
Assessment and Implementation				
4. Assesses patient	☑	☐	☐	☐
a. Pulse:				
(1) Locates site _80_	☑	☐	☐	☐
(2) Measures for at least 15 sec; if pulse irregular, measures for full minute _30 × 2_	☑	☐	☐	☐
(3) Assesses rhythm and quality of pulse	☑	☐	☐	☐
b. Respirations:				
(1) Measures for at least 15 sec _30 12_	☑	☐	☐	☐
(2) Assesses depth and I:E ratio _range 1-2 or 1to3_	☑	☐	☐	☐
(3) Assesses rhythm and quality of respirations	☑	☐	☐	☐
(4) Assesses degree of labored breathing: accessory muscle use, pursed-lip breathing, retractions, nasal flaring, abdominal paradox	☑	☐	☐	☐
(5) Ensures that patient is unaware of assessment	☑	☐	☐	☐
5. Thanks patient for cooperation	☑	☐	☐	☐
Follow-up				
6. Maintains/processes equipment; removes PPE	☑	☐	☐	☐
7. Disposes of infectious waste and washes hands	☑	☐	☐	☐
8. Records pertinent data in chart and departmental records	☑	☐	☐	☐
9. Notifies appropriate personnel and makes any necessary recommendations or modifications to the patient care plan	☑	☐	☐	☐

_____   _____
Signature of Evaluator   Signature of Student

PERFORMANCE RATING SCALE

5 EXCELLENT—FAR EXCEEDS EXPECTED LEVEL, FLAWLESS PERFORMANCE
4 ABOVE AVERAGE—NO PROMPTING REQUIRED, ABLE TO SELF-CORRECT
3 AVERAGE—THE MINIMUM COMPETENCY LEVEL, NO CRITICAL ERRORS
2 IMPROVEMENT NEEDED—PROBLEM AREAS EXIST; CRITICAL ERRORS, CORRECTIONS NEEDED
1 POOR AND UNACCEPTABLE PERFORMANCE—GROSS INACCURACIES, POTENTIALLY HARMFUL

PERFORMANCE CRITERIA	SCALE				
1. DISPLAYS KNOWLEDGE OF ESSENTIAL CONCEPTS	5	4	3	2	1
2. DEMONSTRATES THE RELATIONSHIP BETWEEN THEORY AND CLINICAL PRACTICE	5	4	3	2	1
3. FOLLOWS DIRECTIONS, EXHIBITS SOUND JUDGMENT, AND DEMONSTRATES ATTENTION TO SAFETY AND DETAIL	5	4	3	2	1
4. EXHIBITS THE REQUIRED MANUAL DEXTERITY	5	4	3	2	1
5. PERFORMS PROCEDURE IN A REASONABLE TIME FRAME	5	4	3	2	1
6. MAINTAINS STERILE OR ASEPTIC TECHNIQUE	5	4	3	2	1
7. INITIATES UNAMBIGUOUS GOAL-DIRECTED COMMUNICATION	5	4	3	2	1
8. PROVIDES FOR ADEQUATE CARE AND MAINTENANCE OF EQUIPMENT AND SUPPLIES	5	4	3	2	1
9. EXHIBITS COURTEOUS AND PLEASANT DEMEANOR	5	4	3	2	1
10. MAINTAINS CONCISE AND ACCURATE RECORDS	5	4	3	2	1

ADDITIONAL COMMENTS: INCLUDE ERRORS OF OMISSION OR COMMISSION, COMMUNICATIVE SKILLS, AND EFFECTIVENESS OF PATIENT INTERACTION:

SUMMARY PERFORMANCE EVALUATION AND RECOMMENDATIONS

SATISFACTORY PERFORMANCE—Performed without error or prompting, or able to self-correct, no critical errors.

_____ LABORATORY EVALUATION. SKILLS MAY BE APPLIED/OBSERVED IN THE CLINICAL SETTING.

_____ CLINICAL EVALUATION. STUDENT READY FOR MINIMALLY SUPERVISED APPLICATION AND REFINEMENT.

UNSATISFACTORY PERFORMANCE—Prompting required; performed with critical errors, potentially harmful.

_____ STUDENT REQUIRES ADDITIONAL LABORATORY PRACTICE.

_____ STUDENT REQUIRES ADDITIONAL SUPERVISED CLINICAL PRACTICE.

SIGNATURES

STUDENT: _____   EVALUATOR: _____

DATE: _____   DATE: _____

PROCEDURAL COMPETENCY EVALUATION

Name _Celia. Ayala_   Date _6/78/00_

Blood Pressure Measurement

Setting: ☑ Lab   ☐ Clinical   Evaluator: ☐ Peer   ☑ Instructor

Conditions (describe): _____

_____

Equipment Used

_____

_____

	SATISFACTORY	UNSATISFACTORY	NOT OBSERVED	NOT APPLICABLE

Equipment and Patient Preparation

	SATISFACTORY	UNSATISFACTORY	NOT OBSERVED	NOT APPLICABLE
1. Selects, gathers, and assembles the necessary equipment:				
a. Stethoscope	☑	☐	☐	☐
b. Sphygmomanometer	☑	☐	☐	☐
c. Correct size cuff and inflation bulb	☑	☐	☐	☐
2. Washes hands and applies standard precautions and transmission-based isolation procedures as appropriate	☑	☐	☐	☐
3. Identifies patient, introduces self and department	☑	☐	☐	☐
4. Explains purpose of the procedure and confirms patient understanding	☑	☐	☐	☐

Assessment and Implementation

	SATISFACTORY	UNSATISFACTORY	NOT OBSERVED	NOT APPLICABLE
5. Positions patient	☑	☐	☐	☐
6. Wraps sphygmomanometer cuff snugly around patient's arm	☑	☐	☐	☐
7. Positions mercury manometer at eye level; if using aneroid gauge, keeps at level of arm with arm at heart level	☑	☐	☐	☐
8. Has patient relax arm	☑	☐	☐	☐
9. Palpates brachial pulse and inflates cuff approximately 30 mm Hg above level at which pulse disappears; deflates slowly until pulse reappears; notes pressure at that point	☑	☐	☐	☐
10. Places stethoscope in ears and places bell of stethoscope over the brachial pulse, slightly distal to or partially under cuff	☑	☐	☐	☐
11. Reinflates cuff 30 mm Hg above expected systolic pressure	☑	☐	☐	☐
12. Deflates cuff slowly, observes manometer; notes systolic and diastolic pressures	☑	☐	☐	☐
13. Completely deflates cuff and removes	☑	☐	☐	☐
14. Records the blood pressure	☑	☐	☐	☐

Follow-up

	SATISFACTORY	UNSATISFACTORY	NOT OBSERVED	NOT APPLICABLE
15. Maintains/processes equipment	☑	☐	☐	☐
16. Disposes of infectious waste and washes hands	☑	☐	☐	☐
17. Records pertinent data in chart and departmental records	☑	☐	☐	☐
18. Notifies appropriate personnel and makes any necessary recommendations or modifications to the patient care plan	☑	☐	☐	☐

_____   _____
Signature of Evaluator   Signature of Student

PERFORMANCE RATING SCALE

5 EXCELLENT—FAR EXCEEDS EXPECTED LEVEL, FLAWLESS PERFORMANCE
4 ABOVE AVERAGE—NO PROMPTING REQUIRED, ABLE TO SELF-CORRECT
3 AVERAGE—THE MINIMUM COMPETENCY LEVEL, NO CRITICAL ERRORS
2 IMPROVEMENT NEEDED—PROBLEM AREAS EXIST; CRITICAL ERRORS, CORRECTIONS NEEDED
1 POOR AND UNACCEPTABLE PERFORMANCE—GROSS INACCURACIES, POTENTIALLY HARMFUL

PERFORMANCE CRITERIA		SCALE			
1. DISPLAYS KNOWLEDGE OF ESSENTIAL CONCEPTS	5	4	3	2	1
2. DEMONSTRATES THE RELATIONSHIP BETWEEN THEORY AND CLINICAL PRACTICE	5	4	3	2	1
3. FOLLOWS DIRECTIONS, EXHIBITS SOUND JUDGMENT, AND DEMONSTRATES ATTENTION TO SAFETY AND DETAIL	5	4	3	2	1
4. EXHIBITS THE REQUIRED MANUAL DEXTERITY	5	4	3	2	1
5. PERFORMS PROCEDURE IN A REASONABLE TIME FRAME	5	4	3	2	1
6. MAINTAINS STERILE OR ASEPTIC TECHNIQUE	5	4	3	2	1
7. INITIATES UNAMBIGUOUS GOAL-DIRECTED COMMUNICATION	5	4	3	2	1
8. PROVIDES FOR ADEQUATE CARE AND MAINTENANCE OF EQUIPMENT AND SUPPLIES	5	4	3	2	1
9. EXHIBITS COURTEOUS AND PLEASANT DEMEANOR	5	4	3	2	1
10. MAINTAINS CONCISE AND ACCURATE RECORDS	5	4	3	2	1

ADDITIONAL COMMENTS: INCLUDE ERRORS OF OMISSION OR COMMISSION, COMMUNICATIVE SKILLS, AND EFFECTIVENESS OF PATIENT INTERACTION:

SUMMARY PERFORMANCE EVALUATION AND RECOMMENDATIONS

SATISFACTORY PERFORMANCE—Performed without error or prompting, or able to self-correct, no critical errors.

_____ LABORATORY EVALUATION. SKILLS MAY BE APPLIED/OBSERVED IN THE CLINICAL SETTING.

_____ CLINICAL EVALUATION. STUDENT READY FOR MINIMALLY SUPERVISED APPLICATION AND REFINEMENT.

UNSATISFACTORY PERFORMANCE—Prompting required; performed with critical errors, potentially harmful.

_____ STUDENT REQUIRES ADDITIONAL LABORATORY PRACTICE.

_____ STUDENT REQUIRES ADDITIONAL SUPERVISED CLINICAL PRACTICE.

SIGNATURES

STUDENT: _____   EVALUATOR: _____

DATE: _____   DATE: _____

PROCEDURAL COMPETENCY EVALUATION

Name _Celia Ayala_   Date _7/13/00 7/20/00_

Physical Assessment of the Chest

Setting: ☑ Lab   ☐ Clinical   Evaluator: ☐ Peer ☑ Instructor

Conditions (describe): _____

_____

Equipment Used

_____

_____

	SATISFACTORY	UNSATISFACTORY	NOT OBSERVED	NOT APPLICABLE

Equipment and Patient Preparation

1. Washes hands and applies standard precautions and transmission-based isolation procedures as appropriate — ☑ ☐ ☐ ☐
2. Ensures room is well lit — ☑ ☐ ☐ ☐
3. Identifies patient, introduces self and department — ☑ ☐ ☐ ☐
4. Explains purpose of the procedure and confirms patient understanding — ☑ ☐ ☐ ☐
5. Positions the patient in the Fowler's position and ensures patient modesty and privacy — ☑ ☐ ☐ ☐   *90° angle.*

Assessment and Implementation

6. Observes the patient for overall appearance, age, sex, and weight — ☑ ☐ ☐ ☐
7. Stands directly in front of the patient and observes the chest for the following:
   a. General shape and appearance — ☑ ☐ ☐ ☐
   b. Anterior to posterior diameter — ☑ ☐ ☐ ☐
   c. Sternal deformities — ☑ ☐ ☐ ☐
   d. Surgical or other scars — ☑ ☐ ☐ ☐
   e. Symmetrical expansion — ☑ ☐ ☐ ☐
8. Observes for any paradoxical or unequal expansion — ☑ ☐ ☐ ☐
9. Observes for the presence of chest tubes — ☑ ☐ ☐ ☐
10. Observes for the presence of spinal curvature — ☑ ☐ ☐ ☐
11. Observes the skin for cyanosis, pallor, mottling, diaphoresis, swelling, bruises, or erythema — ☑ ☐ ☐ ☐
12. Observes the skin for any obvious masses, lesions, or nodules — ☑ ☐ ☐ ☐
13. Assesses the respiratory pattern by observing regularity, rate, and depth of breathing and patient positioning and accessory muscle use during breathing — ☑ ☐ ☐ ☐
14. Observes for retractions, pursed-lip breathing, and nasal flaring — ☑ ☐ ☐ ☐
15. Performs palpation:
   a. Palpates the position of the trachea — ☑ ☐ ☐ ☐
   b. Palpates the skin for the presence of subcutaneous emphysema — ☑ ☐ ☐ ☐
   c. Places the hands in the "butterfly" position and palpates for equal bilateral expansion — ☑ ☐ ☐ ☐
   d. Palpates the chest wall over each of the lung lobes for tactile fremitus while the patient says "ninety-nine" — ☑ ☐ ☐ ☐
   e. Palpates for spinal curvature — ☑ ☐ ☐ ☐

passage of the fluids (usually blood) thru the body to determine → to produce sound to determine the size / position or density of the underlying structures.

	S A T I S F A C T O R Y	U N S A T I S F A C T O R Y	N O T O B S E R V E D	N O T A P P L I C A B L E
16. Assesses peripheral perfusion by palpating pulses and capillary refill	☑	☐	☐	☐
17. Performs diagnostic chest percussion; places hands and fingers in the proper position	☑	☐	☐	☐
a. Percusses over and identifies the liver margin	☑	☐	☐	☐
b. Percusses over lung tissue and compares the notes made bilaterally	☑	☐	☐	☐
c. Percusses over the stomach	☑	☐	☐	☐
d. Estimates diaphragmatic excursion	☑	☐	☐	☐

Follow-up

18. Repositions the patient and returns the lighting to the original level	☐	☐	☐	☐
19. Disposes of any infectious waste and washes hands	☐	☐	☐	☐
20. Records pertinent data in chart and departmental records	☐	☐	☐	☐
21. Notifies appropriate personnel and makes any necessary recommendations or modifications to the patient care plan	☐	☐	☐	☐

_____
Signature of Evaluator

_____
Signature of Student

PERFORMANCE RATING SCALE

5 EXCELLENT—FAR EXCEEDS EXPECTED LEVEL, FLAWLESS PERFORMANCE
4 ABOVE AVERAGE—NO PROMPTING REQUIRED, ABLE TO SELF-CORRECT
3 AVERAGE—THE MINIMUM COMPETENCY LEVEL, NO CRITICAL ERRORS
2 IMPROVEMENT NEEDED—PROBLEM AREAS EXIST; CRITICAL ERRORS, CORRECTIONS NEEDED
1 POOR AND UNACCEPTABLE PERFORMANCE—GROSS INACCURACIES, POTENTIALLY HARMFUL

PERFORMANCE CRITERIA		SCALE			
1. DISPLAYS KNOWLEDGE OF ESSENTIAL CONCEPTS	5	4	3	2	1
2. DEMONSTRATES THE RELATIONSHIP BETWEEN THEORY AND CLINICAL PRACTICE	5	4	3	2	1
3. FOLLOWS DIRECTIONS, EXHIBITS SOUND JUDGMENT, AND DEMONSTRATES ATTENTION TO SAFETY AND DETAIL	5	4	3	2	1
4. EXHIBITS THE REQUIRED MANUAL DEXTERITY	5	4	3	2	1
5. PERFORMS PROCEDURE IN A REASONABLE TIME FRAME	5	4	3	2	1
6. MAINTAINS STERILE OR ASEPTIC TECHNIQUE	5	4	3	2	1
7. INITIATES UNAMBIGUOUS GOAL-DIRECTED COMMUNICATION	5	4	3	2	1
8. PROVIDES FOR ADEQUATE CARE AND MAINTENANCE OF EQUIPMENT AND SUPPLIES	5	4	3	2	1
9. EXHIBITS COURTEOUS AND PLEASANT DEMEANOR	5	4	3	2	1
10. MAINTAINS CONCISE AND ACCURATE RECORDS	5	4	3	2	1

ADDITIONAL COMMENTS: INCLUDE ERRORS OF OMISSION OR COMMISSION, COMMUNICATIVE SKILLS, AND EFFECTIVENESS OF PATIENT INTERACTION:

SUMMARY PERFORMANCE EVALUATION AND RECOMMENDATIONS

SATISFACTORY PERFORMANCE—Performed without error or prompting, or able to self-correct, no critical errors.

_____ LABORATORY EVALUATION. SKILLS MAY BE APPLIED/OBSERVED IN THE CLINICAL SETTING.

_____ CLINICAL EVALUATION. STUDENT READY FOR MINIMALLY SUPERVISED APPLICATION AND REFINEMENT.

UNSATISFACTORY PERFORMANCE—Prompting required; performed with critical errors, potentially harmful.

_____ STUDENT REQUIRES ADDITIONAL LABORATORY PRACTICE.

_____ STUDENT REQUIRES ADDITIONAL SUPERVISED CLINICAL PRACTICE.

SIGNATURES

STUDENT: _____   EVALUATOR: _____

DATE: _____   DATE: _____

PROCEDURAL COMPETENCY EVALUATION

Name _Cevia· Ayala·_ Date _7/20/00_

Auscultation

Setting: ☑ Lab ☐ Clinical   Evaluator: ☐ Peer ☑ Instructor

Conditions (describe): _____

_____

Equipment Used

_____

_____

	S A T I S F A C T O R Y	U N S A T I S F A C T O R Y	N O T O B S E R V E D	N O T A P P L I C A B L E

Equipment and Patient Preparation

1. Selects, gathers, and assembles the necessary equipment: stethoscope, alcohol pads — ☑ ☐ ☐ ☐

2. Washes hands and applies standard precautions and transmission-based isolation procedures as appropriate — ☑ ☐ ☐ ☐

3. Prepares and tests equipment:

   a. Cleans earpieces of stethoscope — ☑ ☐ ☐ ☐

   b. Cleans and disinfects diaphragm and bell — ☑ ☐ ☐ ☐

   c. Tests equipment and corrects malfunctions if needed — ☑ ☐ ☐ ☐

4. Identifies patient, introduces self and department — ☑ ☐ ☐ ☐

5. Explains purpose of the procedure and confirms patient understanding — ☑ ☐ ☐ ☐

Assessment and Implementation

6. Positions patient:

   a. Has patient sit upright leaning forward (if possible), facing away — ☑ ☐ ☐ ☐

   b. If patient is unable to sit upright, gets assistance to turn patient to side to auscultate posterior chest — ☑ ☐ ☐ ☐

7. Auscultates the anterior chest in at least six positions, comparing sounds bilaterally — ☑ ☐ ☐ ☐

8. Auscultates the lateral chest bilaterally — ☑ ☐ ☐ ☐

9. Auscultates the posterior chest in at least six positions, comparing sounds bilaterally — ☑ ☐ ☐ ☐

10. Ensures patient safety and comfort — ☑ ☐ ☐ ☐

11. Properly identifies normal or abnormal and adventitious sounds — ☑ ☐ ☐ ☐

Follow-up

12. Maintains/processes equipment — ☑ ☐ ☐ ☐

13. Disposes of infectious waste and washes hands — ☑ ☐ ☐ ☐

14. Records pertinent data in chart and departmental records — ☑ ☐ ☐ ☐

15. Notifies appropriate personnel and makes any necessary recommendations or modifications to the patient care plan — ☑ ☐ ☐ ☐

_____   _____
Signature of Evaluator   Signature of Student

PERFORMANCE RATING SCALE

5 EXCELLENT—FAR EXCEEDS EXPECTED LEVEL, FLAWLESS PERFORMANCE
4 ABOVE AVERAGE—NO PROMPTING REQUIRED, ABLE TO SELF-CORRECT
3 AVERAGE—THE MINIMUM COMPETENCY LEVEL, NO CRITICAL ERRORS
2 IMPROVEMENT NEEDED—PROBLEM AREAS EXIST; CRITICAL ERRORS, CORRECTIONS NEEDED
1 POOR AND UNACCEPTABLE PERFORMANCE—GROSS INACCURACIES, POTENTIALLY HARMFUL

PERFORMANCE CRITERIA		SCALE			
1. DISPLAYS KNOWLEDGE OF ESSENTIAL CONCEPTS	5	4	3	2	1
2. DEMONSTRATES THE RELATIONSHIP BETWEEN THEORY AND CLINICAL PRACTICE	5	4	3	2	1
3. FOLLOWS DIRECTIONS, EXHIBITS SOUND JUDGMENT, AND DEMONSTRATES ATTENTION TO SAFETY AND DETAIL	5	4	3	2	1
4. EXHIBITS THE REQUIRED MANUAL DEXTERITY	5	4	3	2	1
5. PERFORMS PROCEDURE IN A REASONABLE TIME FRAME	5	4	3	2	1
6. MAINTAINS STERILE OR ASEPTIC TECHNIQUE	5	4	3	2	1
7. INITIATES UNAMBIGUOUS GOAL-DIRECTED COMMUNICATION	5	4	3	2	1
8. PROVIDES FOR ADEQUATE CARE AND MAINTENANCE OF EQUIPMENT AND SUPPLIES	5	4	3	2	1
9. EXHIBITS COURTEOUS AND PLEASANT DEMEANOR	5	4	3	2	1
10. MAINTAINS CONCISE AND ACCURATE RECORDS	5	4	3	2	1

ADDITIONAL COMMENTS: INCLUDE ERRORS OF OMISSION OR COMMISSION, COMMUNICATIVE SKILLS, AND EFFECTIVENESS OF PATIENT INTERACTION:

SUMMARY PERFORMANCE EVALUATION AND RECOMMENDATIONS

SATISFACTORY PERFORMANCE—Performed without error or prompting, or able to self-correct, no critical errors.

_____ LABORATORY EVALUATION. SKILLS MAY BE APPLIED/OBSERVED IN THE CLINICAL SETTING.

_____ CLINICAL EVALUATION. STUDENT READY FOR MINIMALLY SUPERVISED APPLICATION AND REFINEMENT.

UNSATISFACTORY PERFORMANCE—Prompting required; performed with critical errors, potentially harmful.

_____ STUDENT REQUIRES ADDITIONAL LABORATORY PRACTICE.

_____ STUDENT REQUIRES ADDITIONAL SUPERVISED CLINICAL PRACTICE.

SIGNATURES

STUDENT: _____ EVALUATOR: _____

DATE: _____ DATE: _____

CHAPTER 3

Bedside Assessment of Pulmonary Mechanics

INTRODUCTION

Often the respiratory care practitioner is called to the bedside to obtain data relevant to the state of the patient's ability to breathe. Simple bedside measurements can be performed. These data are essential, in conjunction with clinical assessment, when making decisions regarding initiation, modification, or discontinuance of respiratory modalities and procedures, especially mechanical ventilation.

These studies include, but are not limited to, the following parameters:

1. Tidal volume (V_T), minute ventilation ($\dot{V}_E$), and alveolar ventilation ($\dot{V}_A$)
2. Maximum inspiratory pressure (MIP)
3. Maximum expiratory pressure (MEP)
4. Slow vital capacity (SVC)
5. Peak expiratory flow rate (PEFR)

OBJECTIVES
Upon completion of this chapter, the student will be able to:

1. Perform bedside assessment of pulmonary mechanics in the laboratory and clinical settings.
2. Select, use, and maintain the equipment necessary to perform bedside assessment of pulmonary mechanics, including **vane** and electronic respirometers.
3. Apply infection control guidelines and standards associated with each piece of equipment, according to OSHA regulations, CDC guidelines, and American Thoracic Society (ATS) standards.
4. Given a patient scenario, select the appropriate tests and relate the clinical significance of the measured parameters to treatment decisions.
5. Explain alternative ways of obtaining data when dealing with patients with limited mental or functional capacity or language barriers.
6. Practice communication skills needed to instruct patients in the performance of pulmonary mechanics testing.
7. Practice medical charting for the documentation of performance of bedside pulmonary mechanics procedures.

KEY TERMS

atmospheric temperature and pressure, saturated (ATPS)	pressure, saturated (BTPS)	facilitate	spirometer
body temperature and	compliance	flow rate	transducer
	deadspace	laminar	turbulent
	elastance	lumen	vane
		resistance	vortex

EQUIPMENT REQUIRED

- Watch with a second hand
- Pressure manometer with positive and negative ranges
- Electronic and vane respirometers
- Peak flowmeters (disposable or permanent)
- One-way valves
- Inspiratory force adaptors

- Masks
- Disposable mouthpieces
- Corrugated tubing
- Noseclips
- Briggs adaptors
- Intubated or tracheostomized airway management trainer
- Disposable gloves

● EXERCISES

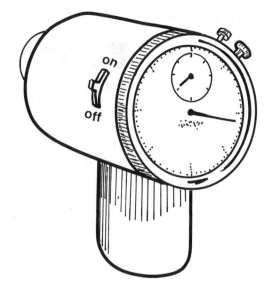

FIGURE 3.1   A vane respirometer.

These exercises require students to work in groups of two. The students may carry out all the exercises with the same partner, or the instructor may want to change pairs to enhance the ability of each student to communicate and explain the procedure to a different person.

In an actual clinical situation, the patient may be receiving supplemental oxygen via mask or may be on a ventilator. To obtain bedside pulmonary mechanics, the patient would have to be removed from these devices and an alternative mode of oxygen delivery instituted. In these circumstances, the practitioner should monitor the patient carefully for signs of hypoxia while the parameters are being obtained. This includes observation of the patient, use of pulse oximetry, and cardiac monitors. Placing the patient on a nasal cannula may be one alternative. The therapist should consult with the physician or follow departmental policies under these circumstances. If the patient is on a ventilator, the practitioner must ensure that the ventilator connector is handled aseptically. The ventilator alarms may need to be temporarily bypassed, but the practitioner must ensure they are reset and functional once the procedure is concluded. The patient must be immediately returned to the ventilator if there is any indication that the patient is not tolerating the testing. Results of the testing may be interpreted based on normal and critical values, shown in Table 3.1.

EXERCISE 3.1 Obtaining V_T, $\dot{V}_E$, and $\dot{V}_A$

This exercise requires data to be obtained using a device called a respirometer. The two major types of respirometers are a rotating vane **spirometer,** as shown in Figure 3.1, and an electronic ultrasonic **vortex** flow sensor, as shown in Figure 3.2.

1. Gather the necessary equipment: watch with a second hand, spirometer, disposable noseclips, mouthpieces, one-way valves, and tubing to prevent cross-contamination with the spirometer.

    A one-way valve should be used each time this procedure is performed. The one-way valve is for single-patient use only.

2. Wash hands and apply standard precautions and transmission-based isolation procedures as appropriate.

3. Assemble the equipment as shown in Figure 3.3.
    a. Attach a single length of large-bore corrugated tubing to the T-piece opening. Attach the mouthpiece to the opposite end of the corrugated tubing.

    b. Attach a single length of corrugated tubing to the expiratory side of the T-piece one-way valve assembly. Place a 22 mm outer diameter (OD)/15 mm inner diameter (ID) adaptor to the opposite end of the corrugated tubing.
    c. Attach the respirometer to the expiratory side of the 22 mm OD/15 mm ID adaptor.
    d. Verify the appropriate direction of flow by ensuring that one-way valves allow for inspiration from the room and expiration into the respirometer.

4. Introduce yourself. *Record your partner's name, age, sex, height, and weight on your laboratory report.*

5. Explain the procedure and the purpose of the testing to your partner. Demonstrate if necessary.

6. Instruct your partner to put the mouthpiece into his or her mouth. Emphasize the importance of maintaining a tight seal around the mouthpiece. Explain the purpose of using the noseclips.

7. Allow your partner to stabilize, or "get used to," breathing through the mouthpiece and spirometer.

TABLE 3.1   **Normal and Critical Values for Bedside Spirometry**

Parameter	Normal Value	Minimal Acceptable Value
Tidal volume	5–7 ml/kg	—
Vital capacity	50–70 ml/kg	10–15 ml/kg
Minute ventilation	6–10 lpm	—
Peak flow	300–600 lpm	80–100 lpm
Negative inspiratory force	−60 to −100 cm H_2O	−20 to −25 cm H_2O
Maximum expiratory pressure	+60 to +100 cm H_2O	+20 to +25 cm H_2O

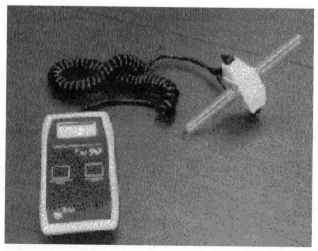

FIGURE 3.2   Electronic ultrasonic vortex flow-sensing respirometer.

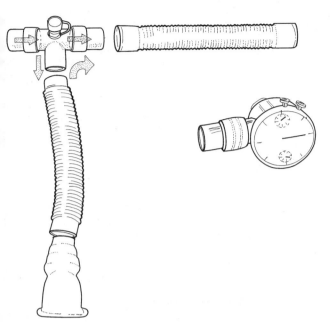

FIGURE 3.3   Assembly of one-way valve monitoring circuit.

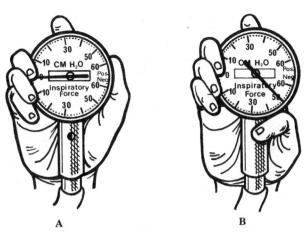

A   **B**

FIGURE 3.4   Inspiratory force meter. (From Pilbeam, SP: Mechanical Ventilation: Physiological and Clinical Applications, ed 2. Mosby-Year Book, St. Louis, 1992, p. 315, with permission.)

8. Turn the spirometer on. Activate the spirometer by pressing the "Reset" button to zero the dial, and begin recording your partner's exhaled volumes.

9. Simultaneously, count your partner's breath rate.

10. Measure these parameters for *one full minute.* At the end of precisely one minute, press the "Stop" or "Off" button to stop the recording and preserve the data.

11. *Record the data on your laboratory report.*

12. Disassemble and properly clean the equipment.
    a. In the event that multiple measurements are required on an individual patient, the one-way valve assembly may be aseptically stored in the patient's room. Otherwise the assembly should be discarded after use.
    b. The respirometer should be wiped down with a 70 percent isopropyl alcohol solution between patients.
    c. For patients with active tuberculosis or any other disorder requiring airborne or droplet isolation precautions, the respirometer should be sterilized between patients.

EXERCISE 3.2 Obtaining Negative Inspiratory Force and Maximum Expiratory Pressure

1. Gather the necessary equipment: mask or mouthpiece and noseclips, disposable inspiratory force adaptor with one-way valve, and pressure manometer (Fig. 3.4).

2. Wash your hands and apply standard precautions and transmission-based isolation procedures as appropriate.

3. Assemble the equipment as shown in Figure 3.5.
   a. Attach the small-bore tubing to the nipple on the inspiratory force meter.
   b. Attach the opposite end of the small-bore tubing to the inspiratory force adaptor or the port on the one-way valve setup.
   c. The inspiratory force adaptor will fit directly onto an endotracheal or tracheostomy tube. For nonintubated patients, attach the adaptor to a mask or mouthpiece.

4. Explain the procedure to your partner. Demonstrate if necessary.

5. Completely occlude the opening on the inspiratory force adaptor with your finger, and instruct your partner to inhale as hard as possible from the normal resting exhalation position. If the one-way valve is used, no occlusion is needed. Note the maximum negative pressure achieved.

6. Repeat the procedure two more times.

7. *Record the data from the three trials on your laboratory report.*

8. Using the same equipment, completely occlude the opening of the adaptor, instruct your partner to take a deep breath, and then to exhale as hard as possible.

9. Repeat the procedure two more times.

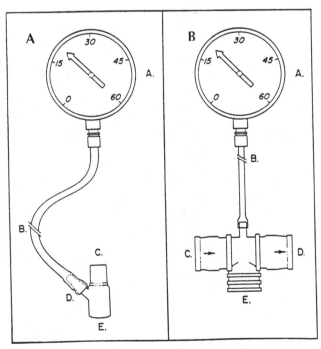

FIGURE 3.5   Assembled equipment for inspiratory force measurement. (From Black, LF and Hyatt, RE: Am Rev Respir Dis 103: 641–650, 1971, with permission.)

10. *Record the data from the three trials on your laboratory report.*

EXERCISE 3.3 Obtaining a Slow Vital Capacity

NOTE: If a vane-type spirometer, such as a Wright respirometer, is used, high **flow rates** will warp the vanes. Do not perform a forced vital capacity (FVC) with this device!

1. Gather and assemble the necessary equipment: respirometer, one-way valves, mouthpiece or mask, and noseclips as in Exercise 3.1.

2. Wash hands and apply standard precautions and transmission-based isolation procedures as appropriate.

3. Turn the spirometer on and reset to zero.

4. Explain the procedure by instructing your partner to take in the deepest breath possible and then exhale *slowly* and completely into the spirometer. Demonstrate if necessary.

5. Ensure a tight seal by making sure that the mouthpiece is secure, that noseclips are in place, or, if using a mask, that there are no leaks.

6. Coach the patient throughout the procedure. Turn off the respirometer or press the "Stop" button when exhalation is complete.

7. Repeat the procedure two more times and *record the data on your laboratory report.*

EXERCISE 3.4 Obtaining Peak Expiratory Flow Rate Measurements

1. Obtain a peak flowmeter and a mouthpiece (Fig. 3.6). The use of noseclips is recommended.

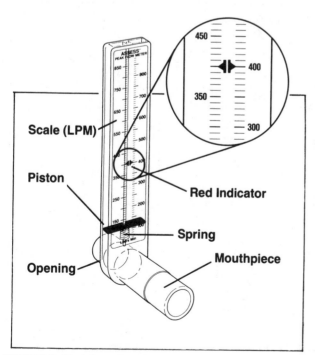

FIGURE 3.6 Peak flowmeter. (From HealthScan Products Inc., Cedar Grove, NJ 07009, with permission.)

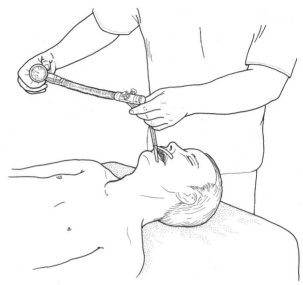

FIGURE 3.7 Attaching monitoring equipment to an artificial airway.

2. Wash hands and apply standard precautions and transmission-based isolation procedures as appropriate.

3. Instruct your partner to take in a deep breath and then to blow as hard as possible into the peak flowmeter. Ensure a tight seal. Exhalation down to residual volume is not necessary. Demonstrate if necessary.

4. Repeat the procedure two more times and *record the data on your laboratory report.*

EXERCISE 3.5 Obtaining Data on Patients with Artificial Airways

1. Obtain one-way valves, corrugated tubing, and Briggs adaptors.

2. Assemble the equipment as previously described.

3. Wash your hands and apply standard precautions and transmission-based isolation procedures as appropriate.

4. Attach equipment to the adaptor of the artificial airway as shown in Figure 3.7.

   NOTE: Because an intubated mannequin cannot breathe spontaneously, no measurements can be obtained at this time.

Related Readings

Eubanks, DH and Bone, RC: Principles and Applications of Cardiorespiratory Care Equipment. Mosby, St Louis, 1994.

Madama, V: Pulmonary Function Testing and Cardiopulmonary Stress Testing. Delmar, Albany, 1993.

McPherson, S: Respiratory Care Equipment, ed 5. Mosby, St Louis, 1995.

Ruppel, G: Manual of Pulmonary Function Testing, ed 6. Mosby, St Louis, 1994.

Scanlan, C et al (eds): Egan's Fundamentals of Respiratory Care, ed 6. Mosby, St Louis, 1995.

Wanger, J: Pulmonary Function Testing. Williams & Wilkins, Baltimore, 1992.

West, J: Respiratory Physiology: The Essentials, ed 5. Williams & Wilkins, Baltimore, 1995.

Wilkins, R, Sheldon, R and Krider, S: Clinical Assessment in Respiratory Care, ed 3. Mosby, St Louis, 1995.

Selected Journal Articles

American Association for Respiratory Care: AARC Clinical Practice Guideline: Spirometry. Respir Care 36:1414–1417, 1991.

American Association for Respiratory Care: AARC Clinical Practice Guideline: Spirometry, 1996 Update. Respir Care 41:629–636, 1996.

American Thoracic Society: Standardization of spirometry: 1994 update. Am J Respir Crit Care Med 152:1107–1136, 1995.

Branson, RD et al: Measurement of maximal inspiratory pressure: A comparison of three methods. Respir Care 34:789–794, 1989.

Centers for Disease Control and Prevention: Guidelines for preventing the transmission of *Mycobacterium tuberculosis* in health-care facilities, 1994. US Department of Health and Human Services, Atlanta, 43:RR-13, pp 33–34.

Centers for Disease Control and Prevention: Guidelines for prevention of nosocomial pneumonia. Respir Care 39:1191–1236, 1994.

Chatburn, R: Decontamination of respiratory care equipment: What should be done, what can be done. Respir Care 34:98–110, 1989.

Chatham, K et al: Inspiratory pressures in adult cystic fibrosis. Physiotherapy 80:748–752, 1994.

Gardner, RM: Quality assurance in spirometry. Choices in Respiratory Management 19:88–97, 1989.

Hankinson, J: Quality control in the pulmonary function laboratory. Respir Care 27:830–833, 1982.

Ilsley, AH et al: Evaluation of five small turbine-type respirometers used in adult anesthesia. J Clin Monit 9:196–201, 1993.

OSHA: Regulations for bloodborne pathogens. Federal Register, January, 1992.

LABORATORY REPORT

CHAPTER 3: ASSESSMENT OF BEDSIDE PULMONARY MECHANICS

Name _____   Date _____

Course/Section _____   Instructor _____

Data Collection

Laboratory partner: _____

Age: _____   Sex: _____   Height: _____   Weight: _____

EXERCISE 3.1   Obtaining V_T, $\dot{V}_E$, and $\dot{V}_A$

Minute ventilation: _____

Breath rate: _____

Calculate your partner's average tidal volume using the following formula: $V_T = \dot{V}_E/f$.

Tidal volume: _____

Calculate your partner's alveolar ventilation using the following formula: $\dot{V}_A = (V_T - V_D)f$.
NOTE: Anatomic **deadspace** (V_D) is estimated as 1 ml/lb or 2.2 ml/kg of ideal body weight.

Anatomic deadspace: _____

Alveolar ventilation: _____

EXERCISE 3.2   Obtaining Negative Inspiratory Force and Maximum Expiratory Pressure

	Trial 1	Trial 2	Trial 3
Negative inspiratory force:	_____	_____	_____
Maximum expiratory force:	_____	_____	_____

Circle the value to be reported.

EXERCISE 3.3   Obtaining a Slow Vital Capacity

	Trial 1	Trial 2	Trial 3
Slow vital capacity:	_____	_____	_____

Circle the value to be reported.

EXERCISE 3.4   Obtaining Peak Expiratory Flow Rate Measurements

	Trial 1	Trial 2	Trial 3
Peak flow rate:	_____	_____	_____

Circle the value to be reported.

CRITICAL THINKING QUESTIONS

1. Calculate the missing values. Show your work!

Weight	200 lb	60 kg	140 lb
V_T	400 ml	_____	_____
f	14	20	15
$\dot{V}_E$	_____	12.6 L	_____
V_D	_____	_____	_____
$\dot{V}_A$	_____	_____	6.0 L

2. Why is it necessary to obtain at least three trials? Which trial(s) would you report to the physician?

3. Which measurement(s) require the most cooperation from your partner to obtain results?

4. Dr. Shah asks you to perform a bedside evaluation on Mrs. Hernandez, a 29-year-old, 150-lb woman admitted with a diagnosis of myasthenia gravis. As you begin to explain the procedure, you realize that she speaks and understands only Spanish.

    How would you alter your instructions or actions to the patient in order to obtain the data under these circumstances?
    What is the clinical significance of monitoring these parameters in a patient with Mrs. Hernandez's condition?

5. You are able to obtain the following parameters:

    Tidal volume: 300 ml   _____

    Respiratory rate: 25/min   _____

    Minute ventilation: 7.7 lpm   _____

    Negative inspiratory force: −40 cm H_2O _____

    Slow vital capacity: 1.5 lpm   _____

    Peak flow: 200 lpm   _____

    For each of these parameters, indicate whether it is within normal limits, abnormal, or a critical value.
    What is your overall impression and interpretation of these results?
    What would be your recommendations to the physician regarding evaluation and treatment of this patient?
    Which of these parameters is indicative of the patient's ability to cough and deep breathe?
    Which of these parameters is most indicative of respiratory muscle strength?

6. Dr. Shah now tells you that she suspects that Mrs. Hernandez has diplococcal pneumonia. What infection control procedures related to the patient, the equipment, and yourself did you practice to ensure that the infection will not be spread to you or to other patients?

    What, if any, additional procedures would you follow if Mrs. Hernandez was suspected of having tuberculosis?

7. Two hours later, the bedside evaluation is repeated and the following data are obtained: V_T, 200 mL; respiratory rate, 40/min. Based on these data, which of the following would most likely be increased above normal? Circle as many as are appropriate.
    a. Minute ventilation ($\dot{V}_E$)
    b. Alveolar ventilation ($\dot{V}_A$)
    c. Deadspace ventilation (V_D)
    d. $PaCO_2$

8. In a patient with an artificial airway, which test(s), if any, could not be performed?
    What parameters could not be obtained in a comatose patient?

PROCEDURAL COMPETENCY EVALUATION

Name _____ Date _____

Bedside Pulmonary Mechanics

Setting: ☐ Lab   ☐ Clinical   Evaluator: ☐ Peer   ☐ Instructor

Conditions (describe): _____

_____

Equipment Used

_____

_____

	SATISFACTORY	UNSATISFACTORY	NOT OBSERVED	NOT APPLICABLE
Equipment and Patient Preparation				
1. Verifies, interprets, and evaluates physician's order or protocol	☐	☐	☐	☐
2. Scans chart for diagnosis and any other pertinent data and notes	☐	☐	☐	☐
3. Selects, gathers, and assembles the necessary equipment	☐	☐	☐	☐
4. Washes hands and applies standard precautions and transmission-based isolation procedures as appropriate	☐	☐	☐	☐
5. Identifies patient, introduces self and department	☐	☐	☐	☐
6. Explains purpose of the procedure and confirms patient understanding	☐	☐	☐	☐
Assessment and Implementation				
7. Assesses patient's pulse, respiratory rate, and respiratory pattern	☐	☐	☐	☐
8. Positions patient	☐	☐	☐	☐
9. Assembles one-way valve monitoring adaptor and connects it to the respirometer	☐	☐	☐	☐
10. Instructs the patient to breathe normally	☐	☐	☐	☐
11. Applies noseclips	☐	☐	☐	☐
12. Connects patient to the monitoring system	☐	☐	☐	☐
13. Measures minute ventilation	☐	☐	☐	☐
14. Simultaneously measures respiratory rate	☐	☐	☐	☐
15. Assesses patient's tolerance of the procedure	☐	☐	☐	☐
16. Disconnects the noseclips and respirometer	☐	☐	☐	☐
17. Instructs patient in the performance of a slow vital capacity	☐	☐	☐	☐
18. Applies noseclips and connects the patient to the respirometer	☐	☐	☐	☐
19. Measures the slow vital capacity	☐	☐	☐	☐
20. Assesses patient performance and tolerance	☐	☐	☐	☐
21. Repeats the slow vital capacity at least two more times, allowing for adequate recovery between attempts	☐	☐	☐	☐
22. Removes the respirometer and noseclips	☐	☐	☐	☐
23. Instructs the patient in the performance of a maximal inspiratory and expiratory pressure	☐	☐	☐	☐
24. Assembles adaptors and manometer	☐	☐	☐	☐
25. Applies noseclips or mask	☐	☐	☐	☐

	S A T I S F A C T O R Y	U N S A T I S F A C T O R Y	N O T O B S E R V E D	N O T A P P L I C A B L E
26. Measures maximal inspiratory and expiratory pressures	☐	☐	☐	☐
27. Assesses patient's performance and tolerance	☐	☐	☐	☐
28. Allows adequate recovery time	☐	☐	☐	☐
29. Instructs the patient in the performance of a peak flow maneuver	☐	☐	☐	☐
30. Applies noseclips and positions mouthpiece properly	☐	☐	☐	☐
31. Measures peak flow	☐	☐	☐	☐
32. Assesses patient performance and tolerance	☐	☐	☐	☐
33. Repeats peak flow measurement at least two more times	☐	☐	☐	☐
34. Allows for adequate recovery between attempts	☐	☐	☐	☐
35. Assesses patient and makes sure the patient is returned to pretesting status	☐	☐	☐	☐

Follow-up

36. Corrects measured values for **body temperature and pressure, saturated (BTPS)**	☐	☐	☐	☐
37. Maintains/processes equipment	☐	☐	☐	☐
38. Disposes of infectious waste and washes hands	☐	☐	☐	☐
39. Calculates V_T	☐	☐	☐	☐
40. Reviews data for the presence of critical values	☐	☐	☐	☐
41. Records best data in chart and departmental records	☐	☐	☐	☐
42. Notifies appropriate personnel and makes any necessary recommendations or modifications to the patient care plan	☐	☐	☐	☐

_____

Signature of Evaluator

_____

Signature of Student

PERFORMANCE RATING SCALE

5 EXCELLENT—FAR EXCEEDS EXPECTED LEVEL, FLAWLESS PERFORMANCE
4 ABOVE AVERAGE—NO PROMPTING REQUIRED, ABLE TO SELF-CORRECT
3 AVERAGE—THE MINIMUM COMPETENCY LEVEL, NO CRITICAL ERRORS
2 IMPROVEMENT NEEDED—PROBLEM AREAS EXIST; CRITICAL ERRORS, CORRECTIONS NEEDED
1 POOR AND UNACCEPTABLE PERFORMANCE—GROSS INACCURACIES, POTENTIALLY HARMFUL

PERFORMANCE CRITERIA		SCALE			
1. DISPLAYS KNOWLEDGE OF ESSENTIAL CONCEPTS	5	4	3	2	1
2. DEMONSTRATES THE RELATIONSHIP BETWEEN THEORY AND CLINICAL PRACTICE	5	4	3	2	1
3. FOLLOWS DIRECTIONS, EXHIBITS SOUND JUDGMENT, AND DEMONSTRATES ATTENTION TO SAFETY AND DETAIL	5	4	3	2	1
4. EXHIBITS THE REQUIRED MANUAL DEXTERITY	5	4	3	2	1
5. PERFORMS PROCEDURE IN A REASONABLE TIME FRAME	5	4	3	2	1
6. MAINTAINS STERILE OR ASEPTIC TECHNIQUE	5	4	3	2	1
7. INITIATES UNAMBIGUOUS GOAL-DIRECTED COMMUNICATION	5	4	3	2	1
8. PROVIDES FOR ADEQUATE CARE AND MAINTENANCE OF EQUIPMENT AND SUPPLIES	5	4	3	2	1
9. EXHIBITS COURTEOUS AND PLEASANT DEMEANOR	5	4	3	2	1
10. MAINTAINS CONCISE AND ACCURATE RECORDS	5	4	3	2	1

ADDITIONAL COMMENTS: INCLUDE ERRORS OF OMISSION OR COMMISSION, COMMUNICATIVE SKILLS, AND EFFECTIVENESS OF PATIENT INTERACTION:

SUMMARY PERFORMANCE EVALUATION AND RECOMMENDATIONS

SATISFACTORY PERFORMANCE—Performed without error or prompting, or able to self-correct, no critical errors.

_____ LABORATORY EVALUATION. SKILLS MAY BE APPLIED/OBSERVED IN THE CLINICAL SETTING.

_____ CLINICAL EVALUATION. STUDENT READY FOR MINIMALLY SUPERVISED APPLICATION AND REFINEMENT.

UNSATISFACTORY PERFORMANCE—Prompting required; performed with critical errors, potentially harmful.

_____ STUDENT REQUIRES ADDITIONAL LABORATORY PRACTICE.

_____ STUDENT REQUIRES ADDITIONAL SUPERVISED CLINICAL PRACTICE.

SIGNATURES

STUDENT: _____   EVALUATOR: _____

DATE: _____   DATE: _____

Oxygen Supply Systems

INTRODUCTION

Most respiratory therapy devices require some type of pressurized gas source. The gas source and its system are considered *primary equipment,* and the delivery devices (such as oxygen masks) are *secondary equipment.*[1] Primary systems include cylinders, piped systems, and bulk gas and liquid systems. Primary systems are too often overlooked by respiratory care practitioners, but a thorough understanding of them is necessary for safe patient care. To illustrate this point, in an issue of *Respiratory Care Manager,* a critical incident was reported in which oxygen was contaminated with trichloroethylene, a toxic substance; this may have contributed to the deaths of five patients.[2] Although the practitioner may have an advanced comprehension of pathophysiology and the goals of medical gas therapy, he or she must also have a sound working knowledge of the capabilities and safe handling of the related equipment. If these systems fail, thorough knowledge would enable a quick and effective response by the respiratory care practitioner.[1]

OBJECTIVES

Upon completion of this chapter, the student will be able to:

1. Identify the contents of medical gas cylinders.
2. Identify the markings on a medical gas cylinder as defined by the Department of Transportation (DOT).
3. Differentiate between the **American Standard Safety System (ASSS)** index for large cylinders, the **Diameter Index Safety System (DISS),** and the **Pin Index Safety System (PISS)** for small cylinders.
4. Demonstrate the safe handling, transport, and storage of medical gas cylinders.
5. Identify the components of a bulk liquid system.
6. Identify the components of a reserve system.
7. Demonstrate the safe handling and refilling of a portable liquid oxygen system.
8. Identify the component parts and troubleshoot an oxygen concentrator.
9. Operate and troubleshoot an air compressor.
10. Identify the components of a single-stage and a multistage **regulator.**
11. Identify the components of a Bourdon gauge regulator.
12. Identify the components of a Thorpe tube flowmeter.
13. Differentiate between a **compensated** and a noncompensated flowmeter.
14. Calculate the duration of flow of a cylinder.
15. Set up and safely operate a blender.
16. Locate and identify zone valves in a health care facility.
17. Identify and safely use wall outlet quick connect systems.

KEY TERMS

ambient
American Standard Safety System (ASSS)
boiling point
combustible
compensation
critical pressure
critical temperature

density
Diameter Index Safety System (DISS)
evaporation
flammable
fractional distillation
frangible
fusible

Joint Commission on Accreditation of Healthcare Organizations (JCAHO)
melting point
Pin Index Safety System (PISS)
pounds per square inch (psi)

pounds per square inch gauge (psig)
reducing valve
regulator
reservoir
specific gravity
sublimation
volatile

EQUIPMENT REQUIRED

- H- and E-sized oxygen and other types of medical gas cylinders
- Cylinder trucks and circle stands
- Adjustable wrenches
- E cylinder keys
- Portable liquid oxygen tanks
- Oxygen concentrator
- Pocket flow measuring device (Erie flowmeter)
- Air compressor
- Single-stage and multistage regulators
- Bourdon gauge regulators
- Thorpe tube flowmeters, with and without regulators
- Blender with high-pressure hoses
- Samples of quick connect adaptors and wall plates

● EXERCISES

EXERCISE 4.1 Medical Gas Cylinders

EXERCISE 4.1.1 Safe Storage of Cylinders

In this exercise, the instructor has prepared a scenario in which medical gas cylinders are being stored improperly. Carefully observe the area. Identify and correct the safety violations. *Record each safety violation observed and corrective actions taken on your laboratory report.*

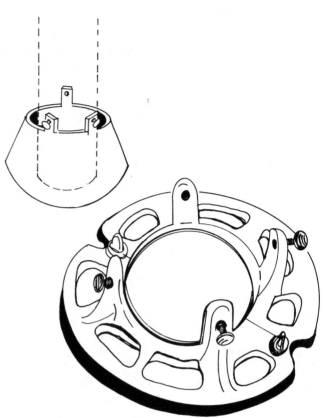

FIGURE 4.2 Circle stand. (From Eubanks, DH and Bone, RC: Comprehensive Respiratory Care: A Learning System. Mosby-Year Book, St. Louis, 1990, p. 136, with permission.)

EXERCISE 4.1.2 Safe Handling and Transport of Cylinders

1. Wheel an H cylinder on its truck (Fig. 4.1) from one side of the laboratory to the other.
2. Take the H cylinder off of its truck. Carefully walk it across the room and safely secure it in a circle stand (Fig. 4.2).
3. Repeat steps 1 and 2 for an E cylinder.

EXERCISE 4.1.3 Cylinder Markings

Your instructor will supply you with two different types and sizes of medical gas cylinders. Observe the cylinder markings, as shown in Figure 4.3. *Record the following data on your laboratory report:*
- Size of each cylinder *E*
- Contents of each cylinder *O₂*
- Safety system of each cylinder outlet
- Date of manufacture of each cylinder
- Retest date of each cylinder
- Ownership of each cylinder
- Serial number
- Filling pressure

EXERCISE 4.1.4 Safety System Connections

1. Obtain an H cylinder with a regulator and an E cylinder with a regulator. Observe the gas outlets and points of regulator

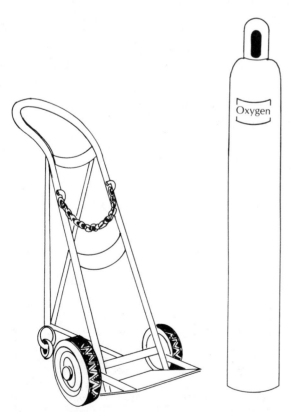

FIGURE 4.1 H cylinder and truck. (From Eubanks, DH and Bone, RC: Comprehensive Respiratory Care: A Learning System. Mosby-Year Book, St. Louis, 1990, p. 136, with permission.)

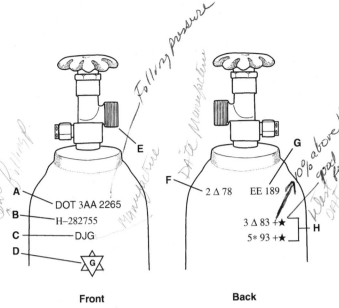

Front   **Back**

FIGURE 4.3   Location of cylinder markings.

Front labels: A DOT 3AA 2265, B H–282755, C DJG, D (hexagram with G)

Back labels: F 2 △ 78, EE 189, G, 3 △ 83 +★, 5* 93 +★, H

(handwritten) Following pressure / Date of Manufacture / 10% above

attachments. Differentiate between the Compressed Gas Association–American Standard Safety System (ASSS), the Diameter Index Safety System (DISS), and the Pin Index Safety System (PISS). Identify the safety systems shown in Figure 4.4. *Record the corresponding letter from the diagram on your laboratory report.*

2. Using the H cylinder, identify the location of the **frangible** disk or **fusible** plug pressure relief valves on the valve stem. *Record the corresponding letter from Figure 4.4 on your laboratory report.*

EXERCISE 4.2 Reducing Valves, Regulators, and Flowmeters

EXERCISE 4.2.1 Reducing Valves

1. Identify the components of the reducing valve shown in Figure 4.5, and *record the labeled parts on your laboratory report.*
   High-pressure inlet
   Gas outlet

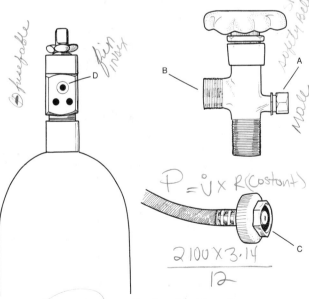

(handwritten) $P = \dot{V} \times R \ (constant)$

$\dfrac{2100 \times 3.14}{12}$

FIGURE 4.4   Identification of safety systems.

(handwritten at bottom) uncompensated ball will not pop up

Manometer reading cylinder pressure
Pressure relief valve(s)
Manometer reading outlet pressure
Outlet pressure adjusting valve

2. Determine whether the reducing valve is adjustable or preset. *Record your observation on your laboratory report.*

3. "Crack" the cylinder by quickly opening and closing the main valve so that a brief blast of gas is released. Make sure no one is facing the gas outlet while this is being done. Then attach the regulator to the cylinder. Turn on the cylinder and *record the pressure on your laboratory report.*

EXERCISE 4.2.2 Bourdon Gauge Regulator

1. Identify the components of a Bourdon gauge regulator, as shown in Figure 4.6, and *record the labeled parts on your laboratory report.*
   Gas inlet
   Gas outlet
   Pressure manometer
   Bourdon flow control
   Flow needle valve
   Pressure relief valve
   Gasloc seal

2. Attach the Bourdon gauge regulator to an H or E cylinder, as available.
   a. Turn on the cylinder completely. *Record the pressure on your laboratory report.*
   b. Turn the flow to 5 lpm. Occlude the orifice with your finger. *Record your observations on your laboratory report.*

3. Obtain an E cylinder. Replace the Gasloc seal (washer) on the regulator and reattach it. If an H cylinder was used for step 2, set the Bourdon gauge flowmeter on this E cylinder to 5 lpm. *Record the pressure on your laboratory report.*

4. Turn the flowmeter off. Turn the regulator off. "Bleed" the pressure from the regulator by turning the flowmeter on until the pressure gauge returns to zero. Turn the flowmeter off.

EXERCISE 4.2.3 Thorpe Tube Flowmeters

1. Identify the components of a Thorpe tube flowmeter, as shown in Figure 4.7, and *record the labeled parts on your laboratory report.*
   High-pressure gas inlet
   Gas outlet
   Thorpe tube
   Flowmeter needle valve
   50 psi outlet
   Flow indicator ball

2. Attach a Thorpe tube flowmeter with a regulator to an H cylinder. Turn the cylinder on. *Record the pressure and your observations on your laboratory report.*

3. Turn the flow up to 8 lpm. Completely occlude the orifice with your finger. *Record your observations on your laboratory report.*

4. Turn the flowmeter off. Turn the regulator off. "Bleed" the pressure from the regulator by turning the flowmeter on until the pressure gauge returns to zero. Turn the flowmeter off.

(handwritten) Compensated ball pop up and it will say calibrated, compensated.

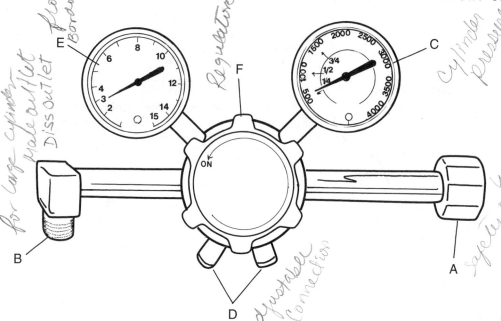

Handwritten annotations:
Bourdon gauge
flow
E
Diss outlet
For large cylinder male outlet
B
Regulator
F
ON
adjustable connection
D
Cylinder pressure
C
large cylinder connector
safety connector ASSS
A

FIGURE 4.5 Components of a reducing valve.

EXERCISE 4.2.4 Calculation of Cylinder Duration

For the pressures and flows recorded in Exercises 4.2.2 and 4.2.3, calculate the duration of flow for the E and H cylinder using the following formula and the appropriate conversion factor from Table 4.1:

$$\text{Duration of flow} = \frac{\text{Pressure in cylinder} \times \text{Cylinder factor}}{\text{Flow rate}}$$

Remember, this will give you the duration of flow in minutes. You must divide by 60 to obtain duration in hours. Show your work!

EXERCISE 4.3 Air Compressors

DO NOT Need to know

1. Identify the following components of an air compressor, as shown in Figure 4.8. *Record the labeled parts on your laboratory report.*
   Electrical cord
   Pressure outlets
   Pressure manometer
   Pressure adjustment
   Filter
   On/off switch

2. Turn on the compressor. What is the operating pressure of the device? How long did it take the compressor to achieve

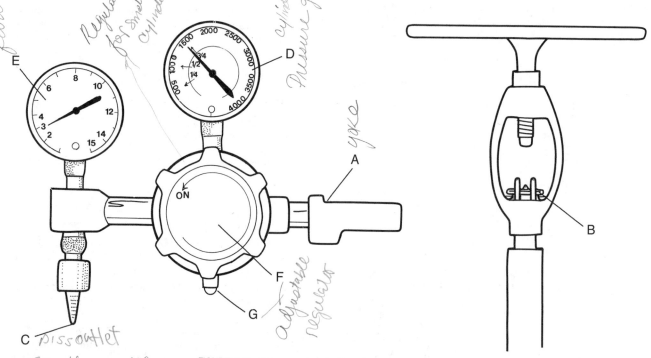

Handwritten annotations:
Bourdon flow gauge
E
Regulator for smaller cylinder
cylinder pressure gauge
D
yoke
A
ON
F
adjustable regulator
G
C Diss outlet small cylinder
B

FIGURE 4.6 Components of a Bourdon gauge regulator.

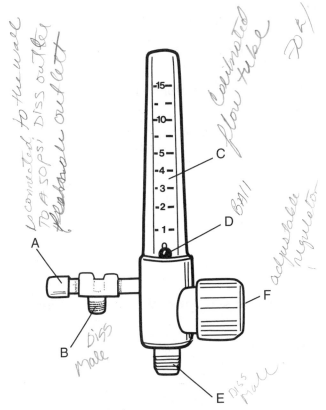

connected to the wall to 50 PSI, DISS outlet pressure outlet

calibrated flow tube

B2/1

adjustable regulator

A

B · *DISS male*

C

D

E · *DISS male*

F

FIGURE 4.7 Components of a Thorpe tube flowmeter.

the operating pressure? *Record the pressure and time on your laboratory report.*

EXERCISE 4.4 Blenders

1. Identify the components of an air/oxygen blender as shown in Figure 4.9.
   Air inlet
   Oxygen inlet
   Gas outlet
   Alarm
   F_IO_2 adjustment
2. Connect the pressure hoses to the appropriate connections. Identify the safety system. Turn on the gas supplies. Adjust the F_IO_2 to 0.40. *Record your observations, if any, on your laboratory report.*
3. Disconnect the air pressure hose. *Record your observations on your laboratory report.*
4. Reattach the air hose. Disconnect the oxygen hose. *Record your observations on your laboratory report.*

TABLE 4.1 **Cylinder Conversion Factors**

Cylinder Size	Conversion Factor
D	0.16
E	0.28
G	2.41
H or K	3.14

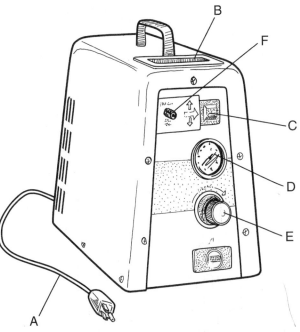

B

F

C

D

E

A

FIGURE 4.8 Components of an air compressor.

EXERCISE 4.5 Bulk Storage Systems

EXERCISE 4.5.1 Liquid Storage System

1. Identify the components of a liquid bulk storage system, as shown in Figure 4.10, and *record the labeled parts on your laboratory report.*
   Liquid container: carbon steel–protected outer shell
   Gas vent valve
   Vaporizer panels

blender to blend mix gases is to adjust you hook up to 50 PSI Air 50 PSI O2

BIRD®
Air-Oxygen Blender
$O_2\%$
50 60 70
40   80
30   90
   E   100
PATENT 3985642

D

C

A

B

FIGURE 4.9 Components of an air/oxygen blender. (Courtesy of Bird Products Corporation, Palm Springs, CA.)

possition air 1 & 5

DISS is found in the E cylinder (only)
Pin index safety System The possition for O2 is
1 6   0 6
20 0 5
30 0 4   2-5

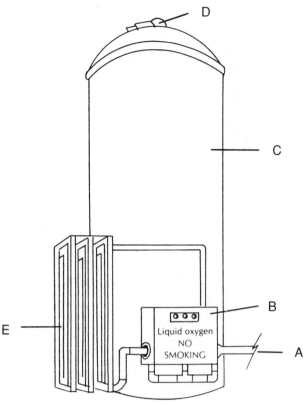

FIGURE 4.10   Components of a bulk liquid oxygen system. (Adapted from Eubanks, DH and Bone, RC: Principles and Applications of Cardiorespiratory Care Equipment, Mosby-Year Book, St. Louis, 1994, p. 9.)

Control panel
Main line to hospital

EXERCISE 4.5.2 Bank and Reserve Systems

1. Identify the components of a bank system, as shown in Figure 4.11, and *record the labeled parts on your laboratory report.*
   Gas cylinders
   Connecting pipes
   Main line pressure alarm
   Bank manometers
   Main supply line
   Switch over
   Check valves
   Main supply manometer

EXERCISE 4.6 Portable Liquid Systems

1. Identify the components of the portable liquid system, as shown in Figure 4.12, and *record the labeled parts on your laboratory report.*
   Continuous demand flow switch
   Vent valve
   Oxygen level indicator
   Fill connector location
   Carrying strap
   Inspiration sensor connector
   Oxygen tube connector
   Flow control knob

2. Connect and refill a portable cylinder from the main cylinder.

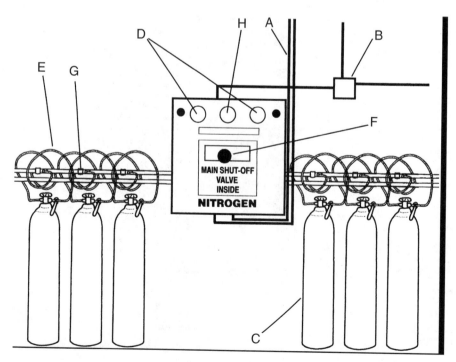

FIGURE 4.11   Components of a bank system.

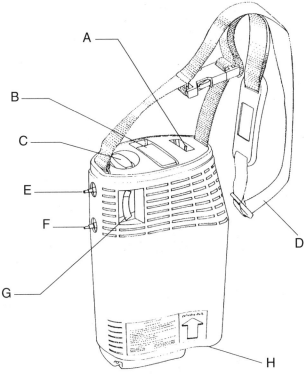

FIGURE 4.12 Components of a portable liquid oxygen system. (Reprinted by permission of Nellcor Puritan Bennett, Pleasanton, CA.)

a. Check the **reservoir** contents indicator to ensure an ample supply.
b. Check the pressure gauge on the reservoir to be sure that the needle is in the "normal" region.
c. Turn the flow control to zero.
d. Remove the dust cap from the reservoir fill connector. Check for presence of moisture. If moisture exists, wipe it with a lint-free cloth.
e. Lower the unit into position so that the unit connector enters the reservoir connector.

f. Rotate the unit in a clockwise direction until the roller gently drops into the slot in the reservoir connector.
g. Move the vent valve into the open position. This will result in a loud hissing noise. The unit is now filling.
h. When the hissing changes sound and a dense white vapor surrounds the cover, close the vent valve.
i. Disengage the unit.

No need to know

EXERCISE 4.7 Oxygen Concentrators

1. Identify the following components of an oxygen concentrator, as shown in Figure 4.13, and *record the labeled parts on your laboratory report.*
   Electrical connector
   On/off switch
   Alarm (not shown)
   Flowmeter
   Filter
   Battery for the alarm (not shown)
   Oxygen connection
2. Turn the concentrator on. Turn the flowmeter to 3 lpm. Attach an Erie test flowmeter to the concentrator flowmeter and *record the reading on your laboratory report.*
3. With the concentrator still turned on, unplug it and *record your observations on your laboratory report.*

need to know

EXERCISE 4.8 Zone Valves and Wall Outlets

This exercise may need to be performed in the clinical setting because of the lack of availability of the necessary equipment in the laboratory.

1. Locate two zone valves (Fig. 4.14) in the health care facility. Determine what rooms or units would be affected by shutting off these valves. *Record this information on your laboratory report.*
2. Identify the types of wall outlet quick connect systems, as shown in Figure 4.15.

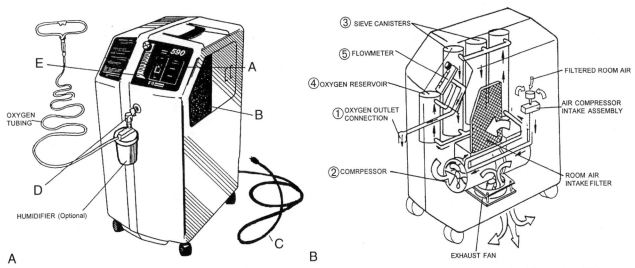

FIGURE 4.13 Components of an oxygen concentrator. (Reprinted by permission of Nellcor Puritan Bennett, Pleasanton, CA.)

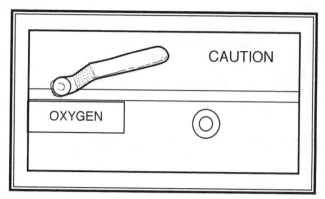

FIGURE 4.14   Zone valve.

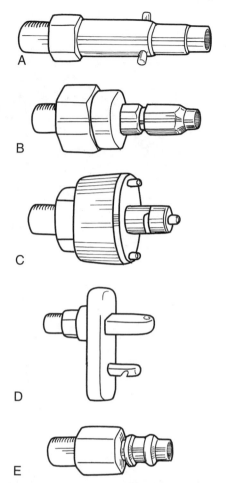

FIGURE 4.15   Types of wall outlet quick-connect systems. *(A)* Oxyquip '07 O.E.S., *(B)* Schrader, *(C)* Ohmeda, *(D)* Chemetron, *(E)* Puritan-Bennett.

3. Locate and identify the types of wall outlet quick connects used at the clinical site. Obtain a flowmeter with the same type of connection. Practice engaging and disengaging the flowmeter. *Record the type of wall outlet quick connects and your observations on your laboratory report.* If different types are used, compare and contrast the ease of use.

References

1. McPherson, S: Respiratory Care Equipment, ed 5. Mosby, St Louis, 1995, p 24.
2. Tainted O_2 linked to ICU deaths. Respiratory Care Manager 5:4, 1996.

Related Readings

Eubanks, DH and Bone, RC: Principles and Applications of Cardiorespiratory Care Equipment. Mosby, St Louis, 1994.
McPherson, S: Respiratory Care Equipment, ed 5. Mosby, St Louis, 1995.
Scanlan, C et al (eds): Egan's Fundamentals of Respiratory Care, ed 6. Mosby, St Louis, 1995.

Selected Journal Articles

American Association for Respiratory Care: AARC clinical practice guideline: Oxygen therapy in the acute care hospital. Respir Care 36:1410–1413, 1991.
American Association for Respiratory Care: AARC clinical practice guideline: Oxygen therapy in the home or extended care facility. Respir Care 37:918–922, 1992.
American Association for Respiratory Care: AARC clinical practice guideline: Selection of an oxygen delivery device for neonatal and pediatric patients. Respir Care 41:637–646, 1996.
ECRI: Medical gas and vacuum system. Health Devices 23:4–53, 1994.
Maxwell, DL et al: Hazards of domicillary oxygen therapy. Respir Med 87:225–226, 1993.
Oxygen concentrators. Health Devices 22:485–497, 1993.
West, GA and Primo, P: Nonmedical hazards of long-term oxygen therapy. Respir Care 28:906–912, 1983.

LABORATORY REPORT

CHAPTER 4: OXYGEN SUPPLY SYSTEMS

Name _____   Date _____

Course/Section _____   Instructor _____

Data Collection

EXERCISE 4.1   Medical Gas Cylinders

EXERCISE 4.1.1   Safe Storage of Cylinders

Identify the safety violations and corrective actions taken:

1. _____
   _____

2. _____
   _____

3. _____
   _____

4. _____
   _____

5. _____
   _____

EXERCISE 4.1.3   Cylinder Markings

	Cylinder A	*Cylinder B*
Size	_____	_____
Contents	_____	_____
Safety system	_____	_____
Date of manufacture	_____	_____
Retest date	_____	_____
Ownership	_____	_____
Serial number	_____	_____
Filling pressure	_____	

EXERCISE 4.1.4   Safety System Connections

Identify the corresponding letter from Figure 4.4:

ASSS _____

DISS _____

PISS _____

Pressure relief valve(s) _____

EXERCISE 4.2   Reducing Valves, Regulators, and Flowmeters
EXERCISE 4.2.1   Reducing Valves

A. _____

B. _____

C. _____

D. _____

E. _____

F. _____

Adjustable or preset? _____

Pressure recorded: _____

EXERCISE 4.2.2   Bourdon Gauge Regulator

A. _____

B. _____

C. _____

D. _____

E. _____

F. _____

G. _____

Pressure in the cylinder: _____

What occurred when the orifice became obstructed?

_____

EXERCISE 4.2.3   Thorpe Tube Flowmeters

A. _____

B. _____

C. _____

D. _____

E. _____

F. _____

G. _____

What occurred immediately when the cylinder was turned on?

_____

Pressure in the cylinder: _____

What happened when you occluded the orifice of the Thorpe tube? _____

EXERCISE 4.2.4   Calculation of Cylinder Duration

Duration of E cylinder: _____

Duration of H cylinder: _____

Show your work!

EXERCISE 4.3   Air Compressors

A. _____

B. _____

C. _____

D. _____

E. _____

F. _____

Operating pressure reading from the compressor: _____

Time until operating pressure was achieved: _____

EXERCISE 4.4   Blenders

A. _____

B. _____

C. _____

D. _____

E. _____

Observations: _____

_____

_____

_____

_____

EXERCISE 4.5   Bulk Storage Systems
EXERCISE 4.5.1   Liquid Storage Systems

A. _____

B. _____

C. _____

D. _____

E. _____

EXERCISE 4.5.2   Bank and Reserve Systems

A. _____

B. _____

C. _____

D. _____

E. _____

F. _____

G. _____

H. _____

EXERCISE 4.6   Portable Liquid Systems

A. _____

B. _____

C. _____

D. _____

E. _____

F. _____

G. _____

H. _____

EXERCISE 4.7   Oxygen Concentrators

A. _____

B. _____

C. _____

D. _____

E. _____

Reading from the Erie flowmeter: _____

What occurred when the device was unplugged? _____

_____

EXERCISE 4.8   Zone Valves and Wall Outlets

Location of zone valves and areas controlled by each: _____

_____

_____

_____

_____

Type of wall outlet quick connects: _____

_____

_____

CRITICAL THINKING QUESTIONS

1. What are the purposes of zone valves?

2. What safety factors must be considered when storing and handling compressed gas cylinders?
    Stored separate empty container from full, cooled dry place, local & state & federal regulations,

3. Why is it necessary to "crack" a cylinder before attaching a regulator?
    Remove any dust particle because the dust will explode in a fire

4. How many ways are there to determine if a flowmeter is compensated? Identify each.
    when you open the valve the ball will pop off, located will compensated, or will be calibrated at 50 psi,

5. What precautions must be taken when using a Bourdon gauge flowmeter? Explain the rationale for each.
    when using w/ an attach machine it will false higher reading
    Ex. when attached to a jet neubulizer the flow will read false flow.

6. Describe the maintenance procedures and safety checks that can be done on an oxygen concentrator and an air compressor.

Check the filters

7. Identify the following (flammability must be categorized as "flammable," "nonflammable," or "supports combustion"):

Symbol	Gas	Color Code	Combustion
O_2	Oxygen	Green or white	NF /SC
$O_2 + N_2$	Oxygen Nitrogen	Green & black	N.F S/C
CO_2	Carbon dioxide	gray	NF S/C
CO_2/O_2	Carbon Dioxide /oxide	Gray /Green	SC
N_2	Nitrogen	black	NF
He	Helium	Brown	NF
He/O_2	Helium /oxygen	Brown/Green	SC because it has O_2
N_2O	Nitrous Oxide	Blue	NF
NO	Nitrogen Oxide.	Black green	NF
$(CH_2)_3$			
ETO			

8. Mr. Butinsky is using a nasal cannula at 3 lpm. The nurse calls you and tells you that the patient must go to x-ray. Describe the specific equipment required to transport this patient to x-ray.

Use an E-cylinder c̄ a Bourdon gauge because is used for transport

for this week
oxy mixture

PROCEDURAL COMPETENCY EVALUATION

Name _Celia Ayala_ Date _6/9/00 / 6/15/00_

Gas Pressure and Flow Regulation

Setting: ☑ Lab ☐ Clinical   Evaluator: ☐ Peer ☑ Instructor

Conditions (describe): _____

	S A T I S F A C T O R Y	U N S A T I S F A C T O R Y	N O T O B S E R V E D	N O T A P P L I C A B L E
	☑	☐	☐	☐
	☑	☐	☐	☐
...solation pro-	☑	☐	☐	☐
D BAND	☑	☐	☐	☐
	☑	☐	☐	☐
	☑	☐	☐	☐
	☑	☐	☐	☐
...lators, and	☑	☐	☐	☐
	☑	☐	☐	☐
	☑	☐	☐	☐
	☑	☐	☐	☐
	☑	☐	☐	☐
	☑	☐	☐	☐
	☑	☐	☐	☐
	☑	☐	☐	☐
	☑	☐	☐	☐
	☑	☐	☐	☐
...d regulator	☑	☐	☐	☐
	☑	☐	☐	☐
	☑	☐	☐	☐
...r modifi-	☑	☐	☐	☐

Celia Ayala
Signature of Student

...new regulator.
...reduce pressure to 50 psi

Overlapping handwritten note (rotated):

24 - 1:25
80 - 1:10
30 - 1:8
35 - 1:5
40 - 1:3
45 - 1:3
50 - 1:1.1
60 - 1:1
70 - 0.6:1
80 - 0.3:1
100 - 0:1

60 mixing
ex
90 → 50 psi
40 - 1:1.9
- 1:10
60 - 1:1
35 - 1:5

Ratios - Charts

PERFORMANCE RATING SCALE

5 EXCELLENT—FAR EXCEEDS EXPECTED LEVEL, FLAWLESS PERFORMANCE
4 ABOVE AVERAGE—NO PROMPTING REQUIRED, ABLE TO SELF-CORRECT
3 AVERAGE—THE MINIMUM COMPETENCY LEVEL, NO CRITICAL ERRORS
2 IMPROVEMENT NEEDED—PROBLEM AREAS EXIST; CRITICAL ERRORS, CORRECTIONS NEEDED
1 POOR AND UNACCEPTABLE PERFORMANCE—GROSS INACCURACIES, POTENTIALLY HARMFUL

PERFORMANCE CRITERIA		SCALE			
1. DISPLAYS KNOWLEDGE OF ESSENTIAL CONCEPTS	5	4	3	2	1
2. DEMONSTRATES THE RELATIONSHIP BETWEEN THEORY AND CLINICAL PRACTICE	5	4	3	2	1
3. FOLLOWS DIRECTIONS, EXHIBITS SOUND JUDGMENT, AND DEMONSTRATES ATTENTION TO SAFETY AND DETAIL	5	4	3	2	1
4. EXHIBITS THE REQUIRED MANUAL DEXTERITY	5	4	3	2	1
5. PERFORMS PROCEDURE IN A REASONABLE TIME FRAME	5	4	3	2	1
6. MAINTAINS STERILE OR ASEPTIC TECHNIQUE	5	4	3	2	1
7. INITIATES UNAMBIGUOUS GOAL-DIRECTED COMMUNICATION	5	4	3	2	1
8. PROVIDES FOR ADEQUATE CARE AND MAINTENANCE OF EQUIPMENT AND SUPPLIES	5	4	3	2	1
9. EXHIBITS COURTEOUS AND PLEASANT DEMEANOR	5	4	3	2	1
10. MAINTAINS CONCISE AND ACCURATE RECORDS	5	4	3	2	1

ADDITIONAL COMMENTS: INCLUDE ERRORS OF OMISSION OR COMMISSION, COMMUNICATIVE SKILLS, AND EFFECTIVENESS OF PATIENT INTERACTION:

SUMMARY PERFORMANCE EVALUATION AND RECOMMENDATIONS

SATISFACTORY PERFORMANCE—Performed without error or prompting, or able to self-correct, no critical errors.

_____ LABORATORY EVALUATION. SKILLS MAY BE APPLIED/OBSERVED IN THE CLINICAL SETTING.

_____ CLINICAL EVALUATION. STUDENT READY FOR MINIMALLY SUPERVISED APPLICATION AND REFINEMENT.

UNSATISFACTORY PERFORMANCE—Prompting required; performed with critical errors, potentially harmful.

_____ STUDENT REQUIRES ADDITIONAL LABORATORY PRACTICE.

_____ STUDENT REQUIRES ADDITIONAL SUPERVISED CLINICAL PRACTICE.

SIGNATURES

STUDENT: _____   EVALUATOR: _____

DATE: _____   DATE: _____

Oxygen Analysis

Determination of the **accuracy** of the delivered F_1O_2 is an important part of oxygen administration. The only way to verify the concentration being delivered is by oxygen analysis. Four different types of analyzers are available, each working on one of three different physical principles (**paramagnetic,** electromechanical, and electrochemical). The most commonly used types work by the electrochemical principle and include the **polarographic** analyzer, or Clark electrode, and the **galvanic** fuel cell analyzer.

OBJECTIVES
Upon completion of this chapter, the student will be able to:

1. Given a specific oxygen analyzer, identify the type and its component parts.
2. Calibrate both the polarographic analyzer and the galvanic fuel cell analyzer on room air and 100 percent oxygen.
3. Given an oxygen delivery apparatus, analyze the F_1O_2.
4. Perform routine maintenance procedures such as fuel cell or electrode replacement and battery check.
5. Describe the effects of moisture buildup and pressure on the measured F_1O_2 of a polarographic or galvanic analyzer.

KEY TERMS

accuracy	diffusion	galvanic	polarographic
calibration	efficacy	paramagnetic	sensor
	gain	permeability	

EQUIPMENT REQUIRED

- Oxygen analyzers: polarographic and galvanic fuel cell
- In-line adaptors
- Fuel cell cap
- Oxygen gas source—H or E cylinders
- Large wrench
- Cylinder stands
- Regulator with flowmeter
- Oxygen nipple adaptors
- Oxygen connection tubing
- Large-bore corrugated tubing
- Large volume jet nebulizer
- Sterile water
- Plastic bag
- Small screwdriver
- Scissors
- Spare batteries (see manufacturer's specifications)

● EXERCISES

EXERCISE 5.1 Identification of Oxygen Analyzers

For each of the following devices, examine the device and identify the component parts, as shown in the accompanying figures. Depending on the type of analyzer and its manufacturer, the component parts may vary. Refer to the individual operating manual for specifics.

1. Polarographic analyzer (Fig. 5.1):
   Analog scale or light-emitting diode (LED) readout
   Calibration knob
   On/off switch
   Sensor or electrode
   Batteries (not shown)
   Alarms (if applicable)
   In-line adaptor

2. Galvanic fuel cell (Fig. 5.2):
   Analog scale or LED readout
   Calibration knob
   Sensor plug
   Sensor
   Batteries (not shown)
   Alarms (if applicable)
   In-line adaptor

EXERCISE 5.2 Calibration of Oxygen Analyzers

Regular calibration of oxygen analyzers is required to ensure the accuracy of measured F_1O_2. All oxygen delivery systems should be checked at least once daily. More frequent checks by calibrated analyzers may be necessary in specific types of systems (see AARC clinical practice guidelines for details).[1] The frequency of analysis, whether con-

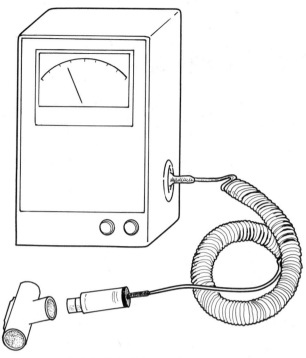

FIGURE 5.1 Polarographic analyzer.

tinuous or intermittent, determines how often calibration is needed.

1. Obtain the analyzer.

2. Set up the oxygen source by attaching a regulator with a Thorpe tube flowmeter to an H cylinder.

3. Attach an oxygen nipple adaptor to the DISS connection of the flowmeter outlet.

4. Secure the oxygen connecting tubing to the oxygen nipple adaptor.

5. Check that the analyzer is in good operating condition. Make sure that the analog scale/LED, sensor cable, and electrode or fuel cell are intact.

6. Prepare analyzer for use.
   a. For the polarographic electrode analyzer, turn or press the on/off switch.
   b. For the galvanic fuel cell analyzer, attach the sensor cable to the analyzer. Some types of fuel cell analyzers may also have on/off switches for the alarms and LED readings.

7. With the sensor exposed to room air, adjust the calibration knob to read 21 percent oxygen.

8. Place the sensor inside a plastic bag, as shown in Figure 5.3. Place the oxygen connecting tubing inside the bag with the sensor. Turn on the flowmeter to 10 lpm (flow needed may vary depending on the size of the bag used). Loosely hold the bag closed.

9. Allow the analyzer reading to stabilize. This may take 20 to 30 sec depending on the type of analyzer. *Excessively long stabilization time or failure to reach greater than 80 percent oxygen may indicate that the sensor must be replaced.*

10. While the sensor is exposed to 100 percent oxygen, adjust the calibration knob (**gain**) to read 100 percent.

11. Shut off the oxygen. Remove the sensor from the bag. Relocate the analyzer to a different part of the room and recheck at 21 percent calibration. Adjust if necessary.

12. After the calibration procedure is performed, the analyzer is now ready for use.

13. Cap and unplug the sensor when not in use. Turn off the analyzer when not in use.

EXERCISE 5.3 Oxygen Analysis

For this exercise, assembly of the oxygen delivery system to be analyzed is required. See Figure 5.4 for the placement of the analyzer in line in a setup of a large volume jet nebulizer.

1. Cut a single length of large-bore tubing (6 inches) from a roll, if it is not already available.

2. Place the analyzer sensor into an in-line adaptor. Make sure it fits tightly.

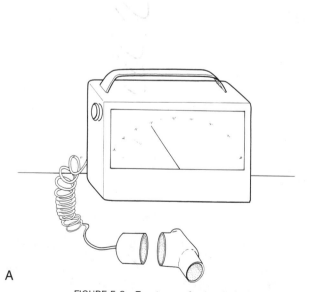

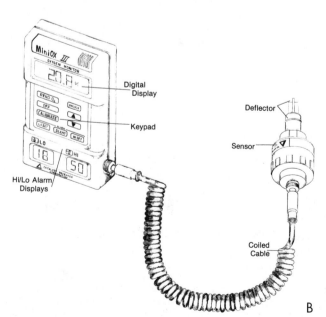

FIGURE 5.2 Two types of galvanic fuel cell analyzers. (*[B]* Courtesy of Mine Safety Appliances, Pittsburgh, PA.)

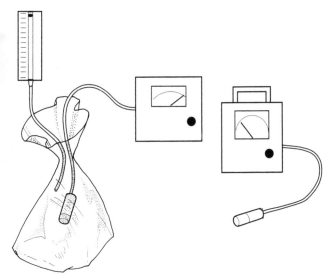

FIGURE 5.3   Calibration of an oxygen analyzer.

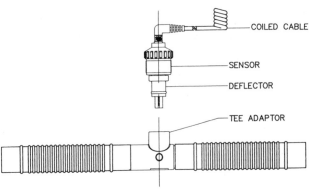

FIGURE 5.5   In-line placement of analyzer sensor. (Courtesy of Mine Safety Appliances, Pittsburgh, PA.)

3. Attach a single length of large-bore tubing to one end of the in-line adaptor.

4. Fill the nebulizer with sterile water. Adjust the nebulizer to an F_IO_2 of 0.40. Turn the flowmeter on to 10 lpm.

5. Attach the in-line adaptor with sensor at the end of the aerosol tubing as close to the delivery device (mask or T-piece) as possible.

6. Position the sensor so that moisture cannot collect on the surface of the membrane. The sensor should be facing down, as shown in Figure 5.5. Make sure the sensor and adaptor are secured tightly in the circuit.

7. Allow the reading to stabilize. *Record the results on your laboratory report.*

8. If a disposable nebulizer is used, the F_IO_2 setting may not be accurate. If the reading on the analyzer does not match the set F_IO_2, adjust the *nebulizer* setting to the prescribed F_IO_2. Note any necessary adjustment. *Record the actual nebulizer setting on your laboratory report.*

9. Repeat the procedure for an F_IO_2 of 0.60. *Record the results on your laboratory report.*

10. Cap and unplug the galvanic sensor. Turn off the analyzer when not in use.

EXERCISE 5.4 Maintenance of Oxygen Analyzers

The following exercises may be considered optional or for demonstration purposes only. *Check with your instructor before proceeding.*

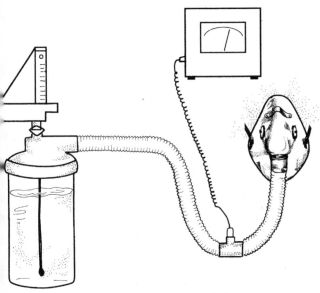

FIGURE 5.4   Oxygen analysis.

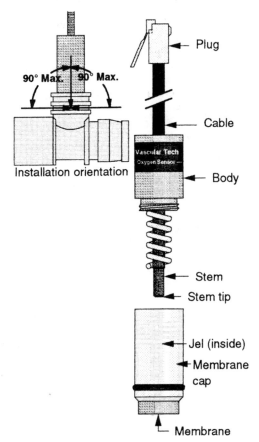

FIGURE 5.6   Maintenance of a polarographic electrode. (Courtesy of Vascular Technology Inc., Chelmsford, MA.)

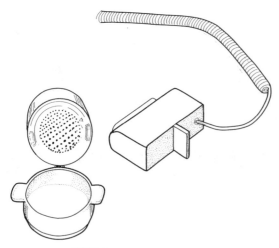

FIGURE 5.7   Galvanic fuel cell.

EXERCISE 5.4.1 Maintenance of Polarographic Analyzers

1. Turn off the analyzer.

2. Depending on the manufacturer or type of electrode, it may be necessary only to unscrew the entire sensor from the coiled cable, remove the new sensor from the sealed package, and reattach it. These types of sensors are sealed units that contain electrolyte solution. *If a leak develops, discard it immediately.*

3. If the sensor requires maintenance, unscrew the membrane cap from the sensor body. This should be done with the cap facing down to prevent electrolyte from spilling (Fig. 5.6).

4. In the clinical setting, if the membrane must be replaced, the entire membrane cap will be discarded. For the purposes of this laboratory, the membrane cap will be reused. The membrane can be damaged by attempting to clean or touch it.

5. Discard the electrolyte fluid from the cap. Check for leaks or cracks in the membrane.

6. Refill the cap with fresh electrolyte fluid up to within one-fourth inch from the top.

7. Reattach the membrane cap securely to the sensor body.

8. Turn the analyzer on. Allow time for the sensor to stabilize.

9. Debubble the sensor by positioning the membrane down and gently tapping the side of the sensor probe cap near the membrane.

10. Check the batteries. Some brands have a low battery indicator or alarm, or you may notice improper operation. To replace the batteries, open the door to the battery compartment, remove the old batteries, and insert new ones. Each battery usually can be installed in only one direction.

11. Recalibrate the analyzer.

EXERCISE 5.4.2 Maintenance of Galvanic Fuel Cell Analyzers

Depending on the manufacturer or type of fuel cell, it may be necessary only to unscrew the entire fuel cell, open the sealed bag, and reattach the new fuel cell. *Never open the fuel cell.*

Other types of fuel cells may require a more detailed procedure. Using a small flat-head screwdriver, unscrew the screen holding the fuel cell in place (Fig. 5.7).

1. Detach the sensor probe cable from the analyzer.

2. Remove the screen.

3. Gently and slowly remove the fuel cell from its compartment (Fig. 5.8). Be careful not to remove the cell too far from the compartment because the cell has two wire connections.

4. Note the position and color of the connecting wires to the fuel cell.

5. Remove the wire connections from the fuel cell.

6. For some analyzers, the fuel cell may come in a plastic bag. Remove the fuel cell from the sealed package. Remove the metal clip, and inspect the base of the cell for any damage or defects before use.

7. Insert the new fuel cell, making sure to reconnect the wires properly by color.

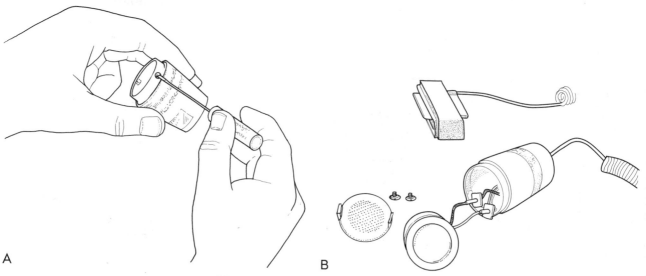

A   B

FIGURE 5.8   Maintenance of galvanic fuel cell.

8. Replace the screen and screws.
9. Reattach the sensor probe to the analyzer and recalibrate.
10. Cap and unplug the sensor when not in use. Turn off the analyzer when not in use.

Reference

1. American Association for Respiratory Care: The AARC clinical practice guideline: Oxygen therapy in the acute care hospital. Respir Care 36:1410–1413, 1991.

Related Readings

Eubanks, DH and Bone, RC: Principles and Applications of Cardiorespiratory Care Equipment. Mosby, St Louis, 1994.
Madama, V: Pulmonary Function Testing and Cardiopulmonary Stress Testing. Albany, Delmar, 1993.
McPherson, S: Respiratory Care Equipment, ed 5. Mosby, St Louis, 1995.
Scanlan, C et al (eds): Egan's Fundamentals of Respiratory Care, ed 6. Mosby, St Louis, 1995.
Shapiro, B et al: Clinical Application of Blood Gases, ed 5. Mosby, Chicago, 1994.

Selected Journal Articles

American Association for Respiratory Care: AARC clinical practice guideline: Oxygen therapy in the acute care hospital. Respir Care 36:1410–1413, 1991.
American Association for Respiratory Care: AARC clinical practice guideline: Oxygen therapy in the home or extended care facility. Respir Care 37:918–922, 1992.
American Association for Respiratory Care: AARC clinical practice guideline: Selection of an oxygen delivery device for neonatal and pediatric patients. Respir Care 41:637–646, 1996.

LABORATORY REPORT

CHAPTER 5: OXYGEN ANALYZERS

Name _____   Date _____

Course/Section _____   Instructor _____

Data Collection

EXERCISE 5.3   Oxygen Analysis

1. Analysis of 40%

   a. Initial reading: _____

   b. Adjusted nebulizer setting: _____

2. Analysis of 60%

   a. Initial reading: _____

   b. Adjusted nebulizer setting: _____

CRITICAL THINKING QUESTIONS

1. Do the electrochemical analyzers measure partial pressure or true oxygen concentration?

   partial pressure

2. How would decreased barometric pressure or increased altitude affect the reading of a polarographic or galvanic analyzer? Why?

   ↓ PO₂   *decrease a reading cause P P O₂ is decrease*

3. How would moisture or condensation buildup on the sensor membrane affect the measured F_IO_2? What measures can be taken to prevent this?

   Condensation will cause decrease FiO₂
   Sensor face down
   The Faces should be down position so the no moisture builds up
   Fio decreases

4. How would positive pressure ventilation affect the measured F_IO_2?

   back pressure will go up if there is an obstruction (FiO₂ goes ↑ due to the obstruction)
   back press FiO₂ ↑
   no Obstruction to flow FiO will remain constant

5. Why is it important to keep the galvanic cell capped or the polarographic analyzer off when not in use?

   The polarographic battery runs down
   galvanic damage due sensitive to condensation
   cell on

6. State two circumstances that indicate that the fuel cell or sensor should be replaced. *after checking the battery.*

   polographic ↓ FiO₂
   , inacurate FiO₂ reading
   , slow FiO₂ reading
   , failed Calibration

PROCEDURAL COMPETENCY EVALUATION

Name _Celia Ayals_　　Date _6/73/00_

Oxygen Analysis

Setting: ☐ Lab　☑ Clinical　　　　Evaluator: ☐ Peer　☑ Instructor

Conditions (describe): _____

_____

Equipment Used

_____

_____

	SATISFACTORY	UNSATISFACTORY	NOT OBSERVED	NOT APPLICABLE

Equipment and Patient Preparation

1. Verifies, interprets, and evaluates physician's order or protocol　☑ ☐ ☐ ☐
2. Scans chart for diagnosis and other pertinent data and notes　☑ ☐ ☐ ☐
3. Selects, gathers, and assembles the necessary equipment　☑ ☐ ☐ ☐
4. Washes hands and applies standard precautions and transmission-based isolation procedures as appropriate　☑ ☐ ☐ ☐
5. Identifies patient, introduces self and department　☑ ☐ ☐ ☐
6. Explains purpose of the procedure and confirms patient understanding　☑ ☐ ☐ ☐

Assessment and Implementation

7. Assesses patient　☑ ☐ ☐ ☐
8. Identifies the following types of oxygen analyzers: electrochemical, polarographic, and galvanic　☑ ☐ ☐ ☐
9. States the operating principle of each type of analyzer　☑ ☐ ☐ ☐
10. Sets up oxygen source and attaches oxygen nipple adaptor to the DISS connection of the flowmeter outlet　☑ ☐ ☐ ☐
11. Secures the oxygen connecting tubing to the oxygen nipple adaptor　☑ ☐ ☐ ☐
12. Checks that the analyzer is in good operating condition; makes sure that the analog scale/LED, sensor cable, and electrode or fuel cell are intact　☑ ☐ ☐ ☐
13. Prepares analyzer for use:
    a. For the polarographic electrode analyzer, turns or presses the on/off switch　☑ ☐ ☐ ☐
    b. For the galvanic fuel cell, attaches the sensor cable to the analyzer　☐ ☐ ☐ ☑
14. With the sensor exposed to room air, adjusts the calibration knob to read 21 percent oxygen　☐ ☐ ☐ ☑
15. Places sensor inside a plastic bag; places oxygen connecting tubing inside the bag with the sensor; turns on the flowmeter to 10 lpm (flow needed may vary depending on the size of the bag used); loosely holds the bag closed　☑ ☐ ☐ ☐
16. Allows analyzer reading to stabilize　☑ ☐ ☐ ☐
17. Adjusts calibration knob to read 100 percent　☑ ☐ ☐ ☐
18. Relocates the analyzer to a different part of the room and rechecks 21 percent calibration; ~~adjusts if necessary~~　☑ ☐ ☐ ☐

Follow-up

19. Caps and unplugs the sensor when not in use　☑ ☐ ☐ ☐
20. Maintains/processes equipment　☑ ☐ ☐ ☐

	S A T I S F A C T O R Y	U N S A T I S F A C T O R Y	N O T O B S E R V E D	N O T A P P L I C A B L E
21. Washes hands	☑	☐	☐	☐
22. Records pertinent data in chart and departmental records	☑	☐	☐	☐
23. Notifies appropriate personnel, makes modifications and recommendations to patient care plan	☑	☐	☐	☐

_____
Signature of Evaluator

_____
Signature of Student

PERFORMANCE RATING SCALE

5 EXCELLENT—FAR EXCEEDS EXPECTED LEVEL, FLAWLESS PERFORMANCE
4 ABOVE AVERAGE—NO PROMPTING REQUIRED, ABLE TO SELF-CORRECT
3 AVERAGE—THE MINIMUM COMPETENCY LEVEL, NO CRITICAL ERRORS
2 IMPROVEMENT NEEDED—PROBLEM AREAS EXIST; CRITICAL ERRORS, CORRECTIONS NEEDED
1 POOR AND UNACCEPTABLE PERFORMANCE—GROSS INACCURACIES, POTENTIALLY HARMFUL

PERFORMANCE CRITERIA	SCALE				
1. DISPLAYS KNOWLEDGE OF ESSENTIAL CONCEPTS	5	4	3	2	1
2. DEMONSTRATES THE RELATIONSHIP BETWEEN THEORY AND CLINICAL PRACTICE	5	4	3	2	1
3. FOLLOWS DIRECTIONS, EXHIBITS SOUND JUDGMENT, AND DEMONSTRATES ATTENTION TO SAFETY AND DETAIL	5	4	3	2	1
4. EXHIBITS THE REQUIRED MANUAL DEXTERITY	5	4	3	2	1
5. PERFORMS PROCEDURE IN A REASONABLE TIME FRAME	5	4	3	2	1
6. MAINTAINS STERILE OR ASEPTIC TECHNIQUE	5	4	3	2	1
7. INITIATES UNAMBIGUOUS GOAL-DIRECTED COMMUNICATION	5	4	3	2	1
8. PROVIDES FOR ADEQUATE CARE AND MAINTENANCE OF EQUIPMENT AND SUPPLIES	5	4	3	2	1
9. EXHIBITS COURTEOUS AND PLEASANT DEMEANOR	5	4	3	2	1
10. MAINTAINS CONCISE AND ACCURATE RECORDS	5	4	3	2	1

ADDITIONAL COMMENTS: INCLUDE ERRORS OF OMISSION OR COMMISSION, COMMUNICATIVE SKILLS, AND EFFECTIVENESS OF PATIENT INTERACTION:

SUMMARY PERFORMANCE EVALUATION AND RECOMMENDATIONS

SATISFACTORY PERFORMANCE—Performed without error or prompting, or able to self-correct, no critical errors.

_____ LABORATORY EVALUATION. SKILLS MAY BE APPLIED/OBSERVED IN THE CLINICAL SETTING.

_____ CLINICAL EVALUATION. STUDENT READY FOR MINIMALLY SUPERVISED APPLICATION AND REFINEMENT.

UNSATISFACTORY PERFORMANCE—Prompting required; performed with critical errors, potentially harmful.

_____ STUDENT REQUIRES ADDITIONAL LABORATORY PRACTICE.

_____ STUDENT REQUIRES ADDITIONAL SUPERVISED CLINICAL PRACTICE.

SIGNATURES

STUDENT: _____   EVALUATOR: _____

DATE: _____   DATE: _____

CHAPTER 6

Oxygen Administration Devices

INTRODUCTION

Oxygen is one of the most commonly administered respiratory drugs. Although administration of oxygen requires relatively simple skills, it is often misused or abused. The competent respiratory care practitioner must be well versed in the variety of devices that can be used to deliver oxygen, the limitations of these devices, and the indications and hazards of oxygen therapy. The primary **goal** of oxygen therapy is to reduce **morbidity** and **mortality.** Proper administration can have significant impact on patient outcomes.

OBJECTIVES

Upon completion of this chapter, the student will be able to:

1. Identify and assemble various oxygen delivery devices such as the nasal cannula, simple mask, partial rebreathing and nonrebreathing mask, air **entrainment (Venturi)** masks, oxygen hoods, and oxygen tents.
2. Classify each oxygen delivery device as high flow or low flow.
3. Estimate the F_IO_2 for an oxygen delivery device, given the operating flow rate.
4. Given a patient scenario, select and administer the indicated oxygen device.
5. Demonstrate effective communication skills needed for patient-practitioner interaction.
6. Calculate inspiratory flow demands and total flows delivered for a given F_IO_2, using air-to-oxygen mixing ratios.
7. Analyze the F_IO_2 achieved with various oxygen devices.
8. Assess a patient for response to oxygen therapy.
9. Identify and correct common problems associated with oxygen delivery devices.

KEY TERMS

acute	contraindication	hypercarbia	mechanical deadspace
adverse	diffusion	hyperventilation	morbidity
anatomic deadspace	dysrhythmia	hypoventilation	mortality
anoxia	entrainment	hypoxemia	neutral thermal
chronic	epistaxis	hypoxia	environment
cold stress	flip-flop phenomenon	indication	optimum
compensatory	goal	insufflation	refractory
	hypercapnea	jet	Venturi

EQUIPMENT REQUIRED

- Watch with a second hand
- Oxygen analyzer
- In-line adaptor
- Oxygen connection tubing
- Oxygen gas source: H or E cylinders
- Blenders
- Compressed air source
- Wrenches
- Cylinder stands
- Oxygen nipple adaptors
- Prefilled bubble humidifiers
- Nasal cannulas
- Simple masks
- Partial rebreathing masks
- Nonrebreathing masks
- Venturi masks, various brands
- Oxygen hood
- Pulse oximeter
- Vane respirometer
- One-way valves
- Temperature probe
- Large-volume heated nebulizer
- Corrugated tubing
- Sterile water
- Water traps
- Oxygen tent and canopies
- Bed (optional)
- Sheets or towels

- Water feed system (optional)
- Oxygen conserving devices: reservoir or pendant cannula and pulsed-dose system
- Transtracheal oxygen catheter (SCOOP)
- "No Smoking" signs
- Plastic bag
- Infant mannequin
- Gloves

● EXERCISES

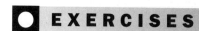

Students should perform these exercises in groups of two. Students may carry out all the exercises with the same partner, or the instructor may want to change pairs to enhance the ability of each student to communicate and explain the procedure to a different person.

EXERCISE 6.1 Oxygen Device Identification

Examine each of the following devices, identify all component parts, and *record the corresponding letters (if shown) on your laboratory report.*

EXERCISE 6.1.1 Nasal Cannula (Fig. 6.1)

Nasal prongs
Elastic strap or lariat ear tubes
Oxygen connecting tube

EXERCISE 6.1.2 Oxygen Conserving Devices

Reservoir cannula (Fig. 6.2)
Pendant cannula (Fig. 6.3)

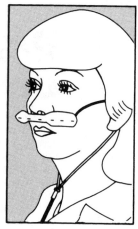

FIGURE 6.2   Oxygen-conserving devices: reservoir cannula. (Courtesy of Chad Therapeutics, Inc., Chatsworth, CA.)

EXERCISE 6.1.3 Simple Mask (Fig. 6.4)

Transparent plastic mask
Oxygen inlet
Exhalation ports
Malleable metal nosepiece

EXERCISE 6.1.4 Partial Rebreathing Mask (Fig. 6.5)

Gas inlet
Exhalation ports
Reservoir bag
Malleable metal nosepiece

EXERCISE 6.1.5 Nonrebreathing Mask (Fig. 6.6)

Gas inlet
Nonrebreathing one-way valve
Exhalation ports and valve
Reservoir bag

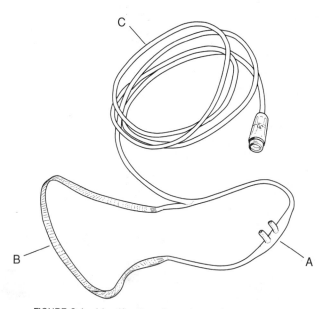

FIGURE 6.1   Identification of nasal cannula components.

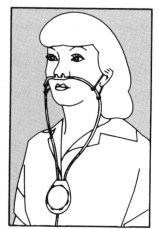

FIGURE 6.3   Oxygen-conserving devices: pendant cannula. (Courtesy of Chad Therapeutics, Inc., Chatsworth, CA.)

Friday lab
Nasal O₂ cannula
non-rebreathing mask
air-entrainment Mask.

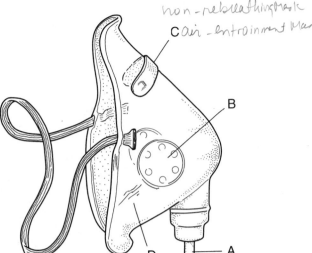

FIGURE 6.4 Identification of simple mask components.

EXERCISE 6.1.6 Air Entrainment (Venturi) Mask (Fig. 6.7)

Oxygen inlet
Jet
Air entrainment port
Exhalation valve
Venturi tube

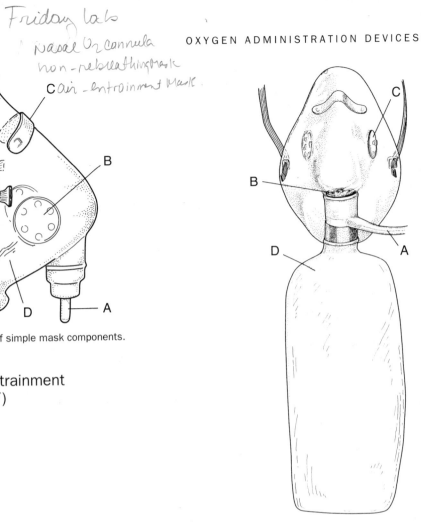

FIGURE 6.6 Identification of nonrebreathing mask components.

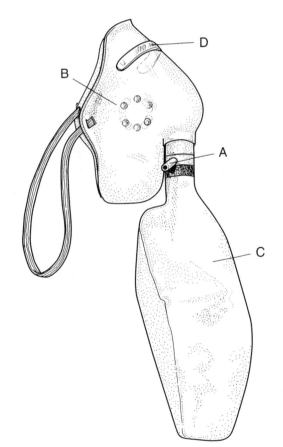

FIGURE 6.5 Identification of partial rebreathing mask components.

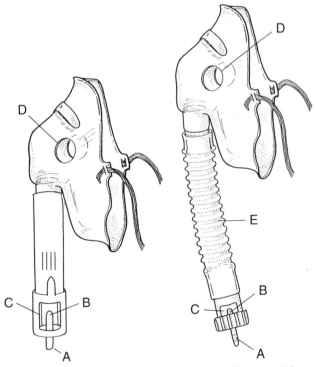

FIGURE 6.7 Identification of air entrainment mask components.

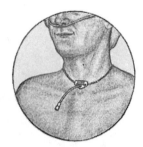

FIGURE 6.8   Transtracheal oxygen catheter. (Permission granted by Transtracheal Systems, Inc., Englewood, CO, USA.)

Not doing

EXERCISE 6.1.7 Transtracheal Oxygen Catheter (Fig. 6.8)

EXERCISE 6.1.8 Oxygen Tent (Fig. 6.9)

Circulation unit or refrigeration unit
Nebulizer
Gas inlet connection (not shown)
Frame
"No Smoking" sign (not shown)
Filter
Canopy
Condensation collection bottle

EXERCISE 6.1.9 Oxygen Hood (Fig. 6.10)

no

Analyzer port
Nebulizer (not shown)
Large-bore tubing connection
Temperature probe
Hood

EXERCISE 6.2 Administration of Oxygen Delivery Devices

EXERCISE 6.2.1 Nasal Cannula (Table 6.1)

1. Verify "physician's" order or protocol.

2. Obtain the following equipment:
   a. Nasal cannula
   b. H cylinder (or piped-in oxygen gas source)
   c. Regulator or flowmeter
   d. Bubble humidifier
   e. Oxygen nipple adaptor
   f. "No Smoking" signs

3. Wash your hands and apply standard precautions and transmission-based isolation procedures as appropriate.

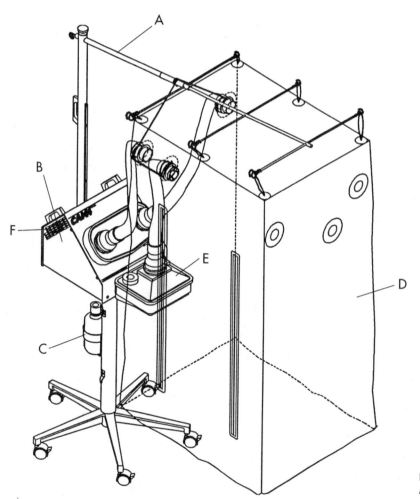

FIGURE 6.9   Oxygen tent. (Courtesy of Timeter, Allied Healthcare Products, Inc., St. Louis, MO.)

a. Introduce yourself, verify your patient's identification, explain the procedure, and verify patient understanding.

b. Assess your patient before beginning oxygen therapy by measuring pulse, respiratory rate, quality of respirations, and color. A pulse oximeter may be used. Interview the patient to determine if dyspnea is present. *Record the results on your laboratory report.*

c. Explain safety considerations regarding smoking and electrical devices and other possible hazards pertinent to the home environment to your patient. Verify patient understanding.

5. Set up the equipment as in Exercise 6.2.1.

6. Attach a pendant or reservoir cannula to the nipple.

7. Adjust the flow to 1.5 lpm.

8. Place the cannula on your patient.

9. Remove the cannula from your patient. Shut the flowmeter and disconnect it from the reducing valve.

10. Attach the pulsed-dose oxygen device to the 50 psi gas source.

11. Adjust the pulsed-dose oxygen device to 1.5 lpm.

12. Reapply the cannula to your patient, attaching it to the pulsed-dose device outlet.

13. Have the patient breathe normally, and note the operation of the pulsed-dose device.

14. Increase the flow rate to 3 lpm.

15. Compare the sensations of using a pulsed-dose oxygen device to a regular nasal cannula at the same liter flow. *Record your observations on your laboratory report.*

EXERCISE 6.3 Air Entrainment (Venturi) Mask

EXERCISE 6.3.1 Administration of Oxygen via Air Entrainment Device (Table 6.3)

1. Verify "physician's" order or protocol.

2. Obtain the following equipment:
   a. Air entrainment (Venturi) mask, jet, or entrainment port adaptors
   b. H cylinder (or piped-in oxygen gas source)
   c. Regulator or flowmeter
   d. Oxygen nipple adaptor
   e. "No Smoking" signs

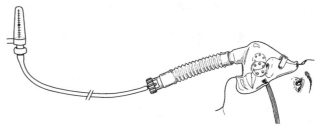

FIGURE 6.15   Air entrainment mask equipment assembly.

3. Wash your hands and apply standard precautions and transmission-based isolation procedures as appropriate.

4. With your laboratory partner acting as your "patient," do the following:
   a. Introduce yourself, verify your patient's identification, explain the procedure, and verify patient understanding.
   b. Assess your patient before beginning oxygen therapy by measuring pulse, respiratory rate, quality of respirations, and color. A pulse oximeter may be used. Interview the patient to determine if dyspnea is present.

5. Set up the equipment as shown in Figure 6.15:
   a. Attach regulator to cylinder as per Chapter 3.
   b. Attach the oxygen nipple to the DISS outlet of the flowmeter.

   NOTE: A bubble humidifier should not be used with this device.

   c. While aseptically keeping the mask in its wrapper, attach the oxygen connecting tubing from the mask to the oxygen nipple. Attach the other end to the mask oxygen inlet connector.
   d. Adjust the flowmeter to the recommended liter flow for the F_IO_2 being used.
   e. Place the mask over the patient's nose and mouth. Adjust the straps and nose bridge for fit. Verify patient comfort.
   f. Reassess the patient after 5 min.

EXERCISE 6.3.2 Accuracy of F_IO_2 with Air Entrainment Devices

1. Set the Venturi device on 40 percent, and adjust the oxygen flow to the manufacturer's recommended setting. *Record the manufacturer brand of mask used on your laboratory report.*

2. Calibrate and set up an oxygen analyzer for use.

3. While the oxygen is on, remove the mask from the Venturi device. Attach an oxygen sensor to an in-line adaptor, and connect the Venturi device to the adaptor. A single length of large-bore corrugated tubing may be required to make this connection.

4. Measure the F_IO_2, allowing time for the reading to stabilize. *Record the liter flow used and the F_IO_2 measured on your laboratory report.*

5. Decrease the oxygen flow rate to any liter flow of your choice below the manufacturer's recommended setting. Measure the F_IO_2, allowing time for the reading to stabilize. *Record the results on your laboratory report.*

6. Increase the oxygen flow rate to any liter flow of your choice above the manufacturer's recommended setting. Measure

TABLE 6.3   **Air:Oxygen Entrainment Mixing Ratios**

Air:Oxygen Ratio	F_IO_2
25:1	24%
10:1	28%
8:1	30%
5:1	35%
3:1	40%
1.7:1	50%
1:1	60%
0.6:1	70%

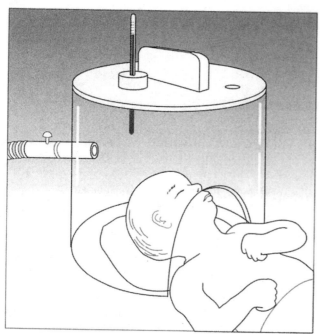

FIGURE 6.16 Oxygen hood equipment assembly. (From Persing, G: Entry-Level Respiratory Care Review: Study Guide and Workbook, ed 2. WB Saunders, Philadelphia, 1996, p. 31, with permission.)

the F_IO_2, allowing time for the reading to stabilize. *Record the results on your laboratory report.*

7. Adjust the Venturi device to another F_IO_2 of your choice.

8. Repeat steps 4, 5, and 6 for this new F_IO_2. *Record the results on your laboratory report.*

9. Place the Venturi device in a plastic bag. Insert an oxygen analyzer sensor into the bag. *Measure the F_IO_2, and record the results on your laboratory report.*

EXERCISE 6.3.3 Adequacy of Flow Rates from an Air Entrainment Device

1. Measure your laboratory partner's minute ventilation using the technique learned in Chapter 3. *Record the results on your laboratory report.*

2. Calculate your partner's estimated inspiratory flow demand. *Record the results on your laboratory report.*

   NOTE: The inspiratory flow demands can be estimated at three times the minute ventilation ($\dot{V}_E$).

3. With the Venturi device set at 40 percent, calculate the total flow being delivered from the mask using the following formula:

   Total flow = (Sum of air:oxygen entrainment ratios) × Flow rate

4. Based on your calculations, adjust the flow rate to meet your laboratory partner's inspiratory flow demand. *Record this flow on your laboratory report.*

EXERCISE 6.4 Oxygen Hood

1. Verify "physician's" order or protocol.

2. Obtain the following equipment to assemble the hood:
   a. Blender and air and oxygen gas sources
   b. Nipple adaptor

c. T-adaptor
d. Oxygen flowmeter
e. Heated large volume nebulizer or wick humidifier
f. Sterile water
g. Large-bore corrugated tubing
h. Oxygen hood
i. Temperature probe
j. Oxygen analyzer

3. Wash your hands and apply standard precautions and transmission-based isolation procedures as appropriate.

4. With your laboratory partner acting as your "patient's parent," do the following:
   a. Introduce yourself, verify your patient's identification, explain the procedure, and verify parent's understanding.
   b. Assess your patient before beginning oxygen therapy by measuring pulse, respiratory rate, quality of respirations, and color. A pulse oximeter may be used. Determine the degree of labored breathing.

5. Set up the blender or air and oxygen flowmeters.

6. Attach the nebulizer or humidifier to the outlet of the flowmeter.

7. Fill the nebulizer with sterile water.

8. Insert the heating probe in the nebulizer and plug it into an electrical outlet.

9. Adjust the blender to the prescribed F_IO_2. Close the air entrainment ports of the nebulizer (set to 100 percent). Set the flowmeter to 10 lpm. If two flowmeters are used, set the nebulizer to 100 percent and adjust the flowmeters to the proper air:oxygen mixing ratio to achieve 60 percent.

10. Attach large-bore tubing to the nebulizer outlet and inlet of the oxygen hood (Fig. 6.16).

11. Insert a temperature probe into the open port on the top of the oxyhood.

12. Insert the infant mannequin into the hood.

13. Analyze the F_IO_2 by placing the sensor at the level of the infant's mouth. Adjust blender or flowmeters if necessary. *Record the results on your laboratory report.*

14. Allow for warm-up time, and then adjust heater so that 37°C temperature or **neutral thermal environment** is achieved (32 to 37°C).

15. Reassess the patient after 5 min.

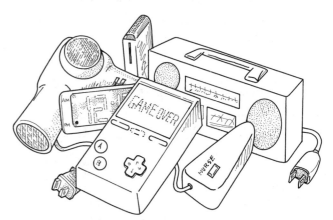

FIGURE 6.17 Hazardous items not to be placed in an oxygen-enriched environment.

EXERCISE 6.5 Oxygen Tent (Croupette)

EXERCISE 6.5.1 Oxygen Tent Setup

1. Verify "physician's" order or protocol.
2. Obtain the following equipment:
   a. Tent frame
   b. Canopy
   c. Oxygen gas source or air compressor
   d. High-pressure hose
   e. Bed
   f. Air or oxygen flowmeter with 50 psi outlet
   g. Nebulizer
   h. Circulation or refrigeration unit
   i. "No Smoking" signs
   j. Gas inlet and outlet hoses
   k. Sheets or towels
   l. Water feed system
3. Wash your hands and apply standard precautions and transmission-based isolation procedures as appropriate.
4. With your laboratory partner acting as your "patient's parent," do the following:
   a. Introduce yourself, verify your patient's identification, explain the procedure, and verify parent's understanding.
   b. Assess your patient before beginning oxygen therapy by measuring pulse, respiratory rate, quality of respirations, and color. A pulse oximeter may be used. Determine the degree of labored breathing present.
5. Attach the canopy to the tent frame.
6. Connect the gas inlet and outlet hoses to the portholes in the canopy.
7. Assemble the nebulizer and fill with sterile water, or connect the water feed system.
8. Turn on the refrigeration or circulation unit.
9. Attach the drain hose to the waste collection bottle.
10. Attach the high-pressure hose to the nebulizer inlet.

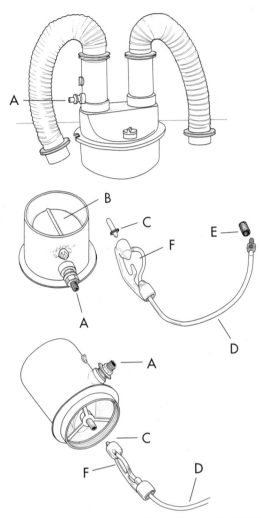

FIGURE 6.19   Identification of the nebulizer unit components.

NOTE: Depending on the brand of tent used, a 50 psi gas source may be used or an oxygen flowmeter and connecting tubing may be used with at least 10 to 15 lpm, depending on the size of the tent.

11. Attach the high-pressure hose to the oxygen flowmeter or the 50 psi DISS outlet. Verify mist production.
12. Ensure that there are no electrical or hazardous items in the tent, as shown in Figure 6.17. Instruct the patient or family members about safety considerations.
13. Post "No Smoking" signs.
14. Place the tent frame over the bed. Flush out tent for 5 min.
15. Place infant in tent and tuck in, using sheets or towels to seal if necessary.
16. After the tent has been in operation for 10 to 15 min, analyze the F_IO_2 at the level of the infant's mouth, as shown in Figure 6.18. *Record the results on your laboratory report.*
17. Reassess the patient after 5 min.

EXERCISE 6.5.2 Comparison of Mist Output

1. Disconnect the high-pressure hose from the 50 psi DISS outlet.

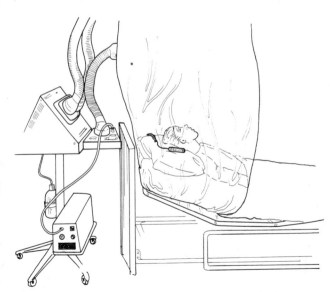

FIGURE 6.18   Analysis of F_IO_2 in an oxygen tent.

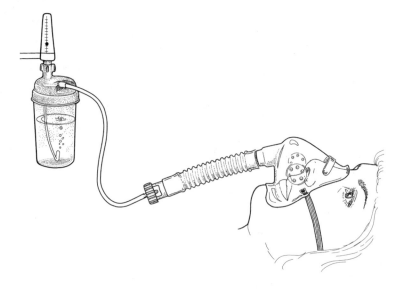

FIGURE 6.20   Troubleshooting oxygen device #1.

2. Connect the hose to an oxygen flowmeter.

3. Turn the flow to 15 lpm.

4. Compare the mist output in this exercise to the mist output in the previous exercise. *Record your observations on your laboratory report.*

EXERCISE 6.5.3 Disassembly of the Nebulizer Unit

1. Turn off and disconnect the gas source from the unit.

2. Unscrew the nebulizer unit from the water reservoir.

3. Disassemble the nebulizer component by unscrewing the nebulizer body from the outer housing.

4. Identify the following components, as shown in Figure 6.19, and *record them on your laboratory report.*
Baffle
Jet
Capillary siphon tube
Entrainment ports
Filter
Oxygen inlet

EXERCISE 6.6 Troubleshooting Common Problems

1. The instructor or your laboratory partner will set up one of the following suggested problems related to oxygen delivery devices. The student will inspect the equipment, identify the problem, and correct it.
a. Incorrect equipment setup
b. Incorrect liter flow used for device
c. Loose humidifier cap
d. Kinked oxygen connecting tubing
e. Tubing disconnection
f. Tent canopy not sealed adequately
g. Inadequate or absent mist from an aerosol tent
h. Water leakage on the floor from an oxygen mist tent
i. Incorrect analyzer placement for hood or tent

Record the problem and corrective action on your laboratory report.

2. Figures 6.20 and 6.21 illustrate one or more problems with the setup of the oxygen delivery systems. Identify the problem(s) and the corrective action to be taken. *Record these on your laboratory report.*

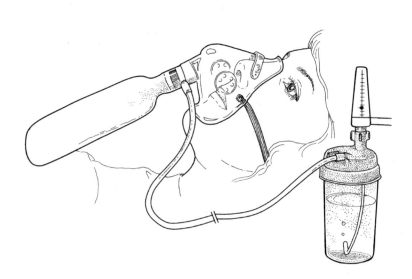

FIGURE 6.21   Troubleshooting oxygen device #2.

Reference

1. Scanlan, C et al (eds): Egan's Fundamentals of Respiratory Care, ed 6. Mosby, St Louis, 1995, p 715.

Related Readings

Eubanks, DH and Bone, RC: Principles and Applications of Cardiorespiratory Care Equipment. Mosby, St Louis, 1994.

McPherson, S: Respiratory Care Equipment, ed 5. Mosby, St Louis, 1995.

Shapiro, B et al: Clinical Application of Blood Gases, ed 5. Mosby, St Louis, 1994.

Scanlan, C et al (eds): Egan's Fundamentals of Respiratory Care, ed 6. Mosby, St Louis, 1995.

Wilkins, R, Sheldon, R and Krider, S: Clinical Assessment in Respiratory Care, ed 3. Mosby, St Louis, 1995.

Selected Journal Articles

Aesbo, U et al: Reversal of sexual impotence in male patients with chronic obstructive lung disease and hypoxemia with long term oxygen therapy. J Steroid Biochem Mol Med 46:799–803, 1993.

American Association for Respiratory Care: AARC clinical practice guideline: Oxygen therapy in the acute care hospital. Respir Care 36:1410–1413, 1991.

American Association for Respiratory Care: AARC clinical practice guideline: Oxygen therapy in the home or extended care facility. Respir Care 37:918–922, 1992.

Barker, AF, Burgher, LW and Plumber, AL: Oxygen conserving methods for adults. Chest 105:248–252, 1994.

Carter, R et al: Evaluation of the pendant oxygen-conserving nasal cannula during exercise. Chest 89:806–810, 1986.

Cottrell, JJ et al: Home oxygen therapy: A comparison of 2 vs 6 month reevaluation. Chest 107:358–361, 1995.

DeGroot, RE et al: A nearly fatal tracheal obstruction resulting from a transtracheal oxygen catheter. Chest 88:2451–2454, 1993.

Dewan, NA and Bell, CW: The effect of low flow and high flow delivery on exercise tolerance and sensation of dyspnea. Chest (April) 105:1061–1965, 1994.

Donlin, NJ and Bryson, PJ: Hyperbaric oxygen therapy. J Wound Care 4:175–178, 1995.

Doyle, D: The rational use of medical oxygen. Emerg Med 15:214–217, 220, 228–229, 1992.

Dubois, PE et al: Prognosis of severe hypoxemic patients under long term oxygen therapy. Chest 105:469–474, 1994.

Fletcher, EC: Controversial indications for long term oxygen therapy. Respir Care 39:333–346, 1994.

Goldhill, DR, Baxter, MK and Nolan, KM: Effect of education on oxygen mask placement. International Journal of Anesthesia 72:234–236, 1994.

Higgenbottam, T and Cremona, G: Acute and chronic hypoxic pulmonary hypertension. Eur Respir J 6:1207–1212, 1993.

Hoffman, LA: Novel strategies for delivering oxygen: Reservoir cannula, demand flow and transtracheal oxygen administration. Respir Care 39:363–377, 1994.

Kollef, MH and Johnson, RC: Transtracheal gas administration and the sensation of dyspnea. Respir Care 35:791–799, 1990.

Pierson, DJ: The toxicity of low flow oxygen therapy. Respir Care 28:889–897, 1983.

Sliwinski, P et al: The adequacy of oxygenation in COPD patients undergoing long term oxygen therapy assessed by pulse oximetry in the home. Eur Respir J 7:274–278, 1994.

Smoker, J et al: A protocol to assess oxygen therapy. Respir Care 31:35–39, 1986.

Spofford, B et al: Transtracheal oxygen therapy: a guide for the respiratory therapist. Respir Care 32:345–352, 1987.

Tiep, BL et al: Evaluation of an oxygen-conserving nasal cannula, Respir Care 30:19–25, 1985.

LABORATORY REPORT

CHAPTER 6: OXYGEN ADMINISTRATION DEVICES

Name _____   Date _____

Course/Section _____   Instructor _____

Data Collection

EXERCISE 6.1   Oxygen Device Identification

EXERCISE 6.1.1   Nasal Cannula

A. _____

B. _____

C. _____

EXERCISE 6.1.3   Simple Mask

A. _____

B. _____

C. _____

D. _____

EXERCISE 6.1.4   Partial Rebreathing Mask

A. _____

B. _____

C. _____

D. _____

EXERCISE 6.1.5   Nonrebreathing Mask

A. _____

B. _____

C. _____

D. _____

EXERCISE 6.1.6   Air Entrainment (Venturi) Mask

A. _____

B. _____

C. _____

D. _____

E. _____

EXERCISE 6.1.8   Oxygen Tent

A. _____

B. _____

C. _____

D. _____

E. _____

F. _____

EXERCISE 6.1.9   Oxygen Hood

A. _____

B. _____

C. _____

D. _____

EXERCISE 6.2   Administration of Oxygen Delivery Devices
EXERCISE 6.2.1   Nasal Cannula

Pulse before oxygen: _____   Pulse after: _____

Respiratory rate *(f)* before oxygen: _____   After: _____

Prescribed liter flow: _____

Estimated F_IO_2: _____

EXERCISE 6.2.2   Simple Mask

Prescribed liter flow: _____

Estimated F_IO_2: _____

EXERCISE 6.2.3   Partial Rebreathing or Nonrebreathing Mask
Partial Rebreather

Liter flow: _____   Estimated F_IO_2: _____

Nonrebreather

Liter flow: _____   Estimated F_IO_2: _____

EXERCISE 6.2.4   Oxygen Conserving Devices

Pulse before oxygen: _____   Pulse after: _____

Respiratory rate *(f)* before oxygen: _____   After: _____

Observations: _____

_____

_____

Explain the rationale for using a pulsed-dose oxygen device: _____

_____

_____

EXERCISE 6.3   Air Entrainment (Venturi) Mask
EXERCISE 6.3.2   Accuracy of F_IO_2 with Air Entrainment Devices

F_IO_2 set: 40%   Recommended liter flow: _____

Measured F_IO_2: _____

Manufacturer and brand: _____

Decreased liter flow: _____

Measured F_IO_2: _____

Increased liter flow: _____

Measured F_IO_2: _____

F_IO_2 set: _____   Recommended liter flow: _____

Measured F_IO_2: _____

Manufacturer and brand: _____

Decreased liter flow: _____

Measured F_IO_2: _____

Increased liter flow: _____

Measured F_IO_2: _____

Measured F_IO_2 of Venturi device in bag: _____

Explain why this result was obtained: _____
_____

EXERCISE 6.3.3. Adequacy of Flow Rates from an Air Entrainment Device

Minute ventilation: _____

Estimated inspiratory flow demand: _____

Total flow at 40%: _____

What adjustment to the liter flow, if any, would you have to make to meet your partner's flow demand? _____
_____
_____

EXERCISE 6.4 Oxygen Hood

Prescribed F_IO_2: _____ F_IO_2 measured: _____

Liter flows (if applicable):   Air _____   Oxygen _____

EXERCISE 6.5 Oxygen Tent (Croupette)
EXERCISE 6.5.1 Oxygen Tent Setup

F_IO_2 measured: _____

EXERCISE 6.5.2 Comparison of Mist Output

Observations: _____
_____

EXERCISE 6.5.3 Disassembly of the Nebulizer Unit

A. _____

B. _____

C. _____

D. _____

E. _____

F. _____

EXERCISE 6.6 Troubleshooting Common Problems

Equipment used: _____

Problem identified: _____

Corrective action: _____

_____

Troubleshooting Diagrams

Identify problem—Figure 6.20: _____

_____

Corrective action: _____

Identify problem—

Corrective action

[handwritten note on card:]
Emotional status
tolerance of ADL
level of dyspnea
Nutrional status

'emogra
QC
Hx present illness

CRITICAL THINKING

Mrs. Plaskowitz is a 60- *[...]* man with COPD who enters the ER via ambulance wearing a nonrebreathing mask at 10 lpm. Mrs. Plaskowitz, who w *[...]* take *[...]* the ambulance *[...]* her up, is now extremely lethargic. The ER physician suggests that you *[...]*

[handwritten: fast rate breath...]

1. Briefly explain the *[cause of the patient's lethargy]* *[...]* ...er field + there was shortage
   [handwritten:] of oxygen *[...]* . was breathing more air
   NOT O_2 The bag collapse   (because too much O_2 being delivered)

2. If the patient were to remain on the nonrebreathing mask for at least 24 hours, what complications or hazards could result from (a) the delivery method and (b) the resulting oxygen concentration?
   [handwritten:]
   a) The pt was going to breath more air + less O_2 const (a) O_2 toxicity
   (closed system)   (low flow)
   (b) The O_2 const. was going to be low

3. What liter flow would you recommend to the physician for the nasal cannula? *[handwritten:]* COP patients generally will get 1, 2, or 3
   [handwritten:] < 5 L/min

4. The pulmonary physician who has been called in on this case requests that you change the delivery device to a Venturi mask at a comparable F_IO_2.
   a. What F_IO_2 should be used for the Venturi mask? *[handwritten:]* % of air entrainment mask, pt vent.   3.4/m
   b. The patient is noted to have a minute ventilation of 15 lpm. What is the minimum liter flow, at this F_IO_2, required to meet the patient's inspiratory flow demands? Show your work!
   [handwritten:] B) TOTAL FLOW of air entrainment DEVICE = SUM PART X INPUT FLOW

5. Why is a minimum flow rate of 5 lpm recommended for oxygen delivery by mask?
   [handwritten:] at a flow less than 5 lpm the mask volume acts as deadspace + loose CO_2 reabreathing

[handwritten at bottom:]
B) 35%
5:1
Insp. Flow = 3 × 15 = 45
45 = 6 × ? = 45/6 = 7   6√45
TOTAL FLOW = SUM PART X INPUT FLOW

6. Explain the difference between a high-flow and a low-flow oxygen delivery system. Give an example of each.

low flow gives the pt partial O2 than   need while

High

7. You observe a patient wearing a nonrebreathing mask and note that the bag completely deflates with each inspiration. What, if any, actions should be taken?

Check The tubing if it is leaking
Change The Mask
Increase The flow

8. What oxygen delivery device would you recommend for a patient who has just been successfully resuscitated and is spontaneously breathing?

partial rebreathing Mask easy to apply 6-10 L/m
quick to apply, No expensive   variable
used For Short term

9. What three environmental factors can be controlled with an oxygen tent?

Temp, oxygen Conct. humidity

10. What is the minimum flow rate that should be used with an oxygen hood?

> 7 L/m to prevent accumulation of CO2 10-15 L/m To maintain high
Stable Conct.

11. List at least three factors that will affect the F_IO_2 delivered by a low-flow oxygen system.

High O2 output increase FIO2   Low tidal volume ↓ FIO2
Mouth close breathing ↑ FIO2   High "   "   ↑ FIO2
*   "   open   "   ↓ FIO2*
The ↑ The Flow the ↑ The Conct O2 you get   The deeper you breath the lower Conct. you get
The ↑ The rate of breathing the

12. List three advantages and three disadvantages of transtracheal oxygenation.

low O2 usage/cost   _Surgical Complications
Eliminates nasal ear irritations   - infections
Increase mobility   - Mucus plugging
Improved compliance   — Lost tract

13. Calculate or fill in the missing parameters. Show your work!

F_IO_2	O₂ Flow Rate	Entrainment Ratio	Total Flow		air:O₂ Ratio	FIO_2
.60	12 lpm	1:1 =2	24 lpm 2×12=24	Table	25:1 →	24%
0.28	8 lpm	10:1 =11	88 11×8=88		10:1 →	28%
0.40	10 L/pm	3:1 =4	40 lpm 4×10=40		8:1 →	30%
.35	6	5:1 = 6	36 lpm 6×7=36		5:1 →	35%
.30	3 lpm	8:1 =9	27		3:1 →	40%
					1.7:1 →	50%
					1:1 →	60%
					0.6:1 →	70%

8:1 = 30%

PROCEDURAL COMPETENCY EVALUATION

Name _Cecelia Ayala_   Date _6/03/00_

Oxygen Therapy

Setting: ☑ Lab ☐ Clinical   Evaluator: ☐ Peer ☑ Instructor

Conditions (describe): _____

Equipment Used

_____

_____

	S A T I S F A C T O R Y	U N S A T I S F A C T O R Y	N O T O B S E R V E D	N O T A P P L I C A B L E

Equipment and Patient Preparation

1. Verifies, interprets, and evaluates physician's order or protocol — ☑ ☐ ☐ ☐

2. Scans chart for diagnosis and any other pertinent data and notes — ☑ ☐ ☐ ☐

3. Selects, gathers, and assembles the necessary equipment, including the appropriate oxygen administration device — ☑ ☐ ☐ ☐

4. Washes hands and applies standard precautions and transmission-based isolation procedures as appropriate — ☑ ☐ ☐ ☐

5. Identifies patient, introduces self and department — ☑ ☐ ☐ ☐

6. Explains purpose of the procedure and confirms patient understanding, including the safety considerations regarding smoking and electrical devices; posts "No Smoking" sign if required by policy — ☑ ☐ ☐ ☐

Assessment and Implementation

The Inner of the mouth, Nail a palm, Hyonosis
most important step

7. Assesses the patient before beginning oxygen therapy by measuring pulse, respiratory rate, quality of respirations, and color; a pulse oximeter may be used; interviews the patient to determine if dyspnea is present — ☑ ☐ ☐ ☐

8. Assembles the equipment as required — *Put equipment together* — ☑ ☐ ☐ ☐

9. Adjusts the flowmeter to the prescribed or adequate level — ☑ ☐ ☐ ☐

10. Verifies flow or concentration *Make sure you put it right* — ☑ ☐ ☐ ☐

11. Places the administration device properly and comfortably on the patient's face — ☑ ☐ ☐ ☐

12. Confirms fit and verifies patient comfort — ☑ ☐ ☐ ☐

13. Reassesses the patient after 5 min *(Increase or reduce dosis, change medication)* — ☑ ☐ ☐ ☐

14. Makes any adjustments in flow if required — ☑ ☐ ☐ ☐

Follow-up

15. Maintains/processes equipment — ☑ ☐ ☐ ☐

16. Disposes of infectious waste and washes hands — ☑ ☐ ☐ ☐

17. Records pertinent data in chart and departmental records — ☑ ☐ ☐ ☐

18. Notifies appropriate personnel and makes any necessary recommendations or modifications to the patient care plan — ☑ ☐ ☐ ☐

_____
Signature of Evaluator

_____
Signature of Student

PERFORMANCE RATING SCALE

5 EXCELLENT—FAR EXCEEDS EXPECTED LEVEL, FLAWLESS PERFORMANCE
4 ABOVE AVERAGE—NO PROMPTING REQUIRED, ABLE TO SELF-CORRECT
3 AVERAGE—THE MINIMUM COMPETENCY LEVEL, NO CRITICAL ERRORS
2 IMPROVEMENT NEEDED—PROBLEM AREAS EXIST; CRITICAL ERRORS, CORRECTIONS NEEDED
1 POOR AND UNACCEPTABLE PERFORMANCE—GROSS INACCURACIES, POTENTIALLY HARMFUL

PERFORMANCE CRITERIA	SCALE				
1. DISPLAYS KNOWLEDGE OF ESSENTIAL CONCEPTS	5	4	3	2	1
2. DEMONSTRATES THE RELATIONSHIP BETWEEN THEORY AND CLINICAL PRACTICE	5	4	3	2	1
3. FOLLOWS DIRECTIONS, EXHIBITS SOUND JUDGMENT, AND DEMONSTRATES ATTENTION TO SAFETY AND DETAIL	5	4	3	2	1
4. EXHIBITS THE REQUIRED MANUAL DEXTERITY	5	4	3	2	1
5. PERFORMS PROCEDURE IN A REASONABLE TIME FRAME	5	4	3	2	1
6. MAINTAINS STERILE OR ASEPTIC TECHNIQUE	5	4	3	2	1
7. INITIATES UNAMBIGUOUS GOAL-DIRECTED COMMUNICATION	5	4	3	2	1
8. PROVIDES FOR ADEQUATE CARE AND MAINTENANCE OF EQUIPMENT AND SUPPLIES	5	4	3	2	1
9. EXHIBITS COURTEOUS AND PLEASANT DEMEANOR	5	4	3	2	1
10. MAINTAINS CONCISE AND ACCURATE RECORDS	5	4	3	2	1

ADDITIONAL COMMENTS: INCLUDE ERRORS OF OMISSION OR COMMISSION, COMMUNICATIVE SKILLS, AND EFFECTIVENESS OF PATIENT INTERACTION:

SUMMARY PERFORMANCE EVALUATION AND RECOMMENDATIONS

SATISFACTORY PERFORMANCE—Performed without error or prompting, or able to self-correct, no critical errors.

_____ LABORATORY EVALUATION. SKILLS MAY BE APPLIED/OBSERVED IN THE CLINICAL SETTING.

_____ CLINICAL EVALUATION. STUDENT READY FOR MINIMALLY SUPERVISED APPLICATION AND REFINEMENT.

UNSATISFACTORY PERFORMANCE—Prompting required; performed with critical errors, potentially harmful.

_____ STUDENT REQUIRES ADDITIONAL LABORATORY PRACTICE.

_____ STUDENT REQUIRES ADDITIONAL SUPERVISED CLINICAL PRACTICE.

SIGNATURES

STUDENT: _____   EVALUATOR: _____

DATE: _____   DATE: _____

PROCEDURAL COMPETENCY EVALUATION

Name _____ Date _____

Oxygen Tent

Setting: ☐ Lab ☐ Clinical   Evaluator: ☐ Peer ☐ Instructor

Conditions (describe): _____

_____

Equipment Used

_____

_____

	SATISFACTORY	UNSATISFACTORY	NOT OBSERVED	NOT APPLICABLE
Equipment and Patient Preparation				
1. Verifies, interprets, and evaluates physician's order or protocol	☐	☐	☐	☐
2. Scans chart for diagnosis and any other pertinent data and notes	☐	☐	☐	☐
3. Selects, gathers, and assembles the necessary equipment	☐	☐	☐	☐
4. Washes hands and applies standard precautions and transmission-based isolation procedures as appropriate	☐	☐	☐	☐
5. Identifies patient, introduces self and department	☐	☐	☐	☐
6. Explains purpose of the procedure and confirms patient or patient's parent understanding, including safety considerations.	☐	☐	☐	☐
Assessment and Implementation				
7. Assesses the patient before beginning oxygen therapy by measuring pulse, respiratory rate, quality of respirations, and color; a pulse oximeter may be used; determines the degree of labored breathing present	☐	☐	☐	☐
8. Attaches the canopy to the tent frame	☐	☐	☐	☐
9. Connects the gas inlet and outlet hoses to the portholes in the canopy	☐	☐	☐	☐
10. Assembles the nebulizer and fills the reservoir with sterile water or connects the feed system	☐	☐	☐	☐
11. Turns on the refrigeration unit if present	☐	☐	☐	☐
12. Attaches the drain hose to the waste collection bottle	☐	☐	☐	☐
13. Attaches the high-pressure hose to the nebulizer inlet	☐	☐	☐	☐
14. Attaches the high-pressure hose to the oxygen flowmeter or 50 psi DISS outlet	☐	☐	☐	☐
15. Verifies mist production	☐	☐	☐	☐
16. Ensures that there are no electrical or hazardous items in the tent	☐	☐	☐	☐
17. Posts "No Smoking" signs if required by policy	☐	☐	☐	☐
18. Places the tent frame over the bed and flushes the tent for 5 min	☐	☐	☐	☐
19. Places infant or child in the tent and tucks in the canopy	☐	☐	☐	☐
20. Analyzes the F_IO_2	☐	☐	☐	☐
21. Reassesses the patient after 5 min	☐	☐	☐	☐
Follow-up				
22. Maintains/processes equipment	☐	☐	☐	☐
23. Disposes of infectious waste and washes hands	☐	☐	☐	☐

	S A T I S F A C T O R Y	U N S A T I S F A C T O R Y	N O T O B S E R V E D	N O T A P P L I C A B L E
24. Records pertinent data in chart and departmental records	☐	☐	☐	☐
25. Notifies appropriate personnel and makes any necessary recommendations or modifications to the patient care plan	☐	☐	☐	☐

_____
Signature of Evaluator

_____
Signature of Student

PERFORMANCE RATING SCALE

5 EXCELLENT—FAR EXCEEDS EXPECTED LEVEL, FLAWLESS PERFORMANCE
4 ABOVE AVERAGE—NO PROMPTING REQUIRED, ABLE TO SELF-CORRECT
3 AVERAGE—THE MINIMUM COMPETENCY LEVEL, NO CRITICAL ERRORS
2 IMPROVEMENT NEEDED—PROBLEM AREAS EXIST; CRITICAL ERRORS, CORRECTIONS NEEDED
1 POOR AND UNACCEPTABLE PERFORMANCE—GROSS INACCURACIES, POTENTIALLY HARMFUL

PERFORMANCE CRITERIA		SCALE			
1. DISPLAYS KNOWLEDGE OF ESSENTIAL CONCEPTS	5	4	3	2	1
2. DEMONSTRATES THE RELATIONSHIP BETWEEN THEORY AND CLINICAL PRACTICE	5	4	3	2	1
3. FOLLOWS DIRECTIONS, EXHIBITS SOUND JUDGMENT, AND DEMONSTRATES ATTENTION TO SAFETY AND DETAIL	5	4	3	2	1
4. EXHIBITS THE REQUIRED MANUAL DEXTERITY	5	4	3	2	1
5. PERFORMS PROCEDURE IN A REASONABLE TIME FRAME	5	4	3	2	1
6. MAINTAINS STERILE OR ASEPTIC TECHNIQUE	5	4	3	2	1
7. INITIATES UNAMBIGUOUS GOAL-DIRECTED COMMUNICATION	5	4	3	2	1
8. PROVIDES FOR ADEQUATE CARE AND MAINTENANCE OF EQUIPMENT AND SUPPLIES	5	4	3	2	1
9. EXHIBITS COURTEOUS AND PLEASANT DEMEANOR	5	4	3	2	1
10. MAINTAINS CONCISE AND ACCURATE RECORDS	5	4	3	2	1

ADDITIONAL COMMENTS: INCLUDE ERRORS OF OMISSION OR COMMISSION, COMMUNICATIVE SKILLS, AND EFFECTIVENESS OF PATIENT INTERACTION:

SUMMARY PERFORMANCE EVALUATION AND RECOMMENDATIONS

SATISFACTORY PERFORMANCE—Performed without error or prompting, or able to self-correct, no critical errors.

_____ LABORATORY EVALUATION. SKILLS MAY BE APPLIED/OBSERVED IN THE CLINICAL SETTING.

_____ CLINICAL EVALUATION. STUDENT READY FOR MINIMALLY SUPERVISED APPLICATION AND REFINEMENT.

UNSATISFACTORY PERFORMANCE—Prompting required; performed with critical errors, potentially harmful.

_____ STUDENT REQUIRES ADDITIONAL LABORATORY PRACTICE.

_____ STUDENT REQUIRES ADDITIONAL SUPERVISED CLINICAL PRACTICE.

SIGNATURES

STUDENT: _____   EVALUATOR: _____

DATE: _____   DATE: _____

PROCEDURAL COMPETENCY EVALUATION

Name _____ Date _____

Oxygen Hood

Setting: ☐ Lab ☐ Clinical

Evaluator: ☐ Peer ☐ Instructor

Conditions (describe): _____

_____

Equipment Used

_____

_____

	SATISFACTORY	UNSATISFACTORY	NOT OBSERVED	NOT APPLICABLE
Equipment and Patient Preparation				
1. Verifies, interprets, and evaluates physician's order or protocol	☐	☐	☐	☐
2. Scans chart for diagnosis and any other pertinent data and notes	☐	☐	☐	☐
3. Selects, gathers, and assembles the necessary equipment	☐	☐	☐	☐
4. Washes hands and applies standard precautions and transmission-based isolation procedures as appropriate	☐	☐	☐	☐
5. Identifies patient, introduces self and department	☐	☐	☐	☐
6. Explains purpose of the procedure and confirms parental understanding	☐	☐	☐	☐
Assessment and Implementation				
7. Assesses the patient before beginning oxygen therapy by measuring pulse, respiratory rate, quality of respirations, and color; a pulse oximeter may be used; determines the degree of labored breathing	☐	☐	☐	☐
8. Connects the blender or air and oxygen flowmeters	☐	☐	☐	☐
9. Attaches the nebulizer or humidifier	☐	☐	☐	☐
10. Fills the nebulizer or humidifier with sterile water	☐	☐	☐	☐
11. Inserts the heater in the nebulizer and plugs it into an electrical outlet	☐	☐	☐	☐
12. Adjusts the blender to the prescribed F_IO_2	☐	☐	☐	☐
13. Sets the flowmeter to 7 lpm or greater	☐	☐	☐	☐
14. Attaches the large-bore tubing to the nebulizer outlet and inlet of the oxygen hood	☐	☐	☐	☐
15. Inserts a temperature probe into the open port on the top of the oxyhood	☐	☐	☐	☐
16. Inserts the infant mannequin into the hood	☐	☐	☐	☐
17. Analyzes the F_IO_2 at the level of the infant's mouth	☐	☐	☐	☐
18. Allows for warm-up time, adjusts heater if necessary, and ensures a neutral thermal environment	☐	☐	☐	☐
19. Reassesses the patient after 5 min	☐	☐	☐	☐
Follow-up				
20. Maintains/processes equipment	☐	☐	☐	☐
21. Disposes of infectious waste and washes hands	☐	☐	☐	☐
22. Records pertinent data in chart and departmental records	☐	☐	☐	☐
23. Notifies appropriate personnel and makes any necessary recommendations or modifications to the patient care plan	☐	☐	☐	☐

_____
Signature of Evaluator

_____
Signature of Student

PERFORMANCE RATING SCALE

5 EXCELLENT—FAR EXCEEDS EXPECTED LEVEL, FLAWLESS PERFORMANCE
4 ABOVE AVERAGE—NO PROMPTING REQUIRED, ABLE TO SELF-CORRECT
3 AVERAGE—THE MINIMUM COMPETENCY LEVEL, NO CRITICAL ERRORS
2 IMPROVEMENT NEEDED—PROBLEM AREAS EXIST; CRITICAL ERRORS, CORRECTIONS NEEDED
1 POOR AND UNACCEPTABLE PERFORMANCE—GROSS INACCURACIES, POTENTIALLY HARMFUL

PERFORMANCE CRITERIA   SCALE

1. DISPLAYS KNOWLEDGE OF ESSENTIAL CONCEPTS	5	4	3	2	1
2. DEMONSTRATES THE RELATIONSHIP BETWEEN THEORY AND CLINICAL PRACTICE	5	4	3	2	1
3. FOLLOWS DIRECTIONS, EXHIBITS SOUND JUDGMENT, AND DEMONSTRATES ATTENTION TO SAFETY AND DETAIL	5	4	3	2	1
4. EXHIBITS THE REQUIRED MANUAL DEXTERITY	5	4	3	2	1
5. PERFORMS PROCEDURE IN A REASONABLE TIME FRAME	5	4	3	2	1
6. MAINTAINS STERILE OR ASEPTIC TECHNIQUE	5	4	3	2	1
7. INITIATES UNAMBIGUOUS GOAL-DIRECTED COMMUNICATION	5	4	3	2	1
8. PROVIDES FOR ADEQUATE CARE AND MAINTENANCE OF EQUIPMENT AND SUPPLIES	5	4	3	2	1
9. EXHIBITS COURTEOUS AND PLEASANT DEMEANOR	5	4	3	2	1
10. MAINTAINS CONCISE AND ACCURATE RECORDS	5	4	3	2	1

ADDITIONAL COMMENTS: INCLUDE ERRORS OF OMISSION OR COMMISSION, COMMUNICATIVE SKILLS, AND EFFECTIVENESS OF PATIENT INTERACTION:

SUMMARY PERFORMANCE EVALUATION AND RECOMMENDATIONS

SATISFACTORY PERFORMANCE—Performed without error or prompting, or able to self-correct, no critical errors.

_____ LABORATORY EVALUATION. SKILLS MAY BE APPLIED/OBSERVED IN THE CLINICAL SETTING.

_____ CLINICAL EVALUATION. STUDENT READY FOR MINIMALLY SUPERVISED APPLICATION AND REFINEMENT.

UNSATISFACTORY PERFORMANCE—Prompting required; performed with critical errors, potentially harmful.

_____ STUDENT REQUIRES ADDITIONAL LABORATORY PRACTICE.

_____ STUDENT REQUIRES ADDITIONAL SUPERVISED CLINICAL PRACTICE.

SIGNATURES

STUDENT: _____   EVALUATOR: _____

DATE: _____   DATE: _____

Humidity Devices

The major functions of the upper airway are to warm, filter, and humidify the air that is breathed. Many conditions, such as artificial airways, **dehydration,** fever, and the breathing of **anhydrous** gases, alter the efficiency of the upper airway in performing these functions. The respiratory care practitioner, in these circumstances, may deliver adjunctive humidity therapy to patients to prevent secretions from becoming **inspissated.** The safe operation and use of these devices requires an understanding of their capabilities and limitations.

OBJECTIVES

Upon completion of this chapter, the student will be able to:

1. Identify the components of the heat and moisture exchanger (HME) and bubble, cascade, and wick humidifiers.
2. Differentiate between the types of humidifiers, including their clinical uses, advantages, and disadvantages.
3. Assemble and operate the various types of humidifiers.
4. Perform monitoring, maintenance, and troubleshooting techniques.
5. Relate, according to AARC clinical practice guidelines, the proper amount of humidification for patients with artificial airways.

KEY TERMS

adhesion	colloid	facilitate	neutral thermal
ambient	condensate	hydration	environment
anhydrous	crystalloid	hygrometer	osmosis
anion	dehydration	hygroscopic	relative humidity
calorie	density	hypertonic	solute
cation	desiccation	hypotonic	solution
cold stress	epithelium	inspissated	solvent
	evaporation	isotonic	

EQUIPMENT REQUIRED

- Bubble humidifier
- Heat and moisture exchanger
- Cascade humidifier
- Wick humidifier
- Sterile water
- Continuous fill system
- Corrugated tubing
- Scissors
- Temperature probe with adaptor
- Compressed gas source
- Regulator with flowmeter
- Manual resuscitator
- Lung simulator (optional)
- Beaker or graduated cylinder
- Clean towels

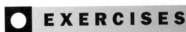 **EXERCISES**

EXERCISE 7.1 Bubble Humidifier

EXERCISE 7.1.1 Identification of Components

Identify the components of a bubble humidifier, as shown in Figure 7.1, and *record the following on your laboratory report:*

DISS connection
Outlet
Capillary inlet tube
Pop-off valve
Bubble diffuser

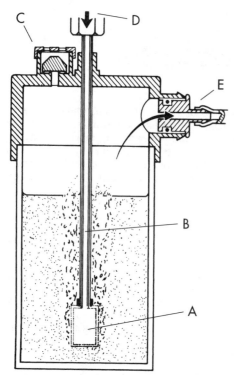

FIGURE 7.1 Identification of bubble humidifier components. (From Burton, GG, Hodgkin, JE and Ward, JJ: Respiratory Care: A Guide to Clinical Practice, ed 3. JB Lippincott, Philadelphia, 1991, p. 368, with permission.)

EXERCISE 7.1.2 Setup of a Bubble Humidifier

1. Connect the bubble humidifier to the DISS outlet of a flowmeter.
2. If a dry humidifier (not prefilled) is used, fill the humidifier to the fill line with sterile water.
3. Adjust the flow rate to 5 lpm.
4. *Record your observations on your laboratory report.*
5. Shut the flowmeter off.
6. Remove the plastic protector from the outlet of the humidifier.
7. Readjust the flowmeter to 5 lpm.
8. Obstruct the outlet of the humidifier.
9. *Record your observations on your laboratory report.*
10. Loosen the cap from the bottle.
11. *Record your observations on your laboratory report.*
12. Tighten the cap. Attach a small-bore oxygen connecting tube to the humidifier outlet.
13. Kink the tubing by bending it in half.
14. *Record your observations on your laboratory report.*
15. Turn the flowmeter to flush.
16. *Record your observations on your laboratory report.*

EXERCISE 7.2 Heat and Moisture Exchanger

Examine a heat and moisture exchanger. Compare HMEs from several manufacturers (Fig. 7.2). Perform the following:

1. Read the manufacturer's insert. *Record the brand used, expected H_2O content, and resistance specifications on your laboratory report.*
2. Ventilate through the HME with a handheld resuscitator. Alternatively, connect the HME to a lung simulator and attempt to bag through the HME. *Record your observations on your laboratory report.*
3. Fill the HME with water. Let it stand for 5 min, and then drain the excess water.
4. Ventilate through the HME with a handheld resuscitator. Alternatively, connect the HME to a lung simulator and attempt to bag through the HME.
5. *Record your observations on your laboratory report.*

EXERCISE 7.3 Cascade Humidifier

EXERCISE 7.3.1 Components of a Cascade Humidifier

Identify the components, as shown in Figure 7.3, of the cascade humidifier by disassembling and reassembling the unit. *Record on your laboratory report.*

Gas inlet
Gas outlet
Temperature control
Sensing port ——or thermostat the two tubes inside
Tower
One-way valve
Grid & the plastic thing inside
Safety shutoff
Heating element
Thermal wells and shunt

EXERCISE 7.3.2 Continuous Feed Assembly

Assemble the unit with a continuous feed system, as shown in Figure 7.4.

1. Connect the cascade to the flowmeter using the adaptor, ensuring that the unit is plugged in.
2. Connect 12 six-inch lengths or sections of corrugated tubing to the outlet of the humidifier.
3. Aseptically fill the humidifier with sterile water.
4. Attach a temperature probe at the end of the tubing using a monitoring adaptor.
5. Turn the flowmeter to 8 lpm.
6. Turn the heater setting to 6.
7. Hold your hand by the end of the corrugated tubing, and *record your observations on your laboratory report.*
8. After 15 min, drain the condensate away from the unit and measure.
9. *Record the temperature and the amount of condensate on your laboratory report.*

EXERCISE 7.4 Wick Humidifier

EXERCISE 7.4.1 Components of a Wick Humidifier

Identify the components of a wick humidifier, as shown in Figure 7.5, and *record them on your laboratory report.*

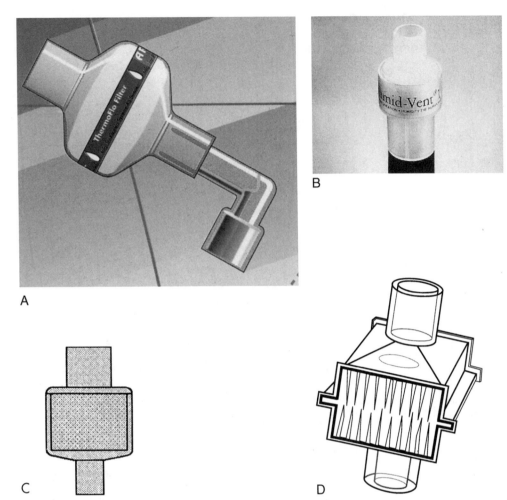

FIGURE 7.2   Heat and moisture exchangers. (Courtesy of *[A]* ARC Medical Inc., Scottdale, GA; *[B]* Gibeck Inc., Indianapolis, IN; *[C]* Mallinckrodt Inc., St. Louis, MO; *[D]* Pall Biomedical Products, East Hills, NY.)

c̄ lower the hemidifier becomes simple pass over ^Blow hemidifier

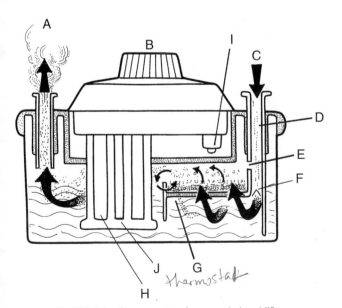

FIGURE 7.3   Components of a cascade humidifier.

thermostat

Inlet
Outlet
Heating element
Wick
On/off switch
Temperature probe

EXERCISE 7.4.2 Assembly of a Wick Humidifier

1. Connect the humidifier to the outlet of a flowmeter; ensure that the unit is plugged in.
2. Connect 12 lengths of corrugated tubing to the outlet of the humidifier.
3. Aseptically fill the humidifier with sterile water.
4. Attach a temperature probe at the end of the tubing using a monitoring adaptor.
5. Turn the flow to 8 lpm, and adjust the temperature setting to 37° C.
6. Hold your hand by the end of the corrugated tubing, and *record your observations on your laboratory report.*

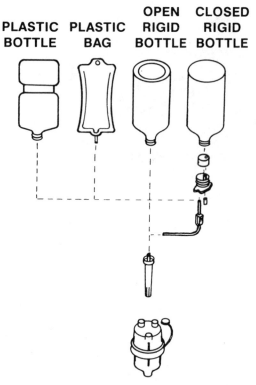

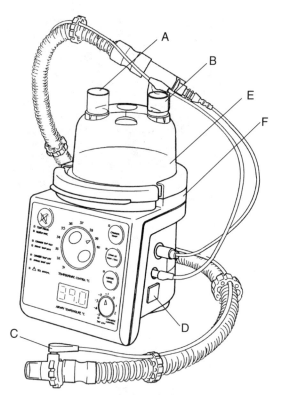

FIGURE 7.4   Setup of a continuous feed system. (Courtesy of Timeter, Allied Healthcare Products Inc., St. Louis, MO.)

FIGURE 7.5   Components of a wick humidifier. (Courtesy of Fisher & Paykel Healthcare, Auckland, New Zealand.)

7. After 15 min, drain the condensate away from the unit and measure.

8. *Record the temperature and the amount of condensate on your laboratory report.*

Related Readings

Eubanks, DH and Bone, RC: Principles and Applications of Cardiorespiratory Care Equipment. Mosby, St Louis, 1994.

McPherson, S: Respiratory Care Equipment, ed 5. Mosby, St Louis, 1995.

Scanlan, C et al (eds): Egan's Fundamentals of Respiratory Care, ed 6. Mosby, St Louis, 1995.

Selected Journal Articles

American Association for Respiratory Care: AARC clinical practice guideline: Oxygen therapy in the acute care hospital. Respir Care 36:1410–1413, 1991.

American Association for Respiratory Care: AARC clinical practice guideline: Oxygen therapy in the home or extended care facility. Respir Care 37: 918–922, 1991.

American Association for Respiratory Care: AARC clinical practice guideline: Humidification during mechanical ventilation. Respir Care 37:887–890, 1992.

Branson, R: Humidification: A dry subject, but . . . Respir Care 32:249–254, 1987.

Branson, R and Chatburn, RL: Humidification of inspired gases during mechanical ventilation. Respir Care 38:461–468, 1993.

Branson, R et al: Humidification in the intensive care unit: Prospective study of a new protocol utilizing heated humidification and a hygroscopic condenser humidifier. Respir Care 104:1800–1805, 1993.

Branson, R and Hurst, J: Laboratory evaluation of moisture output of seven airway heat and moisture exchangers. Respir Care 32:741–747, 1987.

Cahill, C and Heath, J: Sterile water used for humidification in low-flow oxygen therapy: Is it necessary? Am J Infect Control 18:13–17, 1990.

Chatburn, R and Primiano, F: A rational basis for humidity therapy. Respir Care 32:249–253, 1987.

Demers, R: Choosing the right humidification device for your mechanically ventilated patient. Current Respiratory Techniques and Therapy 1988.

Henderson, E et al: Prolonged and multipatient use of prefilled disposable oxygen humidifier bottles: Safety and cost. Infect Control Hosp Epidemiol 14:463–468, 1993.

Ploysongsang, Y et al: Effect of flowrate and duration of use on the pressure drop across six artificial noses. Respir Care 34:902–907, 1989.

Seto, W et al: Evaluating the sterility of disposable wall oxygen humidifiers during and between use on patients. Infect Control Hosp Epidemiol 11:604–605, 1990.

Sottiaux, T et al: Comparative evaluation of three heat and moisture exchangers during short-term post-operative mechanical ventilation. Chest 104:220–224, 1993.

Suzukawa, M, Usuda, Y and Numata, K: The effects on sputum characteristics of combining an unheated humidifier with a heat-moisture exchanging filter. Respir Care 34:976–984, 1989.

F. A. Davis Company
1915 Arch Street
Philadelphia, PA 19103

Printed in the United States of America

Last digit indicates print number: 10 9 8 7 6 5 4 3 2

Publisher, Health Professions: Jean-François Vilain
Senior Editor: Lynn Borders Caldwell
Developmental Editor: Marianne Fithian
Cover Designer: Louis J. Forgione

As new scientific information becomes available through basic and clinical research, recommended treatments and drug therapies undergo changes. The authors and publisher have done everything possible to make this book accurate, up to date, and in accord with accepted standards at the time of publication. The authors, editors, and publisher are not responsible for errors or omissions or for consequences from application of the book, and make no warranty, expressed or implied, in regard to the contents of the book. Any practice described in this book should be applied by the reader in accordance with professional standards of care used in regard to the unique circumstances that may apply in each situation. The reader is advised always to check product information (package inserts) for changes and new information regarding dose and contraindications before administering any drug. Caution is especially urged when using new or infrequently ordered drugs.

Library of Congress Cataloging-in-Publication Data

Butler, Thomas J.
    Laboratory exercises for competency in respiratory care / Thomas
J. Butler, Janice Blaer Close, Robert J. Close.
        p.   cm.
    Includes bibliographical references and index.
    ISBN 0-8036-0248-0
    1. Respiratory therapy—Laboratory manuals.   I. Close, Janice
Blaer.   II. Close, Robert J.   III. Title.
    [DNLM: 1. Respiratory Therapy—laboratory manuals.   2. Diagnosis-
-laboratory manuals.   WB 342 B987L   1997]
RC735.I5B88   1997
616.2—dc21
DNLM/DLC
for Library of Congress   97-41975
                                                              CIP

[handwritten: http://home.att.net./~nrodriguez20/]

Laboratory Exercises for Competency in Respiratory Care

[handwritten: To check off for track.]
[handwritten: http://home.att.net/~nrodriguez25/fundamen check off. htm]

Thomas J. Butler, MS, RRT, RPFT
Perinatal/Pediatric Specialist
Education
Respiratory Care Program
Rockland Community College
Suffern, New York

Rehabilitation
New Jersey
Approved Instructor NIOSH Spirometry Training

MA, RRT, RPFT
Perinatal/Pediatric Specialist
Program Director, Respiratory Care
Rockland Community College

Instructor NIOSH Spirometry Training

BS, RRT
Medical Services Administrator
New York

College

OSH Spirometry Training

[handwritten note 1: http://home.att.net/~nrodri-guez 20/ (peak flow) ↓ Level of obstruction]

[handwritten note 2: Normal HR is b/w 60-100. Normal Blood Pressure is 120/80 systolic/diastolic. The difference bw them is called pulse pressure. HTN - hypertension & is b/w 35-40]

[handwritten right margin: Linda 201-659-738. Angelo 718-698-343. Stanton I TINOWA 973-484-928 H973-731-6118. Indication of humidifier 1. heat + moist 2. bypass Nassal com 1. if Pt comf 2. oxy is abo 4 L/min]

F. A. DAVIS COMPANY • Philadelphia

LABORATORY REPORT

CHAPTER 7: HUMIDITY DEVICES

Name _____   Date _____

Course/Section _____   Instructor _____

Data Collection

EXERCISE 7.1   Bubble Humidifier

EXERCISE 7.1.1.   Identification of Components

A. _____

B. _____

C. _____

D. _____

E. _____

EXERCISE 7.1.2   Setup of a Bubble Humidifier

Observations

Plastic protector on, flow rate to 5 lpm:

_____

_____

Obstruct the outlet of the humidifier, flow rate to 5 lpm:

_____

_____

Loosen the cap from the bottle:

_____

_____

Kinked tubing:

_____

_____

Flowmeter to flush:

_____

_____

EXERCISE 7.2   Heat and Moisture Exchanger

Brand used: _____

Expected H_2O content: _____

Resistance specifications: _____

_____

Ventilate through dry HME: _____

Resistance recorded on simulator: _____

HME wet: _____

Resistance recorded on simulator: _____

EXERCISE 7.3   Cascade Humidifier
EXERCISE 7.3.1   Components of a Cascade Humidifier

A. _____

B. _____

C. _____

D. _____

E. _____

F. _____

G. _____

H. _____

I. _____

J. _____

EXERCISE 7.3.2   Continuous Feed Assembly

Temperature: _____

Amount of condensate: _____

Observations

_____

_____

_____

_____

_____

EXERCISE 7.4   Wick Humidifier
EXERCISE 7.4.1   Components of a Wick Humidifier

Brand used: _____

Components identified:

A. _____

B. _____

C. _____

D. _____

E. _____

F. _____

EXERCISE 7.4.2   Assembly of a Wick Humidifier

Temperature: _____

Amount of condensate: _____

Observations

_____

_____

_____

_____

_____

CRITICAL THINKING QUESTIONS

1. What are the limitations of a heat and moisture exchanger? What are the advantages? What effect does moisture have on HME function? ① *If THE HME is not replace can cause damage on The Respiratory tracle ↑ Volume of secretion, Large tide Volume.*
   ② *Maintain normal py siological conetion in the lower airways*
   ③ *Condensation Measuring proper condition of the inspired gas Cross Contamination.*

2. What humidifiers are the most efficient? What effect does temperature have on the efficiency of the unit? According to AARC clinical practice guidelines, what is the minimum water vapor content (mg/L) that must be provided to patients with artificial airways?
   — bubble humidity
   — passover   "
   the greater the temp q a gas the more water varot
   30 mg/L

3. What are the advantages and disadvantage of using a continuous feed system to fill a humidifier?
   safe dependable
   Opportunity of airway contamination Produce
   interfere humidification operation

4. Define *humidity.* What is the purpose of using humidifiers in the clinical setting? What complications can result if inadequate humidification is provided?

5. According to AARC clinical practice guidelines, what are the recommended liter flows when using a bubble humidifier?

6. For each of the following scenarios, identify what type of humidifier you would use. Explain your rationale.
   a. Nasal cannula at 3 lpm
   b. Nasal cannula at 6 lpm
   c. Postoperative patient on short-term mechanical ventilation
   d. Long-term mechanically ventilated patient with inspissated secretions

PROCEDURAL COMPETENCY EVALUATION

Name _____ Date _____

Humidity Therapy

Setting: ☐ Lab ☐ Clinical   Evaluator: ☐ Peer ☐ Instructor

Conditions (describe): _____

_____

Equipment Used

_____

_____

	S A T I S F A C T O R Y	U N S A T I S F A C T O R Y	N O T O B S E R V E D	N O T A P P L I C A B L E
Equipment and Patient Preparation				
1. Verifies, interprets, and evaluates physician's order or protocol	☐	☐	☐	☐
2. Scans chart for diagnosis and any other pertinent data and notes	☐	☐	☐	☐
3. Selects, gathers, and assembles the necessary equipment	☐	☐	☐	☐
4. Identifies the following types of humidifiers: bubble, wick, jet, cascade, HME, HME/F, HCH	☐	☐	☐	☐
5. Washes hands and applies standard precautions and transmission-based isolation procedures as appropriate	☐	☐	☐	☐
6. Identifies patient, introduces self and department	☐	☐	☐	☐
7. Explains purpose of the procedure and confirms patient understanding	☐	☐	☐	☐
Assessment and Implementation				
8. Fills humidifier with sterile H_2O or handles prefilled humidifier aseptically	☐	☐	☐	☐
9. Attaches flowmeter to gas outlet	☐	☐	☐	☐
10. Attaches humidification device to flowmeter	☐	☐	☐	☐
11. Attaches O_2 connecting tubing and O_2 administration device to humidifier	☐	☐	☐	☐
12. Turns gas source on	☐	☐	☐	☐
13. Checks pressure relief valve	☐	☐	☐	☐
14. Verifies proper function of device	☐	☐	☐	☐
15. If using cascade or wick humidifier:				
a. Assembles unit properly on ventilator	☐	☐	☐	☐
b. Fills humidifier to appropriate level	☐	☐	☐	☐
c. Ensures proper function of continuous feed system if used	☐	☐	☐	☐
d. Verifies proper function of device	☐	☐	☐	☐
Follow-up				
16. Maintains/processes equipment	☐	☐	☐	☐
17. Disposes of infectious waste and washes hands	☐	☐	☐	☐
18. Records pertinent data in chart and departmental records	☐	☐	☐	☐
19. Notifies appropriate personnel and makes any necessary recommendations or modifications to the patient care plan	☐	☐	☐	☐

_____   _____
Signature of Evaluator   Signature of Student

PERFORMANCE RATING SCALE

5 EXCELLENT—FAR EXCEEDS EXPECTED LEVEL, FLAWLESS PERFORMANCE
4 ABOVE AVERAGE—NO PROMPTING REQUIRED, ABLE TO SELF-CORRECT
3 AVERAGE—THE MINIMUM COMPETENCY LEVEL, NO CRITICAL ERRORS
2 IMPROVEMENT NEEDED—PROBLEM AREAS EXIST; CRITICAL ERRORS, CORRECTIONS NEEDED
1 POOR AND UNACCEPTABLE PERFORMANCE—GROSS INACCURACIES, POTENTIALLY HARMFUL

PERFORMANCE CRITERIA	SCALE				
1. DISPLAYS KNOWLEDGE OF ESSENTIAL CONCEPTS	5	4	3	2	1
2. DEMONSTRATES THE RELATIONSHIP BETWEEN THEORY AND CLINICAL PRACTICE	5	4	3	2	1
3. FOLLOWS DIRECTIONS, EXHIBITS SOUND JUDGMENT, AND DEMONSTRATES ATTENTION TO SAFETY AND DETAIL	5	4	3	2	1
4. EXHIBITS THE REQUIRED MANUAL DEXTERITY	5	4	3	2	1
5. PERFORMS PROCEDURE IN A REASONABLE TIME FRAME	5	4	3	2	1
6. MAINTAINS STERILE OR ASEPTIC TECHNIQUE	5	4	3	2	1
7. INITIATES UNAMBIGUOUS GOAL-DIRECTED COMMUNICATION	5	4	3	2	1
8. PROVIDES FOR ADEQUATE CARE AND MAINTENANCE OF EQUIPMENT AND SUPPLIES	5	4	3	2	1
9. EXHIBITS COURTEOUS AND PLEASANT DEMEANOR	5	4	3	2	1
10. MAINTAINS CONCISE AND ACCURATE RECORDS	5	4	3	2	1

ADDITIONAL COMMENTS: INCLUDE ERRORS OF OMISSION OR COMMISSION, COMMUNICATIVE SKILLS, AND EFFECTIVENESS OF PATIENT INTERACTION:

SUMMARY PERFORMANCE EVALUATION AND RECOMMENDATIONS

SATISFACTORY PERFORMANCE—Performed without error or prompting, or able to self-correct, no critical errors.

———— LABORATORY EVALUATION. SKILLS MAY BE APPLIED/OBSERVED IN THE CLINICAL SETTING.

———— CLINICAL EVALUATION. STUDENT READY FOR MINIMALLY SUPERVISED APPLICATION AND REFINEMENT.

UNSATISFACTORY PERFORMANCE—Prompting required; performed with critical errors, potentially harmful.

———— STUDENT REQUIRES ADDITIONAL LABORATORY PRACTICE.

———— STUDENT REQUIRES ADDITIONAL SUPERVISED CLINICAL PRACTICE.

SIGNATURES

STUDENT: _____   EVALUATOR: _____

DATE: _____   DATE: _____

CHAPTER 8	# Aerosol Generators

INTRODUCTION

An **aerosol** is defined as a suspension of solid or liquid particles in a gas. Aerosols may be administered to deliver medication or to deliver a **bland solution** for the purpose of sputum induction, treatment of upper airway edema, or humidification of a bypassed or compromised upper airway.[1]

There are many devices used by the respiratory care practitioner to generate aerosols for application to the upper or lower airway. These devices include small volume nebulizers (SVNs), large volume nebulizers (LVNs), metered dose inhalers (MDIs) and auxiliary spacing devices, dry powder inhalers (DPIs), hydrodynamic (Babington) nebulizers, and ultrasonic nebulizers (USNs).

The selection and utilization of the most appropriate device is based on the specific clinical application and the desired therapeutic goals. The respiratory care practitioner should consider several factors in this selection, including the intended target area of the respiratory tract to be treated; the proven efficacy of the technique being used; patient preference, coordination, and cooperation; availability of medications; convenience; and patient tolerance.[2] Before one can apply these devices in the clinical setting, the operating principles, advantages, and limitations of each device must be understood.

This chapter focuses on aerosol delivery devices used for continuous aerosol therapy. Chapter 9 emphasizes medication delivery devices and techniques.

OBJECTIVES

Upon completion of this chapter, the student will be able to:

1. Differentiate between the types of aerosol generators by operating principle.
2. Given a specific clinical situation, select and apply the appropriate aerosol delivery device.
3. Discuss the limitations of each type of aerosol delivery device.
4. List the hazards and complications associated with aerosol delivery.
5. Practice communication skills needed to explain the application of an aerosol device to a patient and confirm patient understanding.
6. Practice medical charting for the therapeutic application of an aerosol delivery device.
7. Apply infection control guidelines and standards associated with aerosol delivery equipment and procedures, according to OSHA regulations and CDC guidelines.

KEY TERMS

aerosol	density	nebulizer	solution
amplitude	deposition	particulate	solvent
atomizer	expectoration	penetration	tandem
baffle	hypertonic	piezoelectric	titrate
bland	hypotonic	pneumatic	tonicity
couplant	impaction	prophylactic	
	isotonic	solute	

EQUIPMENT REQUIRED

- Large volume **nebulizer**
- Heating elements
- Temperature probes and in-line adaptors
- Ultrasonic nebulizer
- Hydrodynamic nebulizer
- Small particle aerosol generator (SPAG) II
- Face tents
- Aerosol masks
- Tracheostomy collars
- Briggs adaptors (T-pieces)
- Corrugated tubing
- Sterile water
- Scissors
- Compressed gas sources (oxygen and air)
- Flowmeters
- Nipple adaptors
- Oxygen analyzer and in-line adaptor
- Water traps
- Normal saline vials (3 ml)
- Y-connectors
- Oxygen supply tubing
- Intubated and tracheostomized airway management trainer
- Stethoscope
- Watch with second hand

● EXERCISES

EXERCISE 8.1 Large Volume Nebulizer

1. Examine a large volume nebulizer and identify the components shown in Figure 8.1.
   - DISS connection
   - Air entrainment ports
   - F_1O_2 adjustment (entrainment selector)
   - Jet
   - **Baffle** (not shown)
   - Capillary tube
   - Pressure pop-off (not shown)
   - Filter
   - Outlet

2. Assemble the nebulizer according to the manufacturer's instructions.

3. Aseptically fill the nebulizer with sterile water. If a prefilled nebulizer is used, be sure not to contaminate the internal surfaces.

4. Attach the heating element and adjust the settings, if possible, to achieve 37°C.

5. Attach the nebulizer to the DISS outlet of a flowmeter.

6. Adjust the F_1O_2 by turning the entrainment selector to the 100 percent setting.

7. Turn the flow to 8 lpm and observe the mist density and output, the total flow, and the size of the entrainment port.

8. Set the entrainment selector to 35 percent oxygen. Note any changes in the mist density and output, the total flow,

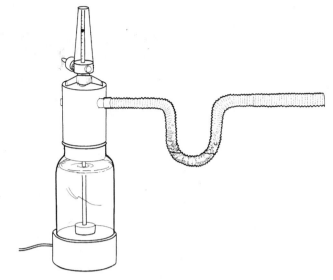

FIGURE 8.2   Water in the corrugated tubing.

and the size of the entrainment port. *Record your observations on your laboratory report.*

9. Set the entrainment selector in between any two oxygen settings.

10. Attach 10 lengths of corrugated tubing.

11. Place temperature probe adaptor one tubing length from the patient interface. Insert the temperature probe.

12. Place another temperature probe adaptor about halfway between the nebulizer and the patient interface. Insert the temperature probe.

13. *Record the beginning temperature on both probes. Note the time.*

14. Measure the time it takes for the temperature to reach 37°C on each probe. *Record the times and final temperatures on your laboratory report.*

15. Analyze the F_1O_2 and *record it on your laboratory report.*

16. Adjust the F_1O_2 by turning the entrainment selector to 0.40. Analyze the F_1O_2 and readjust the entrainment

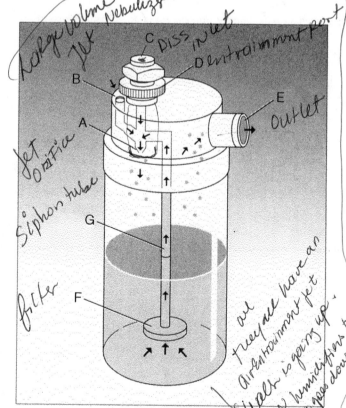

FIGURE 8.1   Components of a large volume nebulizer. (From Persing, G: Entry-Level Respiratory Care Review, ed 2. WB Saunders, Philadelphia, 1996, p. 41, with permission.)

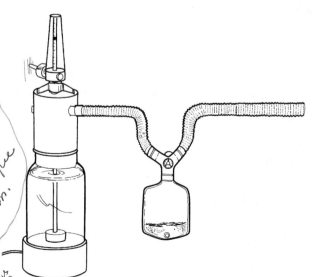

FIGURE 8.3   Insertion of a water trap in a nebulizer setup.

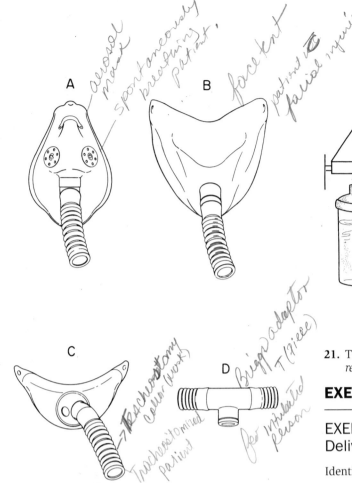

[handwritten annotations: aerosol mask / spontaneously breathing patient; face tent / patient with facial injuries; Tracheostomy collar (mask) / Tracheostomized patient; Briggs adaptor / T (piece) / for intubated person]

FIGURE 8.4 Aerosol delivery devices. (From Kacmarek, RM: Methods of oxygen delivery in the hospital. Problems in Respiratory Care, 3:564–574, 1990, with permission.)

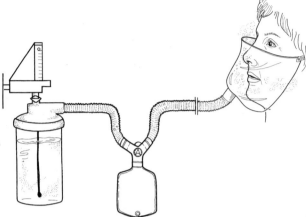

FIGURE 8.6 Aerosol setup with a face tent.

selector if necessary to ensure that the nebulizer is delivering 40 percent oxygen.

17. Put water in the corrugated tubing so that the lumen of the tube is occluded in the loop, or "belly," of the tubing, as shown in Figure 8.2.

18. Analyze the F_IO_2 and *record it on your laboratory report.*

19. Drain the water from the tubing by "milking" the tubing away from the device and into a waste receptacle.

20. Attach a water trap by cutting the corrugated tubing in the belly of the tubing and attaching the trap to the ends of the tubing, as shown in Figure 8.3.

21. Turn the liter flow to 5 lpm. Observe the mist output and *record your observations on your laboratory report.*

EXERCISE 8.2 Aerosol Delivery Devices

EXERCISE 8.2.1 Identification of Aerosol Delivery Devices

Identify the following devices shown in Figure 8.4:

Face tent
Aerosol mask
Tracheostomy collar (mask)
Briggs adaptor (T-piece)

EXERCISE 8.2.2 Application of an Aerosol Generating Device

For these exercises, the students are divided into groups of two. The students may do all the exercises with the same partner, or the instructor might want to change the pairs to enhance the ability of each student to communicate and explain the procedure to a different person. Using your laboratory partner as a patient, set up and deliver a heated aerosol at an F_IO_2 of 0.40 (unless otherwise specified by your instructor) for each of the following scenarios: a spontaneously breathing patient (Fig. 8.5); a spontaneously breathing patient with facial injuries; (Fig. 8.6); a tracheostomized patient (Fig. 8.7); and an intubated patient (Fig. 8.8).

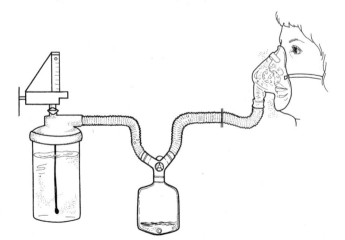

FIGURE 8.5 Aerosol setup with a face mask.

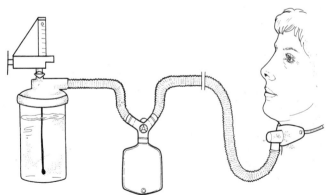

FIGURE 8.7 Aerosol setup with a tracheostomy collar.

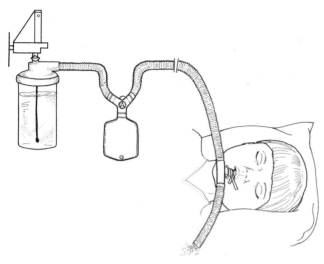

FIGURE 8.8   Aerosol setup with a Briggs adaptor.

1. Check the chart
   a. To verify the physician's order or protocol for mode of delivery and F_IO_2.
   b. For the patient's diagnosis.
2. Gather the necessary equipment:
   a. Large volume nebulizer
   b. Corrugated tubing
   c. Sterile water
   d. Heating element
   e. Temperature probe and in-line adaptor
   f. Oxygen flowmeter and gas source
   g. Water trap
   h. Scissors
   i. Appropriate aerosol delivery device (mask, T-piece, tracheostomy collar, or face tent)
3. Wash your hands. Apply standard precautions and transmission-based isolation procedures as appropriate.

4. Introduce yourself and your department. Verify the patient's identification. Explain the procedure to the patient and confirm patient understanding.
5. Assemble the equipment.
6. Adjust the gas source to the appropriate flow rate for adequate flow to meet the patient's inspiratory demand. In most cases this is between 8 and 12 lpm. For oxygen concentrations of 60 percent or above, a tandem or double setup may be needed. This is demonstrated in Exercise 8.7.
7. Attach the delivery device to the patient. Ensure patient comfort.
8. Analyze the F_IO_2 and adjust the entrainment selector if necessary.
9. Document the procedure appropriately. *"Chart" your therapy on your laboratory report.*

EXERCISE 8.3 Ultrasonic Nebulizer (USN)

1. Identify the components of the ultrasonic nebulizer shown in Figure 8.9. *Record them on your laboratory report.*
   Continuous feed inlet
   Couplant chamber
   Diaphragm
   Amplitude adjustor
   On/off switch

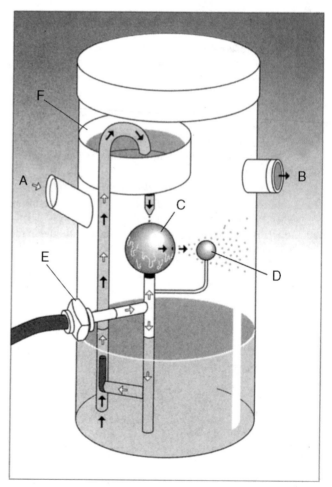

FIGURE 8.10   Components of a hydrodynamic (Babington) nebulizer. (From Persing, G: Entry-Level Respiratory Care Review, ed 2. WB Saunders, Philadelphia, 1996, p. 41, with permission.)

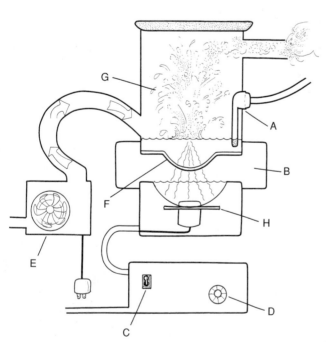

FIGURE 8.9   Components of an ultrasonic nebulizer.

Blower
Medication chamber
Piezoelectric element

2. Fill the **couplant** chamber with tap water.

3. Aseptically fill the medication chamber with 50 ml of sterile water.

4. Plug the unit into an electrical outlet.

5. Turn the unit on with the amplitude at its lowest setting.

6. Note the time, and gradually turn the amplitude to the maximum setting. *Record your observations on your laboratory report.*

7. Record the time required for the unit to go dry, and *record it on your laboratory report.* Refill the medication chamber.

8. Insert an in-line adaptor to **titrate** oxygen into the gas flow. Attach one end of a small-bore oxygen tube to the adaptor and the other end to a flowmeter. Adjust the flow to obtain an F_IO_2 of 0.30.

9. Drain the tap water from the couplant chamber. *Record your observations of USN function on your laboratory report.* Fill it with sterile distilled water. Reassemble the USN and turn it on. *Record your observations of USN function on your laboratory report.*

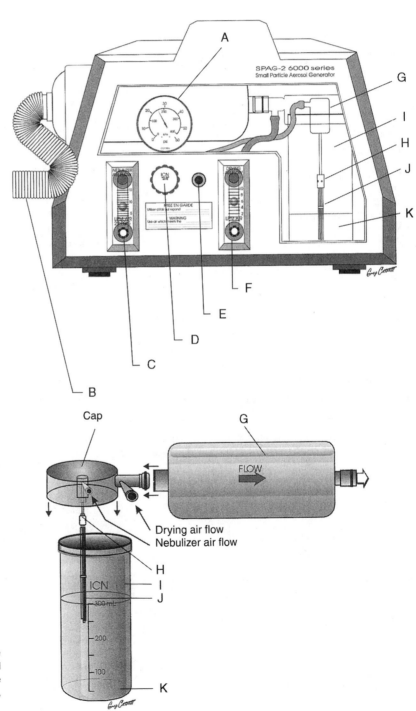

FIGURE 8.11 Components of a small particle aerosol generator (SPAG). (From Cottrel, G and Surkin, H: Pharmacology for Respiratory Care Practitioners. FA Davis, Philadelphia, 1995, p. 25, with permission.)

EXERCISE 8.4 Hydrodynamic Nebulizer

1. Identify the components of the hydrodynamic, or Babington, nebulizer shown in Figure 8.10. *Record them on your laboratory report.*
   DISS connection
   Outlet
   Entrainment port
   Baffle
   Sphere
   Reservoir

2. Assemble the unit and attach it to a flowmeter.

3. Aseptically fill the unit with sterile water.

4. Turn the flowmeter to 8 lpm.

5. Increase the flow rate to 15 lpm. *Record your observations on your laboratory report.*

EXERCISE 8.5 Small Particle Aerosol Generator

1. Identify the components of the small particle aerosol generator shown in Figure 8.11. *Record them on your laboratory report.*
   Drying chamber
   Capillary tube
   Nebulizer flowmeter
   Drying chamber flowmeter
   Medication reservoir
   Aerosol delivery tubing
   Manometer
   Pressure regulator control
   Source gas connection
   Nebulizer jet
   Medication solution

2. Assemble the unit.

3. Connect the drying gas and nebulizer gas to compressed gas sources.

4. Instill 15 mL of normal saline into the medication reservoir.

5. Turn the flowmeters to 7 lpm. *Record your observations on your laboratory report.*

EXERCISE 8.6 Gas Titration

1. Assemble the gas titration system as shown in Figure 8.12 with the nebulizer attached to a compressed gas source.

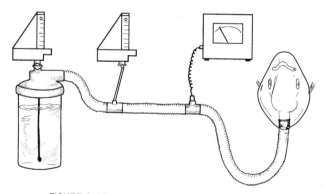

FIGURE 8.12   Setup for titrating to a specific F_IO_2.

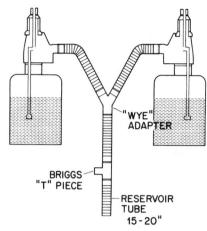

FIGURE 8.13   Tandem nebulizer setup. (From Kacmarek, RM: Methods of oxygen delivery in the hospital. Problems in Respiratory Care, 3:564–574, 1990, with permission.)

2. Turn the flow to 10 lpm.

3. Adjust the oxygen flowmeter to achieve the following values of F_IO_2:
   a. 0.24
   b. 0.30
   c. 0.45

4. *Record your observations and liter flows required on your laboratory report.*

EXERCISE 8.7 Tandem Nebulizer Setup

1. Assemble two large volume nebulizers in **tandem,** as shown in Figure 8.13.

2. Set the flowmeters on each device to 10 lpm.

3. Set the entrainment selector on each nebulizer to the following: 0.50, 0.60, and 0.80. Observe the mist **density** and output and the total flow. *Record your observations for each setting on your laboratory report.*

References

1. American Association for Respiratory Care: AARC clinical practice guideline: Delivery of aerosols to the upper airway. Respir Care 39:803–807, 1992.
2. American Association for Respiratory Care: AARC clinical practice for guideline: Selection of an aerosol delivery device. Respir Care 37:891–897, 1992.

Related Readings

Eubanks, DH and Bone, RC: Principles and Applications of Cardiorespiratory Care Equipment. Mosby, St Louis, 1994.
McPherson, S: Respiratory Care Equipment, ed 5. Mosby, St Louis, 1995.
Scanlan, C et al (eds): Egan's Fundamentals of Respiratory Care, ed 6. Mosby, St Louis, 1995.

Selected Journal Articles

American Association for Respiratory Care: Aerosol consensus statement. Respir Care 36:916–921, 1991.
American Association for Respiratory Care: AARC clinical practice guideline: Selection of an aerosol delivery device. Respir Care 37:891–897, 1992.

American Association for Respiratory Care: AARC clinical practice guideline: Delivery of aerosols to the upper airway. Respir Care 39:803–807, 1994.

American Association for Respiratory Care: AARC clinical practice guideline: Bland aerosol administration. Respir Care 38:1196–1200, 1993.

Bunch, D and Cathcart, M: NIOSH proposes personal safety guidelines for practitioners potentially exposed to tuberculosis. AARC Times 17:52–56, 1993.

Centers for Disease Control and Prevention: Guidelines for preventing the transmission of *Mycobacterium tuberculosis* in health-care facilities, 1994. US Department of Health and Human Services, Atlanta, 43:RR-13, pp 33–34.

Dolovich, M: Physical principles underlying aerosol therapy. J Aerosol Med 2:171–186, 1989.

Kraft-Jacobs, B et al: Aerosolized ribavirin in mechanically ventilated children with respiratory syncytial virus lower respiratory tract disease. Crit Care Med 22:566–572, 1994.

Newman, SP: Aerosol generators and delivery systems. Respir Care 36:939–951, 1991.

Nobel, JJ: Ultrasonic nebulizers. Pediatr Emerg Care 10:251–252, 1994.

Phillips, GD and Millard, FJ: The therapeutic use of ultrasonic nebulizers in acute asthma. Respir Med 88:387–390, 1994.

Waldrep, JC et al: Operating characteristics of 18 different continuous flow jet nebulizers with beclomethasone dipropionate-liposome aerosol. Chest 105:106–110, 1994.

Woo, A, Goetz, A and Yu, V: Transmission of *Legionella* by respiratory equipment and aerosol generating devices. Chest 102:1586–1590, 1992.

LABORATORY REPORT

CHAPTER 8: AEROSOL GENERATORS

Name _____   Date _____

Course/Section _____   Instructor _____

Data Collection

EXERCISE 8.1   Large Volume Nebulizer
Components

A. _____

B. _____

C. _____

D. _____

E. _____

F. _____

G. _____

Observations

Type and brand of nebulizer used: _____

_____

Mist density at 100%: _____

Mist density at 35%: _____

Total flow at 100%: _____

Total flow at 35%: _____

Entrainment port at 100%: _____

Entrainment port at 35%: _____

F_IO_2 set in between _____ and _____

Analyzed at _____

Heating element setting: _____
INITIAL TEMPERATURES

Probe nearest humidifier: _____

Probe nearest patient interface: _____
TIME TO ACHIEVE 37°C

Probe nearest humidifier: _____

Probe nearest patient interface: _____
FINAL TEMPERATURES

Probe nearest humidifier: _____

Probe nearest patient interface: _____

Water in the tubing—F_IO_2 analyzed at _____

5 lpm flow: _____

EXERCISE 8.2   Aerosol Delivery Devices

EXERCISE 8.2.1   Identification of Aerosol Delivery Devices

A. _____

B. _____

C. _____

D. _____

EXERCISE 8.2.2   Application of an Aerosol Generating Device

Chart the procedures for each of the following scenarios:

1. Spontaneously breathing patient

_____

_____

_____

2. Spontaneously breathing patient with facial injuries

_____

_____

_____

3. Intubated patient

_____

_____

_____

4. Tracheostomized patient

_____

_____

_____

EXERCISE 8.3   Ultrasonic Nebulizer

Components

A. _____

B. _____

C. _____

D. _____

E. _____

F. _____

G. _____

H. _____

Observations: Amplitude at Maximum

_____

_____

_____

Time until unit is dry: _____

Liter flow to achieve F_1O_2 of 0.30: _____

Observations: Drained Couplant Chamber

_____

_____

_____

Observations: Couplant Filled with Sterile Water

_____

_____

_____

EXERCISE 8.4 **Hydrodynamic Nebulizer**
Components

A. _____

B. _____

C. _____

D. _____

E. _____

F. _____

Observations

_____

_____

_____

_____

_____

_____

EXERCISE 8.5 **Small Particle Aerosol Generator**
Components

A. _____

B. _____

C. _____

D. _____

E. _____

F. _____

G. _____

H. _____

I. _____

J. _____

K. _____

Observations

_____

_____

_____

_____

_____

EXERCISE 8.6   Gas Titration
Observations

_____

_____

_____

Liter flow required to achieve

1. 0.24: _____

2. 0.30: _____

3. 0.45: _____

EXERCISE 8.7   Tandem Nebulizer Setup
Observations of mist density and total flow:

F_IO_2 0.50: _____

F_IO_2 0.60: _____

F_IO_2 0.80: _____

CRITICAL THINKING QUESTIONS

1. What was the effect on the F_IO_2 of water in the corrugated tubing? Why?

2. What effect did increasing the amplitude of the USN have on the density of the aerosol? What determines the particle size of the USN?

3. The physician orders an ultrasonic treatment to be given to a patient who requires nasal oxygen at 5 lpm. How would you adapt the equipment?

4. What is the purpose of the drying chamber in the SPAG? What medication is delivered via the SPAG?

5. Under what circumstances would it be necessary to set up tandem nebulizers?

PROCEDURAL COMPETENCY EVALUATION

Name _____   Date _____

Aerosol Generators

Setting: ☐ Lab ☐ Clinical   Evaluator: ☐ Peer ☐ Instructor

Conditions (describe): _____

_____

Equipment Used

_____

_____

	SATISFACTORY	UNSATISFACTORY	NOT OBSERVED	NOT APPLICABLE
Equipment and Patient Preparation				
1. Verifies, interprets, and evaluates physician's order or protocol for mode of delivery and F_IO_2	☐	☐	☐	☐
2. Scans chart for diagnosis and any other pertinent data and notes	☐	☐	☐	☐
3. Selects, gathers, and assembles the necessary equipment	☐	☐	☐	☐
4. Washes hands and applies standard precautions and transmission-based isolation procedures as appropriate	☐	☐	☐	☐
5. Identifies patient, introduces self and department	☐	☐	☐	☐
6. Explains purpose of the procedure and confirms patient understanding	☐	☐	☐	☐
7. Selects appropriate aerosol generator and delivery device to achieve therapeutic objectives	☐	☐	☐	☐
Assessment and Implementation				
8. Assembles equipment and verifies function	☐	☐	☐	☐
9. Assesses patient for vital signs, chest palpation, percussion and auscultation, secretions, airway patency, and humidity deficit	☐	☐	☐	☐
10. Adjusts gas source or mist density to the appropriate flow rate for adequate flow to meet the patient's inspiratory demand; for oxygen concentrations 60% or greater, uses a tandem or double nebulizer setup	☐	☐	☐	☐
11. Attaches the delivery device to the patient and ensures patient comfort	☐	☐	☐	☐
12. Analyzes the F_IO_2 and adjusts the entrainment selector or mist density if applicable	☐	☐	☐	☐
Follow-up				
13. Reassesses the patient after application of the aerosol device	☐	☐	☐	☐
14. Collects sputum, labels specimen containers, and sends to lab if indicated	☐	☐	☐	☐
15. Maintains/processes equipment	☐	☐	☐	☐
16. Disposes of infectious waste and washes hands	☐	☐	☐	☐
17. Records pertinent data in chart and departmental records	☐	☐	☐	☐
18. Notifies appropriate personnel and makes any necessary recommendations or modifications to the patient care plan	☐	☐	☐	☐

_____   _____
Signature of Evaluator   Signature of Student

PERFORMANCE RATING SCALE

5 EXCELLENT—FAR EXCEEDS EXPECTED LEVEL, FLAWLESS PERFORMANCE
4 ABOVE AVERAGE—NO PROMPTING REQUIRED, ABLE TO SELF-CORRECT
3 AVERAGE—THE MINIMUM COMPETENCY LEVEL, NO CRITICAL ERRORS
2 IMPROVEMENT NEEDED—PROBLEM AREAS EXIST; CRITICAL ERRORS, CORRECTIONS NEEDED
1 POOR AND UNACCEPTABLE PERFORMANCE—GROSS INACCURACIES, POTENTIALLY HARMFUL

PERFORMANCE CRITERIA	SCALE				
1. DISPLAYS KNOWLEDGE OF ESSENTIAL CONCEPTS	5	4	3	2	1
2. DEMONSTRATES THE RELATIONSHIP BETWEEN THEORY AND CLINICAL PRACTICE	5	4	3	2	1
3. FOLLOWS DIRECTIONS, EXHIBITS SOUND JUDGMENT, AND DEMONSTRATES ATTENTION TO SAFETY AND DETAIL	5	4	3	2	1
4. EXHIBITS THE REQUIRED MANUAL DEXTERITY	5	4	3	2	1
5. PERFORMS PROCEDURE IN A REASONABLE TIME FRAME	5	4	3	2	1
6. MAINTAINS STERILE OR ASEPTIC TECHNIQUE	5	4	3	2	1
7. INITIATES UNAMBIGUOUS GOAL-DIRECTED COMMUNICATION	5	4	3	2	1
8. PROVIDES FOR ADEQUATE CARE AND MAINTENANCE OF EQUIPMENT AND SUPPLIES	5	4	3	2	1
9. EXHIBITS COURTEOUS AND PLEASANT DEMEANOR	5	4	3	2	1
10. MAINTAINS CONCISE AND ACCURATE RECORDS	5	4	3	2	1

ADDITIONAL COMMENTS: INCLUDE ERRORS OF OMISSION OR COMMISSION, COMMUNICATIVE SKILLS, AND EFFECTIVENESS OF PATIENT INTERACTION:

SUMMARY PERFORMANCE EVALUATION AND RECOMMENDATIONS

SATISFACTORY PERFORMANCE—Performed without error or prompting, or able to self-correct, no critical errors.

_____ LABORATORY EVALUATION. SKILLS MAY BE APPLIED/OBSERVED IN THE CLINICAL SETTING.

_____ CLINICAL EVALUATION. STUDENT READY FOR MINIMALLY SUPERVISED APPLICATION AND REFINEMENT.

UNSATISFACTORY PERFORMANCE—Prompting required; performed with critical errors, potentially harmful.

_____ STUDENT REQUIRES ADDITIONAL LABORATORY PRACTICE.

_____ STUDENT REQUIRES ADDITIONAL SUPERVISED CLINICAL PRACTICE.

SIGNATURES

STUDENT: _____   EVALUATOR: _____

DATE: _____   DATE: _____

CHAPTER 9

Aerosol Therapy and Medication Administration

INTRODUCTION

A primary responsibility of the respiratory care practitioner is the delivery of pharmacological agents to the upper and lower airways for a variety of indications, including **bronchodilation,** sputum **induction,** mobilization of secretions, and delivery of anti-inflammatory and anti-infective agents. These medications can be delivered using several different devices, such as dry powder inhalers, metered dose inhalers, small volume nebulizers, continuous nebulizers, and ultrasonic nebulizing devices (see Chapter 8). Techniques for delivery of aerosol medications include short-term intermittent treatments and long-term or continuous nebulization. To effectively deliver medications, the practitioner must be able to recommend and select the appropriate medication and delivery device (Table 9.10), and then mix and prepare the medications. In addition, monitoring and evaluation of therapeutic effectiveness and adverse reactions must be performed and appropriately documented with each procedure.

The practitioner should always be cognizant of potential limitations to these procedures caused by such factors (Fig. 9.11) as device design, use of accessory devices, use of artificial airways, mechanical ventilation, condition or irritation of the airways, medication dosage, inadequate instruction or technique, and patient compliance.

The student is expected to be able to calculate drug dosages as a prerequisite to the exercises in this chapter.

OBJECTIVES

Upon completion of this chapter, the student will be able to:

1. Practice calculation of drug dosages.

2. Select and use various aerosol delivery devices and adjunctive equipment given specific clinical situations.

3. Discuss the indications, advantages, disadvantages, limitations, contraindications, and hazards of each type of aerosol delivery device and method used for medication delivery.

4. Perform patient assessment, and monitor and evaluate patient response to aerosolized medication administration.

5. Obtain a sputum specimen for analysis using sputum induction techniques.

6. Chart an aerosol medication treatment.

7. Practice communication skills needed for the administration of an aerosol medication treatment.

8. Apply infection control guidelines and standards associated with equipment and procedures used for aerosol medication delivery, according to OSHA regulations and CDC guidelines.

KEY TERMS

actuator	antihistamine	decongestant	hypoglycemia
additive	antitussive	diffusion	induction
adrenergic	atopic	diuretic	inotropic
affinity	auxiliary	drugs	interaction
agonist	beta-agonist	dyskinesia	ionization
analgesia	bronchoactive	efficacy	lavage
anaphylaxis	bronchoconstriction	emesis	leukotriene
anesthesia	bronchodilation	enzyme	metabolism
antagonist	catecholamines	excretion	metabolite
anticholinergic	cholinergic	fasciculation	mucokinetic
anticholinesterase	chronotropic	flaccid	mucolytic
	cumulation	hormone	muscarinic

nicotonic	pharmacology	sedation	tachyphylaxis
osteoporosis	pharmacokinetics	solubility	tolerance
parasympatholytic	potency	spacer	topical
parasympathomimetic	potentiation	surfactant	toxicology
parenteral	prophylactic	sympatholytic	vascular
pharmaceutical	protein binding	sympathomimetic	vasoconstriction
pharmacodynamics	racemic	synergism	vasodilation
pharmacognosy	receptor	systemic	

EQUIPMENT REQUIRED

- Dry powder inhaler
- Metered dose inhalers, placebo and sample medications
- **Auxiliary** spacing devices **(spacers)**
- In-line MDI adaptors for ventilator circuits
- Unit-dose **sympathomimetic** bronchodilators, variety
- Unit-dose **parasympatholytic** bronchodilator (Atrovent)
- Multidose vials, sympathomimetic bronchodilators, variety
- Multidose vials, Mucomyst (acetylcysteine)
- Unit-dose normal saline solutions
- Multidose normal saline solution
- Sterile water
- Three-percent hypertonic saline solution (optional)
- Small volume nebulizers, mouthpieces
- Oxygen connecting tubing
- Large-bore aerosol tubing
- Cadema Aero-Tech or Respirgard II nebulizers
- Small particle aerosol generator II nebulizer
- Heart nebulizer for continuous medication delivery
- Scissors
- Compressed gas source, air or oxygen
- Oxygen nipple adaptors
- Ultrasonic nebulizer
- Aerosol masks
- Tracheostomy collars
- T-piece or Briggs adaptor
- Watch with second hand
- Peak flowmeters with disposable mouthpieces
- Stethoscopes
- Sputum specimen cup
- Tissues
- Intubated and trached airway training mannequin

⬤ EXERCISES

EXERCISE 9.1 Review Calculation of Drug Dosages

To calculate percent solutions and dosages, the following formula is most often used:

$$\frac{\text{Original amount, mg}}{\text{Original amount, ml}} = \frac{\text{Desired amount, mg}}{\text{Desired amount, ml}}$$

TABLE 9.1 Frequently Used Pharmacology Conversion Factors

2.2 lb/kg body weight
1000 µg/1 mg
1000 mg/1 g
1000 ml/1 L
5 ml = 1 tsp
1:00 solution = 1% = 10 mg/ml

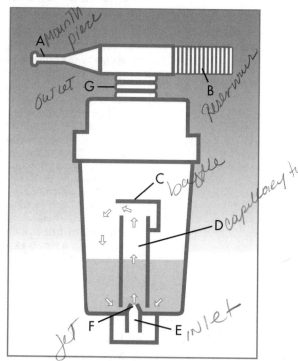

FIGURE 9.1 Components of a small volume nebulizer. (Adapted from Persing, G: Entry-Level Respiratory Care Review, ed 2. WB Saunders, Philadelphia, 1996, p. 42, with permission.)

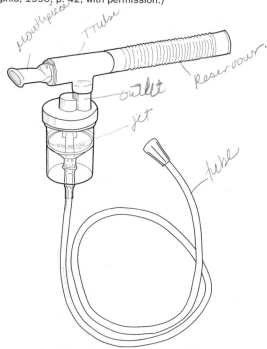

FIGURE 9.2 Assembly of a small volume nebulizer.

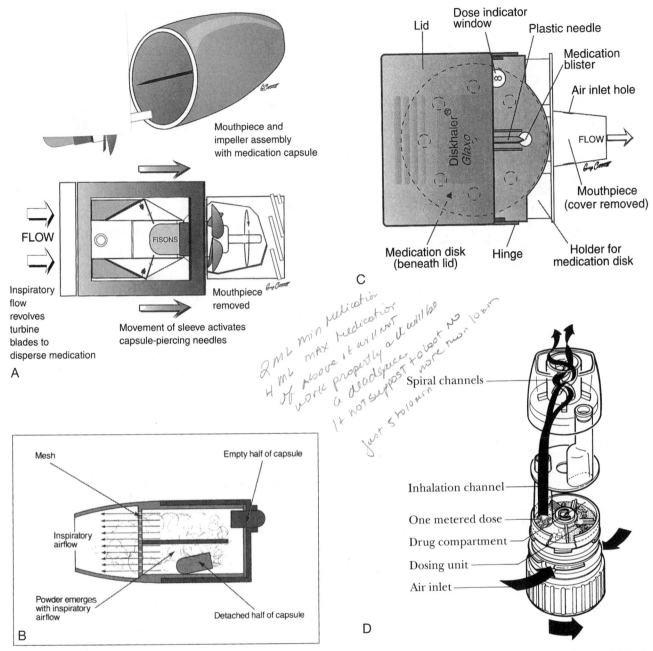

FIGURE 9.3 Components of a dry powder inhaler. (From Cottrel, G and Surkin, H: Pharmacology for Respiratory Care Practitioners. FA Davis, Philadelphia, 1995, pp. 22–23, with permission.)

Table 9.1 identifies frequently used conversion factors required for **pharmacology** calculations.

Calculate the following dosages of commonly used respiratory care medications:

1. A physician orders a 5-ml/kg dose of Exosurf surfactant replacement therapy for a 4.4-lb neonate. You are to administer it one-half dosage at a time. How many milliliters would be required for the initial application? *Show your work and answer on your laboratory report.*

2. A standard dose of 0.3 ml of a 5-percent solution of metaproterenol is given. How many milligrams are being administered? *Show your work and answer on your laboratory report.*

3. A 2.5-mg dose of a 0.5-percent solution of albuterol sulfate is being administered four times daily from a 20-ml multi-dose vial. How many patients could be treated in one day at this dose from this vial? *Show your work and answer on your laboratory report.*

4. Three hundred milligrams of pentamidine are mixed in 6 ml of sterile water. What is the percent solution being administered? How much would need to be administered if a 60-mg dose was ordered? *Show your work and answer on your laboratory report.*

5. Five milliliters of 20-percent Mucomyst are ordered. How many milligrams are being administered? *Show your work and answer on your laboratory report.*

6. Atrovent unit-dose solution comes in a 0.02-percent solution. If the active ingredient is 500 µg, what is the equivalent amount of active ingredient in milliliters? *Show your work and answer on your laboratory report.*

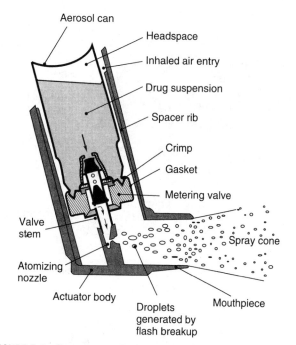

FIGURE 9.4 Components of a metered dose inhaler. (From Witek, TJ Jr and Schachter, EN: Pharmacology and Therapeutics in Respiratory Care. WB Saunders, Philadelphia, 1994, p. 40, with permission.)

7. The unit-dose Atrovent has been back ordered. What drug could you recommend to the physician to substitute for the Atrovent? If this drug came in a 0.4-mg/ml solution and the physician ordered a 1-mg dose, how many milliliters would need to be drawn up to nebulize this dose? *Show your work and answers on your laboratory report.*

8. Alpha dornase (Pulmozyme) has been ordered for a patient with cystic fibrosis. A single 2.5-ml ampule contains a 2.5-mg dose. What is the percent solution of this medication? *Show your work and answer on your laboratory report.*

EXERCISE 9.2 Small Volume Nebulizers

EXERCISE 9.2.1 Identification of Component Parts

Examine the small volume nebulizer and identify the components shown in Figure 9.1.

Capillary tube
Baffle
Jet
Gas source inlet
Outlet
Reservoir tubing
Mouthpiece

EXERCISE 9.2.2 Operation of a Small Volume Nebulizer

1. Assemble a small volume nebulizer as shown in Figure 9.2.

2. Attach the connecting tubing of the nebulizer to the nipple adaptor of a flowmeter or compressor outlet.

3. Aseptically instill 1 ml of normal saline into the medication cup. Do not allow the tip of the saline vial to touch any inside surface of the nebulizer.

4. Turn the flow to 6 lpm. *Record your observations regarding mist density on your laboratory report.*

5. Now instill an additional 2 ml of saline into the medication cup. *Record your observations regarding mist density on your laboratory report.*

6. Turn the flow to 10 lpm. *Record your observations on your laboratory report.*

7. Turn the flow down to 2 lpm. *Record your observations regarding mist density on your laboratory report.*

8. Add an additional 3 ml to the nebulizer and turn the flow to 6 lpm. *Record your observations regarding mist density on your laboratory report.*

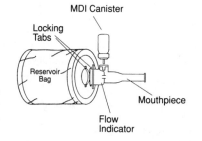

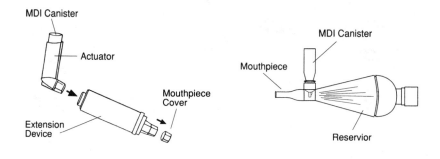

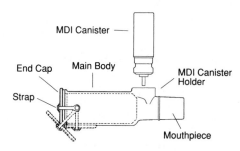

FIGURE 9.5 Auxiliary spacing devices. (From Rau, JL Jr: Respiratory Care Pharmacology, ed 4. Mosby-Year Book, St. Louis, 1994, p. 53, with permission.)

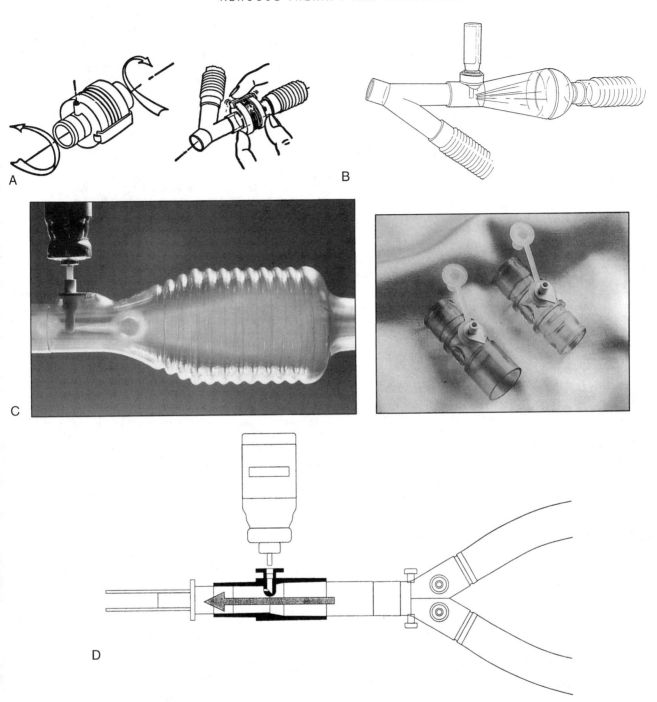

FIGURE 9.6   In-line adaptors for aerosol delivery to ventilator circuits. (Courtesy of *[A]* Monaghan Medical Corporation, Syracuse, NY; *[B]* Diemolding Corp., Diemolding Healthcare Division, Canastota, NY; *[C]* Baxter Health Care, Roundlake, IL; *[D]* Instrumentation Industries, Inc., Bethel Park, PA.)

EXERCISE 9.3 Identification of Component Parts of Additional Delivery Devices

1. Examine the rotohaler and spinhaler dry powder inhalers, and identify the component parts shown in Figure 9.3.
2. Examine a metered dose inhaler, and identify the component parts shown in Figure 9.4.

3. Examine the auxiliary spacing devices (spacers) shown in Figure 9.5.
4. Examine the in-line adaptors for MDI delivery to ventilated patients, as shown in Figure 9.6.
5. Examine the Cadema Aero-Tech and Respirgard nebulizers and identify the component parts shown in Figures 9.7 and 9.8.
   Mouthpiece
   One-way valve

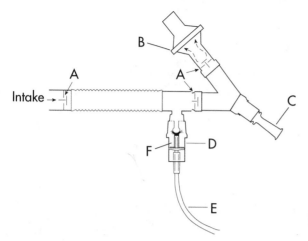

FIGURE 9.7 Respirgard nebulizer. (From Rau, JL Jr: Respiratory Care Pharmacology, ed 4. Mosby-Year Book, St. Louis, 1994, p. 291, with permission.)

Medication reservoir
Nebulizer
Expiratory filter
Connecting tubing

6. Compare the Cadema Aero-Tech and Respirgard nebulizers with a small volume nebulizer and a large volume nebulizer. *Record your comparisons on your laboratory report.*

7. Examine the Heart nebulizer and identify the component parts shown in Figure 9.9. Do the same for the circulaire nebulizer shown in Figure 9.10. Compare these devices with a small volume nebulizer and a large volume nebulizer. *Record your comparisons on your laboratory report.*

EXERCISE 9.4 Aerosol Medication Administration

NOTE: For the following exercises, placebo medications may be used. However, for any student with asthma or reactive airways disease, an actual bronchodilator may be administered with a prescription if the student is agreeable.

EXERCISE 9.4.1 Metered Dose Inhaler Administration

1. Gather the necessary equipment for MDI administration: metered dose inhaler, spacer, peak flowmeter, disposable mouthpiece, and watch with second hand.

2. Check the "chart" for medication order or protocol, diagnosis, history, and other pertinent information.

3. Wash your hands. Apply standard precautions and transmission-based isolation procedures as appropriate.

4. Introduce yourself and your department to your "patient." Verify patient identification. Explain the purpose of the procedure, and verify patient understanding.

5. Position the patient in an upright position.

6. Assess the patient before therapy for heart rate and pattern, respiratory rate and pattern, auscultation, and peak flow measurement.

7. Instruct your patient on MDI administration as follows:
   a. Remove the dust cap and inspect the **actuator** mouthpiece for any foreign objects.
   b. Shake the MDI. Actuate one puff into the air while holding the canister upside down if more than 24 hours have elapsed since the last use.
   c. Place the spacer onto the end of the actuator adaptor.
   d. Place the spacer mouthpiece into the mouth. Keep the tongue relaxed and the teeth out of the way of the opening. Exhale normally (not to residual volume [RV]).
   e. Begin a slow inspiration through the mouth, and activate the MDI as inhalation continues.
   f. Inhale maximally. Maintain inspiratory hold for up to 10 sec if possible.
   g. Wait at least 1 to 2 min between puffs.

8. Recap the mouthpiece.

9. If an inhaled corticosteroid is being used, have the patient rinse mouth and gargle throat with water when finished.

10. Reassess your patient's pulse, respiratory rate, breath sounds, and peak flow.

11. Instruct the patient to rinse the mouthpiece and spacer with warm water at least daily.

12. Instruct the patient on how to determine MDI contents remaining:
    a. Two hundred puffs per MDI.
    b. Floating canister in water. A full canister will sink, an empty canister will float.

13. Once a week, disinfect the mouthpiece assembly in a solution of one-half white vinegar and one-half water for 20 to 30 min. Rinse thoroughly and air dry.

14. *Chart the therapy on your laboratory report.*

EXERCISE 9.4.2 Small Volume Nebulizer Administration

NOTE: For the following exercises, normal saline may be used. However, for any student with asthma or reactive airways disease, an actual bronchodilator may be administered with a prescription if the student is agreeable.

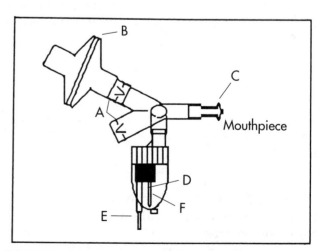

FIGURE 9.8 Cadema Aero-Tech nebulizer. (From Vinciguerra, C and Smaldone, G: Treatment time and patient tolerance for pentamidine delivery by Respirgard II and Aero-Tech II. Respiratory Care 35:11, 1990, p. 1038. With permission of Daedalus Enterprises Inc., Dallas, TX.)

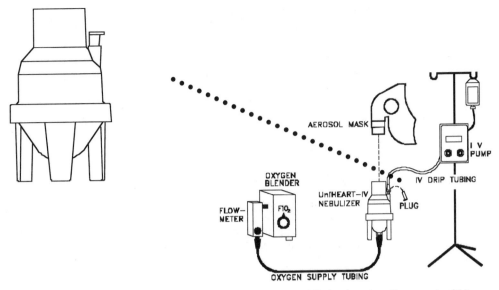

FIGURE 9.9 Heart nebulizer. (Courtesy of VORTRAN Medical Technology, Inc., Sacramento, CA.)

1. Gather the necessary equipment to deliver a medication via small volume nebulizer by mouthpiece: small volume nebulizer, connecting tubing, nipple adaptor, compressed gas source (air or oxygen), mouthpiece, one 6-inch length of large-bore corrugated aerosol tubing, unit-dose normal saline, unit-dose or multidose vial of an aerosolized bronchodilator, watch with second hand, stethoscope, and peak flowmeter.

2. Check the "chart" for order or protocol, diagnosis, history, and other pertinent information.

3. Wash your hands and apply standard precautions and transmission-based isolation procedures as applicable.

4. Assemble the SVN (see Fig. 9.2).

5. Introduce yourself and your department. Verify patient identification, explain the procedure, and verify patient understanding.

6. Position the patient in an upright seated position, if possible.

7. Perform pretreatment assessment of heart rate and pattern, respiratory rate and pattern, auscultation, and peak flow measurement.

8. Aseptically fill the nebulizer with the ordered medication and diluent.

9. Set the compressed gas source to 6 to 8 lpm.

10. Place the mouthpiece in the patient's mouth and instruct the patient to take slow, deep breaths with occasional inspiratory hold as tolerated.

11. Periodically reassess pulse throughout the treatment.

12. Modify the patient's technique as needed based on response, and reinstruct as necessary.

13. Terminate the treatment when complete medication dosage is nebulized or significant adverse reactions occur.

14. Reassess vital signs, breath sounds, and peak flow.

15. Encourage patient to cough and expectorate sputum. Observe for volume, color, consistency, odor, and presence or absence of blood.

16. Rinse the nebulizer with sterile water and air dry. Place it aseptically in a patient treatment bag.

    NOTE: The nebulizer should not be rinsed with tap water because of the possible contamination with *Legionella*.[1]

17. *Chart the therapy on your laboratory report.*

18. Notify appropriate personnel of any adverse reactions or other concerns.

EXERCISE 9.4.3 Aerosol Delivery by Mask

Repeat Exercise 9.4.2 using an aerosol mask in place of the mouthpiece for administration, as shown in Figure 9.12.

EXERCISE 9.4.4 Aerosol Delivery by Tracheostomy Collar

Repeat Exercise 9.4.2 using a tracheostomy collar, as shown in Figure 9.13.

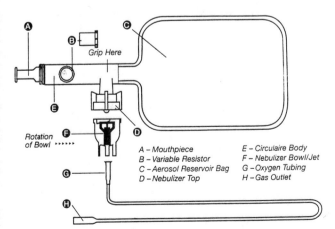

A – Mouthpiece
B – Variable Resistor
C – Aerosol Reservoir Bag
D – Nebulizer Top
E – Circulaire Body
F – Nebulizer Bowl/Jet
G – Oxygen Tubing
H – Gas Outlet

FIGURE 9.10 Circulaire nebulizer. (Courtesy of Westmed, Inc., Tucson, AZ.)

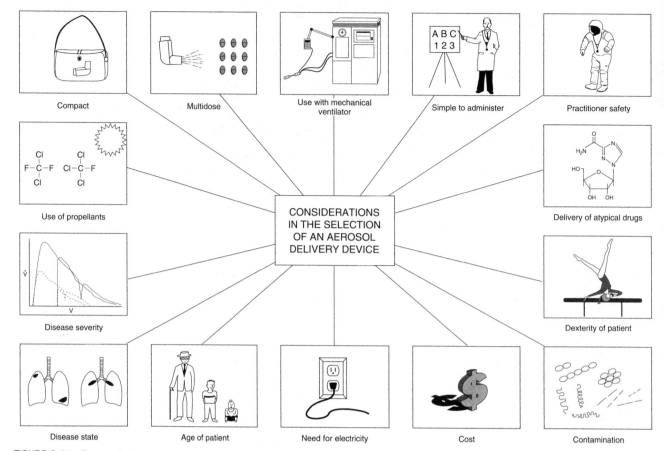

FIGURE 9.11 Factors in the selection of an aerosol delivery device. (From Witek, TJ Jr and Schachter, EN: Pharmacology and Therapeutics in Respiratory Care, WB Saunders, Philadelphia, 1994, p. 47, with permission.)

EXERCISE 9.4.5 Aerosol Delivery by T-Piece or Briggs Adaptor

Repeat Exercise 9.4.2 using a T-piece or Briggs adaptor, as shown in Figure 9.14.

EXERCISE 9.5 Respirgard/Cadema Nebulizers

1. Obtain a Respirgard or Cadema nebulizer and assemble the component parts.
2. Aseptically instill 3 ml of normal saline into the medication cup.

TABLE 9.2 **Factors in Determining Mode of Aerosol Delivery**

SVN: Unable to follow directions, poor vital capacity (VC), inspiratory capacity (IC), incapable of breath hold, tachypnea >25 breaths/ min, medication available in solution only

MDI: Oriented, cooperative, coordinated patient, >900 ml VC, f < 25/min, needs drug in MDI form

DPI: If poor MDI coordination, sensitive to chlorofluorocarbon (CFC) propellant, needs accurate dose counting, if drug available in DPI form

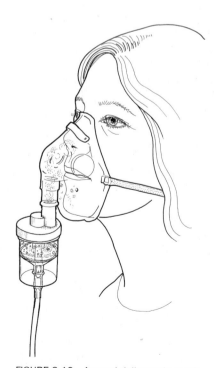

FIGURE 9.12 Aerosol delivery via mask.

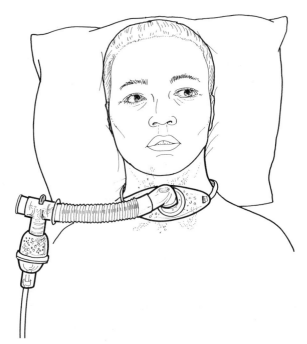

FIGURE 9.13   Aerosol delivery via tracheostomy.

3. Turn the flow to 6 lpm. *Record your observations of the density, particle size, and release of particles into the atmosphere on your laboratory report.*

4. Turn the flow to 10 lpm. *Record your observations of the density, particle size, and release of particles into the atmosphere on your laboratory report.*

EXERCISE 9.6 Sputum Induction

NOTE: For best results in inducing sputum, a 3-percent hypertonic saline solution is used. However, because of its irritating nature and the possibility of adverse reactions, the instructor may wish to use sterile water or saline for this exercise. Caution should always be taken with any student who has asthma or reactive airways disease.

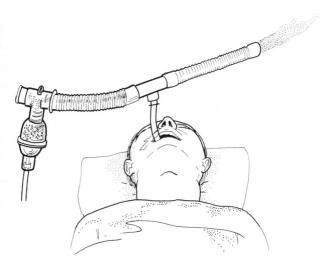

FIGURE 9.14   Aerosol delivery via endotracheal tube.

1. Gather the necessary equipment for sputum induction via ultrasonic nebulizer: ultrasonic nebulizer, electrical outlet, aerosol mask, several lengths of large-bore corrugated aerosol tubing, bottle of sterile water or saline, watch with second hand, and stethoscope.

2. Check the "chart" for order or protocol, diagnosis, history, and other pertinent information.

3. Wash your hands and apply standard precautions and transmission-based isolation procedures as applicable.

4. Introduce yourself and your department. Verify patient identification, explain the procedure, and verify patient understanding.

5. Position the patient in an upright seated position if possible.

6. Perform pretreatment assessment by measuring heart rate and pattern, respiratory rate and pattern, and auscultation.

7. Assemble the ultrasonic nebulizer. Fill the couplant chamber with tap water. Plug the unit into an electrical outlet.

8. Attach the large-bore corrugated tubing to the nebulizer outlet, and attach the aerosol mask to the end of the tubing.

9. Aseptically fill the medication chamber of the nebulizer with the ordered medication.

10. Turn the unit on and adjust the output control.

11. Place the mask comfortably on the patient's face and instruct the patient to take slow, deep breaths with occasional inspiratory hold as tolerated.

12. Periodically reassess vital signs and breath sounds throughout the treatment.

13. Modify technique and reinstruct the patient as needed based on patient response.

14. Terminate treatment after 15 to 30 min, if significant adverse reactions occur, or when sputum specimen has been obtained.

15. Reassess vital signs and breath sounds.

16. Encourage the patient to cough and expectorate sputum into specimen cup. Observe for volume, color, consistency, odor, and presence or absence of blood.

17. Label the specimen container with patient identification and information (including name, room number, identification number, physician, antibiotic therapy, source of specimen, and date and time of collection) and deliver to the appropriate personnel.

18. *Chart the therapy on your laboratory report.*

19. Notify appropriate personnel of any adverse reactions or other concerns and make any necessary recommendations or modifications to the patient care plan.

Reference

1. Woo, AH, Goetz, A and Yu, VL: Transmission of *Legionella* by respiratory equipment and aerosol generating devices. Chest 102: 1586–1589, 1992.

Related Readings

Cottrell, GP and Surkin, SB: Pharmacology for Respiratory Care Practitioners. FA Davis, Philadelphia, 1995.

Eubanks, DH and Bone, RC: Principles and Applications of Cardiorespiratory Care Equipment. Mosby, St Louis, 1994.

McPherson, S: Respiratory Care Equipment, ed 5. Mosby, St Louis, 1995.

Madama, V: Pulmonary Function Testing and Cardiopulmonary Stress Testing. Delmar Publishers, Albany, 1993.

Rau, J: Respiratory Care Pharmacology, ed 4. Mosby, St. Louis, 1994.

Scanlan, C et al (eds): Egan's Fundamentals of Respiratory Care, ed 6. Mosby, St Louis, 1995.

Selected Journal Articles

American Association for Respiratory Care: Aerosol consensus statement. Respir Care 36:916–921, 1991.

American Association for Respiratory Care: AARC clinical practice guideline: Assessing response to bronchodilator therapy at point of care. Respir Care 40:1300–1307, 1995.

American Association for Respiratory Care: AARC clinical practice guideline: Bland aerosol administration. Respir Care 38:1196–1200, 1993.

American Association for Respiratory Care: AARC clinical practice guideline: Delivery of aerosols to the upper airway. Respir Care 39:803–807, 1994.

American Association for Respiratory Care: AARC clinical practice guideline: Selection of aerosol delivery device. Respir Care 37:891–897, 1992.

American Association for Respiratory Care: AARC clinical practice guideline: Selection of an aerosol delivery device for neonatal and pediatric patients. Respir Care 40:1325–1335, 1995.

American Association for Respiratory Care: AARC clinical practice guideline: Selection of a device for delivery of aerosol to the lung parenchyma. Respir Care 41:647–653, 1996.

Barnes, NC: Effects of corticosteroids in acute severe asthma. Thorax 47:582–583, 1992.

Barnes, P: A new approach to the treatment of asthma. N Engl J Med 321:1517–1527, 1989.

Benham, DC: Ribavirin for pediatric patients on mechanical ventilation. Choices in Respiratory Management 19:81–87, 1989.

Bowton, DL: Metered-dose inhalers versus hand-held nebulizers: Some answers and new questions. Chest 101:298–300, 1992.

Burrows, B and Lebowitz, M: The B-agonist dilemma. N Engl J Med 1992.

Byron, P, Phillips, E and Kuhn, R: Ribavirin administration by inhalation: Aerosol-generation factors controlling drug delivery to the lung. Respir Care 33:1011–1019, 1988.

Colacone, A et al: A comparision of albuterol administered by metered dose inhaler and holding chamber or wet nebulizer in acute asthma. Chest, 104:835–841, 1993.

Corkery, KJ et al: Pentamidine: Aerosolized pentamidine for treatment and prophylaxis of *Pneumocystis carinii* pneumonia with AIDS. Respir Care 33:676–685, 1988.

Diot, P and Lemarie, E: Wet nebulizers vs. metered dose inhalers (letter). Chest 106:980, 1994.

Ferguson, G and Cherniack, R: Current concepts: Management of chronic obstructive pulmonary disease. N Engl J Med 328:1017–1022, 1993.

Greer, K: Common sense needed in giving pentamidine treatment. RT Advance 2:29, 1989.

Hardy, W et al: A controlled trial of trimethoprim-sulfamethorxazole or aerosolized pentamidine for secondary prophylaxis of *Pneumocystis carinii* pneumonia in patients with the acquired immunodeficiency syndrome. N Engl J Med 327:1842–1847, 1992.

Herman, J: Therapist involvement in drug choices. Respiratory Management 19:6–12, 1989.

Jobe, A: Pulmonary surfactant therapy. N Engl J Med 328:861–868, 1993.

Kemp, J: Approaches to asthma management. Arch Intern Med 153:805–811, 1993.

Larsen, JS et al: Evaluation of conventional press-and-breathe-metered-dose-inhaler technique in 501 patients. J Asthma 31:193–199, 1994.

Leoung, G, Feigal, D and Montgomery, B: Aerosolized pentamidine for prophylaxis against *Pneumocystis carinii* pneumonia. N Engl J Med 323:769–775, 1990.

Levy, S: Bronchodilators in COPD to the max. Chest 99:793–794, 1991.

Makker, HK et al: Airway effects of local challenge with hypertonic saline in exercise-induced asthma. Am J Respir Crit Care Med 149:1012–1019, 1994.

Malone, RA et al: Optimal duration of nebulized albuterol therapy. Chest 104:1114–1118, 1993.

McCabe, D: Aerosolized pentamidine prophylaxis. Chest 100:1189–1190, 1991.

Merritt, TE: Factors to consider when selecting a surfactant. Neonatal Intensive Care 5:30–34, 1992.

Montgomery, A and Debs, R: Aerosolized pentamidine as sole therapy for *Pneumocystis carinii* pneumonia in patients with acquired immunodeficiency syndrome. Lancet 8:480–483, 1987.

O'Doherty, M et al: Does inhalation of pentaamidine in the supine position increase deposition in the upper part of the lung. Chest 97:1343–1347, 1990.

Page, C: An explanation of the asthma paradox. Am Rev Respir Dis 147:529–530, 1993.

Petty, T: Treatment of patients with asthma in the 1990s. Tex Med 88:58–62, 1992.

Reed, CE: Aerosol steroids as primary treatment of mild asthma. N Engl J Med 1991.

Shepherd, KE and Johnson, DC: Bronchodilator testing: An analysis of paradoxical responses. Respir Care 33:667–671, 1988.

Thompson, J et al: Misuse of metered dose inhalers in hospitalized patients. Chest 105:715–717, 1994.

Witek, TJ Jr, Schachter, EN and Zuskin, E: Paradoxical bronchoconstriction following inhalation of isoetharine: A case report . . . the carrier solution. Respir Care 32:29–31, 1987.

Zamary, R and Gross, N: Anticholinergic drugs for obstructive pulmonary disease. Choices in Respiratory Management 19:141–146, 1989.

LABORATORY REPORT

CHAPTER 9: AEROSOL THERAPY AND MEDICATION ADMINISTRATION

Name _____ Date _____

Course/Section _____ Instructor _____

Data Collection

EXERCISE 9.1   Review Calculation of Drug Dosages

1. _____

2. _____

3. _____

4. _____

5. _____

6. _____

7. Drug: _____

   Dosage: _____

8. _____

EXERCISE 9.2   Small Volume Nebulizers

EXERCISE 9.2.1   Identification of Component Parts

A. _____

B. _____

C. _____

D. _____

E. _____

F. _____

G. _____

EXERCISE 9.2.2   Operation of a Small Volume Nebulizer

Observations

1 ml normal saline solution (NSS)/6 lpm:

_____

_____

3 ml NSS:

_____

_____

10 lpm:

_____

_____

2 lpm:

_____

_____

6 ml NSS/6 lpm:

_____

_____

EXERCISE 9.3 Identification of Component Parts of Additional Delivery Devices

Components of Respirgard or Cadema nebulizer:

A. _____

B. _____

C. _____

D. _____

E. _____

F. _____

Comparison of Respirgard and Cadema to SVN and LVN:

_____

_____

_____

_____

Comparison of Heart nebulizer and circulaire nebulizer to SVN and LVN:

_____

_____

_____

EXERCISE 9.4 Aerosol Medication Administration

EXERCISE 9.4.1 Metered Dose Inhaler Administration

Chart your therapy:

_____

_____

_____

_____

_____

_____

_____

_____

_____

_____

EXERCISE 9.4.2 Small Volume Nebulizer Administration

Chart your therapy:

_____

_____

_____

_____

_____

_____

_____

_____

_____

_____

EXERCISE 9.5 Respirgard/Cadema Nebulizers

Observations

3 ml NSS/6 lpm—density, particle size, and release of particles into the atmosphere:

_____

_____

_____

10 lpm—density, particle size, and release of particles into the atmosphere:

_____

_____

_____

EXERCISE 9.6 Sputum Induction

Chart your therapy:

_____

_____

_____

_____

_____

_____

_____

_____

_____

_____

TABLE 9.3 **Respiratory Medication Summary**

Trade Name	Generic Name	Percent Solution	Dosage	Class	Hazards
	Racemic epinephrine				
Aerobid					
Alupent					
Atropine					
Atrovent					
Azmacort					
Bronkosol					
Exosurf					
Isuprel					
Mucomyst					
Protozyme					
Proventil, Ventolin					
Serevent					
Survanta					
Terbutaline					
Tornalate					
Vanceril					

CRITICAL THINKING QUESTIONS

Complete Table 9.3. Classify the drugs as one of the following:
A. Sympathomimetic
B. Parasympatholytic
C. Mucokinetic
D. Surface active
E. Antiasthmatic
F. Steroid

Mr. Sullivan is a 55-year-old man who has just arrived at the emergency room. He has a documented history of bronchitis and asthma. The physician has requested that you immediately assess the patient and make a recommendation for treatment. Your initial assessment reveals tachypnea, tachycardia, diaphoresis, audible wheezing, and the use of accessory muscles.

1. What other bedside assessments would be important to perform at this time?

2. What specific treatment(s) would you recommend for this patient?

3. Which specific medication and dosage would you suggest?

4. The physician disagrees with your suggestion and orders 5 mg of albuterol sulfate to be delivered every hour. Briefly describe how you would handle this situation. What further recommendations would you make?

5. The initial aerosol therapy treatment has been started in the emergency room and has been administered for 5 min. Monitoring of the patient indicates that the pulse rate has increased from 112/min to 140/min, and the audible wheezing appears to be improving. Describe your response to this situation.

6. The patient's attending physician has been contacted, and the patient is being admitted. The physician has written *additional* orders for an Atrovent, Azmacort, and Intal inhaler, 2 puffs each, to be administered q4h. In which order should the medications be taken?

7. How do the Respirgard/Cadema, Circulaire, and Heart nebulizers differ from small volume nebulizers? What medication is delivered via Respirgard/Cadema nebulizers?

8. List two hazards or complications of each of the following, and explain how each could be assessed and prevented or treated:
   a. An aerosolized sympathomimetic
   b. A parasympatholytic bronchodilator
   c. A **mucolytic** agent
   d. Three percent hypertonic saline
   e. Aerosolized anti-infective agents

9. Given the following clinical scenarios, select the proper aerosol generator *and* aerosol delivery device:
   a. A 60-year-old obtunded black man who requires treatment with 0.5 ml Proventil and 3.0 ml NSS.
   b. An AIDS patient who requires pentamidine.
   c. A 35-year-old woman in the recovery room after abdominal surgery.
   d. A 55-year-old man with a size 8.0 tracheostomy tube.
   e. A 30-year-old patient with possible pneumonia; a sputum sample is required.
   f. A 4-month-old with respiratory syncytial virus.
   g. An 18-year-old asthmatic who is sensitive to the propellant in the MDI.
   h. Status asthmaticus patient admitted to intensive care. The patient is not responding to q1-2h treatments. The physician requests that you administer high-dose bronchodilator therapy.

Hyperinflation Techniques

INTRODUCTION

Hyperinflation techniques include a variety of basic respiratory care modalities, all of which are designed to promote lung expansion and thereby prevent or reverse atelectasis. This is accomplished by increasing **transpulmonary pressure** and inspiratory volumes.[1] Additional benefits of these modalities as a component of bronchial hygiene therapy include promoting a more effective cough, thereby improving mobilization of secretions.

Incentive spirometry, or sustained maximal inspiration (SMI), techniques primarily prevent atelectasis by mimicking or replacing the normal sigh mechanism and encouraging the patient to take slow, deep breaths with an inspiratory hold. Intermittent **positive-pressure** breathing (IPPB) provides short-term mechanical inflation to **augment** inspiratory volumes, deliver aerosol medication, assist ventilation, and mobilize secretions.[2] IPPB may be applied to spontaneously breathing patients and to those with artificial airways. It is not the first choice for aerosol delivery or augmenting lung expansion when less expensive or less invasive techniques can reliably accomplish these clinical outcomes.[2]

OBJECTIVES

Upon completion of this chapter, the student will be able to:

1. Practice the communication skills needed for the instruction of patients in the techniques of sustained maximal inspiration and hyperinflation therapy.
2. Perform and monitor incentive spirometry therapy using both flow and volume devices.
3. Practice medical charting for the therapeutic procedures of hyperinflation.
4. Identify and compare the component parts and controls of various IPPB devices.
5. Assemble and ensure proper function of IPPB equipment.
6. Perform and monitor volume-oriented IPPB therapy.
7. Evaluate the effects of various control manipulation on the volumes, I:E ratio, and F_IO_2 delivered by IPPB devices.
8. Analyze the effect of altered lung compliance and airway resistance on the volume delivered by IPPB devices.

KEY TERMS

augment	bulla	hysteresis	thoracic pump
bleb	hyperinflation	positive pressure	transpulmonary pressure
	hypostasis	splint	

EQUIPMENT REQUIRED

- Flow- and volume-based incentive spirometry devices
- Respirometers
- One-way valve adaptors
- Peak flowmeter and disposable mouthpieces
- Stethoscopes
- Pillow
- Disposable mouthpieces
- Disposable noseclips
- Flange (lip seal)
- Masks
- Unit-dose normal saline vials
- Disposable IPPB circuits
- IPPB machines, Bird and Bennett
- 50 psi air and oxygen sources
- High-pressure hoses
- Test lungs
- Stopwatch
- Oxygen analyzer with T-adaptor
- Tissues
- Gloves
- Computerized lung simulator, optional

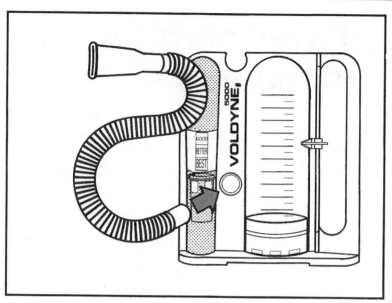

1. Remove components from package.
2. Attach open end of tubing to stem on front side of exerciser.

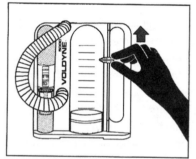

Slide the pointer of unit to prescribed volume level. Hold or stand exerciser in an upright position.

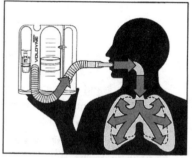

Inhale slowly to raise the white piston in the chamber. When inhaling, maintain top of yellow flow cup in the "Best" flow range.

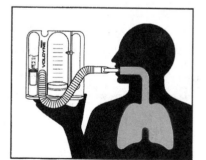

Exhale normally. Then place lips tightly around mouthpiece.

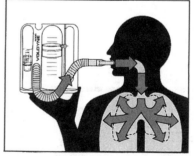

Continue inhaling and try to raise piston to prescribed level.* When inhalation is complete remove mouthpiece, hold breath as prescribed, and exhale normally. Allow piston to return to bottom of chamber, rest and repeat exercise. Frequency of use and recommended inspiratory volumes should be performed at the direction of your physician.

A

FIGURE 10.1   Assembly of *(A)* volume incentive spirometer. (Courtesy of Voldyne, Sherwood, Davis & Geck, St. Louis, MO.)

● EXERCISES

EXERCISE 10.1 Incentive Spirometry

EXERCISE 10.1.1 Sustained Maximal Inspiration Preoperative Instruction

Your laboratory partner will play the role of a preoperative patient who must be instructed in the techniques of SMI. In clinical situations, SMI is most effective when the patient is instructed preoperatively.

1. Gather the necessary equipment for this exercise:
   a. Respirometer
   b. One-way valve adaptor
   c. Flow or volume incentive spirometer device
   d. Pillow
2. Wash your hands and apply standard precautions and transmission-based isolation procedures as applicable.
3. Introduce yourself and your department. Explain the purpose of the therapy to the "patient," and verify patient understanding.
4. Measure the patient's preoperative inspiratory capacity and vital capacity using the respirometer.
5. Assemble the incentive spirometer device as shown in Figure 10.1.

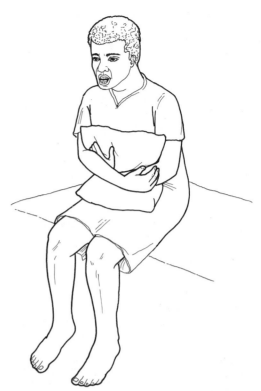

FIGURE 10.2   Splinting an abdominal incision.

6. Instruct the patient on the use and frequency of the incentive spirometer device in the following manner:
   a. Exhale normally.
   b. Insert the mouthpiece into your mouth and inhale *slowly* and *deeply.*
   c. Hold your breath at the end of inspiration to the count of 10 (3 to 5 sec).
   d. Exhale normally.
   e. Repeat the procedure 6 to 10 times per hour. Allow adequate recovery time between breaths to prevent hyperventilation.
7. Instruct the patient on using a pillow to **splint** the incision postoperatively to minimize pain during therapy, as shown in Figure 10.2.
8. Have the patient demonstrate the procedure to you.
9. *Chart your patient's preoperative evaluation and instruction on your laboratory report.*

EXERCISE 10.1.2 Incentive Spirometry Postoperative Therapy

Your laboratory partner will play the role of a postoperative thoracotomy patient who is in mild to moderate discomfort.

1. Gather the necessary equipment:
   a. Stethoscope
   b. Respirometer
   c. One-way valve adaptor
   d. Flow or volume incentive spirometer device
   e. Pillow
2. Wash your hands and apply standard precautions and transmission-based isolation procedures as applicable.
3. Introduce yourself and your department.
4. Explain the purpose of the therapy to the patient, and verify patient understanding.

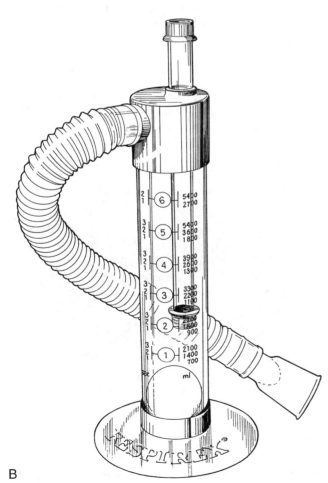

B

FIGURE 10.1   *(B)* Flow incentive spirometer. (Courtesy of Diemolding Corp., Diemolding Healthcare Division, Canastota, NY.)

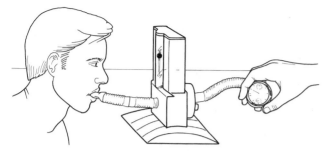

FIGURE 10.3 Measuring inspiratory volumes on an incentive spirometer.

5. Measure the patient's postoperative inspiratory capacity and vital capacity using the respirometer. Your "patient" should simulate a decreased effort for this exercise.

6. Assemble the incentive spirometer device.

7. Assess patient progress by the following:
   a. Pain medication schedule
   b. Chest x-ray report from the "chart"
   c. Change in patient's temperature from the chart
   d. Patient's pulse and respiratory rate
   e. Breath sounds on auscultation

8. Reinstruct the patient on the use and frequency of the incentive spirometer device in the following manner:
   a. Exhale normally.
   b. Insert the mouthpiece into your mouth and inhale *slowly* and *deeply.*
   c. Hold your breath at the end of inspiration to the count of 10 (3 to 5 sec).
   d. Exhale normally.
   e. Repeat the procedure 6 to 10 times per hour. Allow adequate recovery time between breaths to prevent hyperventilation.

9. Assist the patient in using the pillow to splint the incision postoperatively to minimize pain during therapy.

10. Have the patient demonstrate the procedure to you.

11. Measure the achieved volume. For a volume-based device, observe the maximum inspiratory effort achieved. For a flow-based device, the volume can be measured by attaching the respirometer as shown in Figure 10.3.

12. Instruct the patient to cough. Observe for any sputum production. Auscultate the patient.

13. *Chart the therapy on your laboratory report.*

EXERCISE 10.2 Identification of Intermittent Positive-Pressure Breathing Machine Component Parts and Controls

1. Obtain a Bird IPPB machine. Identify the component parts shown in Figure 10.4. *Record the model used and components on your laboratory report.* (If the model used is not the same as the one pictured, identify the controls of the model used and note how the controls differ.)
   Expiratory (apnea) timer
   Manual cycle rod
   Large-bore tubing connection
   Pressure chamber
   Flow rate control
   Gas inlet

Air-mix plunger
Pressure manometer
Sensitivity
Ambient chamber
Pressure limit
Nebulizer/exhalation valve connection

2. Obtain a Bennett IPPB device. Identify the component parts shown in Figure 10.5. *Record the model used and components on your laboratory report.*
   Nebulizer—inspiration
   Control pressure
   Sensitivity
   Air dilution
   Nebulizer—expiration
   System pressure
   Peak flow
   Pressure limit
   Negative pressure
   Expiratory time
   Terminal flow
   Rate
   Bennett valve with dustcover
   Accumulator

3. Remove the dustcover from the Bennett valve. Unscrew and carefully remove and examine the valve. Replace it when you have completed your observation.

EXERCISE 10.3 Intermittent Positive-Pressure Breathing Circuitry Assembly

1. Attach the high-pressure hose to the IPPB machine and then to a 50-psi gas source.

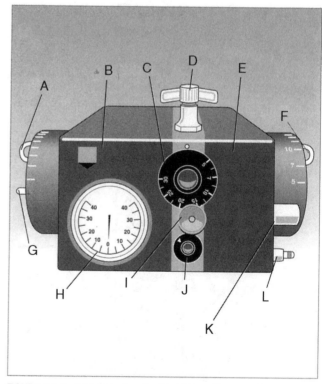

FIGURE 10.4 Components of a Bird intermittent positive-pressure breathing (IPPB) machine. (From Persing, G: Entry-Level Respiratory Care Review, ed 2. WB Saunders, Philadelphia, 1996, p. 27.)

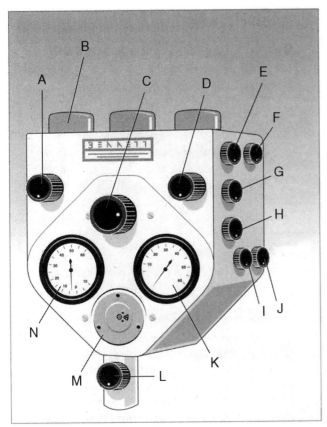

FIGURE 10.5 Components of a Bennett IPPB machine. (From Persing, G: Entry-Level Respiratory Care Review, ed 2. WB Saunders, Philadelphia, 1996, p. 79, with permission.)

2. Assemble an IPPB circuit as shown in Figure 10.6 and attach it to an IPPB machine.

3. Test the function of the machine by adjusting the pressure to maximum, manually cycling the machine on, and aseptically occluding the outlet with a gloved hand or gauze. Ensure that the machine cycles off. If it does not, examine it for any loose connections or a faulty exhalation valve.

4. Attach a test lung to the circuit outlet (where the mouthpiece would normally be attached). Increase the sensitivity adjustment until the machine automatically self-cycles, and then decrease it slightly until autocycling stops. Now squeeze the test lung. The machine should cycle on.

5. Adjust the pressure so that the machine cycles off at 20 cm H_2O.

6. Adjust the flow so that inspiration takes approximately 2 sec.

7. Attach the respirometer to the expiratory outlet of the circuit. Measure the volume achieved, and *record it on your laboratory report.*

EXERCISE 10.4 Manipulation of Intermittent Positive-Pressure Breathing Controls

EXERCISE 10.4.1 Volume and Inspiration:Expiration Ratio Adjustment

Using a test lung attached to the IPPB circuit, make the following adjustments and observe the results. Measure exhaled volumes using a respirometer attached to the expiratory outlet.

1. *Record the current volume, flow, and sensitivity settings on the machine on your laboratory report.* Cycle the machine on, and *record the achieved inspiratory volume on your laboratory report.*

2. Increase the pressure and cycle the machine on. Note and *record the pressure at end inspiration and any change in inspiratory volume and time on your laboratory report.*

3. Set the pressure below the original setting. Note and *record the pressure at end inspiration and any change in inspiratory volume and time on your laboratory report.*

4. Return the pressure to the original setting. Increase the flow setting. Note and *record the pressure at end inspiration and any change in inspiratory volume and time on your laboratory report.*

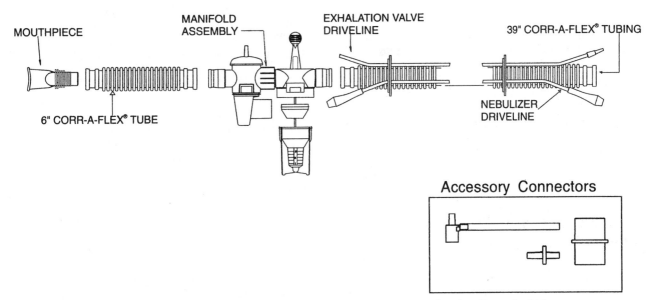

FIGURE 10.6 Assembly and components of an IPPB circuit. (Courtesy of Hudson Respiratory Care Inc., Temecula, CA.)

5. Decrease the flow setting below the original settings. Note and *record the pressure at end inspiration and any change in inspiratory volume on your laboratory report.*

6. Adjust the pressure and flow controls until a tidal volume of 500 ml is achieved. Note and *record the settings needed to achieve this volume and the inspiratory time on your laboratory report.*

7. Adjust the pressure and flow controls until a tidal volume of 700 ml is achieved. Note and *record the settings needed to achieve this volume and the inspiratory time on your laboratory report.*

8. Adjust the pressure and flow controls until a tidal volume of 300 ml is achieved. Note and *record the settings needed to achieve this volume and the inspiratory time on your laboratory report.*

EXERCISE 10.4.2 Sensitivity Control

Set the pressure and flow to the original settings.

1. Increase the sensitivity control, and note what happens when the test lung is squeezed. Note and *record the negative pressure needed to initiate inspiration on your laboratory report.*

2. Increase the sensitivity until the machine autocycles.

3. Decrease the sensitivity setting. Squeeze the test lung, and note and *record the negative pressure needed to initiate inspiration on your laboratory report.*

EXERCISE 10.4.3 F$_I$O$_2$ Control

1. Attach the IPPB machine to a 50-psi oxygen gas source.

2. Calibrate an oxygen analyzer, and insert it between the inspiratory outlet and the test lung.

3. Adjust the rate control so that the machine automatically cycles on at a rate of 12 to 15 breaths per minute.

4. Adjust the oxygen control on the IPPB machine to the "in," or air-mix off, position. Allow the machine to cycle for several breaths, and *record the F$_I$O$_2$ reading on the analyzer on your laboratory report.*

5. Adjust the oxygen control to the "out," or air-mix on, position. Allow the machine to cycle for several breaths, and *record the F$_I$O$_2$ reading on the analyzer on your laboratory report.*

6. Increase the pressure reading. Allow the machine to cycle for several breaths, and *record the F$_I$O$_2$ reading on the analyzer on your laboratory report.*

7. Decrease the pressure setting. Allow the machine to cycle for several breaths, and *record the F$_I$O$_2$ reading on the analyzer on your laboratory report.*

8. Increase the flow setting. Allow the machine to cycle for several breaths, and *record the F$_I$O$_2$ reading on the analyzer on your laboratory report.*

9. Decrease the flow setting. Allow the machine to cycle for several breaths, and *record the F$_I$O$_2$ reading on the analyzer on your laboratory report.*

EXERCISE 10.5 Intermittent Positive-Pressure Breathing Therapy

In this exercise your laboratory partner will act as a patient. Because the therapy will be given with aerosolized normal

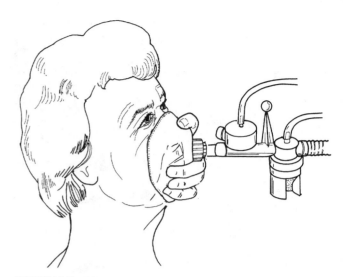

FIGURE 10.7   Administration of an IPPB treatment with a face mask.

saline, caution should be used for any student with hypersensitive airways.

1. Gather the necessary equipment.

2. Wash your hands and apply standard precautions and transmission-based isolation procedures as appropriate.

3. Introduce yourself and your department, explain the procedure, and verify patient understanding.

4. Assess the patient before therapy by measuring pulse rate and pattern, respiratory rate and pattern, and auscultation.

5. Measure the patient's tidal volume, vital capacity, and peak flow rate.

6. Assemble the IPPB circuit with a mouthpiece, and test the function. Adjust the settings initially at a low pressure (approximately 10 cm H$_2$O) and a moderate flow setting. Adjust the sensitivity so that the machine is not autocycling.

7. Aseptically fill the nebulizer with a 3- to 5-ml unit dose of normal saline solution. If a Bennett machine is used, adjust the nebulizer control to achieve a moderate mist.

8. Have the patient insert the mouthpiece into his or her mouth and maintain a tight seal. If the patient has difficulty, noseclips or a mouth flange may be used.

9. Instruct the patient to inhale slightly until the machine triggers on, and allow the machine to augment inspiration. Note the volume achieved during inspiration.

10. Adjust the sensitivity if needed.

11. Adjust the pressure and flow until a maximum possible volume (at least two to three times the tidal volume) is achieved during inspiration without patient discomfort.

12. Instruct the patient to breathe slowly to prevent hyperventilation.

13. Monitor pulse, respirations, and breath sounds during therapy. Observe the patient for any adverse reactions.

14. At the end of the therapy, reassess the patient's vital signs, breath sounds, vital capacity, and peak flow.

15. Instruct the patient to cough. Note any sputum production. Assess volume, color, consistency, and odor.

16. Disassemble the equipment, dispose of any infectious waste in the appropriate containers, and wash your hands.

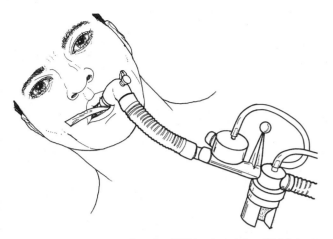

FIGURE 10.8   Administration of an IPPB treatment via artificial airway.

17. *Chart the therapy on your laboratory report.*

18. Repeat the therapy using the mouth flange.

19. Repeat the therapy using a mask, as shown in Figure 10.7.

20. Repeat the therapy using an artificial airway, as shown in Figure 10.8.

EXERCISE 10.6 Computerized Lung Simulator: Effect of Compliance and Resistance Changes on Intermittent Positive-Pressure Breathing Volumes

The following exercise may be performed if a computerized lung simulator is available. If not, an airway management trainer can be used with endotracheal tubes of varying size to simulate resistance changes and manual manipulation of a test lung to simulate compliance changes.

1. Adjust the lung simulator for normal compliance and resistance.

2. Adjust the IPPB machine to achieve a tidal volume of 700 ml. *Record these settings on your laboratory report.*

3. Increase the airway resistance setting (or decrease the size of the endotracheal tube). *Record any changes in achieved tidal volume and inspiratory time on your laboratory report.*

4. Return the resistance to normal. Decrease the compliance below normal on the lung simulator (or manually restrict

the expansion of the test lung). *Record any changes in achieved tidal volume and inspiratory time on your laboratory report.*

5. Increase the compliance above normal. *Record any changes in achieved tidal volume and inspiratory time on your laboratory report.*

References

1. American Association for Respiratory Care: The AARC clinical practice guideline: Incentive spirometry. Respir Care 36:1402–1405, 1991.
2. American Association for Respiratory Care: The AARC clinical practice guideline: Intermittent positive pressure breathing. Respir Care 38:1189–1195, 1993.

Related Readings

Eubanks, DH and Bone, RC: Principles and Applications of Cardiorespiratory Care Equipment. Mosby, St Louis, 1994.
McPherson, S: Respiratory Care Equipment, ed 5. Mosby, St Louis, 1995.
Scanlan, C et al (eds): Egan's Fundamentals of Respiratory Care, ed 6. Mosby, St Louis, 1995.

Selected Journal Articles

American Association for Respiratory Care: The AARC clinical practice guideline: Incentive spirometry. Respir Care 36:1402–1405, 1991.
American Association for Respiratory Care: The AARC clinical practice guideline: Intermittent positive pressure breathing. Respir Care 38:1189–1195, 1993.
DeTroyer, A and Deisser, P: The effects of intermittent positive pressure breathing on patients with respiratory muscle weakness. Am Rev Respir Dis 124:132–137, 1981.
Hall, JC, Tapper, J and Tarala, R: The cost-efficiency of incentive spirometry after abdominal surgery. Aust N Z J Surg 63:356–359, 1993.
Mang, H and Obermayer, A: Imposed work of breathing during sustained maximal inspiration: Comparison of six incentive spirometers. Respir Care 34:1122–1128, 1989.
Scuderi, J and Olsen, JG: Respiratory therapy in the management of postoperative complications. Respir Care 34:281–291, 1989.
Sleszynski, SL and Kelso, AF: Comparison of thoracic manipulation with incentive spirometry in preventing postoperative atelectasis. J Am Osteopath Assoc 93:834–838, 843–845, 1993.
Thomas, JA and McIntosh, JM: Are incentive spirometry, intermittent positive pressure breathing, and deep breathing exercises effective in the prevention of postoperative pulmonary complications after upper abdominal surgery? A systematic overview and meta-analysis. Phys Ther 74:3–10, 1994.

LABORATORY REPORT

CHAPTER 10: HYPERINFLATION TECHNIQUES

Name ———————————————   Date ———————————————

Course/Section ———————————   Instructor ———————————

Data Collection

EXERCISE 10.1   Incentive Spirometry

EXERCISE 10.1.1   Sustained Maximal Inspiration Preoperative Instruction

"Chart" the preoperative patient evaluation and instruction below. Include the patient's preoperative inspiratory, vital capacity, and peak flow measurements.

———————————————————————————————

———————————————————————————————

———————————————————————————————

———————————————————————————————

———————————————————————————————

———————————————————————————————

EXERCISE 10.1.2   Incentive Spirometry Postoperative Therapy

"Chart" the postoperative treatment below as you would on a legal medical record.

———————————————————————————————

———————————————————————————————

———————————————————————————————

———————————————————————————————

———————————————————————————————

———————————————————————————————

———————————————————————————————

———————————————————————————————

EXERCISE 10.2   Identification of Intermittent Positive-Pressure Breathing Machine Component Parts and Controls

1. Bird controls.

   Model of machine used: ———————————

   A. ———————————

   B. ———————————

   C. ———————————

   D. ———————————

   E. ———————————

   F. ———————————

   G. ———————————

    H. _____

    I. _____

    J. _____   (Identify which are the pressure and

    K. _____   ambient chambers.)

    L. _____

2. Bennett controls.

  Model of machine used: _____

    A. _____

    B. _____

    C. _____

    D. _____

    E. _____

    F. _____

    G. _____

    H. _____

    I. _____

    J. _____

    K. _____

    L. _____

    M. _____

    N. _____

Controls on other Bennett machines: _____

_____

_____

_____

_____

EXERCISE 10.3 Intermittent Positive-Pressure Breathing Circuitry Assembly

Volume achieved: _____

EXERCISE 10.4 Manipulation of Intermittent Positive-Pressure Breathing Controls

EXERCISE 10.4.1 Volume and Inspiration:Expiration Ratio Adjustment

A. Original settings:

  Pressure: _____

  Flow: _____

  Sensitivity: _____

  Volume achieved: _____

  Inspiratory time: _____

B. Increased pressure setting:

    Pressure: _____

    Flow: _____

    Sensitivity: _____

    Volume achieved: _____

    Inspiratory time: _____

C. Decreased pressure setting:

    Pressure: _____

    Flow: _____

    Sensitivity: _____

    Volume achieved: _____

    Inspiratory time: _____

D. Increased flow setting:

    Pressure: _____

    Flow: _____

    Sensitivity: _____

    Volume achieved: _____

    Inspiratory time: _____

E. Decreased flow setting:

    Pressure: _____

    Flow: _____

    Sensitivity: _____

    Volume achieved: _____

    Inspiratory time: _____

F. 500 ml:

    Pressure setting: _____

    Flow setting: _____

    Inspiratory time: _____

G. 700 ml:

    Pressure setting: _____

    Flow setting: _____

    Inspiratory time: _____

H. 300 ml:

    Pressure setting: _____

    Flow setting: _____

    Inspiratory time: _____

EXERCISE 10.4.2   Sensitivity Control

1. Increased sensitivity, negative manometer pressure reading: _____

2. Decreased sensitivity, negative manometer pressure reading: _____

EXERCISE 10.4.3 F_IO_2 Control

1. Air mix in; F_IO_2: _____

2. Air mix out; F_IO_2: _____

3. Increased pressure; F_IO_2: _____

4. Decreased pressure; F_IO_2: _____

5. Increased flow; F_IO_2: _____

6. Decreased flow; F_IO_2: _____

EXERCISE 10.5   Intermittent Positive-Pressure Breathing Therapy

"Chart" the IPPB therapy as you would on a legal medical record.

_____

_____

_____

_____

_____

_____

_____

EXERCISE 10.6   Computerized Lung Simulator

1. Original settings:

    Compliance: _____

    Resistance: _____

    Pressure: _____

    Flow: _____

    Volume achieved: _____

    Inspiratory time: _____

2. Increased resistance:

    Compliance: _____

    Resistance: _____

    Pressure: _____

    Flow: _____

    Volume achieved: _____

    Inspiratory time: _____

3. Decreased compliance:

    Compliance: _____

    Resistance: _____

Pressure: _____

Flow: _____

Volume achieved: _____

Inspiratory time: _____

4. Increased compliance:

Compliance: _____

Resistance: _____

Pressure: _____

Flow: _____

Volume achieved: _____

Inspiratory time: _____

CRITICAL THINKING QUESTIONS

Mr. Rodriguez is a 29-year-old man with quadriplegia as a result of a spinal cord injury. He has been having episodes of recurrent atelectasis in the right lower lobe (RLL).

1. What therapeutic hyperinflation technique would you recommend as most appropriate for this patient?

2. Mr. Rodriguez is noted to have a reduced inspiratory and vital capacity.
   a. On the Bird IPPB machine, which control(s) could be adjusted to increase the volume achieved during therapy?
   b. How would you adjust the setting of these control(s) for this purpose?
   c. If a Bennett machine is used, which control(s) could be adjusted to increase the volume? How would the control(s) be adjusted?

3. Mr. Rodriguez is having difficulty initiating inspiration during IPPB. Which control should be adjusted? How should it be adjusted?

4. It is noted during IPPB therapy that the pressure gauge is rising very slowly during the first half of inspiration. What control could be adjusted to correct this situation?

5. The patient complains of light-headedness, paresthesias, and headache during incentive spirometry therapy. What is the most likely cause, and how would you correct this situation?

6. A patient with COPD who is breathing on hypoxic drive is being given an IPPB treatment to prevent impending respiratory failure. How would you adjust the F_IO_2? Describe the difference in this adjustment between a Bird versus a Bennett machine.

7. A Bird IPPB device is noted to be stuck in the inspiratory position. Identify three causes of this problem and what you would need to do to correct each situation.

8. What types of patients would most benefit from incentive spirometry?

9. How can the effectiveness of incentive spirometry therapy be determined?

10. During IPPB therapy, a patient suddenly complains of a sharp, left-sided chest pain. She becomes cyanotic and dyspneic. How would you assess this patient's condition, and what actions should be taken?

PROCEDURAL COMPETENCY EVALUATION

Name _____ Date _____

Intermittent Positive-Pressure Breathing Therapy

Setting: ☐ Lab ☐ Clinical   Evaluator: ☐ Peer ☐ Instructor

Conditions (describe): _____

_____

Equipment Used

_____

_____

	S A T I S F A C T O R Y	U N S A T I S F A C T O R Y	N O T O B S E R V E D	N O T A P P L I C A B L E
Equipment and Patient Preparation				
1. Verifies, interprets, and evaluates physician's order or protocol	☐	☐	☐	☐
2. Scans chart for diagnosis and other pertinent data and notes	☐	☐	☐	☐
3. Selects, gathers, and assembles the necessary equipment	☐	☐	☐	☐
4. Washes hands and applies standard precautions and transmission-based isolation procedures as appropriate	☐	☐	☐	☐
5. Identifies patient, introduces self and department	☐	☐	☐	☐
6. Explains purpose of the procedure and confirms patient understanding	☐	☐	☐	☐
Assessment and Implementation				
7. Assesses the patient before therapy by measuring pulse rate and pattern, respiratory rate and pattern, and auscultation	☐	☐	☐	☐
8. Measures the patient's tidal volume, vital capacity, and peak flow rate	☐	☐	☐	☐
9. Assembles the IPPB circuit and tests the function	☐	☐	☐	☐
10. Adjusts settings initially at a low pressure, moderate flow, and moderate sensitivity (if applicable)	☐	☐	☐	☐
11. Aseptically fills nebulizer with prescribed medication	☐	☐	☐	☐
12. Instructs patient to insert the mouthpiece and maintain a tight seal; applies noseclips, mouth flange, or mask as appropriate	☐	☐	☐	☐
13. Instructs patient to inhale slightly until the machine triggers on, and allows the machine to augment inspiration; notes the volume achieved during inspiration	☐	☐	☐	☐
14. Adjusts the sensitivity if needed	☐	☐	☐	☐
15. Adjusts the pressure and flow until a maximum possible volume (at least two to three times the tidal volume) is achieved during inspiration without patient discomfort	☐	☐	☐	☐
16. Instructs the patient not to exhale forcefully against the exhalation valve	☐	☐	☐	☐
17. Instructs the patient to breathe slowly to prevent hyperventilation	☐	☐	☐	☐
18. Monitors pulse, respirations, and breath sounds during therapy; observes the patient for any adverse reactions	☐	☐	☐	☐
19. Reassess the patient's vital signs, breath sounds, vital capacity, and peak flow	☐	☐	☐	☐
20. Instructs the patient to cough; notes any sputum production and assesses volume, color, consistency, and odor	☐	☐	☐	☐
Follow-up				
21. Maintains/processes equipment	☐	☐	☐	☐
22. Disposes of infectious waste and washes hands	☐	☐	☐	☐
23. Records pertinent data in chart and departmental records	☐	☐	☐	☐
24. Notifies appropriate personnel and makes any necessary recommendations or modifications to the patient care plan	☐	☐	☐	☐

_____   _____
Signature of Evaluator   Signature of Student

PERFORMANCE RATING SCALE

5 EXCELLENT—FAR EXCEEDS EXPECTED LEVEL, FLAWLESS PERFORMANCE
4 ABOVE AVERAGE—NO PROMPTING REQUIRED, ABLE TO SELF-CORRECT
3 AVERAGE—THE MINIMUM COMPETENCY LEVEL, NO CRITICAL ERRORS
2 IMPROVEMENT NEEDED—PROBLEM AREAS EXIST; CRITICAL ERRORS, CORRECTIONS NEEDED
1 POOR AND UNACCEPTABLE PERFORMANCE—GROSS INACCURACIES, POTENTIALLY HARMFUL

PERFORMANCE CRITERIA	SCALE				
1. DISPLAYS KNOWLEDGE OF ESSENTIAL CONCEPTS	5	4	3	2	1
2. DEMONSTRATES THE RELATIONSHIP BETWEEN THEORY AND CLINICAL PRACTICE	5	4	3	2	1
3. FOLLOWS DIRECTIONS, EXHIBITS SOUND JUDGMENT, AND DEMONSTRATES ATTENTION TO SAFETY AND DETAIL	5	4	3	2	1
4. EXHIBITS THE REQUIRED MANUAL DEXTERITY	5	4	3	2	1
5. PERFORMS PROCEDURE IN A REASONABLE TIME FRAME	5	4	3	2	1
6. MAINTAINS STERILE OR ASEPTIC TECHNIQUE	5	4	3	2	1
7. INITIATES UNAMBIGUOUS GOAL-DIRECTED COMMUNICATION	5	4	3	2	1
8. PROVIDES FOR ADEQUATE CARE AND MAINTENANCE OF EQUIPMENT AND SUPPLIES	5	4	3	2	1
9. EXHIBITS COURTEOUS AND PLEASANT DEMEANOR	5	4	3	2	1
10. MAINTAINS CONCISE AND ACCURATE RECORDS	5	4	3	2	1

ADDITIONAL COMMENTS: INCLUDE ERRORS OF OMISSION OR COMMISSION, COMMUNICATIVE SKILLS, AND EFFECTIVENESS OF PATIENT INTERACTION:

SUMMARY PERFORMANCE EVALUATION AND RECOMMENDATIONS

SATISFACTORY PERFORMANCE—Performed without error or prompting, or able to self-correct, no critical errors.

_____ LABORATORY EVALUATION. SKILLS MAY BE APPLIED/OBSERVED IN THE CLINICAL SETTING.

_____ CLINICAL EVALUATION. STUDENT READY FOR MINIMALLY SUPERVISED APPLICATION AND REFINEMENT.

UNSATISFACTORY PERFORMANCE—Prompting required; performed with critical errors, potentially harmful.

_____ STUDENT REQUIRES ADDITIONAL LABORATORY PRACTICE.

_____ STUDENT REQUIRES ADDITIONAL SUPERVISED CLINICAL PRACTICE.

SIGNATURES

STUDENT: _____   EVALUATOR: _____

DATE: _____   DATE: _____

PROCEDURAL COMPETENCY EVALUATION

Name _____ Date _____

Incentive Spirometry

Setting: ☐ Lab ☐ Clinical   Evaluator: ☐ Peer ☐ Instructor

Conditions (describe): _____

_____

Equipment Used

_____

_____

	SATISFACTORY	UNSATISFACTORY	NOT OBSERVED	NOT APPLICABLE
Equipment and Patient Preparation				
1. Verifies, interprets, and evaluates physician's order or protocol	☐	☐	☐	☐
2. Scans chart for diagnosis and other pertinent data and notes	☐	☐	☐	☐
3. Selects, gathers, and assembles the necessary equipment	☐	☐	☐	☐
4. Washes hands and applies standard precautions and transmission-based isolation procedures as appropriate	☐	☐	☐	☐
5. Identifies patient, introduces self and department	☐	☐	☐	☐
6. Explains purpose of the procedure and confirms patient understanding	☐	☐	☐	☐
Assessment and Implementation				
7. Assesses patient progress by the following:				
a. Pain medication schedule	☐	☐	☐	☐
b. Chest x-ray report	☐	☐	☐	☐
c. Patient's temperature	☐	☐	☐	☐
d. Preoperative evaluation of volumes and capacities	☐	☐	☐	☐
e. Patient's pulse and respiratory rate	☐	☐	☐	☐
f. Auscultation of breath sounds	☐	☐	☐	☐
8. Assembles the incentive spirometer	☐	☐	☐	☐
9. Instructs the patient on the use and frequency of the incentive spirometer				
a. Includes breath hold for 5 to 10 sec	☐	☐	☐	☐
b. Repeats the procedure 6 to 10 times per hour; allows adequate recovery time between breaths to prevent hyperventilation	☐	☐	☐	☐
10. Assists patient in using the pillow to splint the incision postoperatively to minimize pain during therapy	☐	☐	☐	☐
11. Has the patient demonstrate the procedure	☐	☐	☐	☐
12. Measures the achieved volume or flow	☐	☐	☐	☐
13. Instructs the patient to cough; observes for any sputum production	☐	☐	☐	☐
14. Reassesses the patient	☐	☐	☐	☐
Follow-up				
15. Maintains/processes equipment	☐	☐	☐	☐
16. Disposes of infectious waste and washes hands	☐	☐	☐	☐
17. Records pertinent data in chart and departmental records	☐	☐	☐	☐
18. Notifies appropriate personnel and makes any necessary recommendations or modifications to the patient care plan	☐	☐	☐	☐

_____   _____
Signature of Evaluator   Signature of Student

PERFORMANCE RATING SCALE

5 EXCELLENT—FAR EXCEEDS EXPECTED LEVEL, FLAWLESS PERFORMANCE
4 ABOVE AVERAGE—NO PROMPTING REQUIRED, ABLE TO SELF-CORRECT
3 AVERAGE—THE MINIMUM COMPETENCY LEVEL, NO CRITICAL ERRORS
2 IMPROVEMENT NEEDED—PROBLEM AREAS EXIST; CRITICAL ERRORS, CORRECTIONS NEEDED
1 POOR AND UNACCEPTABLE PERFORMANCE—GROSS INACCURACIES, POTENTIALLY HARMFUL

PERFORMANCE CRITERIA		SCALE			
1. DISPLAYS KNOWLEDGE OF ESSENTIAL CONCEPTS	5	4	3	2	1
2. DEMONSTRATES THE RELATIONSHIP BETWEEN THEORY AND CLINICAL PRACTICE	5	4	3	2	1
3. FOLLOWS DIRECTIONS, EXHIBITS SOUND JUDGMENT, AND DEMONSTRATES ATTENTION TO SAFETY AND DETAIL	5	4	3	2	1
4. EXHIBITS THE REQUIRED MANUAL DEXTERITY	5	4	3	2	1
5. PERFORMS PROCEDURE IN A REASONABLE TIME FRAME	5	4	3	2	1
6. MAINTAINS STERILE OR ASEPTIC TECHNIQUE	5	4	3	2	1
7. INITIATES UNAMBIGUOUS GOAL-DIRECTED COMMUNICATION	5	4	3	2	1
8. PROVIDES FOR ADEQUATE CARE AND MAINTENANCE OF EQUIPMENT AND SUPPLIES	5	4	3	2	1
9. EXHIBITS COURTEOUS AND PLEASANT DEMEANOR	5	4	3	2	1
10. MAINTAINS CONCISE AND ACCURATE RECORDS	5	4	3	2	1

ADDITIONAL COMMENTS: INCLUDE ERRORS OF OMISSION OR COMMISSION, COMMUNICATIVE SKILLS, AND EFFECTIVENESS OF PATIENT INTERACTION:

SUMMARY PERFORMANCE EVALUATION AND RECOMMENDATIONS

SATISFACTORY PERFORMANCE—Performed without error or prompting, or able to self-correct, no critical errors.

_____ LABORATORY EVALUATION. SKILLS MAY BE APPLIED/OBSERVED IN THE CLINICAL SETTING.

_____ CLINICAL EVALUATION. STUDENT READY FOR MINIMALLY SUPERVISED APPLICATION AND REFINEMENT.

UNSATISFACTORY PERFORMANCE—Prompting required; performed with critical errors, potentially harmful.

_____ STUDENT REQUIRES ADDITIONAL LABORATORY PRACTICE.

_____ STUDENT REQUIRES ADDITIONAL SUPERVISED CLINICAL PRACTICE.

SIGNATURES

STUDENT: _____   EVALUATOR: _____

DATE: _____   DATE: _____

CHAPTER 11

Bronchial Hygiene Techniques

INTRODUCTION

Increased mucus production or impaired cough ability from physical limitations can overwhelm the body's normal clearance mechanisms and lead to retained secretions. Removal of retained secretions and improved cough effort are necessary to prevent atelectasis and infection. Bronchial hygiene incorporates several techniques and therapies, each with unique indications, contraindications, and hazards, to compensate for physical limitations and assist in the removal of secretions. These techniques may be performed either manually or with the use of mechanically assisted devices. By using gravity and mechanical vibrations, secretions can be mobilized to a point at which they may be spontaneously expectorated. If the patient does not have an adequate cough effort, the therapist must incorporate additional procedures to remove the secretions or results may be less than optimal. Responsibilities of the RCP also include instruction of patients and their families in these techniques for home administration.

Bronchial hygiene techniques include the following:

1. Chest physiotherapy (CPT)
   a. Postural drainage
   b. Chest percussion
   c. Expiratory vibration
2. Directed cough and manual assisted cough
3. Positive expiratory pressure (PEP) mask therapy
4. Breathing exercises
5. Inspiratory resistive muscle training

OBJECTIVES
Upon completion of this chapter, the student will be able to:

1. Identify each **lobe** and **segment** of the lungs and the corresponding bronchi on a lung model.
2. Properly position and perform postural drainage, percussion, and vibration techniques for all lung lobes and segments.
3. After reviewing x-ray reports and assessing physical examination results, perform chest physical therapy techniques to the appropriate lobes and segments.
4. Instruct and monitor a patient on coughing, splinting, and pursed-lip breathing.
5. Practice directed cough and manually assisted cough techniques to improve cough effectiveness according to AARC clinical practice guidelines.
6. Instruct and monitor a patient on diaphragmatic, thoracic expansion, and relaxation breathing exercises.
7. Perform PEP mask therapy according to AARC clinical practice guidelines.
8. Perform inspiratory muscle training techniques.

KEY TERMS

abduction	adjunctive	lobe	segment
adduction	fissure	lobule	syncope
	intracranial pressure	orthostatic	

EQUIPMENT REQUIRED

- Segmented lung model and tracheobronchial tree
- Hospital bed, electrical (if available)
- Tilt table (if hospital bed is not available)
- Pillows and pillowcases
- Bedsheets
- Towels
- Adult mannequin
- Infant mannequin
- Blood pressure manometer and cuffs
- Stethoscope
- Watch with second hand
- Tissues

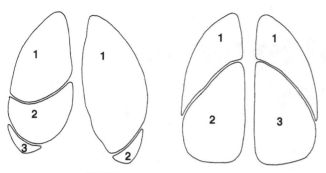

FIGURE 11.1   Lobes of the lung.

- Infectious waste disposal basin
- Mechanical percussor
- Percussion cups, various sizes
- Pulse oximeter and probes
- PEP masks, Thera-Pep, flutter valves
- Nose clips
- Disposable mouthpieces
- Inspiratory resistive muscle-training devices
- Maximum inspiratory pressure manometer
- Inspiratory force adaptors
- Nonsterile gloves

● EXERCISES

EXERCISE 11.1   Identification of Lung Lobes and Segments

Using a segmented lung model and Figure 11.1, identify the lobes of the lung.

Using a segmented lung model and Figure 11.2, identify all the lung segments.

Right Lung

Right upper lobe (RUL)
1   Apical
2   Posterior
3   Anterior
Right middle lobe (RML)
4   Lateral
5   Medial
Right lower lobe (RLL)
6   Superior
7   Medial basal
8   Anterior basal
9   Lateral basal
10   Posterior basal

Left Lung

Left upper lobe (LUL)
1-2   Apical-posterior
3   Anterior

4   Superior lingula
5   Inferior lingula
Left lower lobe (LLL)
6   Superior
7-8   Anteromedial basal
9   Lateral basal
10   Posterior basal

Using the model of the tracheobronchial tree and Figure 11.3, identify the major lobar and segmental bronchi.

EXERCISE 11.2   Postural Drainage

EXERCISE 11.2.1   Postural Drainage Positioning in Adults

Using a laboratory partner or an adult mannequin, practice properly positioning a patient for postural drainage on a bed or table.

NOTE: Because all of the following procedures for mobilization of secretions involve a patient cough effort, local exhaust ventilation and personal protective equipment may be necessary to prevent exposure to droplet nuclei in an actual clinical setting. Standard precautions and transmission-based isolation procedures should be followed.

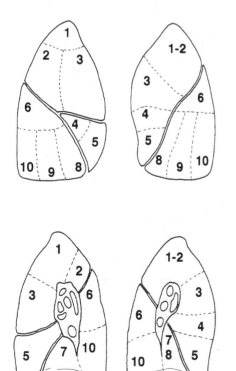

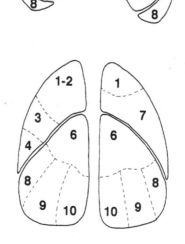

FIGURE 11.2   Lung segments.

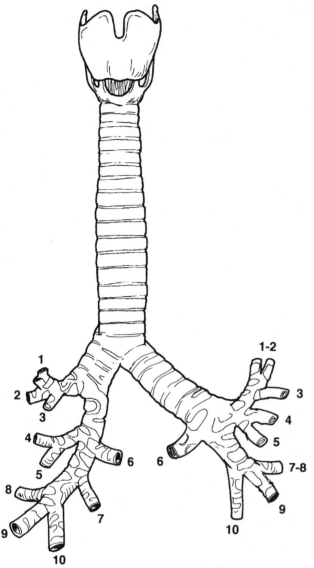

FIGURE 11.3 Tracheobronchial tree.

1. Review any pertinent data on the patient's chart, including physician's orders or protocol, history and physical examination, diagnosis, x-ray results, and any precautions or possible contraindications to performing the procedure.

2. Wash your hands and apply standard precautions and transmission-based isolation procedures as appropriate.

3. Coordinate therapy before meals and tube feedings or one and one-half hours after.

4. Introduce yourself to the patient and explain the procedure.

5. Assess the patient before therapy. Assessment should include the following:
   a. Pulse
   b. Respirations
   c. Blood pressure
   d. Chest symmetry and expansion using palpation
   e. Color
   f. Level of dyspnea
   g. Level of cooperation
   h. Oxygen saturation with pulse oximeter

6. Place the patient in each of the positions for drainage shown in Figure 11.4. Use pillows to support the patient where necessary. Begin with the most dependent segments first. In an adult, this usually means starting from the basilar segments and working up to the apices.

   NOTE: In an actual clinical situation, the patient would remain in each position for a minimum of 3 to 15 min as tolerated, for drainage.[1] In special circumstances, the patient may remain in drainage positions for longer periods of time.

   To drain the anterior basal segments of the lower lobes, two alternative positions have been suggested by different authors.[2,3]

7. The practitioner should always be positioned facing the patient to provide for direct visualization and to permit a rapid response to changing levels of tolerance.

8. Reassess the patient's tolerance in each position by evaluating the following:
   a. Pulse
   b. Respirations
   c. Blood pressure
   d. Color
   e. Level of dyspnea
   f. Level of cooperation
   g. Oxygen saturation with pulse oximeter

9. Allow the patient to sit up and cough after each position. An immediate response does not always result. The practitioner may need to check back with the patient at a later time to determine any sputum production after the treatment.

10. Note the volume, consistency, color, and presence or absence of blood in the sputum. Note which positions are most productive.

11. *"Chart" the therapy on your laboratory report.*

EXERCISE 11.2.2 Postural Drainage Positioning in Infants

Using an infant mannequin, practice the proper positioning of the infant on your lap or pillows for each of the lung segments as shown in Figure 11.5.

EXERCISE 11.3 Chest Percussion

Practice the technique of chest percussion as shown in Figure 11.6, using your laboratory partner as the patient.

1. Cup your hands and allow for relaxed motion from the wrist. Do not stiffen your upper arms. Rhythmically strike the designated area, alternating hands.

2. Practice first on your thigh. Listen for a hollow "clapping" or "galloping" sound. This sound should be audible to someone not in the room, but should not cause pain or discomfort.

3. Remove your jewelry and wash your hands. Apply standard precautions and transmission-based isolation procedures as appropriate.

4. Position the patient for postural drainage (any position may be used for this exercise).

5. Perform chest percussion on the patient for at least 3 min. Remember the following precautions:
   a. Avoid bony processes. Do not percuss on the spine, on clavicles, on scapulae, on breast tissue, over areas of

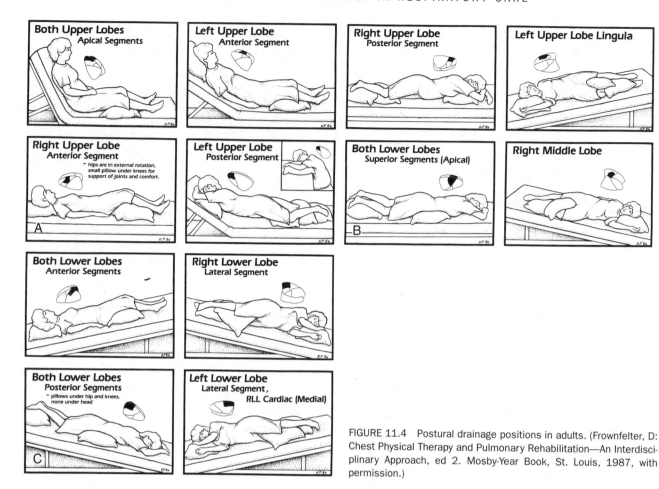

FIGURE 11.4   Postural drainage positions in adults. (Frownfelter, D: Chest Physical Therapy and Pulmonary Rehabilitation—An Interdisciplinary Approach, ed 2. Mosby-Year Book, St. Louis, 1987, with permission.)

incisions, over areas of rib fractures, or below the rib margins.

   b. Do not percuss on bare skin. On an actual patient, use a towel or sheet over the patient's skin.

   c. Remove your jewelry. Do not percuss over any buttons, zippers, or similar items that the subject may have on.

6. Repeat the procedure using a mechanical percussion device (Fig. 11.7). Vary the speed and force to observe the effects. A chest oscillation vest can also be used (Fig. 11.8).

7. Repeat the procedure using percussion cups (Fig. 11.9), one in each hand. Small sizes are available for children and infants, or a small face mask may be used by sealing the opening with tape.

8. Baby G is going to be discharged tomorrow. With your laboratory partner acting as the "parent," instruct the parent on how to perform these procedures.

EXERCISE 11.4 Expiratory Vibration

Practice the technique of expiratory vibration, using your laboratory partner as the patient.

1. Remove jewelry and wash your hands. Apply standard precautions and transmission-based isolation procedures as appropriate.

2. Place the patient in any position for postural drainage in which he or she is lying down.

3. Place one hand over the other on the area to be vibrated, as shown in Figure 11.10.

4. Instruct the patient to take a deep breath and exhale slowly through pursed lips.

5. Apply a gently vibrating motion during exhalation only. Your upper arm muscles should tighten and allow transmission of the vibration to your hands. Do not shake the patient. Repeat the vibration technique two or three times for each segment.

EXERCISE 11.5 Directed Cough

Several techniques are available to help improve the patient's cough effort. Practice patient instruction and monitoring of these techniques, using your laboratory partner as the patient. The sequence of steps in a normal cough is illustrated in Figure 11.11.

EXERCISE 11.5.1 Cough Instruction

1. Wash your hands and apply standard precautions and transmission-based isolation procedures as appropriate.

2. Introduce yourself to the patient, and explain the purpose of an adequate cough effort.

3. Have the patient sit up in a chair or on the bed or table. Patients who cannot tolerate a sitting position can use a side-lying position with knees bent (Fig. 11.12).

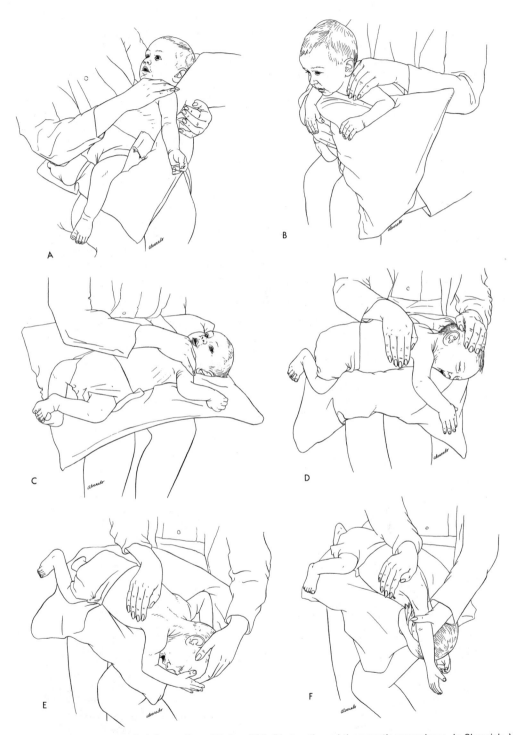

FIGURE 11.5   Postural drainage positions in infants. (From Waring, WW: Diagnostic and therapeutic procedures. In Chernick, V [ed]: Kendig's Disorders of the Respiratory Tract in Children, ed 5. WB Saunders, Philadelphia, 1990, pp. 86–87, with permission.)   *Continued*

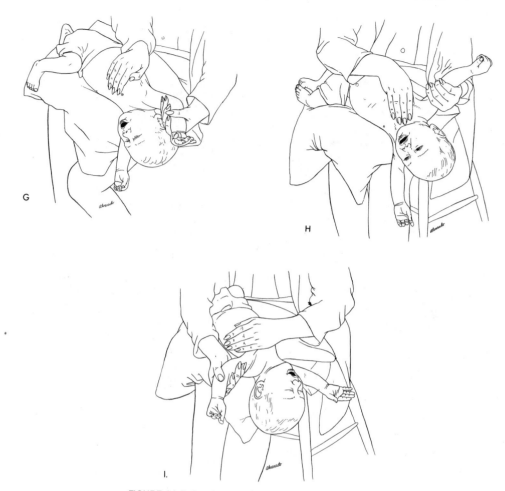

FIGURE 11.5 *Continued*   See legend on previous page.

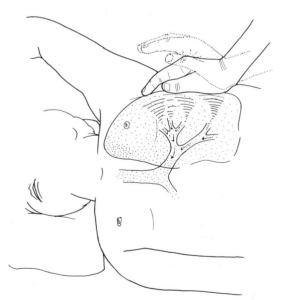

FIGURE 11.6   Chest percussion technique.

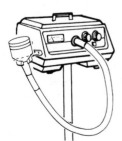

FIGURE 11.7   Mechanical percussor. (Courtesy of General Physiotherapy, Inc., St. Louis, MO.)

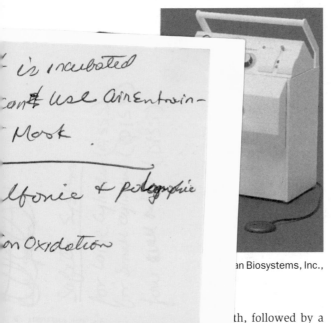

an Biosystems, Inc.,

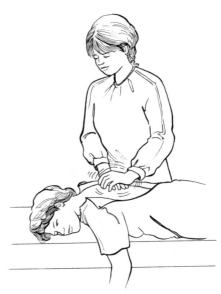

FIGURE 11.10 Expiratory vibration technique. (From Pierce, LNB: Guide to Mechanical Ventilation and Intensive Respiratory Care. WB Saunders, Philadelphia, 1995, p. 143, with permission.)

th, followed by a
slight breath hold, a _____ Have tissues and a waste receptacle readily available. Note the volume, consistency, color, and presence or absence of blood in any sputum expectorated.

5. Using a pillow or your hands, instruct the patient on splinting of any painful areas (Fig. 11.13). Apply gentle pressure over the involved area before deep inspiration, and increase pressure slightly during the forced expiratory phase of the cough. Use standard precautions and transmission-based isolation procedures as appropriate.

EXERCISE 11.5.2 Cough Alternatives

Some patients do not have the capacity or tolerance for a single forceful cough. Alternative methods can be used to improve cough effectiveness, compensate for physical limitations, and provide voluntary control over the cough reflex. Instruct your laboratory partner in each of the following techniques:

1. Wash your hands. Apply standard precautions and transmission-based isolation procedures as appropriate.

2. Introduce yourself to the patient, and explain the purpose of the procedure. Have tissues and a waste receptacle readily available.

3. Instruct the patient in serial coughing techniques. Have the patient take a moderately deep breath, followed by a slight breath hold. Then perform two or three short coughs, one after another. Rest and repeat the procedure.

4. Instruct the patient in a forced expiratory technique (FET), or huffing maneuver.
   a. Have the patient take a moderately deep breath, followed by a short breath hold. Then perform three short forced exhalations with an open glottis. The patient should make a huffing or "Ha-ha-ha" sound on exhalation. Follow this with a period of relaxed, controlled diaphragmatic breathing.
   b. This can be assisted by self-compression of the chest wall by using a brisk **adduction** movement of the upper arms,[4] also known as a "chicken breath," as shown in Figure 11.14.

5. Improvement of the cough effort can be accomplished by providing a manually assisted cough, using epigastric pressure or external lateral compression of the thoracic cage[1] (Fig. 11.15).
   a. Instruct the patient to take a moderately deep breath, followed by a short breath hold. Apply gentle pressure to the epigastric region coordinated with the patient's cough effort, making sure to avoid the xiphoid area. This should not be done after meals.
   b. Instruct the patient to take a moderately deep breath, followed by a short breath hold. Apply pressure to the lateral thoracic cage coordinated with the patient's cough effort.

   NOTE: In a patient with a tracheostomy, a manually assisted deep inspiration can be provided using a manual resuscitator bag in conjunction with manually assisted cough techniques, as shown in Figure 11.16.

EXERCISE 11.6 Breathing Exercises

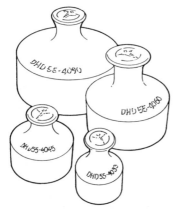

FIGURE 11.9 Percussion cups. (Courtesy of Diemolding Corp., Diemolding Healthcare Division, Canastota, NY.)

Using your laboratory partner as the patient, instruct your patient in the following breathing exercises:

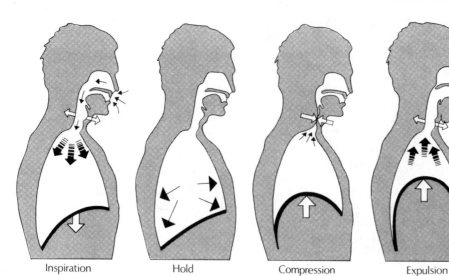

Inspiration Hold Compression Expulsion

FIGURE 11.11 Cough relfex. (From Shapiro, B, Peruzzi, WT and Templin, R: Clinical Application of Respiratory Care, ed 4. Mosby-Year Book, 1991, p. 52, with permission.)

1. Wash your hands and apply standard precautions and transmission-based isolation procedures as appropriate.

2. Introduce yourself, and explain the procedure to the patient.

3. Instruct the patient on pursed-lip breathing technique (Fig. 11.17).
   a. Have the patient take a deep breath through his or her nose.
   b. Instruct the patient to exhale through pursed lips with a slow, steady exhalation at an I:E ratio of at least 1:3.

4. Instruct the patient in abdominal breathing techniques.
   a. Have the patient lie down. For initial instruction, a slight Trendelenburg position is recommended.
   b. Place one hand on the patient's epigastric area and one hand on the upper chest, as shown in Figure 11.18.
   c. Ask the patient to sniff or pant to feel diaphragmatic movement.
   d. Instruct the patient to take a slow, deep breath through the mouth and exhale through pursed lips. Apply firm pressure during inspiration. The patient should push your hand away by protruding the abdomen. The upper chest and shoulders should expand but not move up.
   e. Replace your hands with a light book or other object, and instruct the patient to practice moving the book up on inspiration. A bag of rice or birdseed may be used for this exercise.
   f. The patient can eventually repeat the procedure in a more elevated position as tolerated while sitting and walking, as shown in Figures 11.19, 11.20, and 11.21.

The following relaxation techniques and exercises can be practiced at home on yourself or with a partner as the patient.

1. Have the patient lying in bed with head flexed slightly forward, thoracic spine straight, shoulders rotated inward slightly, elbows flexed, and hips and knees flexed.

2. Instruct the patient to perform the following maneuvers. The patient should close his or her eyes, take slow breaths, and attempt to relax the body part while holding each position for a count of 10.
   Turn head to right.
   Turn head to left.
   Raise head from pillow.
   Push head into pillow.
   Make a fist with both hands.
   Open fists.
   Bend wrists.
   Extend wrists.
   Bend elbows.
   Straighten elbows.
   Reach arms above head.
   Return arms to sides.
   Shrug shoulders.
   Raise the left leg and then lower it.
   Raise the right leg and then lower it.
   Spread legs apart.
   Bring legs together.
   Roll knees in.
   Roll knees out.
   Flex both ankles.
   Extend both ankles.
   Curl toes.
   Straighten toes.

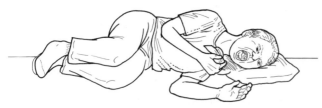

FIGURE 11.12 Side-lying position for cough.

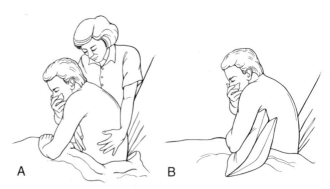

A B

FIGURE 11.13 Splinting techniques. (From Monahan, FD, Drake, T and Neighbors, M: Nursing Care of Adults. WB Saunders, 1994, p. 533, with permission.)

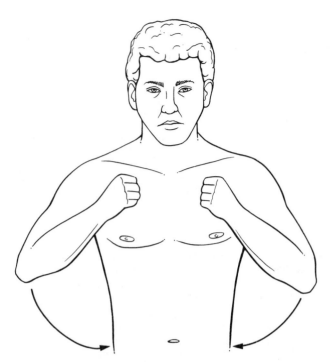

FIGURE 11.14   "Chicken breath" technique for use with huffing. (From Monahan, FD, Drake, T and Neighbors, M: Nursing Care of Adults. WB Saunders, Philadelphia, 1994, p. 474, with permission.)

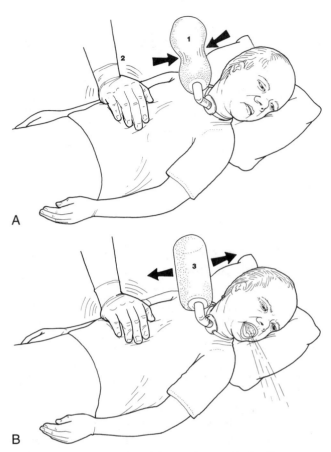

FIGURE 11.16   Assisted cough in a tracheostomized patient.

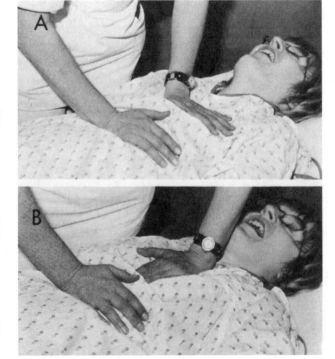

FIGURE 11.15   Quadriplegic cough techniques. (From Frownfelter, D: Chest Physical Therapy and Pulmonary Rehabilitation—An Interdisciplinary Approach, ed 2. Mosby-Year Book, St. Louis, 1987, p. 264, with permission.)

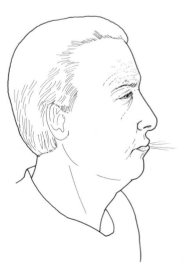

FIGURE 11.17   Pursed-lip breathing technique.

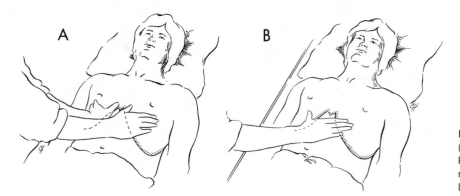

FIGURE 11.18 Diaphragmatic breathing. (Frownfelter, D: Chest Physical Therapy and Pulmonary Rehabilitation—An Interdisciplinary Approach, ed 2. Mosby-Year Book, St. Louis, 1987, p. 237, with permission.)

EXERCISE 11.7 Positive Expiratory Pressure Mask Therapy

Positive expiratory pressure (PEP) mask therapy has received attention as a possible adjunct or alternative to postural drainage and percussion techniques for bronchial hygiene.[5,6] PEP therapy can be performed with a mask or with mouthpiece and nose clips.

1. Obtain the PEP therapy device and set it up as shown in Figure 11.22, with the pressure manometer in line.

2. Wash your hands and apply standard precautions and transmission-based isolation procedures as appropriate.

3. Introduce yourself to the patient, and explain the purpose of the procedure.

4. Assess the patient's vital signs, mental function, skin color, and breath sounds.

5. Adjust the fixed exhalation orifice to the largest setting.

6. Have the patient sit upright with his or her elbows resting comfortably on a table.

7. Place the mask comfortably but tightly over the nose and mouth or adjust nose clips and mouthpiece.

8. Instruct the patient to take a larger than normal breath (but not to total lung capacity) and exhale slowly at an I : E ratio of 1 : 3 or 1 : 4.

9. Observe the pressure generated on the manometer during exhalation. Decrease the size of the fixed orifice until 10 to 20 cm H_2O pressure is generated during exhalation. Note the patient's response.

10. Instruct the patient to take 10 to 20 breaths followed by two or three huffs (FET). In an actual clinical situation, this procedure would be repeated four to eight times for 10 to 20 min. Reassess the patient periodically.

11. Note the quantity, color, and consistency of any sputum expectorated. Note the presence or absence of blood.

12. *"Chart" the therapy on your laboratory report.*

EXERCISE 11.8 Inspiratory Resistive Muscle Training

Inspiratory resistive muscle training is usually performed over a 6-week training period for approximately 30 min/day with a gradual increase in workload.[3]

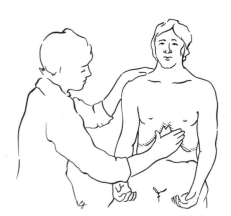

FIGURE 11.19 Abdominal breathing in the sitting position. (From Frownfelter, D: Chest Physical Therapy and Pulmonary Rehabilitation—An Interdisciplinary Approach, ed 2. Mosby-Year Book, St. Louis, 1987, p. 238, with permission.)

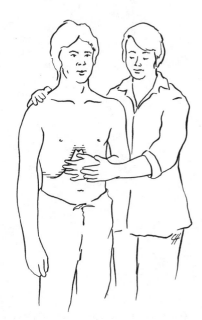

FIGURE 11.20 Abdominal breathing while standing. (From Frownfelter, D: Chest Physical Therapy and Pulmonary Rehabilitation—An Interdisciplinary Approach, ed 2. Mosby-Year Book, St. Louis, 1987, p. 239, with permission.)

1. Wash your hands and apply standard precautions and transmission-based isolation procedures as appropriate.
2. Set up the device as shown in Figure 11.23 or Figure 11.24. A flow-resistive or threshold-resistive device may be used.
3. Measure the patient's maximum inspiratory pressure using a pressure manometer.
4. Select the inspiratory resistive device (colored caps or dial selector) with the largest opening and apply it to the inspiratory port.
5. Attach the pressure manometer in-line to the monitoring adaptor.
6. Place nose clips comfortably on the patient's nose.
7. Have the patient make a tight seal around the mouthpiece.
8. Instruct the patient to inhale and exhale *slowly* through the mouthpiece.
9. Note the manometer pressure during inspiration. Adjust the inspiratory resistive orifice until you are using the resistor that achieves 30 percent of the patient's MIP effort.
10. In an actual clinical situation, this would be repeated for 15 min twice daily.[3]
11. *"Chart" the therapy on your laboratory report.*

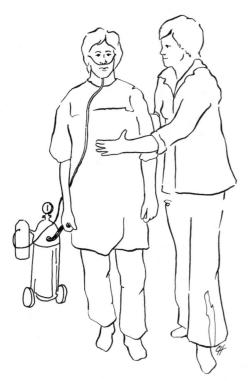

FIGURE 11.21   Breathing retraining while walking with oxygen. (From Frownfelter D: Chest Physical Therapy and Pulmonary Rehabilitation—An Interdisciplinary Approach, ed 2. Mosby-Year Book, St. Louis, 1987, p. 239, with permission.)

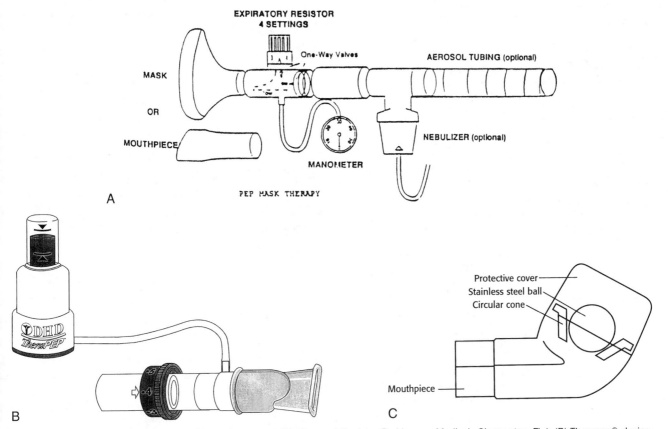

FIGURE 11.22   *(A)* Components of a PEP mask system. (Courtesy of Resistex™, Mercury Medical, Clearwater, FL.) *(B)* Therapep® device. Therapep® is a registered trademark of Diemolding Corp. (Courtesy of Diemolding Corp., DHD Healthcare, Canastota, NY.) *(C)* Flutter valve. (Reprinted by permission of Nellcor Puritan Bennett, Pleasanton, CA.)

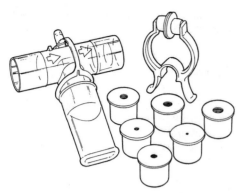

FIGURE 11.23 Flow-resistive inspiratory muscle-training device. (From HealthScan Products, Inc., Cedar Grove, NJ 07009, with permission.)

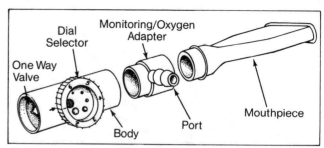

FIGURE 11.24 Threshold-resistive inspiratory muscle-training device. (From HealthScan Products Inc., Cedar Grove, NJ 07009, with permission.)

References

1. American Association for Respiratory Care: AARC clinical practice guideline: Postural drainage therapy. Respir Care 36:1418–1426, 1991.
2. Frownfelter, D: Chest Physical Therapy and Pulmonary Rehabilitation: An Interdisciplinary Approach, ed 2. Mosby, St Louis, 1989.
3. Scanlan, C et al (eds): Egan's Fundamentals of Respiratory Care, ed 6. Mosby, St Louis, 1995.
4. American Association for Respiratory Care: AARC clinical practice guideline: Directed cough. Respir Care 38:495–499, 1993.
5. Mahlmeister, M et al: Positive expiratory pressure mask therapy: Theoretical and practical consideration and a review of the literature. Respir Care 36:1218–1230, 1991.
6. American Association for Respiratory Care: AARC clinical practice guideline: Use of positive airway pressure adjuncts to bronchial hygiene therapy. Respir Care 38:516–521, 1993.

Related Readings

Eubanks, DH and Bone, RC: Principles and Applications of Cardiorespiratory Care Equipment. Mosby, St Louis, 1994.
Frownfelter, D: Chest Physical Therapy and Pulmonary Rehabilitation: An Interdisciplinary Approach, ed 2. Mosby, St Louis, 1989.
McPherson, S: Respiratory Care Equipment, ed 5. Mosby, St Louis, 1995.
Scanlan, C et al (eds): Egan's Fundamentals of Respiratory Care, ed 6. Mosby, St Louis, 1995.

Selected Journal Articles

American Association for Respiratory Care: AARC clinical practice guideline: Postural drainage therapy. Respir Care 36:1418–1426, 1991.

American Association for Respiratory Care: AARC clinical practice guideline: Directed cough. Respir Care 38:495–499, 1993.
American Association for Respiratory Care: AARC clinical practice guideline: Use of positive airway pressure adjuncts to bronchial hygiene therapy. Respir Care 38:516–521, 1993.
Anonymous: Down with the good lung (usually). Respir Care 32:849–850, 1987.
Arens, R et al: Comparison of high frequency chest compression and conventional chest physiotherapy in hospitalized patients with cystic fibrosis. Am J Respir Crit Care Med 150:1154–1157, 1994.
Bach, JR: Mechanical insufflation-exsufflation: Comparison of peak expiratory flows with manually assisted and unassisted coughing techniques. Chest 104:1553–1562, 1993.
Bach, JR: Update and perspective on noninvasive respiratory muscle aids. Part 2: The expiratory aids. Chest 105:1538–1544, 1994.
Bauer, ML, McDougal, J and Schoumacher, RA: Comparison of manual and mechanical chest percussion in hospitalized patients with cystic fibrosis. J Pediatr 124:250–254, 1994.
Breslin, EH: Diaphragm and parasternal muscle recruitment, thoracoabdominal motion, and dyspnea responses to upper extremity exercise with normal breathing and inspiratory resistance breathing. University of California, 1989.
Eid, N et al: Chest physiotherapy in review. Respir Care 36:270–282, 1991.
Lewis, R: Chest physiotherapy: Time for redefinition and renaming. Respir Care 37:419–421, 1992.
Mahler, DA and Horowitz, MB: Clinical evaluation of exertional dyspnea. Clin Chest Med 15:259–269, 1994.
Mahlmeister, M et al: Positive-expiratory pressure mask therapy: Theoretical and practical consideration and a review of the literature. Respir Care 36:1218–1230, 1991.
National Board for Respiratory Care: Positive expiratory pressure therapy. NBRC Horizons 19, 1993.
Preusser, BA, Winningham, ML and Clanton, TL: High vs. low intensity inspiratory muscle interval training in patients with COPD. Chest 106:110–117, 1994.
Reardon, J et al: The effect of comprehensive outpatient pulmonary rehabilitation on dyspnea. Chest 105:1046–1052, 1994.

LABORATORY REPORT

CHAPTER 11: BRONCHIAL HYGIENE TECHNIQUES

Name _____   Date _____

Course/Section _____   Instructor _____

Data Collection

EXERCISE 11.1   Identification of Lung Lobes and Segments

Label Figures 11.25 and 11.26 with the number corresponding to the appropriate lobes and segments.

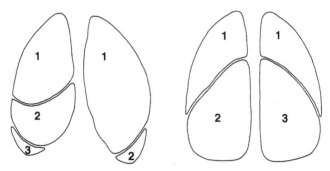

FIGURE 11.25   Label the lobes of the lungs.

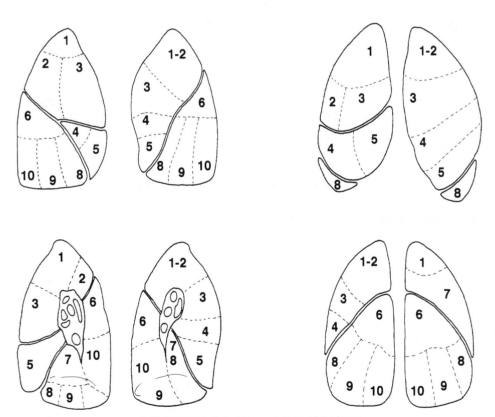

FIGURE 11.26   Label the segments of the lungs.

EXERCISE 11.2   Postural Drainage

EXERCISE 11.2.1   Postural Drainage Positioning in Adults

1. "Chart" the therapy given, including patient assessment and patient response, as you would on a legal medical record.

_____

_____

_____

_____

_____

_____

_____

2. Identify the lobes and segments being drained in Figure 11.27.

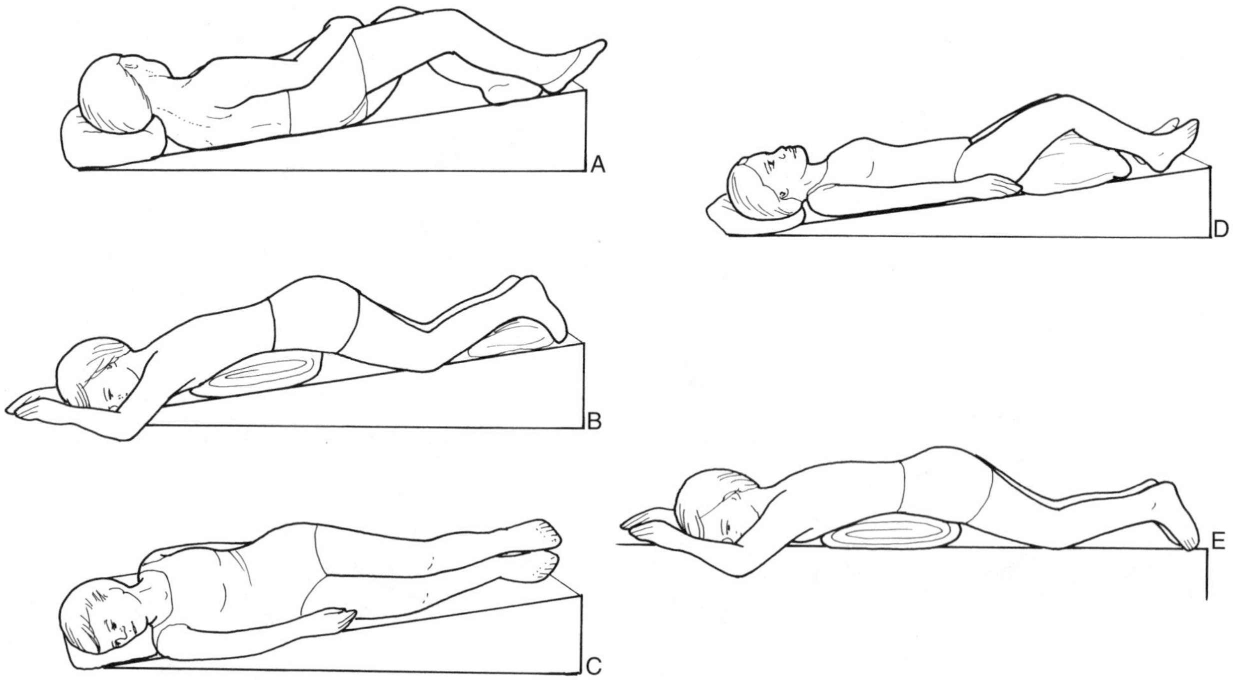

FIGURE 11.27   Label the segments being drained in the positions shown.

EXERCISE 11.7   Positive Expiratory Pressure Mask Therapy

"Chart" the therapy given as you would on a legal medical record. Be sure to include all pertinent data and measurements.

_____

_____

_____

_____

_____

_____

_____

EXERCISE 11.8   Inspiratory Resistive Muscle Training
"Chart" the therapy given below as you would on a legal medical record. Be sure to include all pertinent data and measurements.

_____

_____

_____

_____

_____

_____

_____

CRITICAL THINKING QUESTIONS

1. An 82-year-old woman with a history of osteoporosis who has recently undergone thoracic surgery has been producing large amounts of purulent secretions. The physician has ordered CPT. What recommendations or modifications would you suggest to accomplish this therapy?

2. Identify the possible hazards of PEP mask therapy. State at least one situation in which the procedure may be contraindicated.

3. A physician has ordered chest physical therapy on a postoperative craniotomy patient whose chart indicates that the head of the bed must remain elevated 30°. Identify what modifications to therapy or recommendations you believe are necessary in this situation, and explain why.

4. A 17-year-old girl with cystic fibrosis who has copious sputum production complains of dyspnea and shows signs of mild cyanosis during postural drainage positioning in the Trendelenburg position.
   a. What modifications or recommendations can be made to improve the patient's tolerance of the procedure?
   b. How would you monitor the effectiveness of these modifications?

5. A 65-year-old woman with COPD has begun a breathing exercise regimen. What data, objective and subjective, would indicate beneficial effects of this program?

6. A 25-year-old man with quadriplegia and a tracheostomy has been experiencing recurrent atelectasis in the RML and RLL.
   a. How would you _assess_ what positions to place the patient in for postural drainage?
   b. Describe the appropriate positioning in this situation.
   c. The patient is unable to adequately cough spontaneously after postural drainage. What techniques could be incorporated to improve his cough effort and to remove any mobilized secretions?

PROCEDURAL COMPETENCY EVALUATION

Name _____ Date _____

Directed Cough Techniques

Setting: ☐ Lab ☐ Clinical   Evaluator: ☐ Peer ☐ Instructor

Conditions (describe): _____

_____

Equipment Used

_____

_____

	SATISFACTORY	UNSATISFACTORY	NOT OBSERVED	NOT APPLICABLE
Equipment and Patient Preparation				
1. Verifies, interprets, and evaluates physician's order or protocol	☐	☐	☐	☐
2. Scans chart for diagnosis and any other pertinent data and notes	☐	☐	☐	☐
3. Selects, gathers, and assembles the necessary equipment: pillows, tissues, and waste receptacle	☐	☐	☐	☐
4. Washes hands and applies standard precautions and transmission-based isolation procedures as appropriate	☐	☐	☐	☐
5. Identifies patient, introduces self and department	☐	☐	☐	☐
6. Explains purpose of the procedure and confirms patient understanding	☐	☐	☐	☐
Assessment and Implementation				
7. Assesses patient	☐	☐	☐	☐
8. Positions patient in Fowler's position (or side-lying position with knees bent)	☐	☐	☐	☐
9. Reassesses patient	☐	☐	☐	☐
10. Instructs patient in effective use of diaphragm	☐	☐	☐	☐
11. Demonstrates cough phases	☐	☐	☐	☐
12. Instructs the patient regarding incisional support (postoperative splinting)	☐	☐	☐	☐
13. Encourages deep inspiration, inspiratory hold	☐	☐	☐	☐
14. Ensures forceful contraction of abdominal muscles	☐	☐	☐	☐
15. Observes and corrects common errors	☐	☐	☐	☐
16. Modifies technique as appropriate to patient	☐	☐	☐	☐
17. Reassesses patient and reinstructs as needed	☐	☐	☐	☐
18. Repeats procedure as indicated and tolerated	☐	☐	☐	☐
19. Examines (collects) sputum	☐	☐	☐	☐
20. Instructs the patient in serial coughing techniques				
a. Moderately deep breath, followed by a slight breath hold; then perform two or three short coughs, one after another; rest and repeat the procedure	☐	☐	☐	☐
21. Instructs the patient in a forced expiratory technique or huffing maneuver				
a. Moderately deep breath, followed by a short breath hold; perform three short forced exhalations with an open glottis; the patient should make a huffing or "Ha-ha-ha" sound on exhalation; follow this with a period of relaxed, controlled diaphragmatic breathing	☐	☐	☐	☐

	S A T I S F A C T O R Y	U N S A T I S F A C T O R Y	N O T O B S E R V E D	N O T A P P L I C A B L E

b. Assist by self-compression of the chest wall by using a brisk adduction movement of the upper arms, also known as a "chicken breath" ☐ ☐ ☐ ☐

22. Provides manually assisted cough, using epigastric pressure or external lateral compression of the thoracic cage

a. Instructs the patient to take a moderately deep breath, followed by a short breath hold; applies gentle pressure to the epigastric region coordinated with the patient's cough effort, making sure to avoid the xiphoid area; this should not be done after meals ☐ ☐ ☐ ☐

b. Moderately deep breath, followed by a short breath hold; applies pressure to the lateral thoracic cage coordinated with the patient's cough effort ☐ ☐ ☐ ☐

23. With tracheostomy, provides manually assisted deep inspiration using a manual resuscitator bag in conjunction with manually assisted cough techniques ☐ ☐ ☐ ☐

Follow-up

24. Returns patient to comfortable position ☐ ☐ ☐ ☐

25. Maintains/processes equipment ☐ ☐ ☐ ☐

26. Disposes of infectious waste and washes hands ☐ ☐ ☐ ☐

27. Records pertinent data in chart and departmental records ☐ ☐ ☐ ☐

28. Notifies appropriate personnel and makes any necessary recommendations or modifications to the patient care plan ☐ ☐ ☐ ☐

_____   _____
Signature of Evaluator   Signature of Student

PERFORMANCE RATING SCALE

5 EXCELLENT—FAR EXCEEDS EXPECTED LEVEL, FLAWLESS PERFORMANCE
4 ABOVE AVERAGE—NO PROMPTING REQUIRED, ABLE TO SELF-CORRECT
3 AVERAGE—THE MINIMUM COMPETENCY LEVEL, NO CRITICAL ERRORS
2 IMPROVEMENT NEEDED—PROBLEM AREAS EXIST; CRITICAL ERRORS, CORRECTIONS NEEDED
1 POOR AND UNACCEPTABLE PERFORMANCE—GROSS INACCURACIES, POTENTIALLY HARMFUL

PERFORMANCE CRITERIA	SCALE				
1. DISPLAYS KNOWLEDGE OF ESSENTIAL CONCEPTS	5	4	3	2	1
2. DEMONSTRATES THE RELATIONSHIP BETWEEN THEORY AND CLINICAL PRACTICE	5	4	3	2	1
3. FOLLOWS DIRECTIONS, EXHIBITS SOUND JUDGMENT, AND DEMONSTRATES ATTENTION TO SAFETY AND DETAIL	5	4	3	2	1
4. EXHIBITS THE REQUIRED MANUAL DEXTERITY	5	4	3	2	1
5. PERFORMS PROCEDURE IN A REASONABLE TIME FRAME	5	4	3	2	1
6. MAINTAINS STERILE OR ASEPTIC TECHNIQUE	5	4	3	2	1
7. INITIATES UNAMBIGUOUS GOAL-DIRECTED COMMUNICATION	5	4	3	2	1
8. PROVIDES FOR ADEQUATE CARE AND MAINTENANCE OF EQUIPMENT AND SUPPLIES	5	4	3	2	1
9. EXHIBITS COURTEOUS AND PLEASANT DEMEANOR	5	4	3	2	1
10. MAINTAINS CONCISE AND ACCURATE RECORDS	5	4	3	2	1

ADDITIONAL COMMENTS: INCLUDE ERRORS OF OMISSION OR COMMISSION, COMMUNICATIVE SKILLS, AND EFFECTIVENESS OF PATIENT INTERACTION:

SUMMARY PERFORMANCE EVALUATION AND RECOMMENDATIONS

SATISFACTORY PERFORMANCE—Performed without error or prompting, or able to self-correct, no critical errors.

_____ LABORATORY EVALUATION. SKILLS MAY BE APPLIED/OBSERVED IN THE CLINICAL SETTING.

_____ CLINICAL EVALUATION. STUDENT READY FOR MINIMALLY SUPERVISED APPLICATION AND REFINEMENT.

UNSATISFACTORY PERFORMANCE—Prompting required; performed with critical errors, potentially harmful.

_____ STUDENT REQUIRES ADDITIONAL LABORATORY PRACTICE.

_____ STUDENT REQUIRES ADDITIONAL SUPERVISED CLINICAL PRACTICE.

SIGNATURES

STUDENT: _____   EVALUATOR: _____

DATE: _____   DATE: _____

PROCEDURAL COMPETENCY EVALUATION

Name _____ Date _____

Chest Physiotherapy

Setting: ☐ Lab ☐ Clinical   Evaluator: ☐ Peer ☐ Instructor

Conditions (describe): _____

_____

Equipment Used

_____

_____

	S A T I S F A C T O R Y	U N S A T I S F A C T O R Y	N O T O B S E R V E D	N O T A P P L I C A B L E
Equipment and Patient Preparation				
1. Verifies, interprets, and evaluates physician's order or protocol; determines lobes/segments to be drained by reviewing chest x-ray results, progress notes, and diagnosis; scans chart for any possible contraindications	☐	☐	☐	☐
2. Scans chart for diagnosis and any other pertinent data and notes	☐	☐	☐	☐
3. Selects, gathers, and assembles the necessary equipment: blood pressure manometer, percussor (if needed), and pulse oximeter	☐	☐	☐	☐
4. Coordinates therapy before meals and tube feedings or 1 to 1½ hours after meals	☐	☐	☐	☐
5. Washes hands and applies standard precautions and transmission-based isolation procedures as appropriate	☐	☐	☐	☐
6. Identifies patient, introduces self and department	☐	☐	☐	☐
7. Explains purpose of the procedure and confirms patient understanding	☐	☐	☐	☐
Assessment and Implementation				
8. Assesses patient: pulse, respirations, blood pressure, auscultation, pulse oximetry, level of dyspnea, level of cooperation, and color	☐	☐	☐	☐
9. Instructs (demonstrates) patient in diaphragmatic breathing, segmental expansion, and coughing	☐	☐	☐	☐
10. Positions patient for segmental/lobar drainage, beginning with most dependent portions first	☐	☐	☐	☐
11. Reassesses patient response and tolerance	☐	☐	☐	☐
12. Modifies position to accommodate patient's response, if needed	☐	☐	☐	☐
13. Encourages maintenance of proper breathing pattern	☐	☐	☐	☐
14. Performs percussion over properly identified areas as indicated	☐	☐	☐	☐
15. Performs expiratory vibration over correct area during expiration, if needed	☐	☐	☐	☐
16. Maintains position for appropriate time interval (3 to 15 min) as tolerated	☐	☐	☐	☐
17. Encourages and assists patient with cough expectoration	☐	☐	☐	☐
18. Examines (collects) sputum	☐	☐	☐	☐
19. Repositions patient and repeats procedure as indicated and tolerated	☐	☐	☐	☐
20. Returns patient to comfortable position	☐	☐	☐	☐
21. Reassesses patient	☐	☐	☐	☐

	S A T I S F A C T O R Y	U N S A T I S F A C T O R Y	N O T O B S E R V E D	N O T A P P L I C A B L E

Follow-up

22. Maintains/processes equipment	☐	☐	☐	☐
23. Disposes of infectious waste and washes hands	☐	☐	☐	☐
24. Records pertinent data in chart and departmental records	☐	☐	☐	☐
25. Notifies appropriate personnel and makes any recommendations or modifications to patient care plan as indicated	☐	☐	☐	☐

_____
Signature of Evaluator

_____
Signature of Student

PERFORMANCE RATING SCALE

5 EXCELLENT—FAR EXCEEDS EXPECTED LEVEL, FLAWLESS PERFORMANCE
4 ABOVE AVERAGE—NO PROMPTING REQUIRED, ABLE TO SELF-CORRECT
3 AVERAGE—THE MINIMUM COMPETENCY LEVEL, NO CRITICAL ERRORS
2 IMPROVEMENT NEEDED—PROBLEM AREAS EXIST; CRITICAL ERRORS, CORRECTIONS NEEDED
1 POOR AND UNACCEPTABLE PERFORMANCE—GROSS INACCURACIES, POTENTIALLY HARMFUL

PERFORMANCE CRITERIA		SCALE			
1. DISPLAYS KNOWLEDGE OF ESSENTIAL CONCEPTS	5	4	3	2	1
2. DEMONSTRATES THE RELATIONSHIP BETWEEN THEORY AND CLINICAL PRACTICE	5	4	3	2	1
3. FOLLOWS DIRECTIONS, EXHIBITS SOUND JUDGMENT, AND DEMONSTRATES ATTENTION TO SAFETY AND DETAIL	5	4	3	2	1
4. EXHIBITS THE REQUIRED MANUAL DEXTERITY	5	4	3	2	1
5. PERFORMS PROCEDURE IN A REASONABLE TIME FRAME	5	4	3	2	1
6. MAINTAINS STERILE OR ASEPTIC TECHNIQUE	5	4	3	2	1
7. INITIATES UNAMBIGUOUS GOAL-DIRECTED COMMUNICATION	5	4	3	2	1
8. PROVIDES FOR ADEQUATE CARE AND MAINTENANCE OF EQUIPMENT AND SUPPLIES	5	4	3	2	1
9. EXHIBITS COURTEOUS AND PLEASANT DEMEANOR	5	4	3	2	1
10. MAINTAINS CONCISE AND ACCURATE RECORDS	5	4	3	2	1

ADDITIONAL COMMENTS: INCLUDE ERRORS OF OMISSION OR COMMISSION, COMMUNICATIVE SKILLS, AND EFFECTIVENESS OF PATIENT INTERACTION:

SUMMARY PERFORMANCE EVALUATION AND RECOMMENDATIONS

SATISFACTORY PERFORMANCE—Performed without error or prompting, or able to self-correct, no critical errors.

_____ LABORATORY EVALUATION. SKILLS MAY BE APPLIED/OBSERVED IN THE CLINICAL SETTING.

_____ CLINICAL EVALUATION. STUDENT READY FOR MINIMALLY SUPERVISED APPLICATION AND REFINEMENT.

UNSATISFACTORY PERFORMANCE—Prompting required; performed with critical errors, potentially harmful.

_____ STUDENT REQUIRES ADDITIONAL LABORATORY PRACTICE.

_____ STUDENT REQUIRES ADDITIONAL SUPERVISED CLINICAL PRACTICE.

SIGNATURES

STUDENT: _____   EVALUATOR: _____

DATE: _____   DATE: _____

PROCEDURAL COMPETENCY EVALUATION

Name _____ Date _____

Positive Expiratory Pressure Mask Therapy

Setting: ☐ Lab ☐ Clinical   Evaluator: ☐ Peer ☐ Instructor

Conditions (describe): _____

_____

Equipment Used

_____

_____

	SATISFACTORY	UNSATISFACTORY	NOT OBSERVED	NOT APPLICABLE
Equipment and Patient Preparation				
1. Verifies, interprets, and evaluates physician's order or protocol	☐	☐	☐	☐
2. Scans chart for diagnosis and any other pertinent data and notes	☐	☐	☐	☐
3. Selects, gathers, and assembles the necessary equipment: PEP mask, manometer, adaptors, mask or mouthpiece, noseclips, tissues, and infectious waste receptacle	☐	☐	☐	☐
4. Washes hands and applies standard precautions and transmission-based isolation procedures as appropriate	☐	☐	☐	☐
5. Identifies patient, introduces self and department	☐	☐	☐	☐
6. Explains purpose of the procedure and confirms patient understanding	☐	☐	☐	☐
Assessment and Implementation				
7. Assesses patient's vital signs, mental function, skin color, and breath sounds	☐	☐	☐	☐
8. Adjusts fixed exhalation orifice to the largest setting	☐	☐	☐	☐
9. Positions patient upright, with his or her elbows resting comfortably on a table	☐	☐	☐	☐
10. Places the mask comfortably but tightly over the nose and mouth or adjusts nose clips and mouthpiece	☐	☐	☐	☐
11. Instructs patient to take a larger than normal breath (but not to TLC) and exhale slowly at an I:E ratio of 1:3 or 1:4	☐	☐	☐	☐
12. Observes pressure generated on the manometer during exhalation; decreases size of the fixed orifice until 10 to 20 cm H_2O pressure is generated during exhalation	☐	☐	☐	☐
13. Instructs patient to take 10 to 20 breaths followed by two or three huffs (FET); repeats four to eight times for 10 to 20 min	☐	☐	☐	☐
14. Reassesses patient periodically and reinstructs if necessary	☐	☐	☐	☐
15. Encourages cough periodically, examines/collects sputum	☐	☐	☐	☐
Follow-up				
16. Maintains/processes equipment	☐	☐	☐	☐
17. Disposes of infectious waste and washes hands	☐	☐	☐	☐
18. Records pertinent data in chart and departmental records	☐	☐	☐	☐
19. Notifies appropriate personnel and makes recommendations or modifications to patient care plan	☐	☐	☐	☐

_____   _____
Signature of Evaluator   Signature of Student

PERFORMANCE RATING SCALE

5 EXCELLENT—FAR EXCEEDS EXPECTED LEVEL, FLAWLESS PERFORMANCE
4 ABOVE AVERAGE—NO PROMPTING REQUIRED, ABLE TO SELF-CORRECT
3 AVERAGE—THE MINIMUM COMPETENCY LEVEL, NO CRITICAL ERRORS
2 IMPROVEMENT NEEDED—PROBLEM AREAS EXIST; CRITICAL ERRORS, CORRECTIONS NEEDED
1 POOR AND UNACCEPTABLE PERFORMANCE—GROSS INACCURACIES, POTENTIALLY HARMFUL

PERFORMANCE CRITERIA		SCALE			
1. DISPLAYS KNOWLEDGE OF ESSENTIAL CONCEPTS	5	4	3	2	1
2. DEMONSTRATES THE RELATIONSHIP BETWEEN THEORY AND CLINICAL PRACTICE	5	4	3	2	1
3. FOLLOWS DIRECTIONS, EXHIBITS SOUND JUDGMENT, AND DEMONSTRATES ATTENTION TO SAFETY AND DETAIL	5	4	3	2	1
4. EXHIBITS THE REQUIRED MANUAL DEXTERITY	5	4	3	2	1
5. PERFORMS PROCEDURE IN A REASONABLE TIME FRAME	5	4	3	2	1
6. MAINTAINS STERILE OR ASEPTIC TECHNIQUE	5	4	3	2	1
7. INITIATES UNAMBIGUOUS GOAL-DIRECTED COMMUNICATION	5	4	3	2	1
8. PROVIDES FOR ADEQUATE CARE AND MAINTENANCE OF EQUIPMENT AND SUPPLIES	5	4	3	2	1
9. EXHIBITS COURTEOUS AND PLEASANT DEMEANOR	5	4	3	2	1
10. MAINTAINS CONCISE AND ACCURATE RECORDS	5	4	3	2	1

ADDITIONAL COMMENTS: INCLUDE ERRORS OF OMISSION OR COMMISSION, COMMUNICATIVE SKILLS, AND EFFECTIVENESS OF PATIENT INTERACTION:

SUMMARY PERFORMANCE EVALUATION AND RECOMMENDATIONS

SATISFACTORY PERFORMANCE—Performed without error or prompting, or able to self-correct, no critical errors.

———— LABORATORY EVALUATION. SKILLS MAY BE APPLIED/OBSERVED IN THE CLINICAL SETTING.

———— CLINICAL EVALUATION. STUDENT READY FOR MINIMALLY SUPERVISED APPLICATION AND REFINEMENT.

UNSATISFACTORY PERFORMANCE—Prompting required; performed with critical errors, potentially harmful.

———— STUDENT REQUIRES ADDITIONAL LABORATORY PRACTICE.

———— STUDENT REQUIRES ADDITIONAL SUPERVISED CLINICAL PRACTICE.

SIGNATURES

STUDENT: _____   EVALUATOR: _____

DATE: _____   DATE: _____

PROCEDURAL COMPETENCY EVALUATION

Name _____ Date _____

Inspiratory Resistive Muscle Training

Setting: ☐ Lab ☐ Clinical   Evaluator: ☐ Peer ☐ Instructor

Conditions (describe): _____

_____

Equipment Used

_____

_____

	SATISFACTORY	UNSATISFACTORY	NOT OBSERVED	NOT APPLICABLE
Equipment and Patient Preparation				
1. Verifies, interprets, and evaluates physician's order or protocol	☐	☐	☐	☐
2. Scans chart for diagnosis and any other pertinent data and notes	☐	☐	☐	☐
3. Selects, gathers, and assembles the necessary equipment: muscle training device, mask or mouthpiece and noseclips, and pressure manometer	☐	☐	☐	☐
4. Washes hands and applies standard precautions and transmission-based isolation procedures as appropriate	☐	☐	☐	☐
5. Identifies patient, introduces self and department	☐	☐	☐	☐
6. Explains purpose of the procedure and confirms patient understanding	☐	☐	☐	☐
Assessment and Implementation				
7. Assesses patient, including vital signs and auscultation	☐	☐	☐	☐
8. Measures maximum inspiratory pressure	☐	☐	☐	☐
9. Positions patient	☐	☐	☐	☐
10. Selects inspiratory resistive device or dial selector with least resistance	☐	☐	☐	☐
11. Attaches pressure manometer in-line	☐	☐	☐	☐
12. Comfortably places nose clips	☐	☐	☐	☐
13. Instructs patient to inhale and exhale *slowly* through the mouthpiece, maintaining tight seal	☐	☐	☐	☐
14. Notes manometer pressure during inspiration; adjusts inspiratory resistive orifice to achieve 30 percent of MIP	☐	☐	☐	☐
15. Instructs patient to repeat exercise for 15 min twice daily	☐	☐	☐	☐
16. Reassesses patient periodically and reinstructs if necessary	☐	☐	☐	☐
17. Encourages cough periodically, examines/collects sputum	☐	☐	☐	☐
Follow-up				
18. Maintains/processes equipment	☐	☐	☐	☐
19. Disposes of infectious waste and washes hands	☐	☐	☐	☐
20. Records pertinent data in chart and departmental records	☐	☐	☐	☐
21. Notifies appropriate personnel and makes any necessary recommendations or modifications to the patient care plan	☐	☐	☐	☐

_____   _____
Signature of Evaluator   Signature of Student

PERFORMANCE RATING SCALE

5 EXCELLENT—FAR EXCEEDS EXPECTED LEVEL, FLAWLESS PERFORMANCE
4 ABOVE AVERAGE—NO PROMPTING REQUIRED, ABLE TO SELF-CORRECT
3 AVERAGE—THE MINIMUM COMPETENCY LEVEL, NO CRITICAL ERRORS
2 IMPROVEMENT NEEDED—PROBLEM AREAS EXIST; CRITICAL ERRORS, CORRECTIONS NEEDED
1 POOR AND UNACCEPTABLE PERFORMANCE—GROSS INACCURACIES, POTENTIALLY HARMFUL

PERFORMANCE CRITERIA	SCALE				
1. DISPLAYS KNOWLEDGE OF ESSENTIAL CONCEPTS	5	4	3	2	1
2. DEMONSTRATES THE RELATIONSHIP BETWEEN THEORY AND CLINICAL PRACTICE	5	4	3	2	1
3. FOLLOWS DIRECTIONS, EXHIBITS SOUND JUDGMENT, AND DEMONSTRATES ATTENTION TO SAFETY AND DETAIL	5	4	3	2	1
4. EXHIBITS THE REQUIRED MANUAL DEXTERITY	5	4	3	2	1
5. PERFORMS PROCEDURE IN A REASONABLE TIME FRAME	5	4	3	2	1
6. MAINTAINS STERILE OR ASEPTIC TECHNIQUE	5	4	3	2	1
7. INITIATES UNAMBIGUOUS GOAL-DIRECTED COMMUNICATION	5	4	3	2	1
8. PROVIDES FOR ADEQUATE CARE AND MAINTENANCE OF EQUIPMENT AND SUPPLIES	5	4	3	2	1
9. EXHIBITS COURTEOUS AND PLEASANT DEMEANOR	5	4	3	2	1
10. MAINTAINS CONCISE AND ACCURATE RECORDS	5	4	3	2	1

ADDITIONAL COMMENTS: INCLUDE ERRORS OF OMISSION OR COMMISSION, COMMUNICATIVE SKILLS, AND EFFECTIVENESS OF PATIENT INTERACTION:

SUMMARY PERFORMANCE EVALUATION AND RECOMMENDATIONS

SATISFACTORY PERFORMANCE—Performed without error or prompting, or able to self-correct, no critical errors.

_____ LABORATORY EVALUATION. SKILLS MAY BE APPLIED/OBSERVED IN THE CLINICAL SETTING.

_____ CLINICAL EVALUATION. STUDENT READY FOR MINIMALLY SUPERVISED APPLICATION AND REFINEMENT.

UNSATISFACTORY PERFORMANCE—Prompting required; performed with critical errors, potentially harmful.

_____ STUDENT REQUIRES ADDITIONAL LABORATORY PRACTICE.

_____ STUDENT REQUIRES ADDITIONAL SUPERVISED CLINICAL PRACTICE.

SIGNATURES

STUDENT: _____   EVALUATOR: _____

DATE: _____   DATE: _____

Manual Resuscitators and Manual Ventilation

INTRODUCTION

Manual resuscitators are adjunctive devices used to support short-term artificial ventilation. Situations that may require their use include transport of ventilated patients, application of positive pressure breaths for hyperinflation and oxygenation during suctioning, ventilator malfunction, and cough assisting. These devices can be used to assist the spontaneously breathing patient and to fully support the apneic patient.

One of the most important uses of these devices is to support ventilation during a respiratory or cardiac arrest. The respiratory care practitioner is often one of the first members of the health care team to arrive at a **resuscitation** event and is usually responsible for airway maintenance and ventilation. It is imperative, therefore, that the respiratory care practitioner understand the capabilities and functioning of manual resuscitation devices and be able to troubleshoot them in an emergency situation.

In basic life support procedures, rescue breathing is accomplished by mouth-to-mouth ventilation. In the health care environment, mouth-to-mask ventilation and bag-valve-mask ventilation are used. Bag-valve-mask devices, or manual resuscitators, have changed over the years. Standards for these devices are published by the American Society for Testing and Materials[1] and in the *Journal of the American Medical Association.*[2] These standards include the following:

- Criteria for F_1O_2 delivery
- Prevention of valve malfunction up to flows of 30 lpm
- A valve that is easily cleaned (within 20 sec) if vomitus prevents proper functioning
- A universal 15/22 mm adaptor for the patient connection
- Durability and ability to withstand shock
- An override capability of the pressure relief valve
- A 40 cm H_2O pressure relief valve for neonatal and pediatric bags

Considerations for the practitioner in selecting a resuscitation device should include the following:

- Good "feel" to determine patient's lung compliance
- Quick inflation and refill response
- Adequate ventilating volumes
- Ease of valve opening with the patient's spontaneous breathing efforts
- Durability (if nondisposable)
- Ease of assembly/disassembly

OBJECTIVES
Upon completion of this chapter, the student will be able to:

1. Identify and differentiate the types of patient valves and how each operates during inspiration and expiration.
2. Identify and discuss the advantages and disadvantages of self-filling and flow-filling bags.
3. Assemble and disassemble each type of device.
4. Demonstrate effective manual ventilation techniques with mouth-to-mask devices, bag-valve-mask devices, and bag-valve resuscitators to an artificial airway and a spontaneously breathing subject.
5. Explain the purpose of a pressure relief valve on a manual resuscitator, and demonstrate its operation.
6. Discuss the relationship between resistance, compliance, and the amount of positive pressure necessary to accomplish ventilation.
7. Compare the variability in positive pressure, volume delivery, and F_1O_2 using different ventilation techniques.

KEY TERMS   hyperextension   insufflation   resuscitation

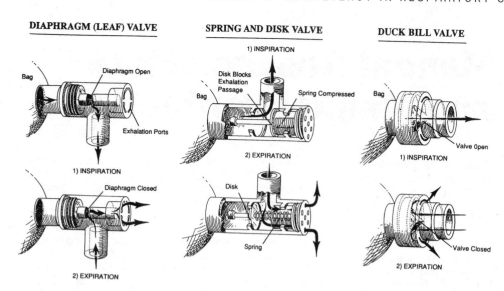

DIAPHRAGM (LEAF) VALVE

SPRING AND DISK VALVE

DUCK BILL VALVE

FIGURE 12.1 Nonrebreathing valves commonly used with manual resuscitators. (From Branson, RD, Hess, DR and Chatburn, RL: Respiratory Care Equipment. JB Lippincott, Philadelphia, 1995, p. 153, with permission.)

EQUIPMENT REQUIRED

- Spring-loaded, duckbill/diaphragm, and diaphragm/leaf types of adult and neonatal/pediatric resuscitators
- Masks of various sizes
- Mouth-valve-mask resuscitation unit (pocket mask)
- Oxygen gas source
- Oxygen connecting tubing
- Intubated and nonintubated mannequins (adult and infant)
- Pressure manometers
- Respirometers
- Oxygen analyzers
- Adaptors and connectors
- Computerized lung simulator or test lungs

● E X E R C I S E S

EXERCISE 12.1 Assembly and Disassembly of Resuscitators

1. Select one of each type of resuscitator: spring-loaded, duckbill/diaphragm, and diaphragm/leaf (Fig. 12.1). Study the type of valves and identify the manufacturers. *Record these on your laboratory report.*

2. Disassemble the unit completely. This step will depend on which bag you are disassembling. See the manufacturer's specifications or refer to an equipment text if needed.

3. Reassemble the units. Make sure there are no leftover parts.

4. Test the unit for proper function by occluding the outlet and squeezing the bag. *Record your observations on your laboratory report.*

5. Carefully observe the operation of the patient valve and oxygen inlet during inspiration and expiration. *Draw a schematic representation of the operation of the valves on your laboratory report.*

6. Repeat steps 2 through 5 for each bag selected.

EXERCISE 12.2 Mouth-to-Mask Ventilation

1. Select a mouth-valve-mask breathing device.

2. Select an adult, unintubated mannequin.

3. Place the head in the proper position using the head-tilt/chin-lift technique learned in BLS, as shown in Figure 12.2.

4. Grasp the mask properly, as shown in Figure 12.3. Place your thumb over the bridge of the mask. Use the index and middle or middle and ring fingers to grasp just above the mask cushion.[3] Seal the mask over the mouth and nose, placing the mask on the bridge of the nose first (Fig. 12.4).

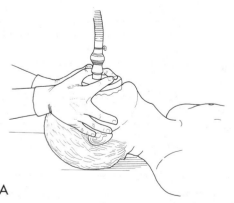

A

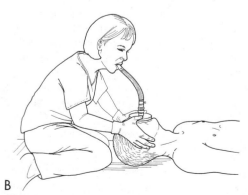

B

FIGURE 12.2 Mouth-to-mask ventilation with a one-way valve.

Using both hands, tilt the head back to reopen the airway, as shown in Figure 12.5.

5. Administer three breaths. Make sure you allow time for exhalation. Observe to see if the chest rises and falls.

6. Seal the mask over the nose using one hand only, without applying pressure on the mask over the chin. Administer three breaths. Observe to see if the chest rises and falls. *Record your observations on your laboratory report.*

7. Place the head in a neutral position without using any airway-opening techniques. Attempt to ventilate. *Record your observations on your laboratory report.*

EXERCISE 12.3 Manual Ventilation with Mask

1. Select adult and infant bag-valve-mask resuscitators.

2. Select infant and adult, unintubated mannequins.

3. Attach the oxygen supply tubing to the oxygen source and turn to 15 lpm.

4. Place the head in the proper position using the head-tilt/chin-lift technique.

5. Place the mask over the mouth and nose using one hand to achieve a seal *while maintaining proper head position.* This can be accomplished by using the last three fingers of your nondominant hand to seal the lower portion of the mask while lifting up on the jaw and using your thumb and index finger to secure the mask over the mouth and nose.

6. Administer ventilations at a rate of 12 breaths per minute for 5 min. Make sure the chest rises and falls, but do not hyperinflate.

7. Repeat these steps using the infant mannequin and resuscitator at a rate of 20 breaths per minute for 1 min. *Remember: do not hyperextend the infant's head to open the airway! Do not overventilate.*

8. *Record your observations on your laboratory report.*

EXERCISE 12.4 Manual Ventilation with an Intubated Mannequin

1. Select adult and infant bag-valve-mask resuscitators.

2. Select infant and adult intubated mannequins.

3. Attach the oxygen supply tubing to the oxygen source and turn to 15 lpm.

4. Connect the patient connector on the resuscitator to the 22/15 connector on the endotracheal tube.

5. Squeeze the bag and give the mannequin three breaths, allowing for sufficient exhalation after each breath. *Record your observations on your laboratory report.*

6. Repeat these steps using the infant mannequin and resuscitator.

7. Examine the pressure relief pop-off on the infant resuscitator. *Record the set pressure release on your laboratory report.*

8. Occlude the outlet of the bag while squeezing it. Observe the function of the pressure pop-off, and *record your observations on your laboratory report.*

9. Bypass the pressure relief mechanism so that it is nonfunctional. According to standards, it should be obvious how to do this. Refer to the manufacturer's literature or your instructor if you have any questions.

10. Occlude the outlet of the bag while squeezing it. Observe the function of the pressure pop-off, and *record your observations on your laboratory report.*

EXERCISE 12.5 Measurement of Pressures, Stroke Volumes, and F_IO_2

1. Using the same equipment as in Exercise 12.4, attach a pressure manometer, respirometer, and oxygen analyzer in-line between the patient valve and the endotracheal tube connection, as shown in Figure 12.6. Make sure you have the oxygen turned up to 15 lpm before proceeding to step 2.

2. Squeeze the bag gently with one hand several times, allowing for sufficient exhalation between breaths. *Record the pressure generated, the F_IO_2, and the volume delivered on your laboratory report.*

3. Repeat the exercise, except this time squeeze the bag vigorously with both hands. *Record the pressure generated, F_IO_2, and the volume delivered on your laboratory report.*

4. Disconnect the reservoir and repeat the measurement.

5. Reattach the reservoir.

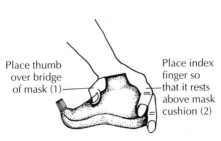

FIGURE 12.3 Proper hand position for resuscitator mask. (From Eubanks, DH and Bone, RC: Comprehensive Respiratory Care: A Learning System, ed 2. Mosby-Year Book, St. Louis, 1990, p. 642, with permission.)

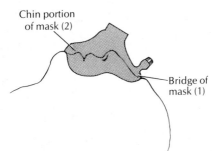

FIGURE 12.4 Mask position on face. (From Eubanks, DH and Bone, RC: Comprehensive Respiratory Care: A Learning System, ed 2. Mosby-Year Book, St. Louis, 1990, p. 642, with permission.)

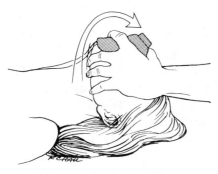

FIGURE 12.5 Performing head-tilt maneuver with mask in place. (From Eubanks, DH and Bone, RC: Comprehensive Respiratory Care: A Learning System, ed 2. Mosby-Year Book, St. Louis, 1990, p. 642, with permission.)

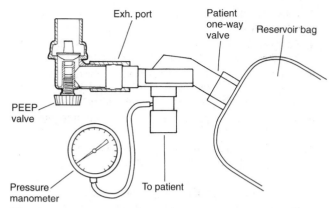

FIGURE 12.6 Monitoring equipment and PEEP valve in-line with manual resuscitator. (Courtesy of Instrumentation Industries, Inc., Bethel Park, PA.)

6. Turn the liter flow down to 8 lpm and repeat the one-handed squeeze and the two-handed squeeze. *Record the F$_I$O$_2$ delivered on your laboratory report.*

7. Disconnect the reservoir and repeat the measurement. *Record the F$_I$O$_2$ delivered on your laboratory report.*

8. Place a positive end-expiratory pressure (PEEP) valve on the exhalation valve of the resuscitator (see Fig. 12.6), and repeat the measurements. Depending on the type of bag being used, a special adaptor may be required. The PEEP valve may be preset or adjustable. *Record the type of valve used and the pressure setting on your laboratory report.*

The following exercises should be done using a lung simulator, if available. If not, a test lung can be adapted to approximate the resistance and compliance changes.

9. Set the resistance at R = 5 (normal resistance) and the compliance at 0.10 L/cm H$_2$O. Deliver three breaths, and *record the pressures and volumes on your laboratory report.* If a lung simulator is not available, use a standard test lung with an 8-mm endotracheal tube.

10. Increase the resistance to R = 50 (high resistance). Deliver three breaths, and *record the pressures and volumes on your laboratory report.* If a lung simulator is not available, use a standard test lung with a 3-mm endotracheal tube.

11. Return the resistance to R = 5 (normal resistance), and change the compliance to 0.01 L/cm H$_2$O. Deliver three breaths, and *record the pressures and volumes on your laboratory report.* If a lung simulator is not available, use a standard test lung with an 8-mm endotracheal tube. Place a rubber band around the center of the test lung.

EXERCISE 12.6 Assisted Manual Ventilation in a Spontaneously Breathing Subject

1. Select an adult bag-valve-mask resuscitator. Apply standard precautions and transmission-based isolation procedures as appropriate.

2. Attach the oxygen supply tubing to the oxygen source and turn to 15 lpm.

3. Using your laboratory partner as the subject, place the head in the proper position using the head-tilt/chin-lift technique.

4. Place the mask over the mouth and nose using one hand to achieve a seal while maintaining proper head position.

5. Allow your partner to breath spontaneously through the bag. Observe the valve operation.

6. Assist your partner's spontaneous ventilations. This is accomplished by timing when you squeeze the bag to synchronize with the early inspiratory phase. Administer a moderately deep ventilation. For your laboratory partner's comfort, do this only for every second or third breath.

7. Place the bags and masks in the designated dirty equipment area when this exercise is completed.

References

1. American Society for Testing and Materials: Standard Specifications for Performance and Safety Requirements for Resuscitators Intended for Use with Humans (F-920-85). Philadelphia, 1985.
2. American Heart Association: Guidelines for cardiopulmonary resuscitation and emergency cardiac care: Recommendations of the 1992 national conference. JAMA 268:2200, 1992.
3. Eubanks, DH and Bone, RC: Comprehensive Respiratory Care: A Learning System, ed 2. Mosby, St Louis, 1990, p 642.

Related Readings

American Society for Testing and Materials Committee on Manual Resuscitators: Standards for Minimal Performance and Safety Requirements for Resuscitators Intended for Use on Humans. American Materials Testing Society, Philadelphia, 1984.
Eubanks, DH and Bone, RC: Principles and Applications of Cardiorespiratory Care Equipment. Mosby, St Louis, 1994.
McPherson, S: Respiratory Care Equipment, ed 5. Mosby, St Louis, 1995.
Scanlan, C et al (eds): Egan's Fundamentals of Respiratory Care, ed 6. Mosby, St Louis, 1995.

Selected Journal Articles

American Association for Respiratory Care: Clinical practice guideline: Transport of the mechanically ventilated patient. Respir Care 38:1169–1172, 1993.
American Association for Respiratory Care: AARC clinical practice guideline: Management of airway emergencies. Respir Care 40:749–760, 1995.
American Association for Respiratory Care: Clinical practice guideline: Resuscitation in acute care hospitals. Respir Care 38:1179–1188, 1993.
Barnes, TA: Emergency ventilation techniques and related equipment. Respir Care 37:673–694, 1992.
Barnes, TA and McGarry, WP III: Evaluation of ten disposable manual resuscitators. Respir Care 35:960–968, 1990.
Barnes, TA and Stockwell, DL: Evaluation of ten manual resuscitators across an operational temperature range of −18 degrees C to 50 degrees C. Respir Care 36:161–172, 1991.
Barnes, TA and Watson, ME: Oxygen delivery performance of four adult resuscitation bags. Respir Care 27:139–146, 1982.
Chatburn, R: Decontamination of respiratory care equipment: What should be done, what can be done. Respir Care 34:98–110, 1989.
National conference on standards for cardiopulmonary resuscitation and emergency cardiac care. JAMA 255:2481, 1986.

LABORATORY REPORT

CHAPTER 12: MANUAL RESUSCITATORS AND MANUAL VENTILATION

Name _____ Date _____

Course/Section _____ Instructor _____

Data Collection

EXERCISE 12.1 Assembly and Disassembly of Resuscitators

Bag 1: Type of valve: _____

Name and manufacturer: _____

Flow or self-filling: _____

Schematic for inspiration:

Schematic for expiration:

Test function observations: _____

_____

Bag 2: Type of valve: _____

Name and manufacturer: _____

Flow or self-filling: _____

Schematic for inspiration:

Schematic for expiration:

Test function observations: _____

_____

Bag 3: Type of valve: _____

Name and manufacturer: _____

Flow or self-filling: _____

Schematic for inspiration:

Schematic for expiration:

Test function observations: _____

_____

EXERCISE 12.2   Mouth-to-Mask Ventilation

Observation of one-handed, nose seal only: _____

_____

Observations with head in neutral position: _____

_____

EXERCISE 12.3   Manual Ventilation with Mask

Observations: _____

_____

_____

EXERCISE 12.4   Manual Ventilation with an Intubated Mannequin

Observations: _____

_____

_____

Pressure relief setting: _____

Observations with occluded outlet: _____

_____

Observations with pressure relief bypassed: _____

_____

EXERCISE 12.5   Measurement of Pressures, Stroke Volumes, and F$_I$O$_2$
One-Hand Squeeze

Pressure: _____

Volume: _____

F$_I$O$_2$ with reservoir: _____

Two-Hand Squeeze

Pressure: _____

Volume: _____

F_IO_2: _____

F_IO_2 without reservoir: _____

Flow at 8 lpm

F_IO_2 with one-handed squeeze: _____

F_IO_2 with two-handed squeeze: _____

F_IO_2 without reservoir: _____

PEEP Valve Attachment

Pressure: _____

Volume: _____

Lung Simulator

Normal resistance ($R_p = 5$):   Pressure _____

Normal compliance 0.10 L/cm H_2O: Volume _____

Increased resistance ($R_p = 50$):   Pressure _____

                                        Volume _____

Resistance ($R_p = 5$):   Pressure _____

Decreased compliance 0.01 L/cm H_2O: Volume _____

CRITICAL THINKING QUESTIONS

1. Based on your observations in Exercise 12.1, how do you know that you assembled the device properly?

2. Identify at least three ways to increase the F_IO_2 delivered by a manual resuscitator.

3. What two additional techniques could be used to improve the patient's PaO_2 during manual ventilation?

4. What are the complications of manual ventilation? Compare and contrast adult ventilation with that of a neonate.

5. How can you initially assess the adequacy of manual ventilation? What limitations are there to ventilating with (a) a mask and (b) an artificial airway?

6. What effect did changes in compliance and resistance have on the volumes and pressures delivered?

7. What clinical situations would imitate the changes in compliance and resistance as demonstrated on the lung simulator?

PROCEDURAL COMPETENCY EVALUATION

Name _____ Date _____

Manual Ventilation

Setting: ☐ Lab ☐ Clinical   Evaluator: ☐ Peer ☐ Instructor

Conditions (describe): _____

_____

Equipment Used

_____

_____

	S A T I S F A C T O R Y	U N S A T I S F A C T O R Y	N O T O B S E R V E D	N O T A P P L I C A B L E
Equipment and Patient Preparation				
1. Selects, gathers, and assembles the necessary equipment: mask, bag-valve-mask, supplemental oxygen, flowmeter, and adaptors	☐	☐	☐	☐
2. Washes hands and applies standard precautions and transmission-based isolation procedures as appropriate	☐	☐	☐	☐
3. Identifies patient, introduces self and department	☐	☐	☐	☐
4. Explains purpose of the procedure and confirms patient understanding if the patient is alert	☐	☐	☐	☐
Assessment and Implementation				
5. Assesses patient for spontaneous breathing	☐	☐	☐	☐
6. Positions the patient's head	☐	☐	☐	☐
7. Adjusts liter flow	☐	☐	☐	☐
8. Applies mask to the face properly; if an artificial airway is employed, attaches the vale to the 22/15 mm adaptor	☐	☐	☐	☐
9. Squeezes the bag to administer a breath; timing with a spontaneous breath if indicated	☐	☐	☐	☐
10. Assesses the adequacy of ventilation: chest expansion and breath sounds	☐	☐	☐	☐
11. Repositions the head and mask if needed	☐	☐	☐	☐
12. Manually ventilates and assesses the adequacy of ventilation: chest expansion and breath sounds	☐	☐	☐	☐
13. Manually ventilates the patient, 12 to 16 breaths per minute; keeps up with the patient's own rate if the patient is spontaneously breathing	☐	☐	☐	☐
14. Reassesses the adequacy of ventilation: chest expansion and breath sounds	☐	☐	☐	☐
Follow-up				
15. Maintains/processes equipment	☐	☐	☐	☐
16. Disposes of infectious waste and washes hands	☐	☐	☐	☐
17. Records pertinent data in chart and departmental records	☐	☐	☐	☐
18. Notifies appropriate personnel and makes any necessary modifications or recommendations to patient care plan	☐	☐	☐	☐

_____   _____
Signature of Evaluator   Signature of Student

PERFORMANCE RATING SCALE

5 EXCELLENT—FAR EXCEEDS EXPECTED LEVEL, FLAWLESS PERFORMANCE
4 ABOVE AVERAGE—NO PROMPTING REQUIRED, ABLE TO SELF-CORRECT
3 AVERAGE—THE MINIMUM COMPETENCY LEVEL, NO CRITICAL ERRORS
2 IMPROVEMENT NEEDED—PROBLEM AREAS EXIST; CRITICAL ERRORS, CORRECTIONS NEEDED
1 POOR AND UNACCEPTABLE PERFORMANCE—GROSS INACCURACIES, POTENTIALLY HARMFUL

PERFORMANCE CRITERIA	SCALE				
1. DISPLAYS KNOWLEDGE OF ESSENTIAL CONCEPTS	5	4	3	2	1
2. DEMONSTRATES THE RELATIONSHIP BETWEEN THEORY AND CLINICAL PRACTICE	5	4	3	2	1
3. FOLLOWS DIRECTIONS, EXHIBITS SOUND JUDGMENT, AND DEMONSTRATES ATTENTION TO SAFETY AND DETAIL	5	4	3	2	1
4. EXHIBITS THE REQUIRED MANUAL DEXTERITY	5	4	3	2	1
5. PERFORMS PROCEDURE IN A REASONABLE TIME FRAME	5	4	3	2	1
6. MAINTAINS STERILE OR ASEPTIC TECHNIQUE	5	4	3	2	1
7. INITIATES UNAMBIGUOUS GOAL-DIRECTED COMMUNICATION	5	4	3	2	1
8. PROVIDES FOR ADEQUATE CARE AND MAINTENANCE OF EQUIPMENT AND SUPPLIES	5	4	3	2	1
9. EXHIBITS COURTEOUS AND PLEASANT DEMEANOR	5	4	3	2	1
10. MAINTAINS CONCISE AND ACCURATE RECORDS	5	4	3	2	1

ADDITIONAL COMMENTS: INCLUDE ERRORS OF OMISSION OR COMMISSION, COMMUNICATIVE SKILLS, AND EFFECTIVENESS OF PATIENT INTERACTION:

SUMMARY PERFORMANCE EVALUATION AND RECOMMENDATIONS

SATISFACTORY PERFORMANCE—Performed without error or prompting, or able to self-correct, no critical errors.

_____ LABORATORY EVALUATION. SKILLS MAY BE APPLIED/OBSERVED IN THE CLINICAL SETTING.

_____ CLINICAL EVALUATION. STUDENT READY FOR MINIMALLY SUPERVISED APPLICATION AND REFINEMENT.

UNSATISFACTORY PERFORMANCE—Prompting required; performed with critical errors, potentially harmful.

_____ STUDENT REQUIRES ADDITIONAL LABORATORY PRACTICE.

_____ STUDENT REQUIRES ADDITIONAL SUPERVISED CLINICAL PRACTICE.

SIGNATURES

STUDENT: _____   EVALUATOR: _____

DATE: _____   DATE: _____

Pharyngeal Airways

Artificial airways are devices that are used to establish and maintain airway patency, facilitate ventilation, and assist in the removal of secretions. These include nasopharyngeal and oropharyngeal airways, laryngeal mask airways, and endotracheal and tracheostomy tubes. The respiratory care practitioner must be able to select the appropriate airway, properly size and insert the airway, and maintain the airway and ventilation.

Nasopharyngeal airways, sometimes called nasal airways or trumpets, are chiefly used to facilitate the suctioning procedure. If the tube is too long, it can interfere with the opening of the epiglottis.

Oropharyngeal tubes are used to prevent the tongue from falling back into the oropharynx and blocking the airway. They are chiefly used to facilitate bag-valve-mask ventilation. They may also be used to maintain airway patency in patients who have adequate respiratory effort but inadequate muscle tone or airway protection reflexes. If the airway selected is too large, it can interfere with the epiglottis. If the airway is too small, it can push the tongue back into the pharynx. According to the AARC practice guideline on resuscitation, the oropharyngeal airway design should incorporate a **flange** and a short bite-block segment.[1] The esophageal obturator airway/esophageal gastric tube airway (EOA/EGTA) was previously commonly used by many paramedic organizations for prehospital airway management. Although some believe it to be a useful second-line airway adjunct, others believe that it is an outdated and undesirable modality.[2,3] Newer tubes, such as the Pharyngeotracheal Lumen (PTL) airway and the Esophageal-Tracheal Combitube, are being used more frequently by prehospital providers.[3] Time needed for training in EOA insertion may be better spent in training for endotracheal intubation or by placing more emphasis on basic airway maintenance and ventilation.[3]

The laryngeal mask airway (LMA) is becoming increasingly popular as an alternative for difficult intubations in the operating room setting. This device provides a low-pressure seal around the glottis and may cause less trauma than endotracheal intubation. However, it does not reliably prevent aspiration.[3,4] It is contraindicated in nonfasting patients and in patients at high risk for aspiration. Its usefulness in an emergency setting has not yet been completely evaluated.

Endotracheal intubation and tracheostomy tubes are discussed in Chapter 14.

OBJECTIVES
Upon completion of this chapter, the student will be able to:

1. Identify various types of airway adjuncts, including oropharyngeal and nasopharyngeal airways, laryngeal mask airway, the Esophageal-Tracheal Combitube, and esophageal obturator/esophageal gastric tube airway.

2. Given a clinical scenario, select the most appropriate airway.

3. Measure a subject for the appropriate size airway.

4. Insert nasopharyngeal, oropharyngeal, esophageal, and esophageal-tracheal airways.

5. Practice insertion of a laryngeal mask airway.

KEY TERMS
flange
laryngospasm

meatus
perforation

pinna
redundancy

tragus
uvula

EQUIPMENT REQUIRED

- Oropharyngeal airways, various sizes
- Nasopharyngeal airways, various sizes
- Laryngeal mask airway
- Esophageal obturator/esophageal gastric tube airway

- Esophageal-Tracheal Combitube™
- Airway management trainers, adult and infant
- Silicone spray lubricant
- Nonsterile gloves
- Manual resuscitators with masks
- Water-soluble lubricant

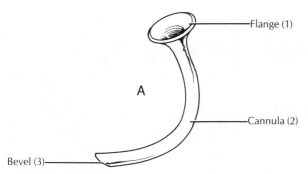

FIGURE 13.1   **A.** (Adapted from Eubanks, DH and Bone, RC: Comprehensive Respiratory Care: A Learning System, ed 2. Mosby-Year Book, St. Louis, p. 548, with permission.)

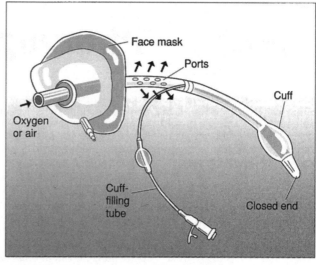

FIGURE 13.4   **D.** (From Persing, G: Advanced Practitioner Respiratory Care Review. WB Saunders, Philadelphia, 1994, p. 53, with permission.)

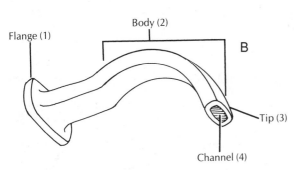

FIGURE 13.2   **B.** (Adapted from Eubanks, DH and Bone, RC: Comprehensive Respiratory Care: A Learning System, ed 2. Mosby-Year Book, St. Louis, p. 548, with permission.)

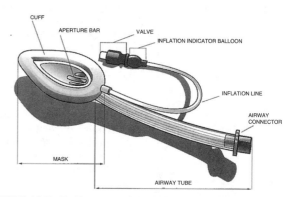

FIGURE 13.5   **E.** (Courtesy of Gensia, Inc., San Diego, CA. Gensia, Inc., is the exclusive distributor of the Laryngeal Mask Airway [LMA] in the United States.)

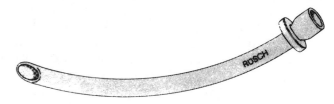

FIGURE 13.6   **F.** (Courtesy of Rüsch Inc., Duluth, GA.)

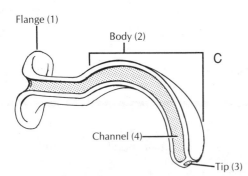

FIGURE 13.3   **C.** (Adapted from Eubanks, DH and Bone, RC: Comprehensive Respiratory Care: A Learning System, ed 2. Mosby-Year Book, St. Louis, p. 548, with permission.)

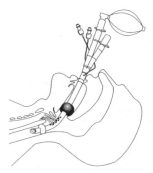

FIGURE 13.7   **G.** (Courtesy of Kendall Healthcare Products Company, Mansfield, MA.)

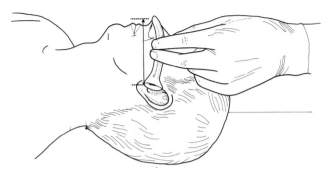

FIGURE 13.8   Sizing of nasopharyngeal airway.

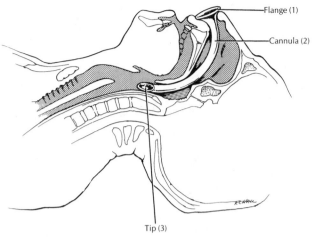

Flange (1)

Cannula (2)

Tip (3)

FIGURE 13.10   Placement of nasopharyngeal airway. (Adapted from Eubanks, DH and Bone, RC: Comprehensive Respiratory Care: A Learning System, ed 2. Mosby-Year Book, St. Louis, 1990, with permission.)

● E X E R C I S E S

EXERCISE 13.1 Identification of Airway Adjuncts

Compare Figures 13.1 through 13.7 with the airways provided in the laboratory. *Identify the type of airway shown for each and record on your laboratory report.*

EXERCISE 13.2 Selection and Insertion of a Nasopharyngeal Airway

1. Select several sizes of nasopharyngeal airways.
2. Determine the proper size airway to use on your laboratory partner, as shown in Figure 13.8, by placing one end of the airway at the tip of the nose of your partner. Now pull the tube toward the ear. If the tube goes past the opening of the ear, it is too large. The tube length should equal the distance from the tip of the nose to the **meatus** (opening) of the ear or from the nose to the **tragus** of the ear plus 1 inch.[5] *Record the size selected on your laboratory report.*

3. Wash your hands and apply standard precautions and transmission-based isolation procedures as appropriate. Put on nonsterile gloves.
4. Lubricate the airway of the airway management training mannequin with the silicone spray. *Note: When inserting an airway into a patient, use a water-soluble lubricant.*
5. Insert the airway into the external naris of the airway management trainer and push the airway gently into place, following the anatomical curve as shown in Figure 13.9. *Never* force an airway into place. If an obstruction is met, try the other naris.
6. The tip of the airway should be just past the uvula, as shown in Figure 13.10.

EXERCISE 13.3 Selection and Insertion of an Oropharyngeal Airway

1. Select several sizes of oropharyngeal airways.
2. Determine the proper size airway for your laboratory partner, as shown in Figure 13.11, by approximating the

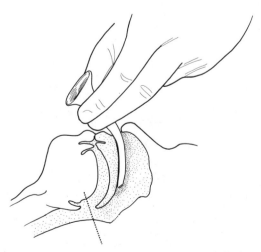

FIGURE 13.9   Insertion of a nasopharyngeal airway.

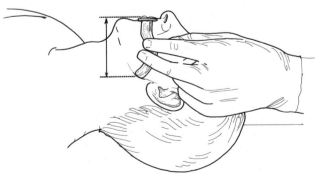

FIGURE 13.11   Sizing of an oropharyngeal airway.

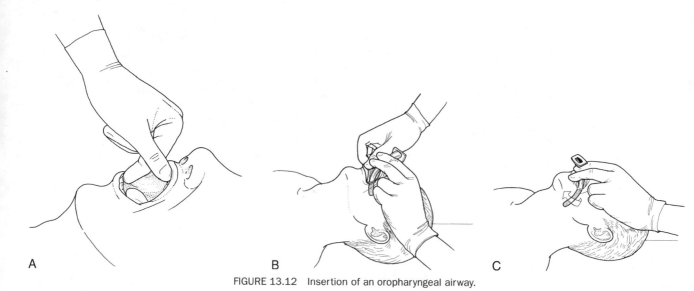

A   B   C

FIGURE 13.12   Insertion of an oropharyngeal airway.

distance from the central incisors (front teeth) to the angle of the mandible.[1] *Record the size and type selected on your laboratory report.*

3. Wash your hands and apply standard precautions and transmission-based isolation procedures as appropriate. Put on nonsterile gloves.

4. Insert the airway into the airway management trainer (Fig. 13.12). Open the mouth using a cross-finger technique, and insert the airway into the mouth rotated 180° (upside down). Continue to advance the airway until it is past the hard palate to the level of the **uvula**. When it is almost completely in, rotate the airway into its final position, so that the curvature of the airway follows the natural curvature of the tongue, keeping it in place. The end of the airway should be just beyond the base of the tongue, as shown in Figure 13.13.

5. Using a bag-valve-mask device, manually ventilate the mannequin with the airway in place for at least 5 min. Ensure that the chest is rising and falling.

References

1. American Association for Respiratory Care: Clinical practice guideline: Resuscitation in acute care hospitals. Respir Care 38:1169–1200, 1993.
2. Kharasch, M and Graff, J: Emergency management of the airway. Crit Care Clin 11:53–67, 1995.
3. American Association for Respiratory Care: AARC clinical practice guideline: Management of airway emergencies. Respir Care 40:749–760, 1995.
4. Sofair, E: Preanesthetic assessment: The professional singer with a difficult airway. Anesthesiology News 1:9, 40, 1993.
5. McPherson, S: Respiratory Care Equipment, ed 5. Mosby, St Louis, 1995, p 117.

Related Readings

Eubanks, DH and Bone, RC: Principles and Applications of Cardiorespiratory Care Equipment. Mosby, St Louis, 1994.
McPherson, S: Respiratory Care Equipment, ed 5. Mosby, St Louis, 1995.
Scanlan, C et al (eds): Egan's Fundamentals of Respiratory Care, ed 6. Mosby, St Louis, 1995.

Selected Journal Articles

American Association for Respiratory Care: AARC clinical practice guideline: Management of airway emergencies. Respir Care 40:749–760, 1995.
American Association for Respiratory Care: Clinical practice guideline: Resuscitation in acute care hospitals. Respir Care 38:1169–1200, 1993.
Demers, RR: Management of the airway in the perioperative period. Respir Care 29:529–539, 1984.
Kharasch, M and Graff, J: Emergency management of the airway. Crit Care Clin 11:53–67, 1995.
Reines, H: Airway management options. Respir Care 37:695–707, 1992.
Sofair, E: Preanesthetic assessment: The professional singer with a difficult airway. Anesthesiology News 1:9, 40, 1993.
Wilson, R: Upper airway problems. Respir Care 37:533–550, 1992.

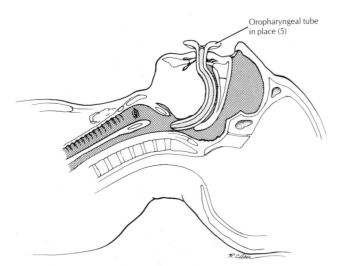

Oropharyngeal tube in place (5)

FIGURE 13.13   Placement of an oropharyngeal airway. (Adapted from Eubanks, DH and Bone, RC: Comprehensive Respiratory Care: A Learning System, ed 2. Mosby-Year Book, St. Louis, 1990, p. 548, with permission.)

LABORATORY REPORT

CHAPTER 13: PHARYNGEAL AIRWAYS

Name _____   Date _____

Course/Section _____   Instructor _____

Data Collection

EXERCISE 13.1   Identification of Airway Adjuncts

A. Figure 13.1: _____

B. Figure 13.2: _____

C. Figure 13.3: _____

D. Figure 13.4: _____

E. Figure 13.5: _____

F. Figure 13.6: _____

G. Figure 13.7: _____

EXERCISE 13.2   Selection and Insertion of a Nasopharyngeal Airway

Size selected: _____

EXERCISE 13.3   Selection and Insertion of an Oropharyngeal Airway

Size selected: _____

Type selected: _____

CRITICAL THINKING QUESTIONS

1. Why is a water-soluble lubricant used for inserting a nasal airway?

2. What complications might arise from the improper insertion of a nasal airway?

3. For each of the following scenarios, indicate what type of airway should be used. State your rationale.
   a. A patient requiring manual ventilation:

   _____

   b. Semiconscious patient in the recovery room:

   _____

   c. An elderly, nonintubated patient who requires frequent suctioning:

   _____

   d. A comatose patient in the intensive care unit (ICU):

   _____

   e. A patient in cardiac arrest in the emergency room receiving basic life support (BLS):

   _____

4. What complications might arise from an improperly sized oropharyngeal airway?

5. A patient is brought into the emergency room with an esophageal obturator in place. The physician wants you to intubate the patient with an endotracheal tube. What is the proper sequence of actions for replacing the EOA?

6. You are called to the recovery room to administer 40-percent oxygen to a patient with a laryngeal mask airway in place. Describe the equipment setup you would employ.

7. The patient in Critical Thinking Question 6 has regained consciousness, and the laryngeal mask airway has been removed. What should you do with the device at this time?

PROCEDURAL COMPETENCY EVALUATION

Name _____ Date _____

Artificial Airway Insertion

Setting: ☐ Lab ☐ Clinical   Evaluator: ☐ Peer ☐ Instructor

Conditions (describe): _____

_____

Equipment Used

_____

_____

	SATISFACTORY	UNSATISFACTORY	NOT OBSERVED	NOT APPLICABLE
Equipment and Patient Preparation				
1. Selects, gathers, and assembles the necessary equipment	☐	☐	☐	☐
2. Washes hands and applies standard precautions and transmission-based isolation procedures as appropriate	☐	☐	☐	☐
3. Identifies patient, introduces self and department	☐	☐	☐	☐
4. Explains purpose of the procedure and confirms patient understanding if the patient is alert	☐	☐	☐	☐
Assessment and Implementation				
5. Assesses patient for the appropriate airway	☐	☐	☐	☐
6. Measures the patient for the appropriate size	☐	☐	☐	☐
7. Lubricates the airway if necessary	☐	☐	☐	☐
8. Positions patient	☐	☐	☐	☐
9. Inserts the airway	☐	☐	☐	☐
10. Assesses the patient for proper placement	☐	☐	☐	☐
11. Reinserts and adjusts if necessary	☐	☐	☐	☐
12. Reassesses if necessary	☐	☐	☐	☐
13. Secures airway	☐	☐	☐	☐
Follow-up				
14. Disposes of infectious waste and washes hands	☐	☐	☐	☐
15. Records pertinent data in chart and departmental records	☐	☐	☐	☐
16. Notifies appropriate personnel and makes any necessary recommendations or modifications to the patient care plan	☐	☐	☐	☐

_____   _____
Signature of Evaluator   Signature of Student

PERFORMANCE RATING SCALE

5 EXCELLENT—FAR EXCEEDS EXPECTED LEVEL, FLAWLESS PERFORMANCE
4 ABOVE AVERAGE—NO PROMPTING REQUIRED, ABLE TO SELF-CORRECT
3 AVERAGE—THE MINIMUM COMPETENCY LEVEL, NO CRITICAL ERRORS
2 IMPROVEMENT NEEDED—PROBLEM AREAS EXIST; CRITICAL ERRORS, CORRECTIONS NEEDED
1 POOR AND UNACCEPTABLE PERFORMANCE—GROSS INACCURACIES, POTENTIALLY HARMFUL

PERFORMANCE CRITERIA		SCALE			
1. DISPLAYS KNOWLEDGE OF ESSENTIAL CONCEPTS	5	4	3	2	1
2. DEMONSTRATES THE RELATIONSHIP BETWEEN THEORY AND CLINICAL PRACTICE	5	4	3	2	1
3. FOLLOWS DIRECTIONS, EXHIBITS SOUND JUDGMENT, AND DEMONSTRATES ATTENTION TO SAFETY AND DETAIL	5	4	3	2	1
4. EXHIBITS THE REQUIRED MANUAL DEXTERITY	5	4	3	2	1
5. PERFORMS PROCEDURE IN A REASONABLE TIME FRAME	5	4	3	2	1
6. MAINTAINS STERILE OR ASEPTIC TECHNIQUE	5	4	3	2	1
7. INITIATES UNAMBIGUOUS GOAL-DIRECTED COMMUNICATION	5	4	3	2	1
8. PROVIDES FOR ADEQUATE CARE AND MAINTENANCE OF EQUIPMENT AND SUPPLIES	5	4	3	2	1
9. EXHIBITS COURTEOUS AND PLEASANT DEMEANOR	5	4	3	2	1
10. MAINTAINS CONCISE AND ACCURATE RECORDS	5	4	3	2	1

ADDITIONAL COMMENTS: INCLUDE ERRORS OF OMISSION OR COMMISSION, COMMUNICATIVE SKILLS, AND EFFECTIVENESS OF PATIENT INTERACTION:

SUMMARY PERFORMANCE EVALUATION AND RECOMMENDATIONS

SATISFACTORY PERFORMANCE—Performed without error or prompting, or able to self-correct, no critical errors.

_____ LABORATORY EVALUATION. SKILLS MAY BE APPLIED/OBSERVED IN THE CLINICAL SETTING.

_____ CLINICAL EVALUATION. STUDENT READY FOR MINIMALLY SUPERVISED APPLICATION AND REFINEMENT.

UNSATISFACTORY PERFORMANCE—Prompting required; performed with critical errors, potentially harmful.

_____ STUDENT REQUIRES ADDITIONAL LABORATORY PRACTICE.

_____ STUDENT REQUIRES ADDITIONAL SUPERVISED CLINICAL PRACTICE.

SIGNATURES

STUDENT: _____ EVALUATOR: _____

DATE: _____ DATE: _____

CHAPTER 14

Suctioning

INTRODUCTION

Suctioning is one of the most frequent procedures performed by the respiratory care practitioner. It may be achieved by insertion of a suction catheter through the nasal passages (nasotracheal suction), by oral suctioning of the pharynx, or via an endotracheal tube. Unfortunately, it is too often treated as a benign procedure, which it most definitely is not. Hypoxemia, cardiac dysrhythmias, nosocomial infection, atelectasis, mucosal trauma, bronchospasm, pulmonary hemorrhage, elevated intracranial pressure, and patient discomfort are some of the more frequently encountered complications of this procedure even when it is performed properly.[1,2] Respiratory or cardiac arrest is always a distinct possibility. Nasotracheal suctioning without an artificial airway may be one of the most dangerous procedures performed by respiratory care practitioners.

It is necessary to perform proper patient assessment before suctioning a patient. Assessing the need for suctioning can be accomplished by auscultation and palpation. "Routine" suctioning should never be done. Endotracheal suctioning may be required at some minimum frequency to ensure artificial airway patency.[1]

Practitioners should always be aware of the possible hazards and complications of these procedures. Care should be taken to ensure patient safety. Considerations include using the proper size catheter, maintenance of aseptic technique, patient preparation (including adequate preoxygenation), and appropriate pressure and time limitations.

OBJECTIVES

Upon completion of this chapter, the student will be able to:

1. Identify the various types of suction devices and accessories, including Yankauer (tonsillar) catheter, Coudé or Bronchitrach-L angle-tip endobronchial catheters, closed suction system devices, and sputum traps.

2. Determine the proper suction catheter size for a given airway.

3. Demonstrate the proper aseptic donning of gloves and handling of the sterile contents of a suction kit.

4. Aseptically perform nasotracheal suctioning on an airway management trainer using appropriate personal protective equipment.

5. Perform endotracheal suctioning on an intubated airway management trainer using appropriate personal protective equipment.

6. Perform tracheobronchial lavage during suctioning.

7. Collect a sputum specimen during suctioning.

8. Demonstrate the proper disposal of contaminated suction equipment.

9. Correlate the physical principles involved in suctioning, such as Poiseuille's law, to suction equipment and procedures.

KEY TERMS

aspiration	irrigation	lubricant	vacuum
flush	instillation	soluble	
	lavage	tenacious	

EQUIPMENT REQUIRED

- Airway management trainers (intubated and unintubated)
- Suction catheter kits
- Coude or Bronchitrach-L angle-tip endobronchial catheter
- Yankauer (tonsillar tip) suction device
- Silicone spray (water-**soluble lubricant**)
- Suction machines
- Goggles
- Sterile gloves
- Nonsterile disposable latex and vinyl gloves, various sizes
- Sputum traps: Lukens and DeLee types
- Closed suction catheter system
- Sterile water or normal saline
- Sterile water-soluble lubricant
- Basins
- Disposal bags
- Oxygen gas source and flowmeter
- Oxygen connecting tubing and nipple adaptors
- T-piece and large-bore corrugated tubing

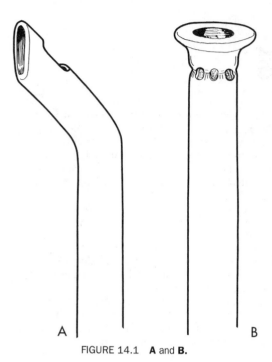

FIGURE 14.1 **A** and **B.**

- Nonrebreathing masks
- Unit-dose saline
- Biohazard transport bags
- Stethoscopes
- Pulse oximeter and probes
- Manual resuscitator with mask

 E X E R C I S E S

EXERCISE 14.1 Suction Equipment Identification

Compare the equipment provided in the laboratory with Figures 14.1 through 14.7. *Identify each item and record it on your laboratory report.*

    Yankauer catheter
    Lukens sputum trap
    DeLee sputum trap
    Suction connecting tubing
    Closed suction system

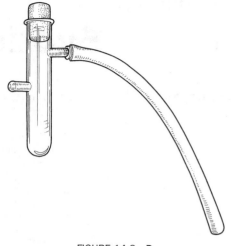

FIGURE 14.3 **D.**

    Murphy-tip catheter
    Bronchitrach-L angle-tip endobronchial catheter
    Beaded-tip catheter

EXERCISE 14.2 Oropharyngeal Suctioning

1. Wash your hands and apply standard precautions and transmission-based isolation procedures as appropriate.
2. Select a Yankauer (tonsillar) suction unit.
3. Put on nonsterile gloves.
4. Attach the Yankauer suction device to the end of the suction connecting tube.
5. Fill a basin with sterile water or normal saline.
6. Turn on the suction unit.

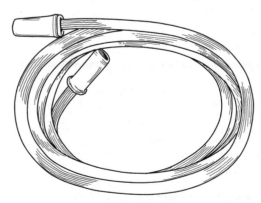

FIGURE 14.2 **C.**

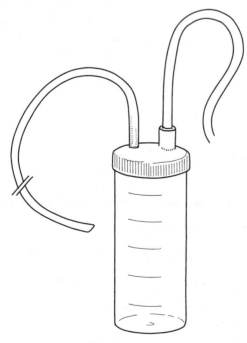

FIGURE 14.4 **E.**

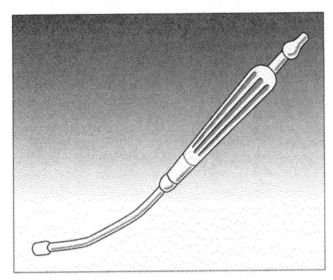

FIGURE 14.5 **F.** (From Persing, G: Entry-Level Respiratory Care Review, ed 2. WB Saunders, Philadelphia, 1996, p. 62, with permission.)

7. Test the unit by suctioning some of the sterile water or normal saline.

8. Introduce the Yankauer suction unit into the mouth of the mannequin and "suction" the mouth of the mannequin.

9. Remove the unit from the mouth of the mannequin and clean it by flushing the unit and the tubing.

10. Disconnect the unit and shut off the machine.

11. Cover the unit with the wrapper.

12. Remove your gloves and wash your hands.

13. Dispose of all infectious waste in the proper receptacles.

EXERCISE 14.3 Suction Kits

This section is designed to practice aseptic technique in handling suction equipment. The actual suctioning procedure will be practiced in the next exercise.

1. Select a suction kit.

2. Open the kit, making sure to maintain the sterility of the contents.

3. Identify the components in the kit by visual inspection. *Do not touch the contents.*
   a. *Record the brand used and contents contained on your laboratory report.*
   b. Depending on the brand of suction kit used, additional items may need to be obtained to complete the procedure. Compare the contents of your kit with the following list, and obtain any additional items needed.

(1) Two sterile gloves
(2) Sterile drape or other surface on which to place equipment
(3) Sterile basin
(4) Sterile water or saline
(5) Sterile suction catheter

4. Put on the gloves using the procedure practiced in Chapter 1.

5. Open the sterile basin and fill the basin with the sterile solution using your nondominant hand, if the basin is not prefilled. Keep in mind that if you are using a separate supply of sterile solution, the container must also be handled aseptically. The bottle of sterile solution should be marked with the date and time when first opened. Solution should be discarded after 24 hours. When opening the solution, the bottle cap should be placed upside down aseptically on a clean surface.

6. Pick up the catheter with your dominant hand, keeping the catheter coiled. Remember that this hand is considered to be the sterile hand and must touch nothing but the catheter.

7. While grasping the catheter in the palm of your hand, remove the glove from your dominant hand by pulling the glove down and completely over the catheter.

8. Remove the other glove and *discard* the gloves into the proper garbage receptacle.

NOTE: For the purpose of laboratory practice, you may be reusing the suction kit and supplies. If so, you should attempt to reorganize the kit in the way in which it was originally found.

EXERCISE 14.4 Nasotracheal Suctioning

1. Wash your hands and apply personal protective equipment as appropriate.

2. Gather the necessary equipment: oxygen gas source, nonrebreathing mask, suction kit, water-soluble lubricant, sterile water or normal saline, and suction machine.

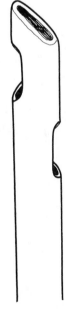

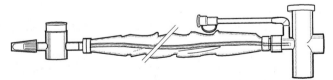

FIGURE 14.6 **G.** (Courtesy of Ballard Medical Products, Draper, UT.)

FIGURE 14.7 **H.**

TABLE 14.1 **Recommended Suction Vacuum Pressures**

	Wall Unit	**Portable Unit**
Adult	−100 to −120 mm Hg (−150 mm Hg maximum may be used)	10–15 in. Hg
Child	−80 to −100 mm Hg	5–10 in. Hg
Infant	−60 to −80 mm Hg	3–5 in. Hg

3. Place the mannequin in the Fowler's position. In an actual clinical situation, you should remove the pillow from behind the patient's head and place the head in a neutral position, avoiding hyperextension.

4. Assemble the nonrebreathing mask and oxygen.

5. Place the mask on the mannequin to hyperoxygenate the "patient" before suctioning. Instruct the patient to take several deep breaths. Patients should be hyperoxygenated before the suction event for at least 30 sec.[1]

6. Assess the patient for adequate oxygenation, including color, respiratory rate and pattern, heart rate and rhythm, and pulse oximetry.

7. Turn on the suction unit.

8. Adjust the suction to the appropriate suction pressure (Table 14.1).

9. Open the water-soluble lubricant.

10. Open the suction kit and put on the gloves as in Exercise 14.2.

11. Connect the suction tubing to the thumb-port connection or Y-connector of the suction catheter, as shown in Figure 14.8.

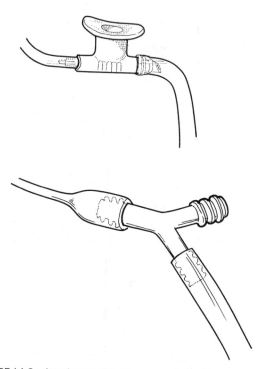

FIGURE 14.8   Attachment of suction source to thumb-port connection or Y-connector of suction catheter.

12. Test the suction by placing the catheter into the sterile solution and occluding the thumb port with the thumb of your nondominant hand. Readjust the suction pressure if necessary.

13. Apply the lubricant to the catheter by either squeezing the tube or packet into the palm of your sterile hand and then pulling the catheter through the jelly to achieve lubrication, or applying the lubricant to the sterile interior of the suction kit and then rotating the catheter through it.

14. Without applying the suction, introduce the catheter into one of the nares, slowly and gently pushing the catheter until it advances into the oropharynx. *Never* force the catheter. If an obstruction is met, attempt to pass the catheter through the other naris.

15. When you notice "fogging" of the catheter (condensation from exhaled air), or you hear a change in the patient's voice, you are entering the trachea. Obviously this will not be apparent on a mannequin. Continue introducing the catheter until an obstruction is met.

16. Once the obstruction is met, withdraw the catheter about one-half inch, and apply the suction with your thumb on the thumb port.

17. Continue to withdraw the catheter until it is removed. The withdrawal procedure and application of suction should not take longer than 10 to 15 sec.[1,2] Frequently assess the patient during the procedure.

18. Reapply the nonrebreathing mask with your nonsterile hand to reoxygenate the patient. Patients should be reoxygenated for at least 1 min before repeating the suction event.[2]

19. **Flush** the catheter and the tubing to clean it by suctioning the sterile solution through the catheter.

20. Reassess the patient and repeat the procedure if needed after a sufficient time for recovery.

21. Remove the nonrebreathing mask.

22. Turn the suction off.

23. Remove gloves and dispose of all equipment properly.

24. Wash your hands.

EXERCISE 14.5 Endotracheal Suctioning

1. Select an intubated mannequin. Note the size of the endotracheal tube being used by looking at the underside of the 15-mm endotracheal tube adaptor. *Record the size of the endotracheal tube on your laboratory report.*

2. Determine the size of the suction catheter to use. The outer diameter (OD) of the suction catheter should not exceed one-half the size of the inner diameter (ID) of the airway.[1] Because the airway is usually measured in millimeters and suction catheters are usually measured in even-numbered French (Fr) sizes, a conversion is necessary. The formula will result in the maximum recommended catheter size:

$$(0.5 \text{ ID mm} \times 3) + 2 = \text{Fr suction catheter size}$$

Record the size of the catheter selected on your laboratory report.

3. Wash your hands and apply personal protective equipment as appropriate. Goggles, gloves, and gown are recommended.[4,5]

4. Gather the necessary equipment: oxygen gas source, manual resuscitator, suction kit, sterile water or normal saline, unit-dose saline, and suction machine.

5. Assemble the manual resuscitator and oxygen. The patient should receive hyperoxygenation by 100-percent oxygen for at least 30 sec before the suction procedure.[1] This may be accomplished by several methods:

   a. Increase the F_1O_2 to 100 percent on the oxygen delivery device, if possible.

   b. A manual resuscitator may be used with maximum F_1O_2. Practitioners should ensure that PEEP levels are maintained.[1]

   c. If the patient is on a mechanical ventilator, the F_1O_2 can be adjusted to 100 percent, or, alternatively, some ventilators have a temporary oxygen enrichment mode available. This method may be more effective than using a manual resuscitator.[1] If this method is used, sufficient time must be allowed for the circuit to be flushed with the 100-percent oxygen before the suction event.

   d. Regardless of the method selected, the practitioner *must* be sure to return the F_1O_2 to the original setting when the procedure is completed.

6. Adjust the suction to the appropriate suction pressure.

7. Loosen the oxygen delivery device connected to the endotracheal tube.

8. Open the suction kit and put on the gloves as described in Exercise 14.2.

9. Connect the suction tubing to the other end of the suction catheter.

10. Test the suction unit as described in Exercise 14.3.

11. With your nonsterile hand, disconnect the oxygen delivery device attached to the endotracheal tube and connect the manual resuscitator. Make sure that you place the oxygen delivery device on a sterile field in order not to contaminate the device.

12. Hyperinflate and hyperoxygenate for at least 30 sec. Assess the patient for adequate oxygenation, including color, respiratory rate and pattern, heart rate and rhythm, electrocardiogram (ECG), and pulse oximetry.

13. Quickly disconnect the oxygen source with your nondominant hand. Be sure not to place the device in a soiled area.

14. Without applying the suction, quickly introduce the catheter into the tube, advancing the catheter until it meets an obstruction.

15. Upon meeting an obstruction, withdraw the catheter about one-half inch, and apply the suction with your thumb on the thumb port.

16. Continue to withdraw the catheter, rotating it between your fingers, until it is removed. The entire procedure should not take longer than 20 sec. The withdrawal procedure and application of suction should not take longer than 10 to 15 sec. Frequently reassess the patient during the procedure. Suction may be applied continuously. Intermittent suction has not demonstrated any significant beneficial effect.[6,7]

17. Reconnect the bag and hyperinflate and hyperoxygenate for at least 1 min.

18. With your nonsterile hand, open one or two unit-dose saline vials.

NOTE: If secretions are particularly **tenacious** or difficult to remove, the patient may be **lavaged** with saline to facilitate secretion removal. Recent studies suggest that a potential for dislodging bacteria into the lower airway and causing nosocomial infection may exist,[5,8] and continued practice is an unresolved issue. At this time, the procedure is still recommended when necessary, but should be abandoned as a routine procedure.[1,9]

19. Disconnect the bag and aseptically instill the saline into the tube.

20. Reconnect and hyperinflate and hyperoxygenate for at least 1 min.

21. Repeat the suction procedure.

22. Reconnect and hyperinflate and hyperoxygenate for at least 1 min.

23. Return the patient to the proper oxygen delivery device and F_1O_2.

24. Flush the catheter and the tubing.

25. Disconnect the catheter from the connecting tubing. Remove gloves around the catheter as previously described, and dispose of all equipment properly.

26. Turn the suction off.

27. Dispose of infectious waste. Wash your hands.

EXERCISE 14.6 Endotracheal Suctioning with a Closed System

1. Select an intubated mannequin.

2. Wash your hands, and then put on nonsterile gloves.

3. Assemble the closed suction system, as shown in Figure 14.9, and attach to the patient connection.

4. Connect the end of the system to the suction tubing.

5. Turn the suction unit on.

6. Turn the thumb control for suction to the on position.

7. Hyperoxygenate and hyperinflate the patient for at least 30 sec. (Note that because these units are most commonly used with a ventilator, hyperinflation and hyperoxygenation are achieved through the ventilator before this step.)

8. Assess the patient for adequate oxygenation, including color, respiratory rate and pattern, heart rate and rhythm, ECG (if available), and pulse oximetry.

9. Introduce the catheter into the airway by sliding it through the plastic sheath until resistance is met.

10. Withdraw the catheter about one-half inch and apply suction as you withdraw the catheter completely, pulling it straight out. Make sure that the tip is visible past the T-connection. Reassess the patient frequently during the procedure.

11. Reoxygenate and hyperinflate for at least 1 min. Repeat the procedure if necessary.

12. Clean the catheter. Some brands have an irrigation port that allows you to inject saline and flush the catheter. Refer to the manufacturer's package insert for brand-specific instructions.

13. Make sure the thumb suction control is returned to the off position.

14. Turn the suction off.

STERI-CATH™ D.L.
CLOSED VENTILATION SUCTION SYSTEM -- DUAL LUMEN
DIRECTIONS FOR USE

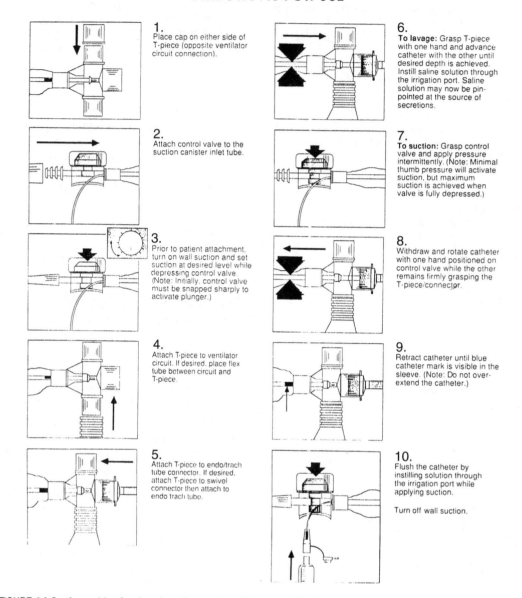

1. Place cap on either side of T-piece (opposite ventilator circuit connection).

2. Attach control valve to the suction canister inlet tube.

3. Prior to patient attachment, turn on wall suction and set suction at desired level while depressing control valve. (Note: Initially, control valve must be snapped sharply to activate plunger.)

4. Attach T-piece to ventilator circuit. If desired, place flex tube between circuit and T-piece.

5. Attach T-piece to endo/trach tube connector. If desired, attach T-piece to swivel connector then attach to endo trach tube.

6. **To lavage:** Grasp T-piece with one hand and advance catheter with the other until desired depth is achieved. Instill saline solution through the irrigation port. Saline solution may now be pinpointed at the source of secretions.

7. **To suction:** Grasp control valve and apply pressure intermittently. (Note: Minimal thumb pressure will activate suction, but maximum suction is achieved when valve is fully depressed.)

8. Withdraw and rotate catheter with one hand positioned on control valve while the other remains firmly grasping the T-piece/connector.

9. Retract catheter until blue catheter mark is visible in the sleeve. (Note: Do not over-extend the catheter.)

10. Flush the catheter by instilling solution through the irrigation port while applying suction.

Turn off wall suction.

FIGURE 14.9   Assembly of a closed suction system. (Courtesy of Smiths Industries Medical Systems, Keene, NH.)

EXERCISE 14.7 Obtaining a Sputum Sample

1. Repeat all the steps in Exercise 14.4, except make sure that you have put a sputum trap in line as shown in Figure 14.10. Do not perform the lavage procedure.

2. After completing the procedure, disconnect the trap from the suction connecting tube. Seal it by interconnecting the tubing to the trap inlet.

3. Label the sample with the appropriate information, and *record this information on your laboratory report.*
   Patient name and identification number
   Room number
   Date
   Time
   Type or source of sample
   Site

4. Place in biohazard transport bag with the "lab slip."

5. Notify the nurse that the sample has been obtained.

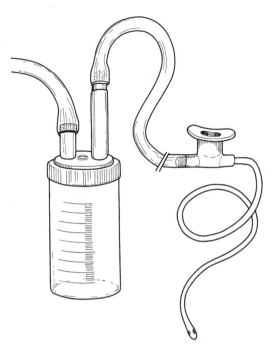

FIGURE 14.10 Assembly of suction-sputum trap equipment.

References

1. American Association for Respiratory Care: AARC clinical practice guideline: Endotracheal suctioning of mechanically ventilated adults and children with artificial airways. Respir Care 36:500–504, 1991.
2. American Association for Respiratory Care: AARC clinical practice guideline: Nasotracheal suctioning. Respir Care 36:898–901, 1991.
3. Chang, DW: Respiratory Care Calculations. Delmar, Albany, 1994, p 245.
4. Centers for Disease Control: Update: Universal precautions for prevention of transmission of human immunodeficiency virus, hepatitis B virus, and other blood-borne pathogens in the health care setting. MMWR 37:377–399, 1988.
5. Centers for Disease Control and Prevention: Guideline for prevention of nosocomial pneumonia. Respir Care 39:1191–1236, 1994.
6. Czarni, R et al: Differential effects of continuous versus intermittent suction on tracheal tissue. Heart Lung 202:144, 1991.
7. Kleiber, C, Krutzfield, N and Rose, E: Acute histologic changes in the tracheobronchial tree associated with different suction catheter insertion techniques. Heart Lung 17:12, 1988.
8. Hagler, DA and Traver, GA: Endotracheal saline and suction catheters: Sources of lower airway contamination. Am J Crit Care 3:444, 1993.
9. Ackerman, MH: The effect of saline lavage prior to suctioning. Am J Crit Care 2:326–330, 1993.

Related Readings

Chang, DW: Respiratory Care Calculations. Delmar, Albany, 1994.
Eubanks, DH and Bone, RC: Comprehensive Respiratory Care: A Learning System, ed 2. Mosby, St Louis, 1990.
Finucane, B and Santora, A: Principles of Airway Management, ed 2. Mosby, St Louis, 1996.
McPherson, S: Respiratory Care Equipment, ed 5. Mosby, St Louis, 1995.
Scanlan, C et al (eds): Egan's Fundamentals of Respiratory Care, ed 6. Mosby, St Louis, 1995.

Selected Journal Articles

Ackerman, MH: The use of bolus normal saline instillations in artificial airways: Is it useful or necessary? Heart Lung 14:505–506, 1985.
Ackerman, MH, Eckland, I and Abu-Jumah, M: A review of normal saline instillation: Implications for practice. Dimensions of Critical Care Nursing 15:31–38, 1996.
American Association for Respiratory Care: AARC clinical practice guideline: Endotracheal suctioning of mechanically ventilated adults and children with artificial airways. Respir Care 36:500–504, 1991.
American Association for Respiratory Care: AARC clinical practice guideline: Use of positive airway pressure adjuncts to bronchial hygiene therapy. Respir Care 36:516–521, 1991.
American Association for Respiratory Care: AARC clinical practice guideline: Nasotracheal suctioning. Respir Care 36:898–901, 1991.
Barnes, CA and Kirchoff, KT: Minimizing hypoxemia due to endotracheal suctioning: A review of the literature. Heart Lung 15:164–178, 1986.
Bishop, MJ: Practice guidelines for airway care during resuscitation. Respir Care 40:393–401, 1995.
Bostick, J and Wendelgass, ST: Normal saline instillation as part of the suctioning procedure: Effects on PaO_2 and amount of secretions. Heart Lung 16:532–537, 1987.
Centers for Disease Control and Prevention: Guideline for prevention of nosocomial pneumonia. Respir Care 39:1191–1236, 1994.
Czarni, R et al: Differential effects of continuous versus intermittent suction on tracheal tissue. Heart Lung 202:144–151, 1991.
DePew, CL et al: Open vs. closed system endotracheal suctioning: A cost comparison. Crit Care Nurse 14:94–108, 1994.
ECRI: Medical gas and vacuum systems. Health Devices 23:4–53, 1994.
Hagler, DS and Traver, GA: Endotracheal saline and suction catheters: sources of lower airway contamination. Am J Crit Care 3:444–447, 1994.
Kleiber, C, Krutzfield, N and Rose, E: Acute histologic changes in the tracheobronchial tree associated with different suction catheter insertion techniques. Heart Lung 17:10–14, 1988.
Martinez, FJ et al: Increased resistance of hygroscopic condenser humidifiers when using a closed suction system. Crit Care Med 22:1668–1673, 1994.

LABORATORY REPORT

CHAPTER 14: SUCTIONING

Name _____   Date _____

Course/Section _____   Instructor _____

Data Collection

EXERCISE 14.1   Suction Equipment Identification

A. _____

B. _____

C. _____

D. _____

E. _____

F. _____

G. _____

H. _____

EXERCISE 14.3   Suction Kits

Brand used: _____

Contents: _____

_____

EXERCISE 14.5   Endotracheal Suctioning

Size of endotracheal tube: _____

Size of the suction catheter *(show your work!)*: _____

EXERCISE 14.7   Obtaining a Sputum Sample
Label Information

Patient name: _____   Room number: _____

Date: _____   Time: _____

Type of sample: _____   Site: _____

CRITICAL THINKING QUESTIONS

1. What hazards and complications of suctioning are unique to the nasotracheal route?

2. Contrast the dysrhythmias one would expect as a result of vagal stimulation during the suctioning procedure versus those that would result from hypoxemia.

3. Is sputum normally considered a high-risk fluid for the transmission of blood-borne pathogens?

4. What is the rationale for personal protective equipment use while performing suctioning?

5. Given the following scenarios, identify all possible causes of the problem and offer at least two alternative solutions to correct each problem.
   a. You turn on an electrical suction machine and it does not work.
   b. In the middle of suctioning a patient, the suction is lost.
   c. You cannot get suction from a wall suction regulator.
   d. While attempting to suction an adult patient with an endotracheal tube, you cannot advance the catheter more than 5 inches.
   e. After suctioning a patient, you hear a honking or high-pitched sound coming from the endotracheal tube.

6. Calculate the maximum catheter sizes that can be used *(show your work!)*:

   a. ID 4.0-mm tracheostomy tube _____

   b. ID 6.0-mm endotracheal tube _____

   c. ID 7.5-mm endotracheal tube _____

   d. ID 10-mm tracheostomy tube _____

7. A patient is suffering from hypoxemia, dysrhythmias, and bronchospasm during suctioning. Identify what methods you used to assess the patient's status during suctioning, and describe what precautions should be taken to prevent each of the hazards mentioned.

PROCEDURAL COMPETENCY EVALUATION

Name _____   Date _____

Endotracheal Suctioning

Setting: ☐ Lab ☐ Clinical   Evaluator: ☐ Peer ☐ Instructor

Conditions (describe): _____

_____

Equipment Used

_____

_____

	SATISFACTORY	UNSATISFACTORY	NOT OBSERVED	NOT APPLICABLE
Equipment and Patient Preparation				
1. Selects, gathers, and assembles the necessary equipment	☐	☐	☐	☐
2. Washes hands and applies standard precautions and transmission-based isolation procedures as appropriate	☐	☐	☐	☐
3. Identifies patient, introduces self and department	☐	☐	☐	☐
4. Explains purpose of the procedure and confirms patient understanding	☐	☐	☐	☐
Assessment and Implementation				
5. Assesses patient for adequate oxygenation, cardiac rhythm, need for suction	☐	☐	☐	☐
6. Adjusts suction to appropriate level	☐	☐	☐	☐
7. Positions patient	☐	☐	☐	☐
8. Puts on sterile gloves	☐	☐	☐	☐
9. Maintains sterile technique throughout procedure	☐	☐	☐	☐
10. Pours sterile water into sterile container	☐	☐	☐	☐
11. Attaches sputum trap to suction source	☐	☐	☐	☐
12. Attaches catheter to suction source	☐	☐	☐	☐
13. Hyperoxygenates and hyperinflates patient for at least 30 sec	☐	☐	☐	☐
14. Reassures patient; disconnects oxygen or ventilator source and places aseptically	☐	☐	☐	☐
15. Inserts catheter into airway and advances until resistance is met	☐	☐	☐	☐
16. Withdraws catheter 1 to 2 cm	☐	☐	☐	☐
17. Applies suction continuously, rotates and withdraws catheter; reassesses patient frequently	☐	☐	☐	☐
18. Lavage with sterile saline, if indicated	☐	☐	☐	☐
19. Hyperoxygenates and hyperinflates patient for at least 1 min	☐	☐	☐	☐
20. Rinses catheter with sterile solution and repeats if necessary	☐	☐	☐	☐
21. Reassesses patient airway and patient periodically; reinstructs if necessary	☐	☐	☐	☐
22. Reassures patient, resumes oxygen or ventilator source	☐	☐	☐	☐
Follow-up				
23. Restores patient to prior status	☐	☐	☐	☐
24. Returns F_1O_2 to prior settings	☐	☐	☐	☐
25. Maintains/processes equipment and supplies	☐	☐	☐	☐

	S A T I S F A C T O R Y	U N S A T I S F A C T O R Y	N O T O B S E R V E D	N O T A P P L I C A B L E
26. Disposes of infectious waste and washes hands	☐	☐	☐	☐
27. Records pertinent data in chart and departmental records	☐	☐	☐	☐
28. Notifies appropriate personnel and makes any necessary recommendations or modifications to the patient care plan	☐	☐	☐	☐

_____
Signature of Evaluator

_____
Signature of Student

PERFORMANCE RATING SCALE

5 EXCELLENT—FAR EXCEEDS EXPECTED LEVEL, FLAWLESS PERFORMANCE
4 ABOVE AVERAGE—NO PROMPTING REQUIRED, ABLE TO SELF-CORRECT
3 AVERAGE—THE MINIMUM COMPETENCY LEVEL, NO CRITICAL ERRORS
2 IMPROVEMENT NEEDED—PROBLEM AREAS EXIST; CRITICAL ERRORS, CORRECTIONS NEEDED
1 POOR AND UNACCEPTABLE PERFORMANCE—GROSS INACCURACIES, POTENTIALLY HARMFUL

PERFORMANCE CRITERIA	SCALE				
1. DISPLAYS KNOWLEDGE OF ESSENTIAL CONCEPTS	5	4	3	2	1
2. DEMONSTRATES THE RELATIONSHIP BETWEEN THEORY AND CLINICAL PRACTICE	5	4	3	2	1
3. FOLLOWS DIRECTIONS, EXHIBITS SOUND JUDGMENT, AND DEMONSTRATES ATTENTION TO SAFETY AND DETAIL	5	4	3	2	1
4. EXHIBITS THE REQUIRED MANUAL DEXTERITY	5	4	3	2	1
5. PERFORMS PROCEDURE IN A REASONABLE TIME FRAME	5	4	3	2	1
6. MAINTAINS STERILE OR ASEPTIC TECHNIQUE	5	4	3	2	1
7. INITIATES UNAMBIGUOUS GOAL-DIRECTED COMMUNICATION	5	4	3	2	1
8. PROVIDES FOR ADEQUATE CARE AND MAINTENANCE OF EQUIPMENT AND SUPPLIES	5	4	3	2	1
9. EXHIBITS COURTEOUS AND PLEASANT DEMEANOR	5	4	3	2	1
10. MAINTAINS CONCISE AND ACCURATE RECORDS	5	4	3	2	1

ADDITIONAL COMMENTS: INCLUDE ERRORS OF OMISSION OR COMMISSION, COMMUNICATIVE SKILLS, AND EFFECTIVENESS OF PATIENT INTERACTION:

SUMMARY PERFORMANCE EVALUATION AND RECOMMENDATIONS

SATISFACTORY PERFORMANCE—Performed without error or prompting, or able to self-correct, no critical errors.

_____ LABORATORY EVALUATION. SKILLS MAY BE APPLIED/OBSERVED IN THE CLINICAL SETTING.

_____ CLINICAL EVALUATION. STUDENT READY FOR MINIMALLY SUPERVISED APPLICATION AND REFINEMENT.

UNSATISFACTORY PERFORMANCE—Prompting required; performed with critical errors, potentially harmful.

_____ STUDENT REQUIRES ADDITIONAL LABORATORY PRACTICE.

_____ STUDENT REQUIRES ADDITIONAL SUPERVISED CLINICAL PRACTICE.

SIGNATURES

STUDENT: _____ EVALUATOR: _____

DATE: _____ DATE: _____

Name _____ Date _____

Nasotracheal Suctioning

Setting: ☐ Lab ☐ Clinical   Evaluator: ☐ Peer ☐ Instructor

Conditions (describe): _____

_____

Equipment Used

_____

_____

	SATISFACTORY	UNSATISFACTORY	NOT OBSERVED	NOT APPLICABLE
Equipment and Patient Preparation				
1. Verifies, interprets, and evaluates physician's order or protocol	☐	☐	☐	☐
2. Selects, gathers, and assembles the necessary equipment	☐	☐	☐	☐
3. Washes hands and applies standard precautions and transmission-based isolation procedures as appropriate	☐	☐	☐	☐
4. Identifies patient, introduces self and department	☐	☐	☐	☐
5. Explains purpose of the procedure and confirms patient understanding	☐	☐	☐	☐
Assessment and Implementation				
6. Assesses patient and patient airway; determines preferred naris	☐	☐	☐	☐
7. Hyperoxygenates and hyperinflates patient for at least 30 sec	☐	☐	☐	☐
8. Adjusts suction to appropriate level; lubricates nasopharyngeal airway with water-soluble lubricant	☐	☐	☐	☐
9. Removes pillow and positions patient's head	☐	☐	☐	☐
10. Puts on sterile gloves and maintains sterile technique throughout procedure	☐	☐	☐	☐
11. Pours sterile water into a sterile container	☐	☐	☐	☐
12. Lubricates catheter with water-soluble lubricant	☐	☐	☐	☐
13. Attaches catheter to suction source	☐	☐	☐	☐
14. Reassures patient; removes oxygen source and places aseptically	☐	☐	☐	☐
15. Inserts catheter into airway	☐	☐	☐	☐
16. Passes catheter into the oropharynx and into trachea; confirms positioning	☐	☐	☐	☐
17. Advances catheter until resistance is met (without suction applied)	☐	☐	☐	☐
18. Applies suction and rotates/withdraws catheter for a maximum of 10 to 15 sec	☐	☐	☐	☐
19. Frequently assesses patient for oxygenation status, including pulse oximetry	☐	☐	☐	☐
20. Hyperoxygenates and hyperinflates patient for at least 1 min	☐	☐	☐	☐
21. Rinses catheter with sterile solution and repeats if necessary	☐	☐	☐	☐
22. Reassesses patient and repeats if necessary	☐	☐	☐	☐
Follow-up				
23. Restores patient to prior status	☐	☐	☐	☐
24. Maintains/processes equipment and supplies	☐	☐	☐	☐
25. Records pertinent data in chart and departmental records	☐	☐	☐	☐
26. Notifies appropriate personnel, makes recommendations or modifications to the patient care plan	☐	☐	☐	☐

_____   _____

Signature of Evaluator   Signature of Student

PERFORMANCE RATING SCALE

5 EXCELLENT—FAR EXCEEDS EXPECTED LEVEL, FLAWLESS PERFORMANCE
4 ABOVE AVERAGE—NO PROMPTING REQUIRED, ABLE TO SELF-CORRECT
3 AVERAGE—THE MINIMUM COMPETENCY LEVEL, NO CRITICAL ERRORS
2 IMPROVEMENT NEEDED—PROBLEM AREAS EXIST; CRITICAL ERRORS, CORRECTIONS NEEDED
1 POOR AND UNACCEPTABLE PERFORMANCE—GROSS INACCURACIES, POTENTIALLY HARMFUL

PERFORMANCE CRITERIA	SCALE				
1. DISPLAYS KNOWLEDGE OF ESSENTIAL CONCEPTS	5	4	3	2	1
2. DEMONSTRATES THE RELATIONSHIP BETWEEN THEORY AND CLINICAL PRACTICE	5	4	3	2	1
3. FOLLOWS DIRECTIONS, EXHIBITS SOUND JUDGMENT, AND DEMONSTRATES ATTENTION TO SAFETY AND DETAIL	5	4	3	2	1
4. EXHIBITS THE REQUIRED MANUAL DEXTERITY	5	4	3	2	1
5. PERFORMS PROCEDURE IN A REASONABLE TIME FRAME	5	4	3	2	1
6. MAINTAINS STERILE OR ASEPTIC TECHNIQUE	5	4	3	2	1
7. INITIATES UNAMBIGUOUS GOAL-DIRECTED COMMUNICATION	5	4	3	2	1
8. PROVIDES FOR ADEQUATE CARE AND MAINTENANCE OF EQUIPMENT AND SUPPLIES	5	4	3	2	1
9. EXHIBITS COURTEOUS AND PLEASANT DEMEANOR	5	4	3	2	1
10. MAINTAINS CONCISE AND ACCURATE RECORDS	5	4	3	2	1

ADDITIONAL COMMENTS: INCLUDE ERRORS OF OMISSION OR COMMISSION, COMMUNICATIVE SKILLS, AND EFFECTIVENESS OF PATIENT INTERACTION:

SUMMARY PERFORMANCE EVALUATION AND RECOMMENDATIONS

SATISFACTORY PERFORMANCE—Performed without error or prompting, or able to self-correct, no critical errors.

_____ LABORATORY EVALUATION. SKILLS MAY BE APPLIED/OBSERVED IN THE CLINICAL SETTING.

_____ CLINICAL EVALUATION. STUDENT READY FOR MINIMALLY SUPERVISED APPLICATION AND REFINEMENT.

UNSATISFACTORY PERFORMANCE—Prompting required; performed with critical errors, potentially harmful.

_____ STUDENT REQUIRES ADDITIONAL LABORATORY PRACTICE.

_____ STUDENT REQUIRES ADDITIONAL SUPERVISED CLINICAL PRACTICE.

SIGNATURES

STUDENT: _____   EVALUATOR: _____

DATE: _____   DATE: _____

Endotracheal Intubation

INTRODUCTION

In previous chapters, you have learned how to manage the airway without inserting an artificial airway into the trachea. A patient's life may depend on the ability of an individual to recognize the need for intubation of the trachea and to place and manage that airway properly. That individual is often the respiratory care practitioner. The practitioner must be able to place the airway properly and must be able to recognize the clinical situations in which one airway is preferred over another.[1] The AARC clinical practice guideline for management of airway emergencies emphasizes the need for the practitioner to be able to identify, use, and maintain the equipment necessary for intubation. Intubation of the trachea is an advanced skill that requires extensive practice. One does not become proficient in intubation by completing these exercises. Further practice in an environment such as an operating room is required.

OBJECTIVES

Upon completion of this chapter, the student will be able to:

1. Identify, select, prepare, and correct malfunctions of equipment necessary for endotracheal intubation of the infant and adult.
2. Identify the different types of endotracheal tubes, component parts, and tube markings.
3. Assess the potential difficulty of intubation using the Mallampati classification.[2,3]
4. Test an artificial airway for cuff leaks.
5. Insert an orotracheal tube into an infant and an adult airway management trainer.
6. Remove an esophageal obturator/esophageal gastric tube airway after intubation.
7. Insert a nasotracheal tube into an adult airway management trainer using direct vision and blind technique.
8. Verify the proper positioning of an artificial airway and secure it in place.
9. Apply infection control guidelines and standards according to OSHA regulations and CDC guidelines while performing endotracheal intubation.

KEY TERMS

adduction	fenestrated	paresis	supraglottic
anastomosis	fistula	perforation	vallecula
denudation	laryngospasm	polyps	
erosion	malacia	stenosis	
	paralysis	subglottic	

EQUIPMENT REQUIRED

- Oropharyngeal airways, various sizes
- Nasopharyngeal airways, various sizes
- Esophageal obturator/esophageal gastric tube airway
- Airway management trainers, adult and infant
- Suction catheter kits
- Basins
- Silicone spray
- Water-soluble lubricant
- Atomizer
- Suction machines
- Goggles or face shields
- Sterile and nonsterile disposable latex and vinyl gloves, various sizes
- Sterile water or normal saline
- Oxygen gas source and flowmeter
- Oxygen connecting tubing and nipple adaptors
- Stethoscopes
- Easy Cap or other spot-check capnography device
- Manual resuscitators with masks, adult and infant
- Laryngoscope blades and handles, Miller (various sizes) and MacIntosh (various sizes)
- Batteries for laryngoscopes
- Replacement laryngoscope bulbs
- Stylets
- Magill forceps
- Yankauer catheter
- Endotracheal tubes, various sizes
- Cloth tape
- Endotracheal tube holders
- 10-ml syringes
- Towels
- Scissors

⬤ **E X E R C I S E S**

EXERCISE 15.1 Intubation Equipment and Preparation

EXERCISE 15.1.1 Identification of Intubation Equipment

Compare the equipment provided in the laboratory with Figures 15.1 through 15.10. *Identify the items and record them on your laboratory report.*

Adult endotracheal tube
Infant endotracheal tube
Carlens catheter
Deane tube
Cole endotracheal tube
Stylet
Laryngoscope handle
Miller laryngoscope blade
MacIntosh laryngoscope blade
Magill forceps

EXERCISE 15.1.2 Identification of the Components of an Endotracheal Tube

Select an endotracheal tube and compare it with Figure 15.11. *Identify the components and record them on your laboratory report.*

15-mm connector
Internal diameter in mm
Radiopaque line
Pilot balloon
Spring-loaded pilot valve
Cuff
Cuff filling tube
Murphy eye
Length markings
Test markings (IT or Z-79)

EXERCISE 15.1.3 Equipment Testing

1. Gather the necessary equipment:
   Laryngoscope handles and blades
   Batteries
   Bulbs
   Basins
   Endotracheal tube
   10-ml syringe
   Sterile solution

2. Assemble the laryngoscope as shown in Figure 15.12.

3. Open the blade and observe whether the light is lit. *Record this observation on your laboratory report.* Loosen the bulb (if not using a fiberoptic system) and observe whether the

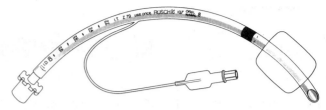

FIGURE 15.2   **B.** (Courtesy of Rüsch Inc., Duluth, GA.)

light goes on. *Record this observation on your laboratory report.* Retighten the bulb.

4. Unscrew the base of the laryngoscope handle and remove the batteries. *Note the size of the batteries on your laboratory report.*

5. Open the blade and observe whether the light is lit. *Record this observation on your laboratory report.*

6. Fill a basin with water or saline solution.

7. Put 5 ml of air into the 10-ml syringe and connect it to the valve on the pilot balloon.

8. Inject the air into the pilot balloon and observe the cuff inflation.

9. Submerge the cuffed end of the endotracheal tube in the basin. Observe the solution for any air bubbles, and *record your observations on your laboratory report.*

10. Add 5 ml more into the cuff. Squeeze the cuff gently and observe the pilot balloon. *Record this observation on your laboratory report.* Place the syringe into the Luer-lok of the pilot valve. Squeeze the cuff gently and observe the pilot balloon and syringe. *Record this observation on your laboratory report.*

11. Remove the tube and deflate the cuff completely.

EXERCISE 15.1.4 Assignment of Mallampati Classification

Frequently the Mallampati classification is employed to help anticipate the difficulty of orotracheal intubation. This is usually done for elective intubations, but it may be of help in an emergency intubation as well. It is not, however, a sole predictor of difficulty.[2,3]

1. Using your laboratory partner as the patient, explain the purpose of this assessment.

2. With your patient seated and head placed in a neutral position, instruct him or her to open the mouth widely and put the tongue out as far as possible.

3. *Visually* inspect the oropharynx and classify it by comparing your observations with Figure 15.13.

4. *Record the Mallampati classification for your patient on your laboratory report.*

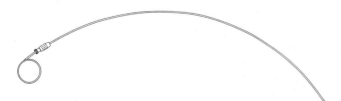

FIGURE 15.1   **A.** (Courtesy of Rüsch Inc., Duluth, GA.)

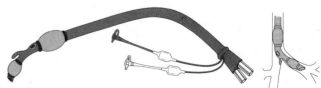

FIGURE 15.3   **C.** (Courtesy of Rüsch Inc., Duluth, GA.)

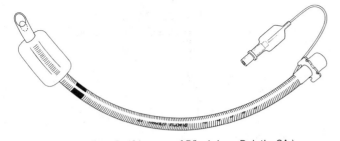

FIGURE 15.4   **D.** (Courtesy of Rüsch Inc., Duluth, GA.)

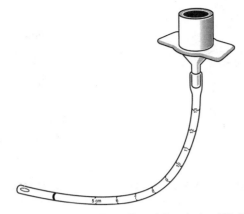

FIGURE 15.9   **I.** (From Barnhart, SL and Czervinske, MP: Perinatal and Pediatric Respiratory Care. WB Saunders, Philadelphia, 1995, p. 241, with permission.)

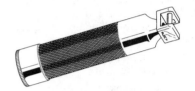

FIGURE 15.5   **E.** (Courtesy of Rüsch Inc., Duluth, GA.)

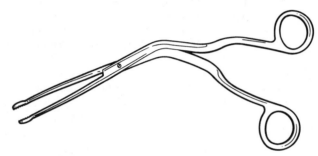

FIGURE 15.10   **J.** (Courtesy of Rüsch Inc., Duluth, GA.)

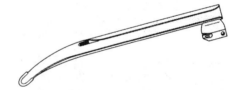

FIGURE 15.6   **F.** (Courtesy of Rüsch Inc., Duluth, GA.)

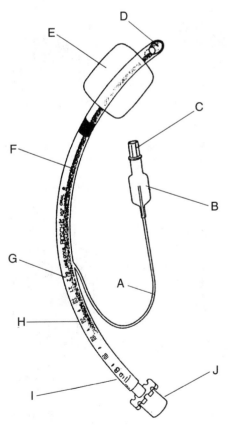

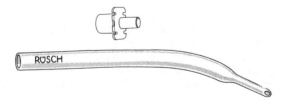

FIGURE 15.7   **G.** (Courtesy of Rüsch Inc., Duluth, GA.)

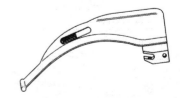

FIGURE 15.8   **H.** (Courtesy of Rüsch Inc., Duluth, GA.)

FIGURE 15.11   Components of an endotracheal tube. (Courtesy of Rüsch Inc., Duluth, GA.)

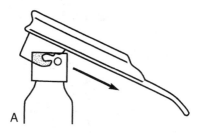
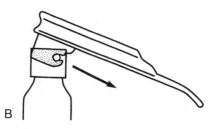
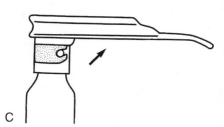

A   B   C

FIGURE 15.12   Assembly of a laryngoscope.

EXERCISE 15.2 Orotracheal Intubation

EXERCISE 15.2.1 Orotracheal Intubation with a MacIntosh Blade

1. Gather the necessary equipment to intubate an adult airway management trainer (make sure that the trainer is properly lubricated with the silicone spray) using the MacIntosh blade. The proper endotracheal tube and blade sizes are shown in Table 15.1.

2. Wash your hands and apply standard precautions and transmission-based isolation procedures as appropriate. The use of goggles is recommended.

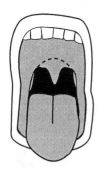
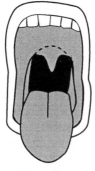

Class I: soft palate, uvula, fauces, pillars visible

No difficulty

Class II: soft palate, uvula, fauces visible

No difficulty

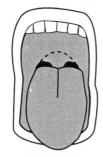
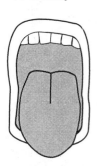

Class III: soft palate, base of uvula visible

Moderate difficulty

Class IV: hard palate only visible

Severe difficulty

FIGURE 15.13   Mallampati classification. (From Whitten, CE: Anyone Can Intubate: A Practical, Step-by-Step Guide for Health Professionals, ed 3. KW Publications, San Diego, 1994, p. 41, with permission.)

3. Open the endotracheal tube package halfway, leaving the cuffed end aseptically protected in the wrapper. Insert a stylet into the tube, making sure that the tip does not protrude from the other end, as shown in Figure 15.14. Bend the top of the stylet (if necessary) over the top of the tube to prevent it from slipping down. Shape the tube so that the curve is maintained.

4. Using the manual resuscitator with bag-valve-mask, pre-oxygenate the patient.

5. Suction the oropharynx.

6. Remove the oropharyngeal airway if one is present.

7. Position the head in the sniffing position as shown in Figure 15.15 by flexing the neck and tilting the head backward. Do not hyperextend. This allows alignment of the mouth, pharynx, and larynx. One or two towels can be used under the neck and shoulders to help achieve this position.

8. Ensure that all equipment is functioning and readily available.

9. Open the mouth using the crossed-finger, or scissor, technique.

10. Holding the laryngoscope in your left hand, insert the blade into the mouth, as shown in Figure 15.16.

11. Pushing aside the tongue to the left, as shown in Figure 15.17, advance the blade until the epiglottis is visualized, as shown in Figure 15.18. Identify the anatomic landmarks and *record the corresponding letters on your laboratory report.*

12. Continue to advance the tip of the blade into the **vallecula,** as shown in Figure 15.19, and indirectly expose the glottis by applying an upward and forward lift with your wrist kept straight, as shown in Figure 15.20. *Do not use the blade as a lever and rest it on the upper teeth. This prying motion will result in cracked or broken teeth.* Sellick's maneuver, the application of pressure on the cricoid cartilage by an assistant, is

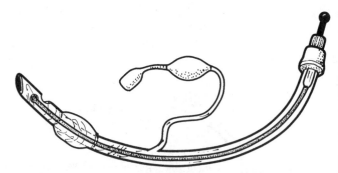

FIGURE 15.14   Insertion of a stylet into an endotracheal tube.

TABLE 15.1 **Endotracheal Tubes, Tracheostomy Tubes, and Laryngoscope Blades (Tube Thickness May Vary with Manufacturer)**

Approximate Age or Weight	Endotracheal Tubes*		
	Internal Diameter (in mm)	External Diameter (in mm)	Length (cm) (avg OD)
Premature infants (2–5 lb)	2.0–3.0	3.7–4.5	8
Newborn infants (5.0–5.5 lb)	3.0	4.5	9
Newborn infants to 3 mo (5.5–11 lb)	3.5–4.0	5.0–5.5	9
3–10 mo (11–18 lb)	4.3	5.7	10
10–12 mo (19–20 lb)	4.5	6.0	11
13–24 mo (20–25 lb)	5.0	6.5	12
2–3 yr (25–33 lb)	5.5	7.0	13
4–5 yr (33–44 lb)	6.0	8.0	14
6–7 yr (44–55 lb)	6.5	8.5	15
8–9 yr (55–70 lb)	7.0	9.0	16
9–10 yr (55–70 lb)	7.0	9.0	16
10–12 yr (70–85 lb)	7.5	9.5	17
12–16 yr (85–130 lb)	7.5	9.5	22.5
Adult females	8.0–9.0	10.0–12.0	19–24
Adult males	8.5–10.0	11.5–13.0	20–28

*Conversion to French scale: 4 × ID or 3 × ED.

Age	Tracheostomy Tubes	
	Jackson Tube Size	OD
Premature to newborn	00	4.5
Newborn to 3 mo	0	5.0
Up to 1 yr	1	5.5
1–3 yr	2	6.0
3–6 yr	3	7.0
6–12 yr	4	8.0
12 yr to adult	5–9	9.0–13.0

Age	Laryngoscope Blades (Type and Size)
Premature	Miller (0)
Infant to 3 mo	Miller (1)
3–12 mo	Miller or MacIntosh (1½)
3–9 yr	MacIntosh (2)
9 yr to adult	MacIntosh (3)

(From Pilbeam, SP: Mechanical Ventilation: Physiological and Clinical Applications, ed 2. Mosby-Year Book, St. Louis, p. 603, with permission.)

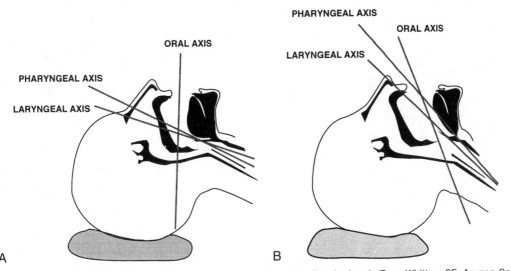

FIGURE 15.15   (A) "Sniffing" position for intubation. (B) The three axes after extending the head. (From Whitten, CE: Anyone Can Intubate: A Practical, Step-by-Step Guide for Health Professionals, ed 3. KW Publications, San Diego, 1994, pp. 52–53, with permission.)

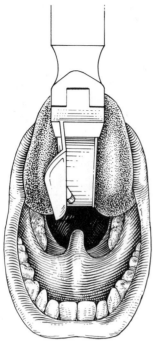

FIGURE 15.16 Insertion of laryngoscope blade into the mouth. (Finucane, BT and Santora, AH: Principles of Airway Management, ed 2. Mosby-Year Book, St. Louis, 1996, p. 168, with permission.)

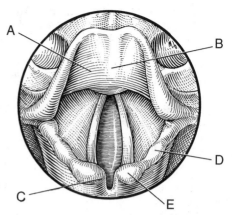

FIGURE 15.18 Visualization of the landmarks for intubation. (Finucane, BT and Santora, AH: Principles of Airway Management, ed 2. Mosby-Year Book, St. Louis, 1996, p. 9, with permission.)

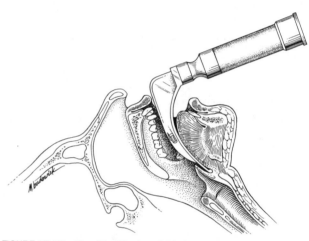

FIGURE 15.19 Tip of the Macintosh blade in the vallecula. (Finucane, BT and Santora, AH: Principles of Airway Management, ed 2. Mosby-Year Book, St. Louis, 1996, p. 168, with permission.)

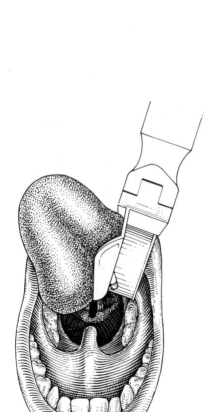

FIGURE 15.17 Displacement of the tongue. (Finucane, BT and Santora, AH: Principles of Airway Management, ed 2. Mosby-Year Book, St. Louis, 1996, p. 168, with permission.)

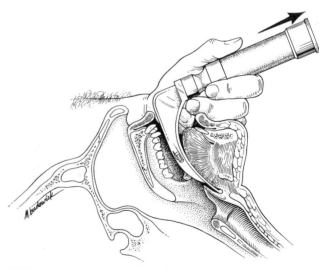

FIGURE 15.20 The upward, forward tilt to expose the glottis. Notice that the blade is not resting on the teeth. (Finucane, BT and Santora, AH: Principles of Airway Management, ed 2. Mosby-Year Book, St. Louis, 1996, p. 169, with permission.)

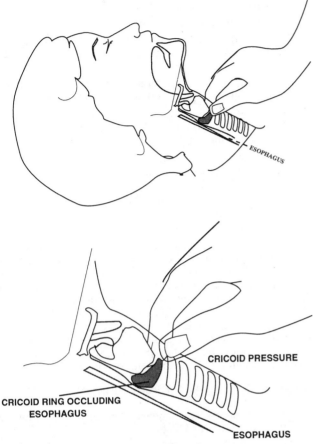

FIGURE 15.21 Applying cricoid pressure. (From Whitten, C: Anyone Can Intubate: A Practical, Step-by-Step Guide for Health Professionals, ed 3. KW Publications, San Diego, 1994, p. 97, with permission.)

sometimes beneficial in visualization, as shown in Figure 15.21.

13. The glottis is now exposed.

14. Identify the anatomical landmarks shown in Figure 15.21.

15. No intubation attempt should last longer than 30 sec. If problems are encountered with the visualization procedure, stop the intubation attempt and reoxygenate the patient with 100-percent oxygen between attempts for at least 1 min.

16. Have your assistant remove the tube from the wrapper without contaminating the cuffed end. Without taking your eyes off the glottis, insert the endotracheal tube into the right side of the mouth, advancing it until the cuff goes just beyond the vocal cords.

17. Holding the tube securely in position, quickly but gently remove the laryngoscope blade from the mouth. Remove the stylet and inflate the cuff with 5 ml of air.

18. Ventilate and oxygenate the patient. Observe for bilateral symmetrical chest expansion.

19. Auscultate for bilateral breath sounds.

20. Auscultate the epigastric region to listen for air in the stomach.

21. If no breath sounds are heard, deflate the cuff, remove the tube, and ventilate with a bag-valve-mask until the procedure is attempted again.

22. If unilateral sounds are heard, deflate the cuff and withdraw the tube gently while continuing to bag the patient until bilateral sounds are heard. Then reinflate the cuff.

    NOTE: In an actual clinical situation, a colorimetric capnometer (e.g., Easy Cap) may be useful to verify tube placement in the trachea.

23. Secure the tube with tape, as shown in Figure 15.22, or with a commercial orotracheal tube holder.

24. Attach the patient to an oxygenation or ventilation device.

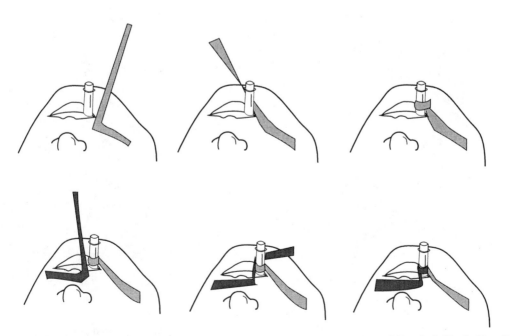

FIGURE 15.22 Securing the endotracheal tube with tape. (From Whitten, C: Anyone Can Intubate: A Practical, Step-by-Step Guide for Health Professionals, ed 3. KW Publications, San Diego, 1994, p. 64, with permission.)

25. Remove your gloves and other personal protective equipment.

26. Wash your hands.

EXERCISE 15.2.2 Orotracheal Intubation with a Miller Blade

1. Replace the MacIntosh blade used in the previous exercise with a Miller blade.

2. Repeat all of the steps in the previous exercise through step 10.

3. Directly expose the glottis by picking up the epiglottis with the tip of the blade, as shown in Figure 15.23.

4. Continue the remaining steps in the previous exercise.

EXERCISE 15.2.3 Intubation When an Esophageal Obturator Airway Is in Place

1. Select an airway management trainer that has an esophageal obturator airway/esophageal gastric tube airway in place.

2. Intubate the trainer as previously described.

3. Remove the EOA once the endotracheal tube is in place.

EXERCISE 15.2.4 Nasotracheal Intubation

1. Gather the necessary equipment.

2. Lubricate the nose of the adult airway management trainer with silicon spray. In the clinical setting a water-soluble jelly is used to lubricate the nasotracheal tube.

3. Wash hands and apply standard precautions and transmission-based isolation procedures as appropriate.

4. Prepare the patient as in Exercise 15.2.1.

5. Insert the tube into one of the nares.

6. Advance the tube into the oropharynx. *Never force a tube.* If an obstruction is met, attempt to pass the tube through the other naris.

7. When the tube is in the oropharynx, insert the laryngoscope blade into the mouth as previously described and expose the glottis.

8. Using the Magill forceps, pick up the tip of the nasotracheal tube before the cuff.

9. Ask your laboratory partner to push on the tube as you direct the tip into the glottis. Steps 8 and 9 are shown in Figure 15.24.

10. Once the tube is in the trachea, gently remove the equipment from the mouth and continue as in the previous exercises.

Blind nasotracheal intubation is sometimes attempted. It is difficult to practice in the laboratory setting because the passing of the tube requires a spontaneously breathing subject.[4] The procedure is basically the same for nasotracheal intubation except that a laryngoscope and forceps are not used. The practitioner must time the insertion of the tube with the opening of the epiglottis. Successful attempts are often indicated by an emission of a harsh sound as the tube passes the vocal cords, the inability of the patient to speak, and the feel of moist air coming from the tube on exhalation.

EXERCISE 15.2.5 Infant Intubation

1. Gather the necessary equipment. Refer to Table 15.1 for the proper size tubes and blades.

2. Select an infant airway management trainer and lubricate the pharynx with silicone spray. (In a clinical setting, tubes would not be lubricated.)

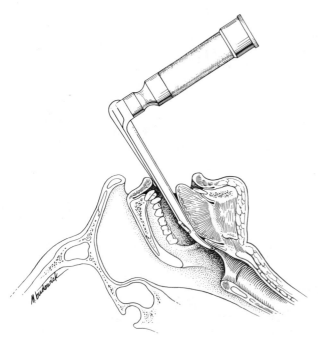

FIGURE 15.23 Exposure of the glottis using the Miller blade. (Finucane, BT and Santora, AH: Principles of Airway Management, ed 2. Mosby-Year Book, St. Louis, 1996, p. 178, with permission.)

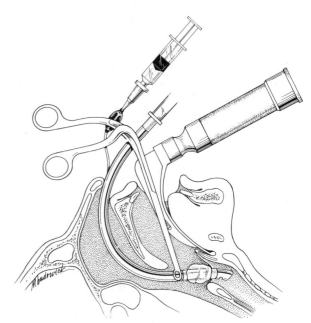

FIGURE 15.24 Nasal intubation using Magill forceps. (Finucane, BT and Santora, AH: Principles of Airway Management, ed 2. Mosby-Year Book, St. Louis, 1996, p. 180, with permission.)

3. Preoxygenate.

4. Position the head in the neutral, or "sniffing," position.

5. Intubate the trainer using the techniques learned in Exercise 15.2.1.

6. Continue the steps as described in Exercise 15.2.1.

EXERCISE 15.3 Securing an Endotracheal Tube

Using the intubated mannequins from the previous exercises, do the following:

1. Have your laboratory partner wash his or her hands, apply standard precautions and transmission-based isolation procedures as appropriate, and hold the endotracheal tube securely in position while you perform the following steps. Note the position of the endotracheal tube.

2. Wash your hands. Apply standard precautions and transmission-based isolation procedures as appropriate. Do not apply gloves until the tape is prepared. Prepare the cloth tape for use to secure the endotracheal tube. Several methods may be used, as shown in Figures 15.25 and 15.26.

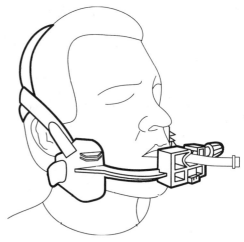

FIGURE 15.26 Securing an endotracheal tube using a commercial endotracheal tube holder. (Courtesy of STI Medical Products Corp., Costa Mesa, CA.)

3. Put on your gloves.

4. To enhance the adhesiveness of the tape, tincture of benzoin may be applied using a 4 × 4 gauze pad to the patient's skin. Do not spray or apply the liquid directly to the patient's face.

5. Apply the tape using one of the previously shown methods. Ensure that the tube position is correct. Secure the tape around the oropharyngeal airway to serve as a bite block. Reassess correct tube placement when finished. *"Chart" the procedure on your laboratory report.*

6. Repeat the exercise using a nasotracheally intubated mannequin.

7. Repeat the exercise using an infant mannequin.

References

1. American Association for Respiratory Care: AARC clinical practice guideline: Management of airway emergencies. Respir Care 40:749–760, 1995.
2. Sofair, E: Preanesthetic assessment: The professional singer with a difficult airway. Anesthesiology News 1:40, 1993.
3. Whitten, CE: Anyone Can Intubate. KW Publications, San Diego, 1996, p. 41.
4. Finucane, BT and Santora, AH: Principles of Airway Management, ed 2. Mosby, St Louis, 1996.

Related Readings

Barnhart, SL and Czervinske, MP: Perinatal and Pediatric Respiratory Care. WB Saunders, Philadelphia, 1995.
Eubanks, DH and Bone, RC: Principles and Applications of Cardiorespiratory Care Equipment. Mosby, St Louis, 1994.
Finucane, BT and Santora, AH: Principles of Airway Management, ed 2. Mosby, St Louis, 1996.
McPherson, S: Respiratory Care Equipment, ed 5. Mosby, St Louis, 1995.
Scanlan, C et al (eds): Egan's Fundamentals of Respiratory Care. Mosby, St Louis, 1995.
Whitten, CE: Anyone Can Intubate. KW Publications, San Diego, 1996.

Selected Journal Articles

American Association for Respiratory Care: AARC clinical practice guideline: Management of airway emergencies. Respir Care 40:749–760, 1995.

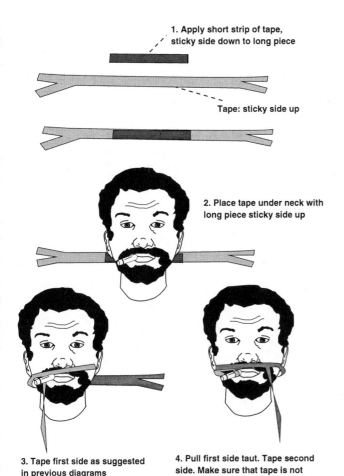

1. Apply short strip of tape, sticky side down to long piece

Tape: sticky side up

2. Place tape under neck with long piece sticky side up

3. Tape first side as suggested in previous diagrams

4. Pull first side taut. Tape second side. Make sure that tape is not tight enough to act as a tournequet.

FIGURE 15.25 Securing the tube in a bearded patient. (From Whitten, CE: Anyone Can Intubate: A Practical, Step-by-Step Guide for Health Professionals, ed 3. KW Publications, San Diego, 1994, p. 66, with permission.)

Bishop, MJ: Practice guidelines for airway care during resuscitation. Respir Care 40:393–401, 1995.

Criswell, J and Parr, M: Emergency airway management in patients with cervical spine injuries. Anaesthesia 49:900–903, 1994.

Dellinger, R: Airway management and nosocomial infection. Crit Care Management 21:1109–1110, 1993.

Kharasch, M and Graff, J: Emergency management of the airway. Crit Care Clin 11:53–67, 1995.

Mizutanti, A et al: Auscultation cannot distinguish esophageal from tracheal passage of a tube. J Clin Monit 7:232–236, 1991.

O'Hanlon, J and Harper, KW: Epistaxis and nasotracheal intubation: Prevention with vasocontrictor spray. Ir J Med Sci 163:58–60, 1994.

Reines, H: Airway management options. Respir Care 37:695–707, 1992.

Scannell, G et al: Orotracheal intubation in trauma patients with cervical fractures. Arch Surg 128:903–905, 1993.

Sklar, D and Tandberg, D: Glass ingestion from the fracture of a laryngoscope bulb. J Emerg Med 10:569–571, 1992.

Wilson, R: Upper airway problems. Respir Care 37:533–550, 1992.

LABORATORY REPORT

CHAPTER 15: ENDOTRACHEAL INTUBATION

Name _____ Date _____

Course/Section _____ Instructor _____

Data Collection

EXERCISE 15.1   Intubation Equipment and Preparation

EXERCISE 15.1.1   Identification of Intubation Equipment

A. _____

B. _____

C. _____

D. _____

E. _____

F. _____

G. _____

H. _____

I. _____

J. _____

EXERCISE 15.1.2   Identification of the Components of an Endotracheal Tube

A. _____

B. _____

C. _____

D. _____

E. _____

F. _____

G. _____

H. _____

I. _____

J. _____

EXERCISE 15.1.3   Equipment Testing

Light observation: _____

Light observation with loosened bulb: _____

If the lamp failed to light, list the items you would check in the order in which you would check them:

_____

_____

_____

Size of batteries: _____

Light observation with blade open: _____

Observations of endotracheal tube cuff testing in solution:

_____

Observations of cuff and pilot balloon:

_____

Observations of the cuff and pilot balloon with syringe in place: _____

EXERCISE 15.1.4 Assignment of Mallampati Classification

Mallampati classification: _____

EXERCISE 15.2   Orotracheal Intubation
EXERCISE 15.2.1   Orotracheal Intubation with a MacIntosh Blade

Identify the anatomic landmarks.

A. _____

B. _____

C. _____

D. _____

E. _____

EXERCISE 15.3   Securing an Endotracheal Tube

Chart the intubation procedure, your assessment of tube placement, and the securing of the endotracheal tube:

_____

_____

_____

_____

_____

_____

_____

_____

CRITICAL THINKING QUESTIONS

1. You have been asked by the nursing supervisor to supply an adult intubation tray for the emergency room. List *all* the equipment that you would recommend.

2. When would a topical anesthetic be indicated during the intubation procedure? What anesthetics can be used?

3. In a restless, fighting patient requiring immediate oral intubation, what pharmacological agent(s) could be used to facilitate intubation?

4. Describe in specific radiologic terms the proper location of an endotracheal tube.

The emergency medical technicians have brought in a 65-year-old victim in cardiac arrest. The patient had been ventilated with a manual resuscitator and mask. As you attempt to ventilate, the patient vomits.

5. What would be your immediate actions?

6. During your next attempt to intubate, you observe a large piece of undigested steak blocking your view of the glottis. How would you clear the airway, and what equipment would be needed?

PROCEDURAL COMPETENCY EVALUATION

Name _____ Date _____

Endotracheal Intubation

Setting: ☐ Lab ☐ Clinical   Evaluator: ☐ Peer ☐ Instructor

Conditions (describe): _____

_____

Equipment Used

_____

_____

	SATISFACTORY	UNSATISFACTORY	NOT OBSERVED	NOT APPLICABLE
Equipment and Patient Preparation				
1. Verifies, interprets, and evaluates physician's order or protocol	☐	☐	☐	☐
2. Selects, gathers, and assembles the necessary equipment	☐	☐	☐	☐
3. Washes hands and applies standard precautions and transmission-based isolation procedures as appropriate	☐	☐	☐	☐
4. Identifies patient, introduces self and department	☐	☐	☐	☐
5. Explains purpose of the procedure and confirms patient understanding	☐	☐	☐	☐
6. Provides for sedation/topical anesthetic or vasocontrictor, if indicated	☐	☐	☐	☐
7. Tests laryngoscope and endotracheal tube cuff	☐	☐	☐	☐
8. Lubricates endotracheal tube/stylet	☐	☐	☐	☐
Assessment and Implementation				
9. Assesses patient	☐	☐	☐	☐
10. Positions patient in sniffing position	☐	☐	☐	☐
11. Clears airway	☐	☐	☐	☐
12. Anesthetizes airway	☐	☐	☐	☐
13. Hyperoxygenates patient	☐	☐	☐	☐
14. Inserts laryngoscope into the oropharynx	☐	☐	☐	☐
15. Exposes and lifts epiglottis; visualizes cords	☐	☐	☐	☐
16. Inserts endotracheal tube between the vocal cords until cuff disappears	☐	☐	☐	☐
17. Inflates the cuff	☐	☐	☐	☐
18. Provides ventilation and hyperoxygenation	☐	☐	☐	☐
19. Observes, auscultates chest for symmetrical ventilation; auscultates stomach	☐	☐	☐	☐
20. Performs capnography or colorimetric capnometry to verify tube placement	☐	☐	☐	☐
Follow-up				
21. Hyperoxygenates between attempts if necessary	☐	☐	☐	☐
22. Marks proximal end of tube	☐	☐	☐	☐
23. Secures and stabilizes tube	☐	☐	☐	☐
24. Aspirates trachea	☐	☐	☐	☐
25. Provides postintubation care	☐	☐	☐	☐

	SATISFACTORY	UNSATISFACTORY	NOT OBSERVED	NOT APPLICABLE
26. Places patient on appropriate oxygen/humidification/ventilation device	☐	☐	☐	☐
27. Provides for postintubation chest x-ray	☐	☐	☐	☐
28. Repositions tube, if needed	☐	☐	☐	☐
29. Maintains/processes equipment	☐	☐	☐	☐
30. Disposes of infectious waste and washes hands	☐	☐	☐	☐
31. Records pertinent data in chart and departmental records	☐	☐	☐	☐
32. Notifies appropriate personnel and makes any necessary recommendations or modifications to patient care plan	☐	☐	☐	☐

_____
Signature of Evaluator

_____
Signature of Student

PERFORMANCE RATING SCALE

5 EXCELLENT—FAR EXCEEDS EXPECTED LEVEL, FLAWLESS PERFORMANCE
4 ABOVE AVERAGE—NO PROMPTING REQUIRED, ABLE TO SELF-CORRECT
3 AVERAGE—THE MINIMUM COMPETENCY LEVEL, NO CRITICAL ERRORS
2 IMPROVEMENT NEEDED—PROBLEM AREAS EXIST; CRITICAL ERRORS, CORRECTIONS NEEDED
1 POOR AND UNACCEPTABLE PERFORMANCE—GROSS INACCURACIES, POTENTIALLY HARMFUL

PERFORMANCE CRITERIA	SCALE				
1. DISPLAYS KNOWLEDGE OF ESSENTIAL CONCEPTS	5	4	3	2	1
2. DEMONSTRATES THE RELATIONSHIP BETWEEN THEORY AND CLINICAL PRACTICE	5	4	3	2	1
3. FOLLOWS DIRECTIONS, EXHIBITS SOUND JUDGMENT, AND DEMONSTRATES ATTENTION TO SAFETY AND DETAIL	5	4	3	2	1
4. EXHIBITS THE REQUIRED MANUAL DEXTERITY	5	4	3	2	1
5. PERFORMS PROCEDURE IN A REASONABLE TIME FRAME	5	4	3	2	1
6. MAINTAINS STERILE OR ASEPTIC TECHNIQUE	5	4	3	2	1
7. INITIATES UNAMBIGUOUS GOAL-DIRECTED COMMUNICATION	5	4	3	2	1
8. PROVIDES FOR ADEQUATE CARE AND MAINTENANCE OF EQUIPMENT AND SUPPLIES	5	4	3	2	1
9. EXHIBITS COURTEOUS AND PLEASANT DEMEANOR	5	4	3	2	1
10. MAINTAINS CONCISE AND ACCURATE RECORDS	5	4	3	2	1

ADDITIONAL COMMENTS: INCLUDE ERRORS OF OMISSION OR COMMISSION, COMMUNICATIVE SKILLS, AND EFFECTIVENESS OF PATIENT INTERACTION:

SUMMARY PERFORMANCE EVALUATION AND RECOMMENDATIONS

SATISFACTORY PERFORMANCE—Performed without error or prompting, or able to self-correct, no critical errors.

_____ LABORATORY EVALUATION. SKILLS MAY BE APPLIED/OBSERVED IN THE CLINICAL SETTING.

_____ CLINICAL EVALUATION. STUDENT READY FOR MINIMALLY SUPERVISED APPLICATION AND REFINEMENT.

UNSATISFACTORY PERFORMANCE—Prompting required; performed with critical errors, potentially harmful.

_____ STUDENT REQUIRES ADDITIONAL LABORATORY PRACTICE.

_____ STUDENT REQUIRES ADDITIONAL SUPERVISED CLINICAL PRACTICE.

SIGNATURES

STUDENT: _____   EVALUATOR: _____

DATE: _____   DATE: _____

Tracheostomies and Artificial Airway Maintenance

INTRODUCTION

Once an artificial tracheal airway is in place, meticulous maintenance and care are needed to prevent infection, airway emergencies, and other complications of prolonged intubation or cannulation. Critical responsibilities of the respiratory care practitioner include securing the tube and maintaining proper position, adequate humidification and secretion clearance, provision for patient communication, providing cuff and **stoma** care, changing **tracheostomy** tubes, and troubleshooting airway-related problems.[1] Although a respiratory care practitioner is not responsible for the actual **tracheotomy** procedure, the practitioner may be called on to assist with the procedure, replace a displaced tracheostomy tube, or change it from one type to another. Detailed knowledge of these tubes is also an essential part of the responsibility of the practitioner.

The respiratory care practitioner qualified to intubate may also extubate patients. The patient must be assessed after **extubation** for laryngeal edema and vocal cord injury. Appropriate oxygenation and humidification must be provided. Administration of racemic epinephrine or steroids may help relieve airway obstruction caused by edema.

Lack of appropriate airway care can lead to short- and long-term complications ranging from minor bleeding or edema to permanent anatomical airway changes or life-threatening emergencies.[2,3] Airway emergencies include inadvertent extubation, cuff leak, and obstructed airway with failure to provide adequate ventilation. Injuries associated with airway placement include tissue pressure **necrosis, granulomas,** tracheoesophageal or arterial **fistula, tracheomalacia,** tracheal **stenosis,** laryngotracheal web formation, vocal cord paralysis, and **paresis.**

OBJECTIVES
Upon completion of this chapter, the student will be able to:

1. Practice communication skills needed for assessing the level of patient comprehension while instructing patients in airway care procedures.
2. Practice medical charting for airway care procedures.
3. Apply infection control guidelines and standards associated with equipment and procedures, according to OSHA regulations and CDC guidelines.
4. Resecure an endotracheal tube in place by changing cloth tape and commercial endotracheal tube holders.
5. Reposition an endotracheal tube and assess the proper size and placement.
6. Perform minimum occluding volume (MOV) and minimal leak technique (MLT) cuff inflation procedures.
7. Measure airway cuff pressures with aneroid and mercury pressure manometers.
8. Extubate a patient and evaluate the patient's respiratory status after extubation.
9. Provide appropriate postextubation airway care, including oxygenation, humidification, and pharmacological treatment.
10. Identify airway emergencies and take appropriate actions to ensure patient ventilation and oxygenation, as well as troubleshoot equipment, including cuff leaks, tube obstructions, tube malpositions, and inadvertent extubation.
11. Identify the various types of tracheostomy tubes, buttons, and adjuncts and their component parts.
12. Perform tracheostomy care, including equipment cleaning and stoma care.
13. Change a tracheostomy tube on an adult airway management trainer.
14. Provide for adequate patient communication with an artificial airway in place.

KEY TERMS

decannulation	extubation	obturator	stoma
dysphagia	fistula	paresis	tracheomalacia
dysphonia	granulomas	phonation	tracheostomy
	necrosis	stenosis	tracheotomy

EQUIPMENT REQUIRED

- Oropharyngeal airways, various sizes
- Airway management trainers, adult and infant
- Silicone spray
- Water-soluble lubricant
- Goggles or face shields
- Sterile and nonsterile disposable latex and vinyl gloves, various sizes
- Oxygen gas source and flowmeter
- Oxygen connecting tubing and nipple adaptors
- Endotracheal tubes, various sizes
- Tracheostomy tubes, various sizes and styles:
  Jackson metal
  Cuffed and cuffless
  Cuffed and cuffless fenestrated
  Disposable and nondisposable inner cannulas
  Fenestrated and nonfenestrated cannulas
  Bivona or Kamen-Wilkinson Fome-Cuff tubes
  Lanz-Maguiness cuff tubes
  Shiley speaking valve with oxygen port
- Tracheal buttons
- Stethoscopes
- Colorimetric capnometry (Easy Cap) or other spot-check capnography device
- Manual resuscitators with masks, adult and infant
- Laryngoscope blades and handles:
  Miller (various sizes)
  MacIntosh (various sizes)
- Batteries for laryngoscopes
- Replacement laryngoscope bulbs
- Stylets
- Suction catheter kits
- Yankauer catheter
- Basins
- Suction machines
- Sterile water or normal saline
- Hydrogen peroxide
- Tracheostomy care kits
- Swivel adaptor and deadspace tubing
- Tracheostomy collars
- Briggs adaptors (T-piece)
- Montgomery tubes
- Passy-Muir or other brand of speaking valves
- Letter board or pad and pen/pencil
- Tracheostomy communication devices
- Cloth tape
- Tincture of benzoin
- Endotracheal tube holders
- Tracheostomy tube holders
- 10-ml syringes
- Towels
- Scissors
- Lemon glycerine swabs
- Toothbrush and toothpaste
- Razor and shaving cream
- Cotton swabs
- 4 × 4 sterile gauze
- Hemostats

- Needles, various sizes
- Pressure manometers (aneroid and mercury)
- Three-way stop cocks
- Posey Cuffalator cuff inflation device
- Large volume nebulizer
- Large-bore corrugated tubing
- Aerosol masks
- Endotracheal tubes with ruptured cuff, malfunctioning pilot balloon, cut pilot tube
- Endotracheal tubes obstructed by Silly Putty, Play-Doh, or material of similar consistency
- Pulse oximeter

● EXERCISES

EXERCISE 16.1 Cuff Care

EXERCISE 16.1.1 Minimal Leak Technique

1. Orally intubate an airway management trainer.
2. Verify correct tube placement as practiced in Chapter 15. *Record the endotracheal tube size and centimeter mark to the mouth on your laboratory report.*
3. While your laboratory partner is manually ventilating the mannequin, use a 10-ml syringe to slowly inject air into the pilot balloon of the endotracheal tube.
4. Continue to inflate the cuff until no leak is heard while auscultating the lateral neck (this will have to be simuated on the mannequin). Withdraw a slight amount of air from the cuff until a small leak is heard above the cuff on the lateral neck during peak inspiration. If air leakage is felt from the nose or mouth, too large a leak has been created.
5. Note the total volume of air used to inflate the cuff, and *record the volume on your laboratory report.*

EXERCISE 16.1.2 Minimum Occluding Volume

1. Orally intubate an airway management trainer.
2. Verify correct tube placement as practiced in Chapter 15. *Record the endotracheal tube size and centimeter mark to the mouth on your laboratory report.*
3. While your laboratory partner is manually ventilating the mannequin, use a 10-ml syringe to slowly inject air into the pilot balloon of the endotracheal tube.
4. Continue to inflate the cuff until no leak is heard while auscultating the lateral neck (this will have to be simulated on the mannequin). Maximum inflation should be done during peak inspiration of positive pressure breath where the seal is needed most.
5. Note the total volume of air used to inflate the cuff, and *record the volume on your laboratory report.*

EXERCISE 16.1.3 Cuff Pressure Measurement

1. Inflate the cuff of an orally intubated mannequin to MOV.

2. Obtain a three-way stopcock (Fig. 16.1). Turn the valve stem so that it is off to the Luer-lok. Observe all three of the openings to determine which two of the ports are open. This would allow air to flow in that particular direction.

3. Turn the valve stem so that it is off to the left port of the three-way stopcock. Observe all three of the openings to determine which two of the ports are open. This would allow air to flow in that particular direction.

4. Turn the valve stem so that it is off to the right port of the three-way stopcock. Observe all three of the openings to determine which two of the ports are open. This would allow air to flow in that particular direction.

5. A mercury manometer, aneroid manometer, or commercial cuff inflation device may be used to measure cuff pressure, as shown in Figure 16.2. Set up a cuff pressure measurement system using the mercury manometer, as shown in Figure 16.2A.

6. Suction any secretions in the pharynx and above the cuff thoroughly.

7. Attach the measurement system to the valve connection on the pilot balloon with the three-way stopcock open to all directions. The cuff will automatically deflate. This will allow equilibration between the manometer, the pilot tube, and the cuff.

8. Pull the syringe barrel back to 10 ml and attach it to the three-way stopcock.

9. Slowly inflate the cuff to MOV during peak inspiration. *Record the peak pressure achieved on the manometer during expiration on your laboratory report.*

10. The maximum cuff pressure should be maintained at less than 20 to 25 mm Hg or 25 to 33 cm H_2O. The pressure increases during exhalation when the tracheal diameter is narrower. Maximum cuff pressures should not be exceeded during the exhalation phase.

11. Turn the stopcock off to the pilot tube. Detach the manometer system.

12. Attach the 10-ml syringe to the pilot tube. Remove the air from the cuff, measure it, and *record the volume on your laboratory report.* Reinsert the air slowly back into the cuff.

13. Repeat steps 6 through 12 using MLT.

14. Repeat steps 6 through 12 using a Posey Cuffalator.

EXERCISE 16.2 Resecuring and Repositioning of an Endotracheal Tube

To perform this exercise, you will need an intubated mannequin with a Briggs adaptor and large-bore tubing attached to simulate a clinical situation. The tube should be secured with tape before the exercise.

1. Have your laboratory partner wash his or her hands, apply standard precautions and transmission-based isolation procedures as appropriate, and hold the endotracheal tube securely in position while you perform the following steps. Note the position of the endotracheal tube.

2. Wash your hands. Apply standard precautions and transmission-based isolation procedures as appropriate. Do not apply gloves until the tape is prepared. Prepare the cloth tape for use to secure the endotracheal tube. Several methods may be used, as shown in Figures 16.3 and 16.4.

3. Put on your gloves. Carefully cut and remove the tape currently securing the endotracheal tube. *Do not cut the pilot tube.* Make sure it is out of your way. Discard the used tape in an infectious waste container. Oral hygiene is crucial in an intubated patient. The teeth may be brushed, or lemon glycerine swabs may be used to clean the mouth. Male patients may also be shaved at this time.

4. Move the endotracheal tube to the opposite side of the mouth. A tongue depressor may be used to assist if the tongue prevents easy repositioning. Insert an oropharyngeal airway into the mouth medially to the endotracheal tube.

5. Clean the patient's face using a wet 4 × 4 gauze pad, removing as much of the previous adhesive as possible.

6. Dry the skin with a clean towel or 4 × 4 gauze pad.

7. To enhance the adhesiveness of the tape, tincture of benzoin may be applied using a 4 × 4 gauze pad to the patient's skin. Do not spray or apply the liquid directly to the patient's face.

8. Apply the tape using one of the previously described methods. Ensure that the tube position is correct. Secure the tape around the oropharyngeal airway to serve as a bite block. Reassess correct tube placement when finished. *"Chart" the procedure on your laboratory report.*

9. Repeat the exercise using a commercial endotracheal tube holder to secure the tube.

EXERCISE 16.3 Extubation

1. Verify a physician's order or protocol or assess patient's readiness for extubation. Check the chart or protocol for the appropriate F_IO_2 after extubation.

2. Gather the necessary equipment:
   Suction and suction kits
   Large volume nebulizer
   Large-bore corrugated tubing
   Aerosol mask

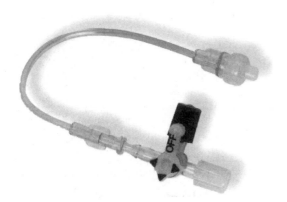

FIGURE 16.1   3-way stopcock. (Courtesy of Smith Industries Medical Systems, Keene, NH.)

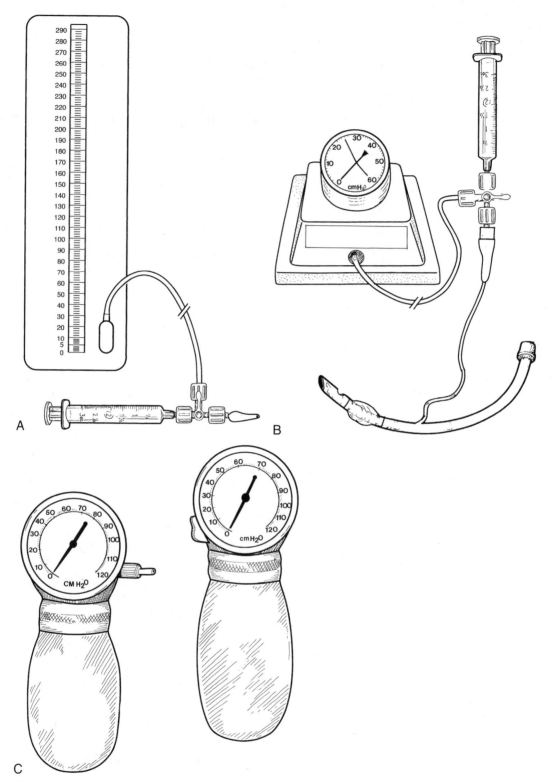

FIGURE 16.2 Cuff pressure measurements *(A)* using a mercury manometer, *(B)* using an aneroid manometer, *(C)* using a Posey Cufflator.

Scissors
10-ml syringe
Intubation tray (see Chapter 15)

3. Assemble the equipment to deliver the appropriate F_IO_2.

4. Using your lab partner as the "patient," explain the procedure and confirm the patient's understanding.

5. Wash your hands and apply standard precautions and transmission-based isolation procedures as appropriate.

6. Assess the patient, including pulse oximetry.

7. Place the patient in a high Fowler's position.

8. Suction the patient's endotracheal tube and pharynx thoroughly, as described in Chapter 14.

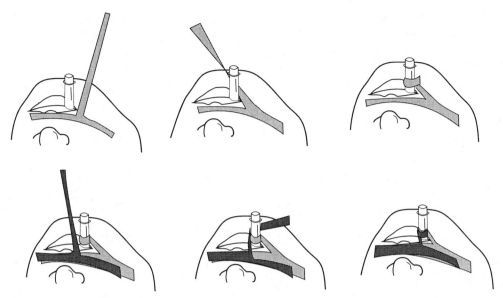

FIGURE 16.3   Securing an endotracheal tube to the maxilla. (From Whitten, CE: Anyone Can Intubate: A Practical, Step-by-Step Guide for Health Professionals, ed 3. KW Publications, San Diego, 1994, p. 63, with permission.)

9. Remove the endotracheal tube tape or securing device and deflate the cuff completely. Alternatively, the pilot tube may then be cut to ensure easy removal of any remaining air during tube withdrawal.[1]

10. Instruct the patient to take a maximum inspiration and remove the tube at peak inspiration so that the vocal cords are completely abducted. An alternative method is to have the patient cough, which will also maximally abduct the vocal cords.[4]

11. Apply the oxygen and humidity device on the patient.

12. Assess the patient. Determine the adequacy of spontaneous ventilation. Make particular note of hoarseness or stridor. If stridor is present, racemic epinephrine aerosol may be administered. If stridor worsens and the patient's clinical situation deteriorates, reintubation may be necessary.

13. *Chart the procedure on your laboratory report.*

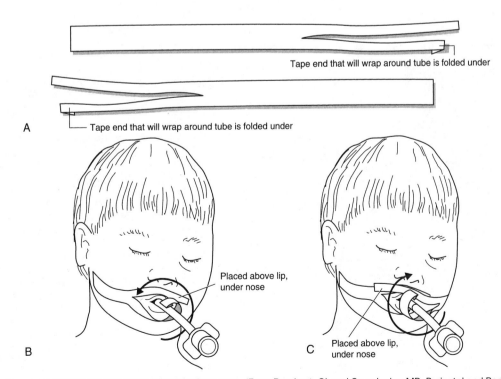

FIGURE 16.4   Recommended method to secure the tube long term. (From Barnhart, SL and Czervinske, MP: Perinatal and Pediatric Respiratory Care. WB Saunders, Philadelphia, 1995, p. 245, with permission.)

EXERCISE 16.4 Airway Emergencies

Your instructor will provide you with an orally intubated mannequin attached to a ventilator swivel adaptor and tubing connection. The mannequin has one of the following airway emergencies simulated:

    Cuff rupture
    Tube obstruction
    Pilot tube leak
    Pilot valve leak

1. Remove the ventilator adaptor and manually ventilate the mannequin. Can you ventilate the mannequin? Does the air go in easily? Is there an air leak around the mouth or nose? *Record your observations on your laboratory report.*

2. Your action plan will depend on the cause of the airway emergency.
    a. If you cannot ventilate or air cannot enter easily and there does *not* appear to be an air leak, the tube is most likely obstructed. Troubleshooting steps for an obstructed airway should be followed:
        (1) Attempt to pass a suction catheter. Suction and lavage the airway to clear the obstruction. Attempt to ventilate. Assess the adequacy of ventilation.
        (2) If it is not possible to clear the obstruction, notify the appropriate personnel. Emergency extubation is a last resort and should not be performed unless all other attempts have failed. The next step in a spontaneously breathing patient is to deflate the cuff and assess for adequate ventilation. If ventilation is adequate, the situation is less emergent and the proper equipment and personnel can be assembled to reintubate under more controlled circumstances.
        (3) If the patient cannot be adequately ventilated, an emergent situation is at hand. The nurse and physi-

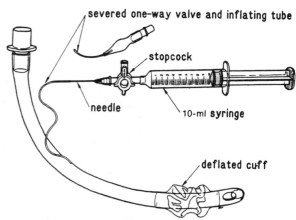

FIGURE 16.6   Temporary inflation device for a damaged pilot valve. (From Sills, J: An emergency cuff inflation technique. Respiratory Care, March, 31:200, 1986, with permission.)

cian should be notified of the situation, and the patient should be extubated. Extubate and manually ventilate the mannequin with a mask while preparations for reintubation are made.

    b. If you are able to squeeze the manual resuscitator without difficulty, but a leak is noted from the mouth or nose, there is a problem with the cuff or the pilot tube or valve. In an actual clinical situation a conscious patient may even be able to vocalize. Troubleshooting steps for a cuff leak should be followed:
        (1) Attempt to reinflate the cuff as previously practiced. If successful, measure the cuff pressure.
        (2) Ventilate and assess for leaks.
        (3) If the leak persists, visually inspect the pilot tube, balloon, and valve for any cuts, nicks, or other signs of damage. If the pilot tube is damaged, refer to step (7).
        (4) Reinflate the cuff and apply a hemostat to the pilot tube as shown in Figure 16.5. Be cautious not to apply excessive pressure so that the tube is not permanently crimped or damaged.
        (5) Ventilate and assess for leaks.
        (6) If clamping the pilot tube in step (4) eliminated the leak, most likely the pilot valve is damaged. Gather the equipment and assemble a temporary inflating device as shown in Figure 16.6 by using an appropriate size needle, three-way stopcock, and syringe. Cut the pilot valve and inflating tube past the point of any damage. Insert the needle into the remaining portion of the pilot tube and attach the inflating device. Tape the entire assembly to a tongue depressor to prevent accidental needle-stick injuries or dislodging of the needle. Reinflate the cuff, measure the cuff pressure, and reassess ventilation.
        (7) If the leak persists, it is likely that the cuff is ruptured. This is the most emergent situation if you cannot achieve adequate ventilation. The nurse and physician should be notified of the situation, and the patient should be extubated. Extubate and manually ventilate the mannequin with a mask while preparations for reintubation are made.

3. *Chart your assessment of the cause of the airway emergency and the corrective actions taken on your laboratory report.*

4. Repeat steps 1 and 2 for the other three airway emergencies.

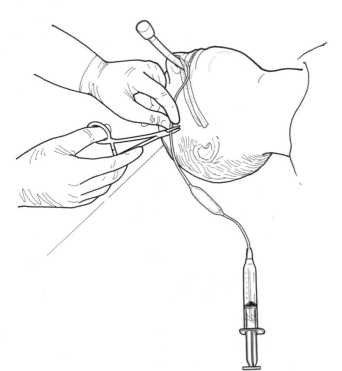

FIGURE 16.5   Clamping the pilot tube.

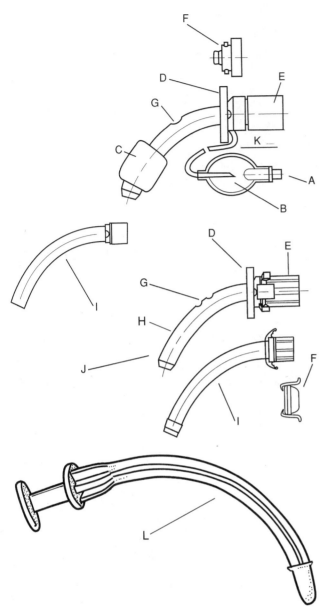

FIGURE 16.7 Components of tracheostomy tubes. (Adapted from Shiley Tracheostomy Products, courtesy of Mallinckrodt Medical, St. Louis, MO, with permission.)

EXERCISE 16.5 Tracheostomy Tubes

EXERCISE 16.5.1 Components and Types of Tracheostomy Tubes

1. Compare the various types and components provided in the laboratory with Figures 16.7 through 16.15. *Identify the items and record them on your laboratory report.*

    Disposable inner cannula
    Nondisposable inner cannula
    Outer cannula
    Pilot balloon
    Pilot valve
    Cuff
    Fenestration
    Cannula cap
    Obturator
    15-mm connector
    Neck plate
    Inflation line
    Montgomery tube
    Tracheostomy button
    Lanz-Maguinness cuff
    Bivona or Kamen-Wilkinson Fome-Cuff
    Passy-Muir valve
    Pitt speaking tube
    Olympic Trach-Talk
    Jackson tracheostomy tube

2. Open a tracheostomy tube box. Examine the contents and the manner in which they are packed. Pay close attention to what is sterile and what is not. *Record the contents of the box on your laboratory report. Include the manufacturer, size, and style of the tube.*

EXERCISE 16.5.2 Tracheostomy Tube Insertion

1. Select a tracheostomized adult airway management trainer.

2. Gather the necessary equipment:
    Tracheostomy tube and components
    Tracheostomy ties or holder
    Suction equipment
    Water-soluble lubricant (silicone spray)
    Sterile water or saline
    Basin
    Sterile gloves

3. Using your laboratory partner as the patient, explain the procedure for changing the tracheostomy tube.

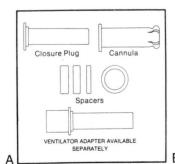

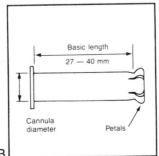

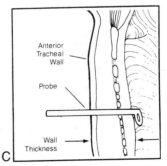

FIGURE 16.8 **M.** (Courtesy of Olympic Medical, Seattle, WA.)

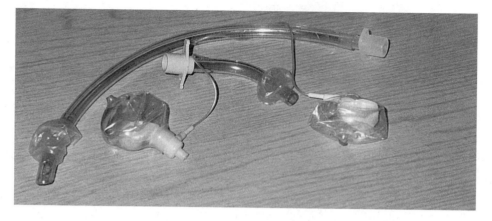

FIGURE 16.9 **N.**

4. Suction the trachea based on patient assessment.

5. Wash your hands, put on sterile gloves, and use other standard precautions and transmission-based isolation procedures as appropriate.

6. Your laboratory partner will now serve as your assistant. Have your partner open the new tracheostomy tube box, remove the tube, and place it on a sterile field.

7. Have your partner fill a basin with sterile solution.

8. While you hold the new tube in your sterile hand, instruct your partner to inject 5 ml of air into the cuff. Remember that your partner *cannot* touch the tube.

9. Check the tube for cuff leaks.

10. If no leaks are present, deflate the cuff completely.

11. Have your partner attach the new, clean tracheostomy ties or holder.

12. Remove the inner cannula and insert the obturator.

13. Lubricate the tip of the tracheostomy tube/obturator.

14. Reassure your patient and position the patient's head. The patient should be seated in a semi-Fowler's position with the neck slightly extended.

15. Have your partner loosen or untie the old tracheostomy ties and deflate the cuff if it is inflated.

16. Remove the oxygen or humidity therapy device and place aseptically.

17. With one hand, remove the old tracheostomy tube.

18. Visually inspect the stoma for bleeding or infection.

19. Insert the new tube as shown in Figure 16.16. Gently introduce the tip of the obturator into the stoma and advance the tube into the trachea with a slightly downward motion. Do not force if resistance is met.

20. Quickly remove the obturator and insert the inner cannula. Make sure that one finger keeps the tracheostomy tube in place until it is secured.

21. Inflate the cuff if ordered.

22. Ensure proper placement by auscultation, feeling airflow through the tube and chest expansion.

23. Tie the tube into place. Remember to place one finger under the tie to prevent overtightening. Velcro tube holders may also be employed.

24. Restore the patient to the previous oxygen or humidity therapy device.

25. Dispose of the dirty tube, ties, and gloves in the proper receptacle.

26. Wash your hands.

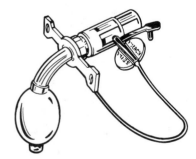

FIGURE 16.10 **O.** (Courtesy of Bivona Medical Technologies, Gary, IN.)

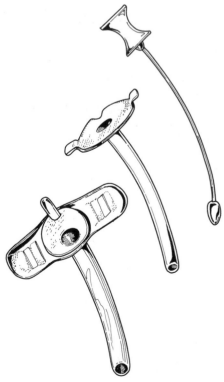

FIGURE 16.11 **P.**

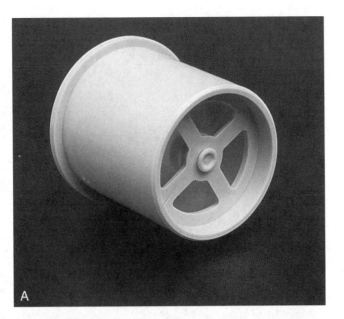

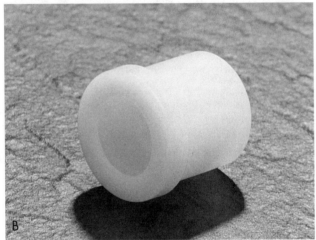

FIGURE 16.12 **Q.** (Courtesy of *[A]* Passy-Muir Inc., Irvine, CA; *[B]* Boston Medical Products, Westborough, MA.)

EXERCISE 16.5.3 Tracheostomy Care and Cleaning

NOTE: Tracheostomy patients should always have a replacement tracheostomy tube at the bedside in case an emergency replacement becomes necessary.

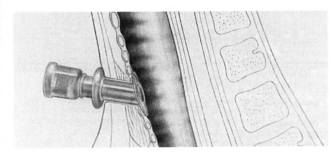

FIGURE 16.13 **R.** (Courtesy of Boston Medical Products, Westborough, MA.)

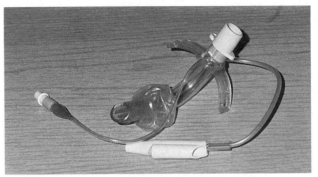

FIGURE 16.14 **S.**

1. Wash your hands and apply standard precautions and transmission-based isolation procedures as appropriate.
2. Gather the necessary equipment:
   Tracheostomy care kit
   Suction kit
   Gloves
   Peroxide
   Sterile water or saline
   Spare inner cannula or disposable cannula
3. Explain the procedure and confirm patient understanding.
4. Suction thoroughly.
5. Remove the old dressing and discard in an infectious waste container.
6. Remove the inner cannula and replace with the spare red-top cannula if a nondisposable cannula is in place.
7. Open the tracheostomy care kit and fill one basin with hydrogen peroxide and the other with sterile saline.
8. Scrub the cannula with a brush in the peroxide and rinse with the sterile saline.
9. Replace the permanent cannula.
10. If a disposable cannula is used, remove the dirty cannula, dispose of it properly, and replace it with a clean disposable cannula.
11. Clean the stoma site and exterior portions of the tube using peroxide, cotton-tipped applicators, and pipe cleaner for the tube crevices.
12. Replace the dressing using a precut 4 × 4 gauze pad.
13. Remove the old ties by cutting them with a scissor. *Be careful not to cut the pilot tube.* Commercial tracheostomy tube holders can be removed and replaced by following the manufacturer's instructions.

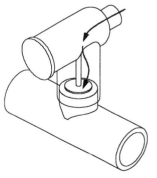

FIGURE 16.15 **T.** (Courtesy of Olympic Medical, Seattle, WA.)

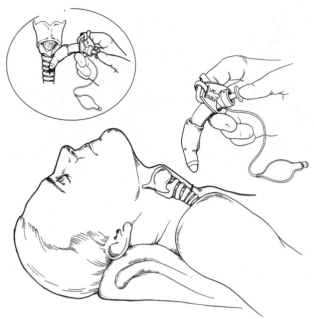

FIGURE 16.16   Insertion of replacement tracheostomy tube. (Courtesy of Shiley Tracheostomy Products, Mallinckrodt Medical, St. Louis, MO.)

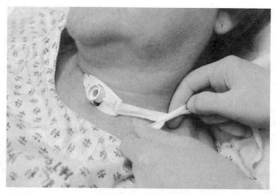

FIGURE 16.17   Retying tracheostomy tapes. (Courtesy of Shiley Tracheostomy Products, Mallinckrodt Medical, St. Louis, MO.)

4. Scanlan, C et al (eds): Egan's Fundamentals of Respiratory Care, ed 6. Mosby, St Louis, 1995, p 575.

Related Readings

Eubanks, DH and Bone, RC: Principles and Applications of Cardiorespiratory Care Equipment. Mosby, St Louis, 1994.
Finucane, B and Santora, A: Principles of Airway Management, ed. 2. Mosby, St Louis, 1996.
McPherson, S: Respiratory Care Equipment, ed 5. Mosby, St Louis, 1995.
Scanlan, C et al (eds): Egan's Fundamentals of Respiratory Care, ed 6. Mosby, St Louis, 1995.
Shiley Tracheostomy Products: Tracheostomy Tube: Adult Home Care Guide. Mallenckrodt Medical, Irvine, CA, 1993.

Selected Journal Articles

American Association for Respiratory Care: The AARC clinical practice guideline: Management of airway emergencies. Respir Care 40:749–760, 1995.
Bach, J and Alba, A: Tracheostomy ventilation: A study of efficacy with deflated cuffs and cuffless tubes. Chest 97:79–89, 1990.
Hoffman, L: Timing of tracheostomy: What is the best approach? Respir Care 9:378–389, 1994.
Kaplow, R and Bookbinder, M: A comparison of four endotracheal tube holders. Heart Lung 23:59–66, 1994.
Kollef, MH, Legare, EJ and Damiano, M: Endotracheal tube misplacement: Incidence, risk factors and impact of a quality improvement program. South Med J 87:248–254, 1994.
Reines, H: Airway management options. Respir Care 37:695–707, 1992.
Santos, PM, Afrassiabi, A and Weymuller, EA: Risk factors associated with prolonged intubation and laryngeal injury. Otolaryngol Head Neck Surg 111:453–459, 1994.
Sills, J: An emergency cuff inflation technique. Respir Care 31:199–201, 1996.
Wilson, R: Upper airway problems. Respir Care 37:533–550, 1992.

14. Attach the tracheostomy twill tape to one end of the tube by making a loop and inserting it into one of the holes on the neck plate. Bring the other end back through the loop and pull. Bring the tape around the patient's neck and insert one end of the tape into the other hole. Tie the tube in place by making a square knot on the side of the neck. Avoid overtightening by placing one finger between the tape and the patient's neck (Fig. 16.17).

15. Ensure that the tube is in the proper position, and reassess the patient.

16. Ensure that all equipment is disposed of in the proper waste container.

17. Remove gloves and wash your hands.

References

1. Scanlan, C et al (eds): Egan's Fundamentals of Respiratory Care, ed 6. Mosby, St Louis, 1995, p 565.
2. Scanlan, C et al (eds): Egan's Fundamentals of Respiratory Care, ed 6. Mosby, St Louis, 1995, p 562.
3. American Association for Respiratory Care: AARC clinical practice guideline: Management of airway emergencies. Respir Care 40:749–760, 1995.

LABORATORY REPORT

CHAPTER 16: TRACHEOSTOMIES AND ARTIFICIAL AIRWAY MAINTENANCE

Name _____   Date _____

Course/Section _____   Instructor _____

Data Collection

EXERCISE 16.1   Cuff Care

EXERCISE 16.1.1   Minimal Leak Technique

Endotracheal tube size: _____

Position: _____ cm

Cuff volume: _____

EXERCISE 16.1.2   Minimal Occluding Volume

Endotracheal tube size: _____

Position: _____ cm

Cuff volume: _____

EXERCISE 16.1.3   Cuff Pressure Measurement

Cuff pressure at MOV: _____

Volume at MOV: _____

Cuff pressure at MLT: _____

Volume at MLT: _____

Cuff pressure using Posey Cuffalator: _____

Volume using Posey Cuffalator: _____

EXERCISE 16.2   Resecuring and Repositioning of an Endotracheal Tube

Chart the procedure:

_____

_____

_____

_____

EXERCISE 16.3   Extubation

Chart the procedure:

_____

_____

_____

_____

EXERCISE 16.4   Airway Emergencies

Can you ventilate? _____

Does air go in easily? _____

Is there an air leak around the mouth and nose? _____

Chart your assessment of the airway emergency and corrective actions taken:

_____

_____

_____

_____

_____

_____

_____

_____

_____

_____

EXERCISE 16.5   Tracheostomy Tubes

EXERCISE 16.5.1   Components and Types of Tracheostomy Tubes

A. _____

B. _____

C. _____

D. _____

E. _____

F. _____

G. _____

H. _____

I. _____

J. _____

K. _____

L. _____

M. _____

N. _____

O. _____

P. _____

Q. _____

R. _____

S. _____

T. _____

Manufacturer: _____

Size of tube: _____

Type of tube: _____

Box contents: _____

_____

CRITICAL THINKING QUESTIONS

1. For the following clinical situations, what type of artificial tracheal airway should be used? If more than one option is indicated, include all appropriate choices with an explanation.
   a. Cardiac arrest
   b. Suspected C-1 fracture
   c. Three-year-old with epiglottitis
   d. Patient with paralyzed vocal cords
   e. Patient with dysphagia and chronic aspiration
   f. Fractured jaw
   g. An alert stroke patient who cannot cough

2. You are called to the surgical ICU to assess Mrs. King, who had open heart surgery and is 20 hours postop. Describe how you would assess her readiness for extubation.

3. Mr. Kee is intubated with a 7.5-mm orotracheal tube. He is in the ICU on a ventilator. The low-exhaled-volume alarm is sounding, and Mr. Kee is phonating. His respiratory rate is 32/min, the heart rate is 122/min, and the pulse oximeter is 89 percent. You measure the cuff pressure to be 30 cm H_2O, and the pilot tube and valve are intact. What would be your recommendations to remedy this situation?

4. You are changing a tracheostomy tube in a patient with no spontaneous respirations who is being mechanically ventilated. You cannot get the new tube in. Describe in detail what you would do.

5. Al Strachen is a 16-year-old quadriplegic with a C-7 fracture caused by a diving accident. He is currently in a rehabilitation facility. He has a size 6 nonfenestrated cuffed tracheostomy tube in place. The physiatrist has requested that the nurse provide a tracheostomy adjunct to allow the patient to speak. The nurse obtained a Passy-Muir valve and attached it to the 15-mm adaptor of the inner cannula. You were then called stat to evaluate the patient for severe respiratory distress. Explain why the patient did not tolerate the procedure and what you would need to do to correct the situation.

PROCEDURAL COMPETENCY EVALUATION

Name _____ _____ Date _____

Extubation

Setting: ☐ Lab ☐ Clinical   Evaluator: ☐ Peer ☐ Instructor

Conditions (describe): _____

_____

Equipment Used

_____

_____

	SATISFACTORY	UNSATISFACTORY	NOT OBSERVED	NOT APPLICABLE
Equipment and Patient Preparation				
NOTE: Equipment and personnel for reintubation should always be available during extubation.				
1. Verifies, interprets, and evaluates physician's order or protocol; checks the chart for the appropriate F_1O_2 after extubation	☐	☐	☐	☐
2. Scans chart for diagnosis and any other pertinent data and notes	☐	☐	☐	☐
3. Selects, gathers, and assembles the necessary equipment	☐	☐	☐	☐
4. Washes hands and applies standard precautions and transmission-based isolation procedures as appropriate	☐	☐	☐	☐
5. Identifies patient, introduces self and department	☐	☐	☐	☐
6. Explains purpose of the procedure and confirms patient understanding	☐	☐	☐	☐
Assessment and Implementation				
7. Assesses patient, including pulse oximetry	☐	☐	☐	☐
8. Positions patient in a high Fowler's position	☐	☐	☐	☐
9. Suctions the patient's endotracheal tube and pharynx thoroughly	☐	☐	☐	☐
10. Removes the endotracheal tube tape or securing device and deflates the cuff completely	☐	☐	☐	☐
11. Instructs the patient to take a maximum inspiration and removes the tube at peak inspiration (an alternative method is to have the patient cough)	☐	☐	☐	☐
NOTE: Do not remove the tube during the suctioning procedure.				
12. Applies the prescribed oxygen and humidity device to the patient	☐	☐	☐	☐
13. Assesses the patient to determine the adequacy of spontaneous ventilation	☐	☐	☐	☐
14. Reassesses the patient periodically	☐	☐	☐	☐
15. Encourages cough periodically	☐	☐	☐	☐
Follow-up				
16. Maintains/processes equipment	☐	☐	☐	☐
17. Disposes of infectious waste and washes hands	☐	☐	☐	☐
18. Records pertinent data in chart and departmental records	☐	☐	☐	☐
19. Notifies appropriate personnel and makes any necessary recommendations or modifications to the patient care plan	☐	☐	☐	☐

_____   _____
Signature of Evaluator   Signature of Student

PERFORMANCE RATING SCALE

5 EXCELLENT—FAR EXCEEDS EXPECTED LEVEL, FLAWLESS PERFORMANCE
4 ABOVE AVERAGE—NO PROMPTING REQUIRED, ABLE TO SELF-CORRECT
3 AVERAGE—THE MINIMUM COMPETENCY LEVEL, NO CRITICAL ERRORS
2 IMPROVEMENT NEEDED—PROBLEM AREAS EXIST; CRITICAL ERRORS, CORRECTIONS NEEDED
1 POOR AND UNACCEPTABLE PERFORMANCE—GROSS INACCURACIES, POTENTIALLY HARMFUL

PERFORMANCE CRITERIA	SCALE				
1. DISPLAYS KNOWLEDGE OF ESSENTIAL CONCEPTS	5	4	3	2	1
2. DEMONSTRATES THE RELATIONSHIP BETWEEN THEORY AND CLINICAL PRACTICE	5	4	3	2	1
3. FOLLOWS DIRECTIONS, EXHIBITS SOUND JUDGMENT, AND DEMONSTRATES ATTENTION TO SAFETY AND DETAIL	5	4	3	2	1
4. EXHIBITS THE REQUIRED MANUAL DEXTERITY	5	4	3	2	1
5. PERFORMS PROCEDURE IN A REASONABLE TIME FRAME	5	4	3	2	1
6. MAINTAINS STERILE OR ASEPTIC TECHNIQUE	5	4	3	2	1
7. INITIATES UNAMBIGUOUS GOAL-DIRECTED COMMUNICATION	5	4	3	2	1
8. PROVIDES FOR ADEQUATE CARE AND MAINTENANCE OF EQUIPMENT AND SUPPLIES	5	4	3	2	1
9. EXHIBITS COURTEOUS AND PLEASANT DEMEANOR	5	4	3	2	1
10. MAINTAINS CONCISE AND ACCURATE RECORDS	5	4	3	2	1

ADDITIONAL COMMENTS: INCLUDE ERRORS OF OMISSION OR COMMISSION, COMMUNICATIVE SKILLS, AND EFFECTIVENESS OF PATIENT INTERACTION:

SUMMARY PERFORMANCE EVALUATION AND RECOMMENDATIONS

SATISFACTORY PERFORMANCE—Performed without error or prompting, or able to self-correct, no critical errors.

———— LABORATORY EVALUATION. SKILLS MAY BE APPLIED/OBSERVED IN THE CLINICAL SETTING.

———— CLINICAL EVALUATION. STUDENT READY FOR MINIMALLY SUPERVISED APPLICATION AND REFINEMENT.

UNSATISFACTORY PERFORMANCE—Prompting required; performed with critical errors, potentially harmful.

———— STUDENT REQUIRES ADDITIONAL LABORATORY PRACTICE.

———— STUDENT REQUIRES ADDITIONAL SUPERVISED CLINICAL PRACTICE.

SIGNATURES

STUDENT: _____   EVALUATOR: _____

DATE: _____   DATE: _____

PROCEDURAL COMPETENCY EVALUATION

Name _____ Date _____

Tracheostomy Care

Setting: ☐ Lab ☐ Clinical   Evaluator: ☐ Peer ☐ Instructor

Conditions (describe): _____

_____

Equipment Used

_____

_____

	SATISFACTORY	UNSATISFACTORY	NOT OBSERVED	NOT APPLICABLE

Equipment and Patient Preparation

NOTE: Tracheostomy patients should always have a replacement tracheostomy tube at the bedside in case an emergency replacement becomes necessary.

	S	U	NO	NA
1. Selects, gathers, and assembles the necessary equipment	☐	☐	☐	☐
2. Washes hands and applies standard precautions and transmission-based isolation procedures as appropriate	☐	☐	☐	☐
3. Identifies patient, introduces self and department	☐	☐	☐	☐
4. Explains purpose of the procedure and confirms patient understanding	☐	☐	☐	☐

Assessment and Implementation

	S	U	NO	NA
5. Assesses patient	☐	☐	☐	☐
6. Positions patient	☐	☐	☐	☐
7. Suctions thoroughly	☐	☐	☐	☐
8. Removes the old dressing and discards properly	☐	☐	☐	☐
9. Removes the inner cannula and replaces with the spare red-top cannula if a nondisposable cannula is in place	☐	☐	☐	☐
10. Opens the tracheostomy care kit and fills one basin with hydrogen peroxide and the other with sterile saline	☐	☐	☐	☐
11. Scrubs the cannula with peroxide and rinses with sterile saline	☐	☐	☐	☐
12. Replaces the permanent cannula	☐	☐	☐	☐
13. If a disposable cannula is used, removes the dirty cannula, disposes of it properly, and replaces it with a clean, disposable cannula	☐	☐	☐	☐
14. Cleans the stoma site and exterior portions of tube using peroxide, cotton-tipped applicators, and pipe cleaners	☐	☐	☐	☐
15. Replaces the dressing using a precut 4 × 4 gauze pad	☐	☐	☐	☐
16. Removes the old ties or tube securing device and replaces with clean ones	☐	☐	☐	☐
17. Ensures that the tube is secured in proper position and reassesses the patient	☐	☐	☐	☐

Follow-up

	S	U	NO	NA
18. Maintains/processes equipment	☐	☐	☐	☐
19. Disposes of infectious waste and washes hands	☐	☐	☐	☐
20. Records pertinent data in chart and departmental records	☐	☐	☐	☐
21. Notifies appropriate personnel and makes any necessary recommendations or modifications to the patient care plan	☐	☐	☐	☐

_____   _____
Signature of Evaluator   Signature of Student

PERFORMANCE RATING SCALE

5 EXCELLENT—FAR EXCEEDS EXPECTED LEVEL, FLAWLESS PERFORMANCE
4 ABOVE AVERAGE—NO PROMPTING REQUIRED, ABLE TO SELF-CORRECT
3 AVERAGE—THE MINIMUM COMPETENCY LEVEL, NO CRITICAL ERRORS
2 IMPROVEMENT NEEDED—PROBLEM AREAS EXIST; CRITICAL ERRORS, CORRECTIONS NEEDED
1 POOR AND UNACCEPTABLE PERFORMANCE—GROSS INACCURACIES, POTENTIALLY HARMFUL

PERFORMANCE CRITERIA	SCALE				
1. DISPLAYS KNOWLEDGE OF ESSENTIAL CONCEPTS	5	4	3	2	1
2. DEMONSTRATES THE RELATIONSHIP BETWEEN THEORY AND CLINICAL PRACTICE	5	4	3	2	1
3. FOLLOWS DIRECTIONS, EXHIBITS SOUND JUDGMENT, AND DEMONSTRATES ATTENTION TO SAFETY AND DETAIL	5	4	3	2	1
4. EXHIBITS THE REQUIRED MANUAL DEXTERITY	5	4	3	2	1
5. PERFORMS PROCEDURE IN A REASONABLE TIME FRAME	5	4	3	2	1
6. MAINTAINS STERILE OR ASEPTIC TECHNIQUE	5	4	3	2	1
7. INITIATES UNAMBIGUOUS GOAL-DIRECTED COMMUNICATION	5	4	3	2	1
8. PROVIDES FOR ADEQUATE CARE AND MAINTENANCE OF EQUIPMENT AND SUPPLIES	5	4	3	2	1
9. EXHIBITS COURTEOUS AND PLEASANT DEMEANOR	5	4	3	2	1
10. MAINTAINS CONCISE AND ACCURATE RECORDS	5	4	3	2	1

ADDITIONAL COMMENTS: INCLUDE ERRORS OF OMISSION OR COMMISSION, COMMUNICATIVE SKILLS, AND EFFECTIVENESS OF PATIENT INTERACTION:

SUMMARY PERFORMANCE EVALUATION AND RECOMMENDATIONS

SATISFACTORY PERFORMANCE—Performed without error or prompting, or able to self-correct, no critical errors.

_____ LABORATORY EVALUATION. SKILLS MAY BE APPLIED/OBSERVED IN THE CLINICAL SETTING.

_____ CLINICAL EVALUATION. STUDENT READY FOR MINIMALLY SUPERVISED APPLICATION AND REFINEMENT.

UNSATISFACTORY PERFORMANCE—Prompting required; performed with critical errors, potentially harmful.

_____ STUDENT REQUIRES ADDITIONAL LABORATORY PRACTICE.

_____ STUDENT REQUIRES ADDITIONAL SUPERVISED CLINICAL PRACTICE.

SIGNATURES

STUDENT: _____ EVALUATOR: _____

DATE: _____ DATE: _____

PROCEDURAL COMPETENCY EVALUATION

Name _____ Date _____

Tracheostomy Tube Change

Setting: ☐ Lab ☐ Clinical   Evaluator: ☐ Peer ☐ Instructor

Conditions (describe): _____

_____

Equipment Used

_____

_____

	SATISFACTORY	UNSATISFACTORY	NOT OBSERVED	NOT APPLICABLE
Equipment and Patient Preparation				
1. Verifies, interprets, and evaluates physician's order or protocol	☐	☐	☐	☐
2. Scans chart for diagnosis and any other pertinent data and notes	☐	☐	☐	☐
3. Selects, gathers, and assembles the necessary equipment	☐	☐	☐	☐
4. Washes hands and applies standard precautions and transmission-based isolation procedures as appropriate	☐	☐	☐	☐
5. Identifies patient, introduces self and department	☐	☐	☐	☐
6. Explains purpose of the procedure and confirms patient understanding	☐	☐	☐	☐
Assessment and Implementation				
7. Assesses patient	☐	☐	☐	☐
8. Suctions the trachea based on assessment	☐	☐	☐	☐
9. Positions patient	☐	☐	☐	☐
10. Opens the new tracheostomy tube box, removes the tube, and places it on a sterile field	☐	☐	☐	☐
11. Checks the tube for cuff leaks	☐	☐	☐	☐
12. Deflates the cuff completely	☐	☐	☐	☐
13. Attaches the new, clean tracheostomy ties or holder	☐	☐	☐	☐
14. Removes the inner cannula and inserts the obturator	☐	☐	☐	☐
15. Lubricates the tip of the tracheostomy tube/obturator	☐	☐	☐	☐
16. Reassures patient and positions in semi-Fowler's position with the neck slightly extended	☐	☐	☐	☐
17. Loosens or unties the old tracheostomy ties and deflates the cuff (if applicable)	☐	☐	☐	☐
18. Removes the oxygen or humidity therapy device and places it aseptically	☐	☐	☐	☐
19. Removes the old tracheostomy tube	☐	☐	☐	☐
20. Visually inspects the stoma for bleeding or infection	☐	☐	☐	☐
21. Inserts the new tube with a slightly downward motion	☐	☐	☐	☐
22. Removes the obturator and inserts the inner cannula; keeps the tracheostomy tube secured in place	☐	☐	☐	☐
23. Periodically reassesses the patient	☐	☐	☐	☐
24. Inflates the cuff if ordered	☐	☐	☐	☐
25. Ensures proper placement	☐	☐	☐	☐

	S A T I S F A C T O R Y	U N S A T I S F A C T O R Y	N O T O B S E R V E D	N O T A P P L I C A B L E
26. Secures the tube in place	☐	☐	☐	☐
27. Restores the patient to the previous oxygen or humidity therapy device	☐	☐	☐	☐

Follow-up

28. Maintains/processes equipment	☐	☐	☐	☐
29. Disposes of infectious waste and washes hands	☐	☐	☐	☐
30. Records pertinent data in chart and departmental records	☐	☐	☐	☐
31. Notifies appropriate personnel and makes any necessary recommendations or modifications to the patient care plan	☐	☐	☐	☐

_____
Signature of Evaluator

_____
Signature of Student

PERFORMANCE RATING SCALE

5 EXCELLENT—FAR EXCEEDS EXPECTED LEVEL, FLAWLESS PERFORMANCE
4 ABOVE AVERAGE—NO PROMPTING REQUIRED, ABLE TO SELF-CORRECT
3 AVERAGE—THE MINIMUM COMPETENCY LEVEL, NO CRITICAL ERRORS
2 IMPROVEMENT NEEDED—PROBLEM AREAS EXIST; CRITICAL ERRORS, CORRECTIONS NEEDED
1 POOR AND UNACCEPTABLE PERFORMANCE—GROSS INACCURACIES, POTENTIALLY HARMFUL

PERFORMANCE CRITERIA	SCALE				
1. DISPLAYS KNOWLEDGE OF ESSENTIAL CONCEPTS	5	4	3	2	1
2. DEMONSTRATES THE RELATIONSHIP BETWEEN THEORY AND CLINICAL PRACTICE	5	4	3	2	1
3. FOLLOWS DIRECTIONS, EXHIBITS SOUND JUDGMENT, AND DEMONSTRATES ATTENTION TO SAFETY AND DETAIL	5	4	3	2	1
4. EXHIBITS THE REQUIRED MANUAL DEXTERITY	5	4	3	2	1
5. PERFORMS PROCEDURE IN A REASONABLE TIME FRAME	5	4	3	2	1
6. MAINTAINS STERILE OR ASEPTIC TECHNIQUE	5	4	3	2	1
7. INITIATES UNAMBIGUOUS GOAL-DIRECTED COMMUNICATION	5	4	3	2	1
8. PROVIDES FOR ADEQUATE CARE AND MAINTENANCE OF EQUIPMENT AND SUPPLIES	5	4	3	2	1
9. EXHIBITS COURTEOUS AND PLEASANT DEMEANOR	5	4	3	2	1
10. MAINTAINS CONCISE AND ACCURATE RECORDS	5	4	3	2	1

ADDITIONAL COMMENTS: INCLUDE ERRORS OF OMISSION OR COMMISSION, COMMUNICATIVE SKILLS, AND EFFECTIVENESS OF PATIENT INTERACTION:

SUMMARY PERFORMANCE EVALUATION AND RECOMMENDATIONS

SATISFACTORY PERFORMANCE—Performed without error or prompting, or able to self-correct, no critical errors.

_____ LABORATORY EVALUATION. SKILLS MAY BE APPLIED/OBSERVED IN THE CLINICAL SETTING.

_____ CLINICAL EVALUATION. STUDENT READY FOR MINIMALLY SUPERVISED APPLICATION AND REFINEMENT.

UNSATISFACTORY PERFORMANCE—Prompting required; performed with critical errors, potentially harmful.

_____ STUDENT REQUIRES ADDITIONAL LABORATORY PRACTICE.

_____ STUDENT REQUIRES ADDITIONAL SUPERVISED CLINICAL PRACTICE.

SIGNATURES

STUDENT: _____   EVALUATOR: _____

DATE: _____   DATE: _____

Electrocardiography

Electrocardiography (ECG) is commonly used for both diagnostic and monitoring purposes. The ECG recording is an integral part of patient assessment for any patient with chest pain or symptoms that suggest myocardial infarction or other cardiac dysfunction. Many procedures performed by respiratory care practitioners can affect cardiac function and electrical conduction. Whether to perform routine ECG recording, to monitor changes in heart rate and rhythm during therapeutic procedures, or to rapidly respond to changes in ECG during emergency procedures, respiratory care practitioners are frequently called on to perform or identify and interpret common abnormalities in electrocardiogram tracings.

OBJECTIVES
Upon completion of this chapter, the student will be able to:

1. Identify normal anatomy of the heart and electrical conduction system.
2. Perform a 12-lead ECG recording.
3. Identify and correct common causes of artifacts that may interfere with the ECG.
4. Analyze and interpret ECG tracings for rate and rhythm, including normal sinus rhythm and common dysrhythmias.
5. Relate the pharmacological treatments of choice according to AHA advanced cardiac life support (ACLS) standards for common life-threatening dysrhythmias.

KEY TERMS

absolute refractory	atrium	fibrillation	systole
arteriosclerosis	cardioversion	isoelectric	unifocal
artifact	defibrillation	multifocal	ventricle
atherosclerosis	depolarization	relative refractory	
	diastole	repolarization	

EQUIPMENT REQUIRED

- Anatomical heart model
- Electrocardiograph (ECG) machine
- ECG recording paper
- Limb and chest leads
- Disposable ECG electrode pads
- Electrode gel
- Alcohol swabs
- Clean towels or washcloths
- 4 × 4 nonsterile gauze
- Bed or table
- Bed linens
- Electrical outlets
- Privacy screen
- ECG calipers
- Ventilator, compressor, or any other large piece of electrical equipment
- Infectious waste container
- ECG monitor or Holter monitoring system, if available

⬤ EXERCISES

EXERCISE 17.1 Cardiac Anatomy

Obtain an anatomical model of the heart. Identify the vessels, coronary circulation chambers, and valves in comparison with Figure 17.1.

Label Figure 17.2, anatomy of the heart. Label Figure 17.3, cardiac conduction system.

EXERCISE 17.2 Identification of Electrocardiograph Machine Controls

Depending on laboratory resources, your instructor will provide you with either a single-channel or a multichannel ECG machine. In either case, certain features are common to all ECG machines.

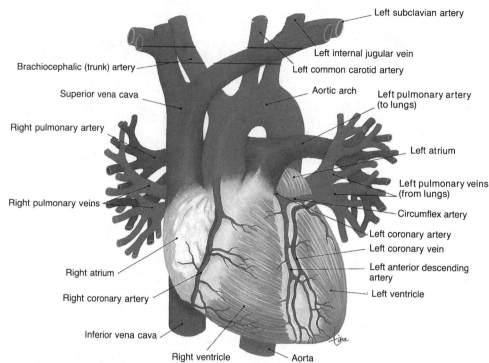

FIGURE 17.1   Anatomy of the heart: vessels and coronary circulation. (From Scanlon, VC and Sanders, T: Essentials of Anatomy and Physiology, ed 2. FA Davis, Philadelphia, 1991, p. 266, with permission.)

Identify the following controls on the ECG machine provided:

1. On/off switch
2. Stylus position
3. Lead marker
4. Calibration standard
5. Lead selector
6. Sensitivity
7. Paper speed

Identify the type of machine used and the specific controls found on this machine. Record on your laboratory report.

EXERCISE 17.3 Preparation and Attachment of Limb Leads

The following exercises will be performed on your laboratory partner or instructor.

1. Gather the necessary equipment:
   ECG machine
   Limb leads
   Disposable electrodes or reusable electrodes and gel
   Alcohol swabs
2. Wash your hands and apply standard precautions and transmission-based isolation procedures as appropriate.
3. Introduce yourself to the subject, verify the subject's identification, and explain the procedure.
4. Have the subject remove all jewelry or metal.
5. Place the subject in a supine position on the bed or table.
6. Plug in the ECG machine. Ensure that there is an adequate paper supply.

7. Apply clean electrodes (Fig. 17.4) to the muscular areas of the arms and legs, as shown in Figure 17.5. The placement should be in a similar location on both arms and legs. Avoid placing the electrodes on any bony prominences.

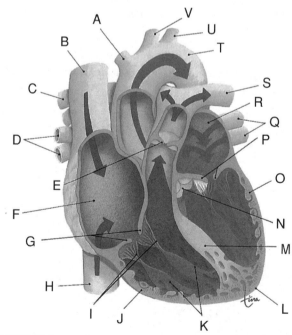

FIGURE 17.2   Label the anatomy of the heart: vessels, valves, and chambers. (From Scanlon, VC and Sanders, T: Essentials of Anatomy and Physiology, ed 2. FA Davis, Philadelphia, 1991, p. 266, with permission.)

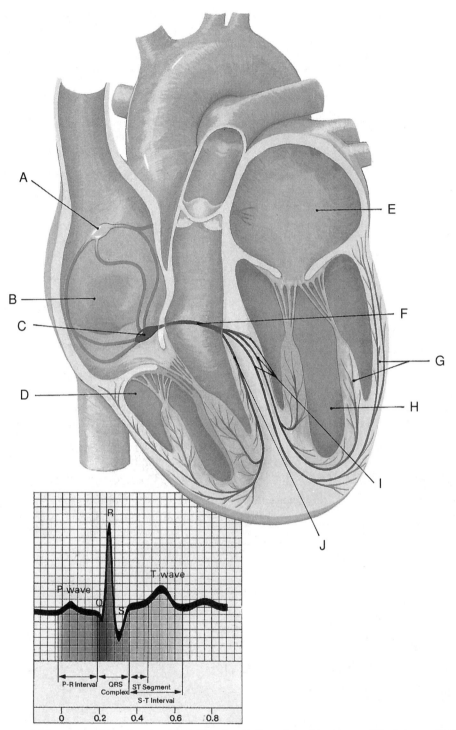

FIGURE 17.3   Cardiac conduction system. (From Scanlon, VC and Sanders, T: Essentials of Anatomy and Physiology, ed 2. FA Davis, Philadelphia, 1991, p. 271, with permission.)

NOTE: In the case of limb deformities or amputation, the electrode should be placed on the torso as close to the point of limb attachment as possible.

It may be necessary to prepare the skin by rubbing it with an alcohol swab before electrode application. Excess body hair may interfere with the contact of an individual electrode; consequently, in a clinical situation, the area may need to be shaved before electrode appli-

cation. For the purposes of this lab, shaving will not be performed.

If disposable electrode pads are used, peel off the backing and stick securely to the subject's skin. If nondisposable electrodes are used, an alcohol swab or electrode gel should be applied to the skin first. Note that the limb leads may be color coded or alphabetically coded as follows:

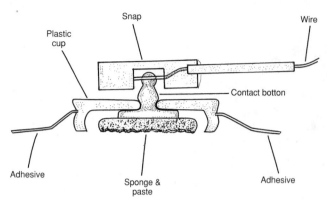

FIGURE 17.4 Cross section of a disposable self-adhesive electrode.

Electrode location	Color
Right arm (RA)	White
Right leg (RL)	Green
Left arm (LA)	Black
Left leg (LL)	Red
Chest	Brown

8. Instruct the subject to attempt to relax completely.

9. If the machine is capable of recording single-channel leads, record the tracings for limb leads I, II, and III, AVR, AVL, and AVF at this time.
   a. Turn the machine on.
   b. Turn to the record position. Check that the stylus is centered on the paper.
   c. Make sure the paper speed is set at 25 mm/sec.
   d. Press the calibration standard mark at the beginning of each tracing (if it is not done automatically). Adjust the sensitivity as necessary so that the size of the complex is not too large or too small.
   e. Run each lead for at least 6 sec (approximately 6 inches). Use the lead marker to identify each lead recorded (if it is not done automatically).

10. Document the subject's name, date, and time of the recording on the ECG tracing when finished.

11. *Attach the ECG tracing to your laboratory report.* If only one subject is used to demonstrate to the class, have the instructor make copies of lead II for each student in the class and attach the copy to your laboratory report. Alternatively, you may run a long strip so that a minimum of a 6-sec strip is available for each student in the laboratory.

You may continue with your partner for Exercise 17.4. However, if you are not performing Exercise 17.4 at this time, you should disconnect and remove the leads from your subject and clean up now. See Exercise 17.5 for directions.

EXERCISE 17.4 Preparation and Attachment of Precordial (Chest) Leads

EXERCISE 17.4.1 Standard Chest Leads

Because the chest leads must be attached to bare skin, it is preferable that a volunteer be used for this exercise. A student should not perform a 12-lead ECG on a female student without the permission of the female student and the instructor. Adequate privacy should be ensured. The chest, or precordial, leads are recorded with either a single electrode or multiple electrodes. If a single chest electrode is used, it must be repositioned before recording each precordial lead.

1. Place a small amount of ECG electrode gel on the skin over the correct position before electrode placement.

2. Place the chest electrodes in the following locations, as shown in Figure 17.6:
   V1: Fourth intercostal space, right sternal margin
   V2: Fourth intercostal space, left sternal margin
   V3: Midway between V2 and V4
   V4: Fifth intercostal space, left midclavicular line (MCL)
   V5: Fifth intercostal space, left anterior axillary line (AAL)
   V6: Sixth intercostal space, left midaxillary line (MAL)

3. Record the ECG tracing for each precordial lead, making sure to mark the calibration standard and lead marker for each lead.

4. If a multichannel 12-lead ECG machine is being used, record the entire 12-lead ECG at this time.

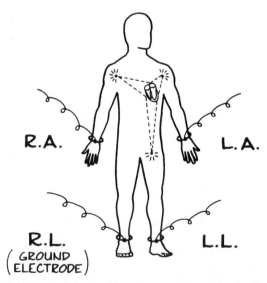

FIGURE 17.5 Limb leads. (From Lipman, BC and Cascio, T: ECG Assessment and Interpretation. FA Davis, Philadelphia, 1994, p. 15, with permission.)

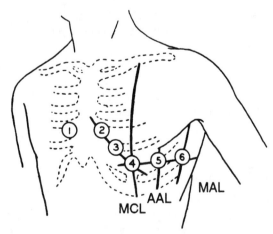

FIGURE 17.6 Precordial chest leads in relation to ribs. (From Lipman, BC and Cascio, T: ECG Assessment and Interpretation. FA Davis, Philadelphia, 1994, p. 16, with permission.)

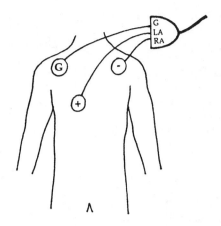

Lead MCL₁

FIGURE 17.7   Modified chest lead MCL₁. (From Lipman, BC and Cascio, T: ECG Assessment and Interpretation. FA Davis, Philadelphia, 1994, p. 20, with permission.)

5. Document the subject's name, the date, and the time of the procedure on the ECG tracing. Attach the tracing to your laboratory report. If only one subject is used to demonstrate to the class, have the instructor make copies of V5 for each student, and attach the copy to your laboratory report.

EXERCISE 17.4.2 Modified Chest Leads

The accompanying figures show modified leads used for continuous ECG monitoring (Fig. 17.7) and for ambulatory or Holter monitoring (Fig. 17.8). If an ECG monitor or Holter monitor is available, students should place electrodes on the chest as shown and run a strip.

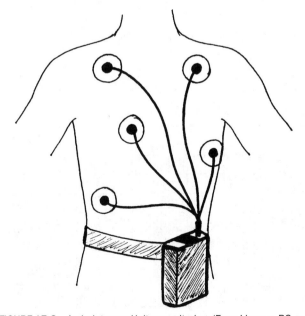

FIGURE 17.8   Ambulatory or Holter monitoring. (From Lipman, BC and Cascio, T: ECG Assessment and Interpretation. FA Davis, Philadelphia, 1994, p. 243, with permission.)

EXERCISE 17.5 Electrocardiograph Artifact

EXERCISE 17.5.1 Identification of Artifact

Match the ECG rhythm strips in Figures 17.9 through 17.12 with the following **artifacts:**
   Wandering baseline
   Muscle tremor
   60-Cycle interference
   Intermittent loss of signal

EXERCISE 17.5.2 Simulation of Artifact

1. Prepare your patient as instructed in Exercise 17.3.
2. Set the ECG machine to record lead II. Have the subject perform the following maneuvers to simulate ECG artifacts while recording the ECG tracing.
   a. Have the subject take deep breaths for several seconds. *Record your observations on, or attach the ECG tracing to, your laboratory report.*
   b. Have the subject tense his or her muscles for several seconds. *Record your observations on, or attach the ECG tracing to, your laboratory report.*
   c. Have the subject move his or her limbs. *Record your observations on, or attach the ECG tracing to, your laboratory report.*
   d. Have the subject touch the metal bed rails or ECG machine while recording. Alternatively, you may plug in another electrical device into the same electrical outlet while recording the ECG. *Record your observations on, or attach the ECG tracing to, the laboratory report.*
3. Loosen the right electrode lead. *Record your observations on, or attach the ECG tracing to, the laboratory report.*
4. Loosen the left electrode lead. *Record your observations on, or attach the ECG tracing to, the laboratory report.*
5. Reverse the right and left electrode leads. *Record your observations on, or attach the ECG tracing to, the laboratory report.*
6. If nondisposable electrodes are used, replace one without using electrode gel or alcohol swab. *Record your observations on, or attach the ECG tracing to, the laboratory report.*

EXERCISE 17.6 Cleanup Procedures

1. Remove the electrodes gently, especially if disposable electrodes are being used over body hair.
2. Clean off the skin using a washcloth or towel.
3. Discard the disposable electrodes in an infectious waste container.
4. Nondisposable electrodes must be thoroughly cleaned and disinfected before storage. Follow manufacturer's recommendations.
5. Neatly store limb leads and other supplies.

EXERCISE 17.7 Rate and Rhythm Interpretation

1. To calculate the heart rate one of three methods may be used.

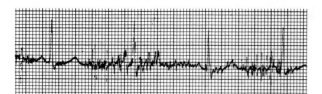

FIGURE 17.9 **Tracing A.** (From Frew, MA, Lane, K and Frew, DR: Comprehensive Medical Assisting, ed 3. FA Davis, Philadelphia, 1995, p. 844, with permission.)

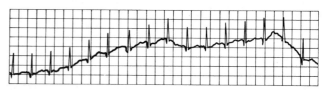

FIGURE 17.10 **Tracing B.** (From Frew, MA, Lane, K and Frew, DR: Comprehensive Medical Assisting, ed 3. FA Davis, Philadelphia, 1995, p. 844, with permission.)

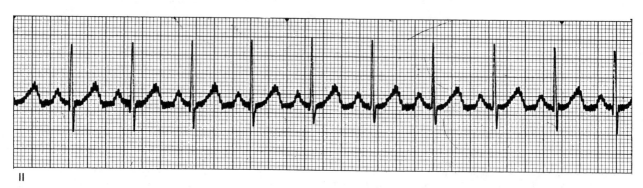

FIGURE 17.11 **Tracing C.** (From Brown, KR and Jacobson, S: Mastering Dysrhythmia: A Problem-Solving Guide. FA Davis, Philadelphia, 1988, p. 164, with permission.)

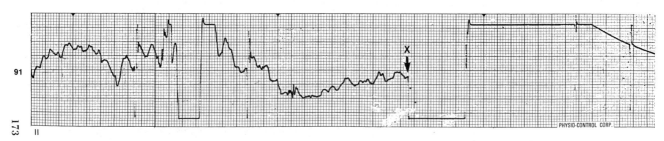

FIGURE 17.12 **Tracing D.** (From Brown, KR and Jacobson, S: Mastering Dysrhythmia: A Problem-Solving Guide. FA Davis, Philadelphia, 1988, p. 173, with permission.)

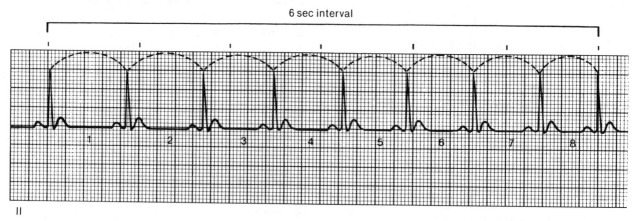

FIGURE 17.13 A 6-second strip. (From Lipman, BC and Cascio, T: ECG Assessment and Interpretation. FA Davis, Philadelphia, 1994, p. 67, with permission.)

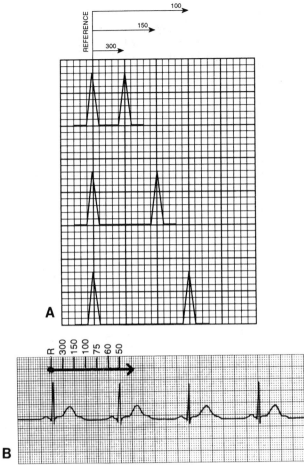

a. An estimation may be determined by counting the number of QRS complexes on a 6-sec strip and multiplying by 10 (Fig. 17.13).

b. The R-R method. First find an R wave in which the peak of the QRS falls on a heavy, dark line. Then find the next QRS. For each dark line between the R waves count backward (300, 150, 100, and so on) until you reach the second QRS, as shown in Figure 17.14.

c. Use the calipers to count the number of small boxes between two R waves, and divide that number into 1500 (Fig. 17.15). This is the most accurate method.

2. Each small box is equal to 0.04 sec. Each large box contains five small boxes across for a duration of 0.20 sec (see Fig. 17.3). Examine the PR intervals and the QRS widths on the rhythm strips obtained from previous exercises. Measure duration of each in seconds, and *record the results on your laboratory report.*

3. To interpret the rhythm, the following systematic approach is recommended:

a. Perform a general inspection of the rhythm strip. Look for possible artifacts.

b. Identify specific waves and intervals.

(1) P waves. Are they present? What is their shape? Are they all alike? Is each followed by a QRS? What is the P-R interval?

(2) QRS. Are they present? What is their shape? Are they all alike? What is the QRS width?

(3) ST segment. Is it baseline? Is it elevated or depressed?

(4) T wave. Is it normal? Is it inverted?

c. Is the rhythm regular or irregular? Using calipers, check the distance between R waves. A regular rhythm should have the same distance (within two small boxes) between all R waves. The conduction ratio is the number of P waves for each QRS complex.

d. Calculate the rate.

e. Identify the rhythm.

FIGURE 17.14 R-R method of calculating rate on an ECG. (From Lipman, BC and Cascio, T: ECG Assessment and Interpretation. FA Davis, Philadelphia, 1994, p. 66, with permission.)

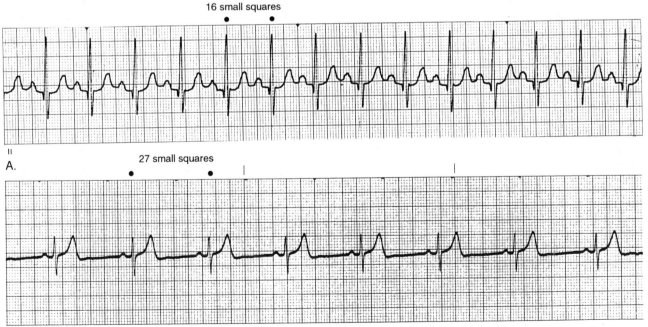

FIGURE 17.15   The 1500 method of calculating rate on an ECG. (From Lipman, BC and Cascio, T: ECG Assessment and Interpretation. FA Davis, Philadelphia, 1994, p. 63, with permission.)

Related Readings

Cottrell, GP and Surkin, HB: Pharmacology for Respiratory Care Practitioners. FA Davis, Philadelphia, 1995.

Dubin, D: Rapid Interpretation of ECGs. Cover Publishing, Tampa, FL, 1994.

McPherson, S: Respiratory Care Equipment, ed 5. Mosby, St Louis, 1995.

Rau, J: Respiratory Care Pharmacology, ed 3. Mosby, St Louis, 1993.

Scanlan, C et al (eds): Egan's Fundamentals of Respiratory Care. Mosby, St Louis, 1995.

Wilkins, R, Sheldon, R and Krider, S: Clinical Assessment in Respiratory Care, ed 3. Mosby, St Louis, 1993.

Selected Journal Articles

American Association for Respiratory Care: AARC clinical practice guideline: Exercise testing for evaluation of hypoxemia and/or desaturation. Respir Care 37:907–912, 1992.

American Association for Respiratory Care: AARC clinical practice guideline: Defibrillation during resuscitation. Respir Care 40:744–748, 1995.

American Association for Respiratory Care: AARC clinical practice guideline: Resuscitation in acute care hospitals. Respir Care 38:1179–1188, 1993.

American Association for Respiratory Care: AARC clinical practice guideline: Resuscitation in acute care hospitals. Respir Care 40:346–363, 1995.

American Heart Association: Guidelines for cardiopulmonary resuscitation and emergency cardiac care: Recommendations of the 1992 national conference. JAMA 268:2171–2302, 1992.

Barnes, TA and Durbin CG, Jr.: ACLS skills for the respiratory therapist: Time for a mandate. Respir Care 37:516–519, 1992.

Grillo, J and Gonzalez, E: Changes in the pharmacotherapy of CPR. Heart Lung 22:548–553, 1993.

Rau, JF: ACLS drugs used during resuscitation. Respir Care 40:404–426, 1995.

LABORATORY REPORT

CHAPTER 17: ELECTROCARDIOGRAPHY

Name _____ Date _____

Course/Section _____ Instructor _____

Data Collection

EXERCISE 17.1 Cardiac Anatomy

Label the heart diagram in Figure 17.2:

A. _____

B. _____

C. _____

D. _____

E. _____

F. _____

G. _____

H. _____

I. _____

J. _____

K. _____

L. _____

M. _____

N. _____

O. _____

P. _____

Q. _____

R. _____

S. _____

T. _____

U. _____

V. _____

Label the conduction system in Figure 17.3:

A. _____

B. _____

C. _____

D. _____

E. _____

F. _____

G. _____

H. _____

I. _____

J. _____

EXERCISE 17.2   Identification of Electrocardiograph Machine Controls

Type of machine used: _____

Controls identified: _____

_____

_____

_____

EXERCISE 17.3   Preparation and Attachment of Limb Leads

Attach the ECG tracing or copy to the laboratory report.

EXERCISE 17.4   Preparation and Attachment of Precordial (Chest) Leads

Attach the ECG tracing or copy to the laboratory report.

EXERCISE 17.5   Electrocardiograph Artifact

EXERCISE 17.5.1   Identification of Artifact

A. Figure 17.9: _____

B. Figure 17.10: _____

C. Figure 17.11: _____

D. Figure 17.12: _____

EXERCISE 17.5.2   Simulation of Artifact

Tracings or Observations

Deep breathing:

_____

_____

Tensing of muscles:

_____

_____

Limb movement:

_____

_____

Touching metal bed rails or ECG machine or plugging in electrical device (record method used):

_____

_____

Loosening the right electrode lead:

_____

_____

Loosening the left electrode lead:

_____

_____

Reversal of the right and left electrode leads:

_____

_____

Replacement of electrode without gel or alcohol swab:

_____

_____

EXERCISE 17.7   Rate and Rhythm Interpretation

Using the tracings obtained from Exercise 17.3 or 17.4, perform the following:

1. General inspection: _____

2. Are all the P waves upright? _____ Are they alike? _____

Is there a P wave for every QRS? _____

3. Measure the PR interval.

Number of small boxes: _____

PR interval duration in seconds: _____

Normal PR interval: _____

4. Look at the QRSs. Are they all alike? _____

Is there a QRS for every P? _____

Measure the QRS width.

Number of small boxes: _____

QRS width in seconds: _____

Normal QRS width: _____

Are all the R-R intervals the same? _____

Is the ST segment baseline, elevated, or depressed? _____

Is the T wave normal? Is it inverted? _____

Is the rhythm regular or irregular? _____

5. Calculate the heart rate by all three methods. _Show your work for each!_

a. 6-sec strip: _____

b. R-R method: _____

c. 1500 method: _____

6. Interpretation: _____

CRITICAL THINKING QUESTIONS

Interpret the following ECG rhythm tracings:

1. A patient was found unconscious at home (Fig. 17.16). Paramedics sent the strip via telemetry.

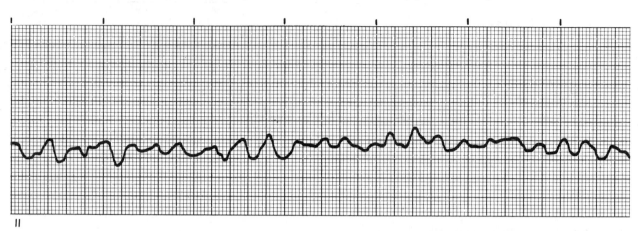

II

FIGURE 17.16   Rhythm strip #1. (From Brown, KR and Jacobson, S: Mastering Dysrhythmias: A Problem-Solving Guide. FA Davis, Philadelphia, 1988, p. 25, with permission.)

Rate: _____

Rhythm: regular or irregular? _____

P waves: present, shape, all alike, followed by normal QRS? _____

P-R interval: _____

QRS: present, shape, all alike? _____

QRS width: _____

ST segment: baseline, elevated, or depressed? _____

T wave: normal or inverted? _____

Identification of rhythm: _____

Pharmacological treatment of choice or other treatment (if applicable): _____

_____

2. An 84-year-old man was seen in the doctor's office complaining of dizziness and light-headedness (Fig. 17.17).

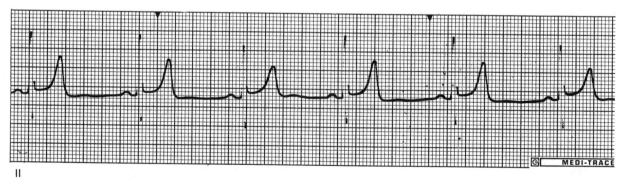

II

FIGURE 17.17   Rhythm strip #2. (From Brown, KR and Jacobson, S: Mastering Dysrhythmias: A Problem-Solving Guide. FA Davis, Philadelphia, 1988, p. 39, with permission.)

Rate: _____

Rhythm: regular or irregular? _____

P waves: present, shape, all alike, followed by normal QRS? _____

P-R interval: _____

QRS: present, shape, all alike? _____

QRS width: _____

ST segment: baseline, elevated, or depressed? _____

T wave: normal or inverted? _____

Identification of rhythm: _____

Pharmacological treatment of choice (if applicable): _____

_____

3. A patient with a history of COPD being treated for an acute exacerbation began complaining of palpitations (Fig. 17.18).

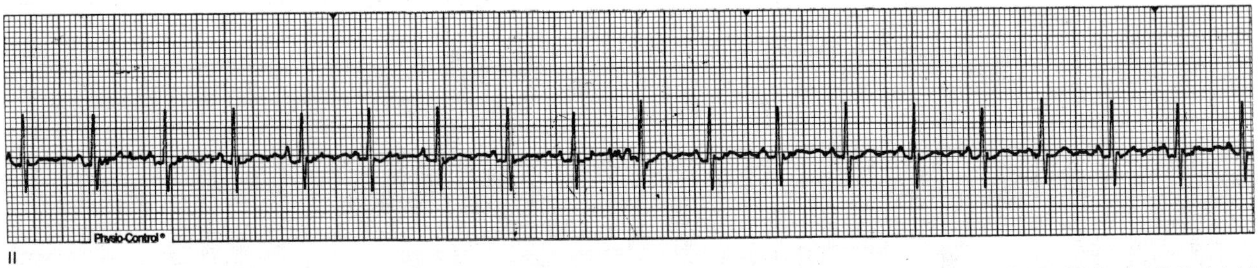

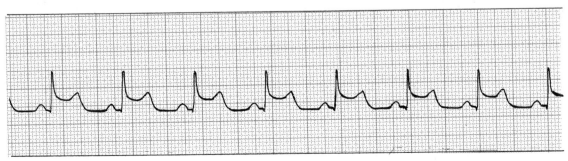

II

FIGURE 17.18   Rhythm strip #3. (From Brown, KR and Jacobson, S: Mastering Dysrhythmias: A Problem-Solving Guide. FA Davis, Philadelphia, 1988, p. 238, with permission.)-

Rate: _____

Rhythm: regular or irregular? _____

P waves: present, shape, all alike, followed by normal QRS? _____

P-R interval: _____

QRS: present, shape, all alike? _____

QRS width: _____

ST segment: baseline, elevated, or depressed? _____

T wave: normal or inverted? _____

Identification of rhythm: _____

Pharmacological treatment of choice (if applicable): _____

_____

4. A 64-year-old woman was brought to the ER with a chief complaint of heaviness in the chest and tightness in the back and left shoulder (Fig. 17.19).

FIGURE 17.19   Rhythm strip #4. (Courtesy of Laerdal Medical Corporation, Wappingers Falls, NY.)

Rate: _____

Rhythm: regular or irregular? _____

P waves: present, shape, all alike, followed by normal QRS? _____

P-R interval: _____

QRS: present, shape, all alike? _____

QRS width: _____

ST segment: baseline, elevated, or depressed? _____

T wave: normal or inverted? _____

Identification of rhythm: _____

Pharmacological treatment of choice (if applicable): _____

_____

5. Figure 17.20 was obtained several days later from the patient in Critical Thinking Question 4.

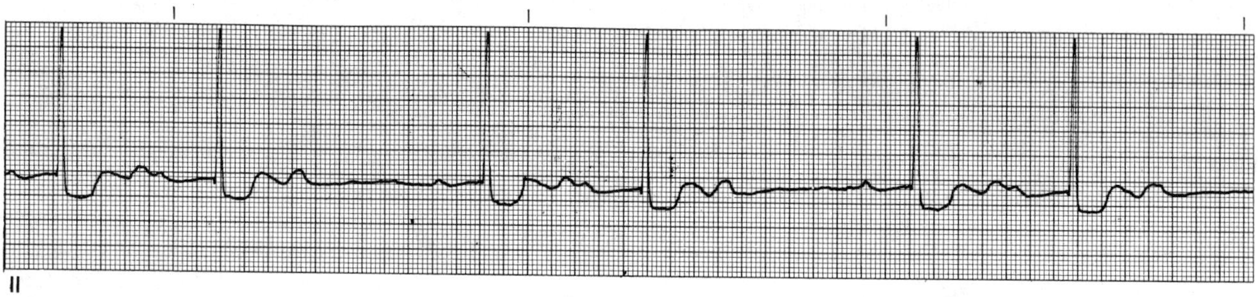

FIGURE 17.20   Rhythm strip #5 (From Brown, KR and Jacobson, S: Mastering Dysrhythmias: A Problem-Solving Guide. FA Davis, Philadelphia, 1988, p. 90, with permission.)

Rate: _____

P waves: present, shape, all alike, followed by normal QRS? _____

P-R interval: _____

QRS: present, shape, all alike? _____

QRS width: _____

ST segment: baseline, elevated, or depressed? _____

T wave: normal or inverted? _____

Rhythm: regular or irregular? _____

Identification of rhythm: _____

Pharmacological treatment of choice (if applicable): _____

_____

You enter a patient's room to perform an arterial blood gas. During preparation for the procedure, you notice the rhythm shown in Figure 17.21 on the ECG monitor.

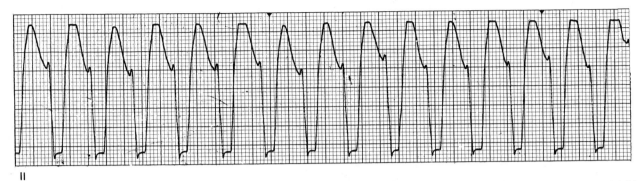

II

FIGURE 17.21   Rhythm strip #6 (From Brown, KR and Jacobson, S: Mastering Dysrhythmias: A Problem-Solving Guide. FA Davis, Philadelphia, 1988, p. 125, with permission.)

6. What should you do first?

7. You have determined that the patient has no respirations or pulse. What would your next action(s) be?

8. Once advanced life support emergency equipment is available, what should be done first to treat this rhythm?

The patient's pulse and blood pressure have returned, and the rhythm shown in Figure 17.22 is noted on the ECG monitor.

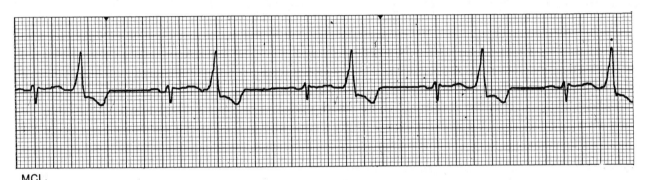

MCL₁

FIGURE 17.22   Rhythm strip #7. (From Brown, KR and Jacobson, S: Mastering Dysrhythmias: A Problem-Solving Guide. FA Davis, Philadelphia, 1988, p. 117, with permission.)

9. What is the most indicated pharmacological treatment for this rhythm?

PROCEDURAL COMPETENCY EVALUATION

Name _____ Date _____

Electrocardiography

Setting: ☐ Lab ☐ Clinical   Evaluator: ☐ Peer ☐ Instructor

Conditions (describe): _____

_____

Equipment Used

_____

_____

	SATISFACTORY	UNSATISFACTORY	NOT OBSERVED	NOT APPLICABLE
Equipment and Patient Preparation				
1. Verifies, interprets, and evaluates physician's order or protocol	☐	☐	☐	☐
2. Scans chart for diagnosis and any other pertinent data and notes	☐	☐	☐	☐
3. Selects, gathers, and assembles the necessary equipment: ECG machine, electrodes, gel, gauze, paper; ensures that the machine has sufficient paper	☐	☐	☐	☐
4. Washes hands and applies standard precautions and transmission-based isolation procedures as appropriate	☐	☐	☐	☐
5. Identifies patient, introduces self and department	☐	☐	☐	☐
6. Explains purpose of the procedure and confirms patient understanding	☐	☐	☐	☐
Assessment and Implementation				
7. Plugs in the machine; ensures that the machine is operating properly and that sufficient supplies are available	☐	☐	☐	☐
8. Places patient appropriately in supine or semi-Fowler's position	☐	☐	☐	☐
9. Has patient remove all jewelry or metal	☐	☐	☐	☐
10. Instructs patient to relax completely	☐	☐	☐	☐
11. Applies clean limb electrodes to muscular areas of arms and legs; places electrodes in similar locations on both arms and legs; places chest leads in proper locations:				
a. V1: Fourth intercostal space, right sternal margin	☐	☐	☐	☐
b. V2: Fourth intercostal space, left sternal margin	☐	☐	☐	☐
c. V3: Midway between V2 and V4	☐	☐	☐	☐
d. V4: Fifth intercostal space, left midclavicular line	☐	☐	☐	☐
e. V5: Fifth intercostal space, left anterior axillary line	☐	☐	☐	☐
f. V6: Sixth intercostal space, left midaxillary line	☐	☐	☐	☐
12. Ensures patient comfort and respects patient privacy and modesty	☐	☐	☐	☐
13. Calibrates machine	☐	☐	☐	☐
14. Runs test strip	☐	☐	☐	☐
15. Inspects rhythm strip for				
a. Wandering baseline	☐	☐	☐	☐
b. 60-Cycle artifact	☐	☐	☐	☐
c. Muscle tremor artifact	☐	☐	☐	☐

	SATISFACTORY	UNSATISFACTORY	NOT OBSERVED	NOT APPLICABLE
d. Disconnected lead or intermittent loss of signal	☐	☐	☐	☐
e. Poor prep (contact) artifact	☐	☐	☐	☐
16. Runs complete 12-lead ECG	☐	☐	☐	☐

Follow-up

	SATISFACTORY	UNSATISFACTORY	NOT OBSERVED	NOT APPLICABLE
17. Removes electrodes and cleans electrode sites	☐	☐	☐	☐
18. Maintains patient's privacy	☐	☐	☐	☐
19. Cleans electrodes and machine	☐	☐	☐	☐
20. Scans cardiogram for any major arrhythmias	☐	☐	☐	☐
21. Records pertinent data in chart and departmental records	☐	☐	☐	☐
22. Measures, analyzes, or interprets				
a. Rhythm	☐	☐	☐	☐
b. Rate	☐	☐	☐	☐
c. P wave	☐	☐	☐	☐
d. P-R interval	☐	☐	☐	☐
e. QRS complex	☐	☐	☐	☐
f. ST segment	☐	☐	☐	☐
g. T wave	☐	☐	☐	☐
h. Rhythm strip interpretation	☐	☐	☐	☐
23. Notifies appropriate personnel and makes any necessary recommendations or modifications to the patient care plan	☐	☐	☐	☐

_____
Signature of Evaluator

_____
Signature of Student

PERFORMANCE RATING SCALE

5 EXCELLENT—FAR EXCEEDS EXPECTED LEVEL, FLAWLESS PERFORMANCE
4 ABOVE AVERAGE—NO PROMPTING REQUIRED, ABLE TO SELF-CORRECT
3 AVERAGE—THE MINIMUM COMPETENCY LEVEL, NO CRITICAL ERRORS
2 IMPROVEMENT NEEDED—PROBLEM AREAS EXIST; CRITICAL ERRORS, CORRECTIONS NEEDED
1 POOR AND UNACCEPTABLE PERFORMANCE—GROSS INACCURACIES, POTENTIALLY HARMFUL

PERFORMANCE CRITERIA		SCALE			
1. DISPLAYS KNOWLEDGE OF ESSENTIAL CONCEPTS	5	4	3	2	1
2. DEMONSTRATES THE RELATIONSHIP BETWEEN THEORY AND CLINICAL PRACTICE	5	4	3	2	1
3. FOLLOWS DIRECTIONS, EXHIBITS SOUND JUDGMENT, AND DEMONSTRATES ATTENTION TO SAFETY AND DETAIL	5	4	3	2	1
4. EXHIBITS THE REQUIRED MANUAL DEXTERITY	5	4	3	2	1
5. PERFORMS PROCEDURE IN A REASONABLE TIME FRAME	5	4	3	2	1
6. MAINTAINS STERILE OR ASEPTIC TECHNIQUE	5	4	3	2	1
7. INITIATES UNAMBIGUOUS GOAL-DIRECTED COMMUNICATION	5	4	3	2	1
8. PROVIDES FOR ADEQUATE CARE AND MAINTENANCE OF EQUIPMENT AND SUPPLIES	5	4	3	2	1
9. EXHIBITS COURTEOUS AND PLEASANT DEMEANOR	5	4	3	2	1
10. MAINTAINS CONCISE AND ACCURATE RECORDS	5	4	3	2	1

ADDITIONAL COMMENTS: INCLUDE ERRORS OF OMISSION OR COMMISSION, COMMUNICATIVE SKILLS, AND EFFECTIVENESS OF PATIENT INTERACTION:

SUMMARY PERFORMANCE EVALUATION AND RECOMMENDATIONS

SATISFACTORY PERFORMANCE—Performed without error or prompting, or able to self-correct, no critical errors.

_____ LABORATORY EVALUATION. SKILLS MAY BE APPLIED/OBSERVED IN THE CLINICAL SETTING.

_____ CLINICAL EVALUATION. STUDENT READY FOR MINIMALLY SUPERVISED APPLICATION AND REFINEMENT.

UNSATISFACTORY PERFORMANCE—Prompting required; performed with critical errors, potentially harmful.

_____ STUDENT REQUIRES ADDITIONAL LABORATORY PRACTICE.

_____ STUDENT REQUIRES ADDITIONAL SUPERVISED CLINICAL PRACTICE.

SIGNATURES

STUDENT: _____   EVALUATOR: _____

DATE: _____   DATE: _____

Basic Chest X-Ray Interpretation

INTRODUCTION

Radiologists and pulmonologists develop x-ray interpretation skills over the course of several years and hundreds of films. Although respiratory care practitioners are not expected to achieve this level of expertise, the ability to identify a normal chest x-ray and common cardiopulmonary abnormalities should be a part of the basic skills an advanced level practitioner can perform. In a critical situation, knowledge of x-ray interpretation can be crucial to patient care. In conjunction with other patient assessment techniques, atelectasis, pneumothorax, or endotracheal tube placement can be confirmed by radiography. Recognition of frequently encountered findings such as hyperinflation, infiltrates, pulmonary edema, and pneumonia is an asset to the practitioner and improves patient care.

The x-ray film is similar to a photographic negative. The x-ray precipitates silver, and an image is created. A cassette is used to enhance this process. It contains a fluorescent screen that, when stimulated by the x-ray, helps darken the film and enhance the image. Therefore objects that are the most dense absorb the x-rays, and the film is not altered photographically. These objects are called radiopaque, or **radiodense,** and appear white to gray depending on the density. Objects that absorb less rays are called **radiolucent.** Air, which allows the rays to pass through, appears black.[1]

One must remember that the image created is a two-dimensional image and the position and distance of the patient relative to the x-ray machine are important. Chest x-rays can be taken in several positions and describe the path or direction in which the ray passes through the patient onto the cassette. The most common view is the posteroanterior (PA) in an ambulatory patient. The anteroposterior (AP) is the usual view of a portable film in a more critically ill patient. The lateral, **lordotic** (used to expose the upper lobes), and decubitus projections are also used.[2]

The proficient interpretation of x-rays by respiratory therapists takes much practice. The learning process can be aided when a systematic approach is used.

Other techniques may also be used to determine lung abnormalities. **Transillumination** of an infant chest may help identify pneumothorax. Ventilation perfusion scans may assist in the diagnosis of pulmonary emboli. The chest x-ray is limited by its two-dimensional nature. Patient complaints and symptomatology sometimes do not correlate with the chest x-ray findings. Advanced techniques such as computerized **tomography** (CT) scans or magnetic resonance imaging (MRI) are then used to define a pulmonary abnormality that might or might not be identifiable on routine chest x-ray. The interpretation of these techniques is well beyond the scope of the respiratory care practitioner.

OBJECTIVES
Upon completion of this chapter, the student will be able to:

1. Differentiate between radiopaque and radiolucent structures.

2. Given a chest x-ray, verify the patient identity, film projection, position, and quality of the film.

3. Identify the major organs and anatomic landmarks on adult and infant chest x-ray films, including the aortic knob and heart shadow, **costophrenic** angles, hemidiaphragms, spinal column, ribs and rib angles, sternum, clavicles, hila, trachea and bifurcation (carina), air bronchogram, stomach bubble, and breast shadows.

4. Confirm the position of an endotracheal tube.

5. Identify the placement of chest tubes and pulmonary artery catheters.

6. Locate the following abnormalities on a chest x-ray: atelectasis, pneumothorax, hyperinflation, pleural effusion, large masses, **infiltrates,** pneumonia, hilar adenopathy, cavitary lesions, respiratory distress syndrome (RDS), epiglottitis, croup, and bronchopulmonary dysplasia (BPD).

7. Differentiate chest deformities from normal chest structure.

KEY TERMS

adenopathy	granuloma	lymphadenopathy	pathology
cardiomegaly	hyperlucent	mass	pathophysiology
caseation	iatrogenic	metastasis	pneumatocele
chylothorax	idiopathic	miliary	radiodense
coalescence	infiltrates	neoplasm	radiolucent
costophrenic	insidious	nodule	tomography
exudate	latent	opacification	transillumination
	lordotic	palliative	transudate

EQUIPMENT REQUIRED

- X-ray view box
- Spare fluorescent bulbs
- Chest x-rays of the following:
  Normal PA and AP view
  Lateral view
  Lordotic view
  Decubitus view
  Pneumothorax
  Atelectasis
  Hyperinflation
  Endotracheal tube in proper placement
  Improperly placed endotracheal tube
  Chest tube placement
  Pulmonary artery catheter placement
  Pleural effusion
  Lung cancer
  Adult respiratory distress syndrome
  Pulmonary edema
  Lobar pneumonia
  Kyphoscoliosis
  Pectus carinatum
  Normal infant chest film
  Epiglottitis
  Respiratory distress syndrome
  Bronchopulmonary dysplasia
  Croup
  Tuberculosis
  Pulmonary fibrosis
  Sarcoidosis
  Bronchiectasis
  Flail chest
  Subcutaneous emphysema
  Congestive heart failure

● EXERCISES

EXERCISE 18.1 Identification of Positions

Identify the position of the film in Figures 18.1 through 18.4 and label each one. *Record the answers on your laboratory report.*

EXERCISE 18.2 Identification of Major Organs and Landmarks

A systematic approach is needed when viewing a chest film. Some authors suggest an alphabetic approach.[3] The following method can be used as a guide. It is helpful to use your index finger to trace along the structure that you are viewing. This helps identify and delineate the object you are viewing.

1. Obtain a normal PA chest x-ray, insert it onto the view box, and turn on the view box.

2. Verify that you have the correct patient's film.

   NOTE: In the laboratory setting, for reasons of patient confidentiality, the patient name should be removed or masked.

3. The film should be placed so that it seems as if the patient is facing you. This is the standard method of viewing.[4] Look for the lead marker.

4. Observe the entire film for symmetry:
   a. Identify the clavicles, scapulae, and ribs.
   b. Identify the spinal column. Is it midline?
   c. Identify the lungs, right and left.
   d. Are there breast shadows?
   e. Locate the stomach air bubble.
   f. Observe the film to ensure that none of the peripheral structures were "clipped," or incompletely shown, because of patient positioning.

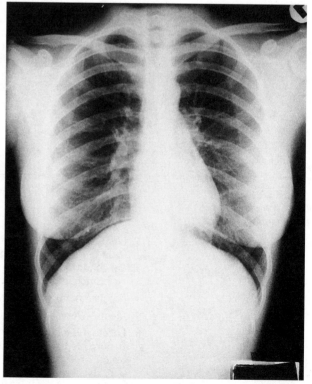

FIGURE 18.1   **Film A.**

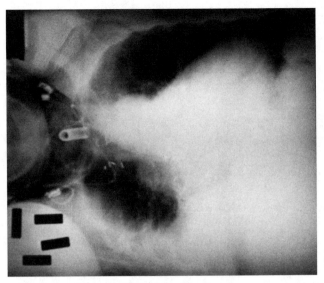

FIGURE 18.2 **Film B.**

5. Observe the film for the quality of the exposure. Is the overall quality too dark or too white? The thoracic spine should be just visible on a routine chest x-ray.[5]

6. Starting in the upper left side, trace your finger along the edge of the lungs down to the edge where the lung meets the diaphragm. This is the costophrenic angle. Is it sharp or blurred (possible fluid), or is it less sharp (blunted)?

7. Note the rib level of the hemi-diaphragms. Chest x-rays are taken at the peak of inspiration, and the diaphragms should be at the level of rib 8 or rib 9. This helps the radiologist determine if the film is of good or poor inspiratory quality.

8. Trace the outline of each rib starting from the sternum and moving outward. Do they go to the edge of the film? Are they continuous or interrupted (indicating a fracture)? Note the angle of the ribs anteriorly. Are they horizontal? Estimate the angle.

9. Observing the center of the film, observe the trachea's position. The trachea appears as a column of air. Is it midline? Follow the trachea to the point of bifurcation.

10. Identify the carina and the mainstem bronchi (the air bronchogram). Count the level of vertebrae and intercostal spaces corresponding to the carina. The carina should be at approximately T5 and between the second and third intercostal space.

11. Examine the hila for size and position. Because of anatomy, the left hilum normally appears higher than the right. The radiopaque image represents the pulmonary vasculature. Trace the lines out. These are the "lung markings" and also represent blood vessels, not airways.

12. In the center of the film, identify the aortic knob and the heart shadow. The cardiothoracic ratio is used to express heart size. If the shadow occupies more than 50 percent it is considered abnormally enlarged.[6] Approximate how much of the film is occupied by the heart shadow, as shown in Figure 18.5, and *record it on your laboratory report.*

NOTE: On AP films, the heart will appear larger than its actual size. Therefore, this projection should not be used to measure heart size.

13. Label the structures on Figure 18.6, and *record them on your laboratory report.*

EXERCISE 18.3 Hyperinflation

1. Obtain an x-ray film already interpreted as hyperinflation, as shown in Figure 18.7, and compare it with the normal film used in Exercise 18.2.

2. Using the technique practiced in the previous exercise, observe and identify the following. *Record them on your laboratory report.*
   a. Projection used.
   b. Patient position.
   c. Flattening of the hemidiaphragms. Note the level of the ribs. Location of the diaphragms at the level of rib 11 is an indicator of hyperinflation.
   d. Horizontal rib margins.
   e. Increased intercostal spaces.
   f. Areas of hyperlucency with decreased lung markings.
   g. Lung size. Compare the size of the lungs.
   h. Increased AP diameter on a lateral film.

EXERCISE 18.4 Pneumothorax

1. Obtain a film with a confirmed pneumothorax, as shown in Figure 18.8, and compare it with the normal film used in Exercise 18.2.

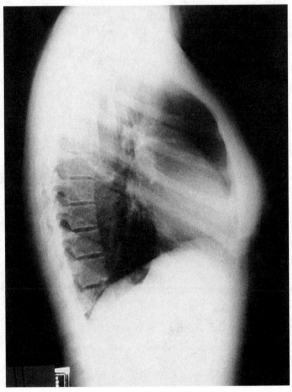

FIGURE 18.3 **Film C.**

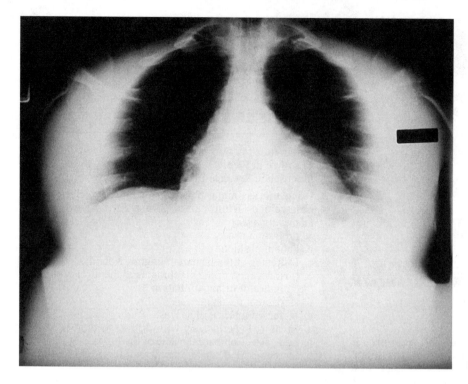

FIGURE 18.4   **Film D.**

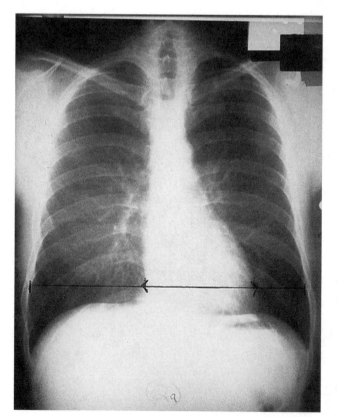

FIGURE 18.5   Measurement of heart size.

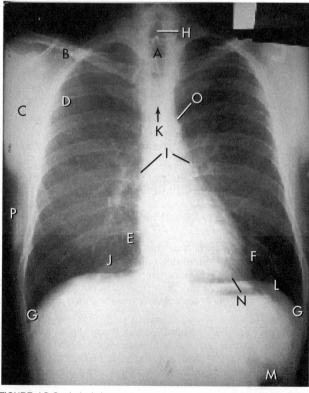

FIGURE 18.6   Label the x-ray, naming the anatomic landmarks and other characteristics.

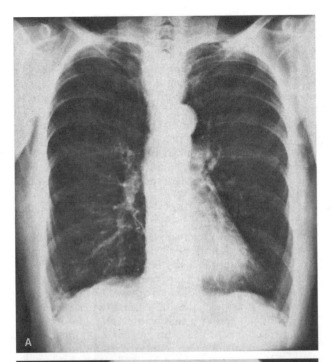

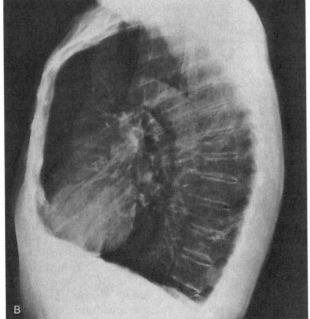

FIGURE 18.7 X-ray typical of emphysema. (From Wilkins, RF and Dexter, JR: Respiratory Disease: Principles of Patient Care. FA Davis, Philadelphia, 1993, p. 48, with permission.)

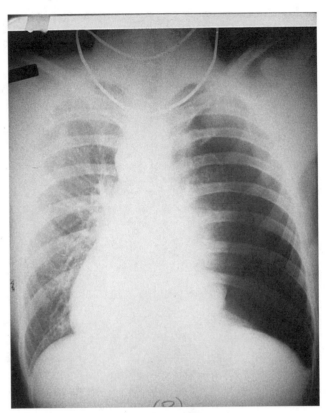

FIGURE 18.8 Pneumothorax.

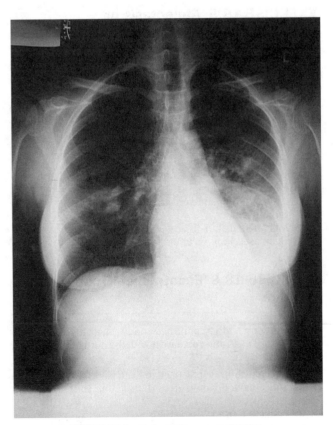

FIGURE 18.9 Atelectasis or consolidation.

2. Using the technique practiced in the previous exercise, observe and identify the following. *Record them on your laboratory report.*
   a. Projection used.
   b. Tracheal or mediastinal shift indicating a tension pneumothorax. Note that not all films display a shift.
   c. Area of darker region without lung markings.
   d. Line of demarcation indicating the edge of the collapsed lung.

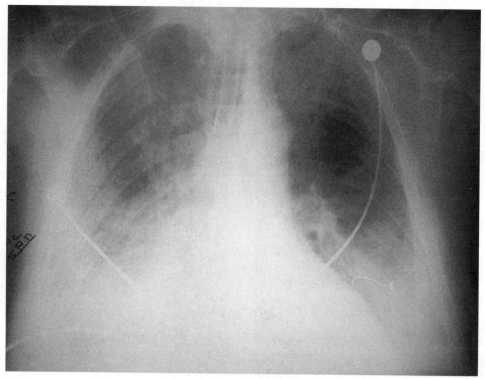

FIGURE 18.10 Endotracheal tube in position.

EXERCISE 18.5 Atelectasis or Consolidation

1. Obtain a film with a confirmed atelectasis or consolidated lung, as shown in Figure 18.9, and compare it with the normal film used in Exercise 18.2.

2. Using the technique practiced in Exercise 18.2, observe and identify the following. *Record them on your laboratory report.*
   a. Projection used
   b. Patient position
   c. Hemidiaphragm positions (relative to normal and relative to each other)
   d. Area of radiopaque image in an area where it should be radiolucent
   e. Mediastinal shift (if any)
   f. Decreased lung volumes

EXERCISE 18.6 Endotracheal Tube Position

1. Obtain a film with a confirmed endotracheal tube, as shown in Figure 18.10, and compare it with the normal film used in Exercise 18.2.

2. Using the technique practiced in Exercise 18.2, observe and identify the following. *Record them on your laboratory report.*
   a. Projection used
   b. The radiopfaque line of the endotracheal tube

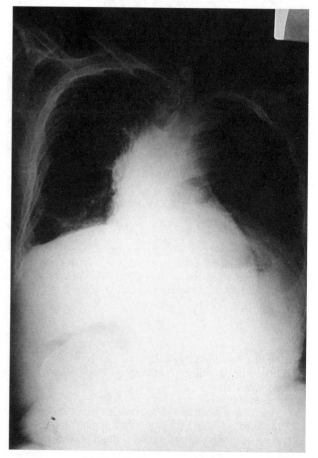

FIGURE 18.11 Kyphoscoliosis.

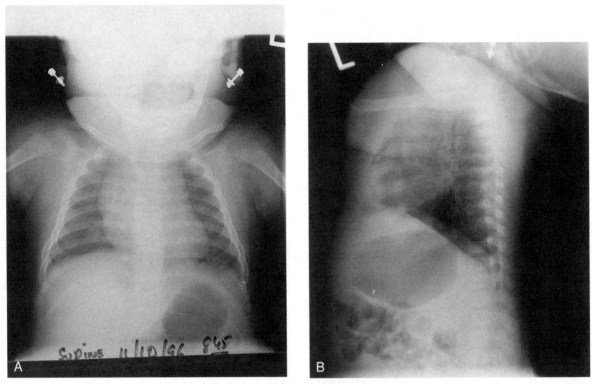

FIGURE 18.12   *(A and B)* Normal infant chest films.

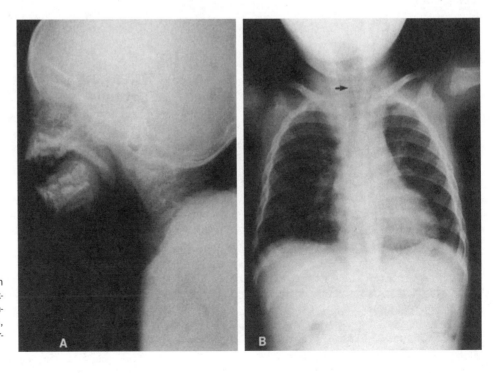

FIGURE 18.13 Steeple sign in croup. (From Wilkins, RF and Dexter, JR: Respiratory Disease: Principles of Patient Care. FA Davis, Philadelphia, 1993, p. 335, with permission.)

c. Tip of the endotracheal tube
d. The carina
e. Aortic knob

3. Once you have identified the structures, identify the following. *Record the answers on your laboratory report.*
   a. Count the ribs. At the level of what rib or intercostal space anteriorly is the tube?
   b. Count the vertebrae. At the level of what vertebra is the tube?
   c. Approximately how far is the tip of the endotracheal tube above the carina?

EXERCISE 18.7 Chest Deformities

1. Obtain a film of Kyphoscoliosis (Fig. 18.11).

2. Using the technique practiced in the previous exercises, compare the abnormalities to a normal chest film. *Record them on your laboratory report.*

EXERCISE 18.8 Infant and Pediatric Films

1. Obtain a normal infant film (Fig. 18.12). Using the technique practiced in the previous exercises, observe the film and compare it with a normal adult chest x-ray. *Record them on your laboratory report.*

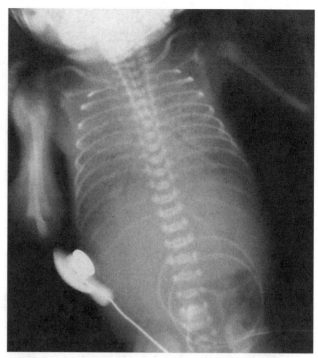

FIGURE 18.15 Infant respiratory distress syndrome. (From Wilkins, RF and Dexter, JR: Respiratory Disease: Principles of Patient Care. FA Davis, Philadelphia, 1993, p. 359, with permission.)

2. Obtain films of the following:
   Steeple sign in croup (Fig. 18.13)
   Thumb sign in epiglottitis (Fig. 18.14)
   RDS (Fig. 18.15)
   BPD (Fig. 18.16)

3. Using the technique practiced in the previous exercises, compare the abnormalities to a normal chest film. *Record them on your laboratory report.*

EXERCISE 18.9 Other Abnormal Patterns

1. Obtain films from your instructor that are consistent with pulmonary edema, cavitary lesion, hilar adenopathy, chest tube, pulmonary artery catheter, and pleural effusion. Compare them with the normal adult film used in Exercise 18.2.

2. Using the technique practiced in the previous exercises, observe and identify the differences in each film. *Record them on your laboratory report.*

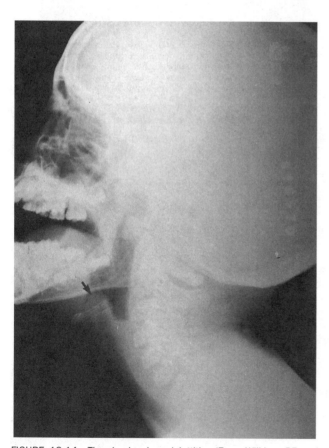

FIGURE 18.14 Thumb sign in epiglottitis. (From Wilkins, RF and Dexter, JR: Respiratory Disease: Principles of Patient Care. FA Davis, Philadelphia, 1993, p. 332, with permission.)

References

1. Squire, LF and Novelline, RA: Fundamentals of Radiology. Harvard University Press, Cambridge, 1988, p 3.
2. Squire, LF and Novelline, RA: Fundamentals of Radiology. Harvard University Press, Cambridge, 1988, p 4.
3. Scanlan, C et al (eds): Egan's Fundamentals of Respiratory Care, ed 6. Mosby, St Louis, 1995, p 435.
4. Squire, LF and Novelline, RA: Fundamentals of Radiology. Harvard University Press, Cambridge, 1988, p 13.
5. Squire, LF and Novelline, RA: Fundamentals of Radiology. Harvard University Press, Cambridge, 1988, p 40–41.

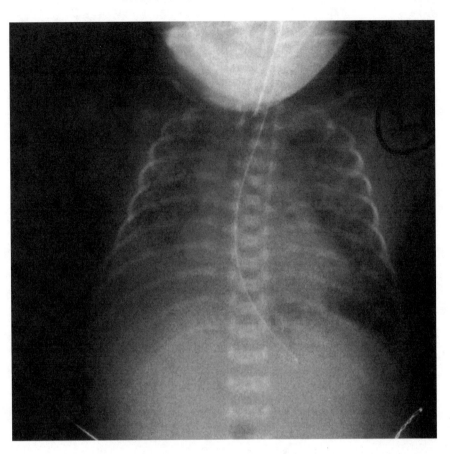

FIGURE 18.16 Bronchopulmonary dysplasia. (From Wilkins, RF and Dexter, JR: Respiratory Disease: Principles of Patient Care. FA Davis, Philadelphia, 1993, p. 373, with permission.)

6. Squire, LF and Novelline, RA: Fundamentals of Radiology. Harvard University Press, Cambridge, 1988, p 129.

Related Readings

Scanlan, C et al (eds): Egan's Fundamentals of Respiratory Care, ed 6. Mosby, St Louis, 1995.
Squire, LF and Novelline, RA: Fundamentals of Radiology. Harvard University Press, Cambridge, 1988.
Wilkins, RL and Dexter, JR. Respiratory Disease: A Case Study Approach to Patient Care, ed 2. FA Davis, Philadelphia, 1997.

Selected Journal Articles

Desai, S and Chan, O: Interpretation of a normal chest X-ray. Nursing Standard 7:38–39, 1992.
Gilbert, T and McGrath, B: Tension pneumothorax: Etiology, diagnosis, pathophysiology and management. J Intensive Care 9:139–150, 1994.
Hall, JB, White, SR and Karrison, T: Efficacy of daily routine chest radiographs in intubated mechanically ventilated patients. Crit Care Med 19:689–693, 1991.
Light, RW: Tension pneumothorax. J Intensive Care Med 20:468–469, 1994.

LABORATORY REPORT

CHAPTER 18: BASIC CHEST X-RAY INTERPRETATION

Name _____   Date _____

Course/Section _____   Instructor _____

Data Collection

EXERCISE 18.1   Identification of Positions

A. _____   C. _____

B. _____   D. _____

EXERCISE 18.2   Identification of Major Organs and Landmarks

Cardiothoracic ratio: _____

Label the chest film on Figure 18.6.

A. _____   G. _____   M. _____

B. _____   H. _____   N. _____

C. _____   I. _____   O. _____

D. _____   J. _____   P. _____

E. _____   K. _____

F. _____   L. _____

EXERCISE 18.3   Hyperinflation

Projection used: _____

Patient position: _____

Flattening of the hemidiaphragms and rib level: _____

_____

Horizontal rib margins present: _____

Increased intercostal spaces: _____

_____

Areas of hyperlucency with decreased lung markings: _____

_____

Comparison of lung size: _____

_____

EXERCISE 18.4   Pneumothorax

Projection used: _____

Patient position: _____

Mediastinal shift: _____

_____

Area of darker region without lung markings: _____

_____

Edge of the collapsed lung: _____

_____

EXERCISE 18.5   Atelectasis or Consolidation

Projection used: _____

Patient position: _____

Hemidiaphragm positions: _____

_____

Area of radiopaque image in an area where it should be radiolucent: _____

_____

Mediastinal shift: _____

_____

Decreased lung volumes: _____

_____

EXERCISE 18.6   Endotracheal Tube Position

Projection used: _____

Patient position: _____

Tip of the endotracheal tube: _____

_____

Carina: _____

_____

Level of the rib: _____

Level of the vertebra: _____

Distance above the carina: _____

EXERCISE 18.7   Chest Deformities
Kyphoscoliosis

Differences observed: _____

_____

_____

EXERCISE 18.8   Infant and Pediatric Films

Comparison of normal infant chest x-ray with a normal adult chest x-ray: _____

_____

Steeple Sign in Croup

Differences observed: _____

_____

_____

Thumb Sign in Epiglottitis

Differences observed: _____

_____

_____

Respiratory Distress Syndrome

Differences observed: _____

_____

_____

Bronchopulmonary Dysplasia

Differences observed: _____

_____

_____

EXERCISE 18.9   Other Abnormal Patterns

Abnormality: _____

Differences observed: _____

_____

_____

Abnormality: _____

Differences observed: _____

_____

_____

Abnormality: _____

Differences observed: _____

_____

_____

Abnormality: _____

Differences observed: _____

_____

_____

Location of the chest tube: _____

Abnormality: _____

Differences observed: _____

_____

_____

Location of the pulmonary artery catheter: _____

Abnormality: _____

Differences observed: _____

_____

_____

CRITICAL THINKING QUESTIONS

1. Why would the patient be asked to remove all necklaces, charms, and medals before a chest x-ray?

2. The physician requires a yearly chest x-ray for his or her patient with COPD. Of what benefit is the previous film?

3. Radiographically, what defines proper endotracheal tube placement?

4. Can the chest x-ray determine if the tube is in the esophagus? Why or why not?

5. What factors might make the interpretation of a film difficult?

6. Given the chest x-rays shown in Figures 18.17 through 18.21, what might the interpretation be?

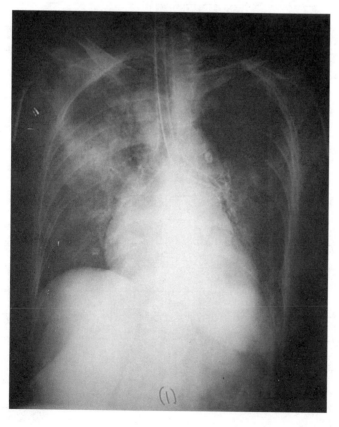

FIGURE 18.17 **Unknown film A.**

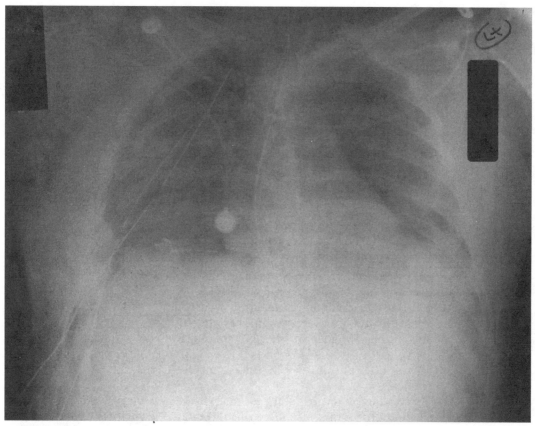

FIGURE 18.18   **Unknown film B.** (From Wilkins, RF and Dexter, JR: Respiratory Disease: Principles of Patient Care. FA Davis, Philadelphia, 1993, p. 207, with permission.)

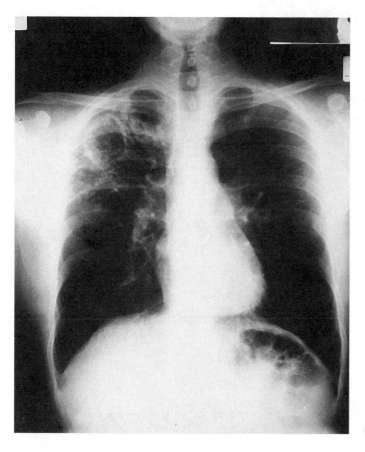

FIGURE 18.19   **Unknown film C.**

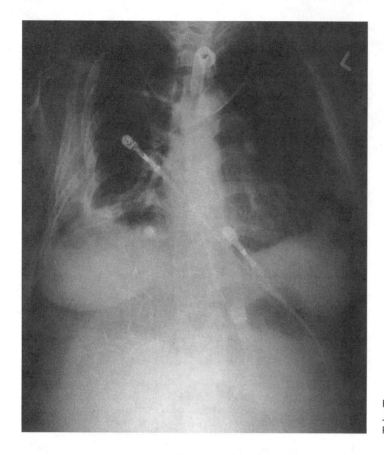

FIGURE 18.20 **Unknown film D.** (From Wilkins, RF and Dexter, JR: Respiratory Disease: Principles of Patient Care. FA Davis, Philadelphia, 1993, p. 212, with permission.)

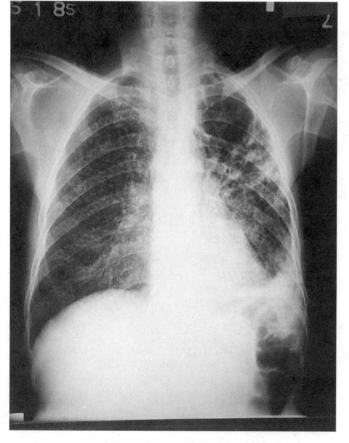

FIGURE 18.21 **Unknown film E.**

PROCEDURAL COMPETENCY EVALUATION

Name _____ Date _____

Chest X-Ray Interpretation

Setting: ☐ Lab ☐ Clinical   Evaluator: ☐ Peer ☐ Instructor

Conditions (describe): _____

_____

Equipment Used

_____

_____

	SATISFACTORY	UNSATISFACTORY	NOT OBSERVED	NOT APPLICABLE
Equipment and Patient Preparation				
1. Reviews the patient's medical record	☐	☐	☐	☐
2. Scans chart for diagnosis and any other pertinent data and notes	☐	☐	☐	☐
3. Washes hands and applies standard precautions and transmission-based isolation procedures as appropriate	☐	☐	☐	☐
4. Identifies patient, introduces self and department	☐	☐	☐	☐
Assessment and Implementation				
5. Assesses the patient	☐	☐	☐	☐
6. Obtains the chest x-ray film; verifies film identification	☐	☐	☐	☐
7. Inserts film onto the view box with the correct orientation and turns on the view box light	☐	☐	☐	☐
8. Identifies the view of the film	☐	☐	☐	☐
9. Observes the entire film for symmetry and identifies				
a. Clavicles, scapulae, and ribs	☐	☐	☐	☐
b. Spinal column (notes whether it is midline)	☐	☐	☐	☐
c. Lungs, right and left	☐	☐	☐	☐
d. Costophrenic angles; notes if they are sharp or blurred (possible fluid) or less sharp (blunted)	☐	☐	☐	☐
e. Level of hemi-diaphragms; notes the rib level to determine if the film is of good or poor inspiratory quality	☐	☐	☐	☐
f. Stomach air bubble	☐	☐	☐	☐
g. Breast shadows	☐	☐	☐	☐
10. Traces the outline of each rib, noting the angle and any fractures or other abnormalities	☐	☐	☐	☐
11. Observes the tracheal position	☐	☐	☐	☐
12. Identifies the carina and the mainstem bronchi	☐	☐	☐	☐
13. Examines the hila for size and position	☐	☐	☐	☐
14. Identifies the lung markings	☐	☐	☐	☐
15. Identifies the aortic knob and the heart shadow	☐	☐	☐	☐
16. Estimates the cardiothoracic ratio	☐	☐	☐	☐
17. Notes the presence and position of any artificial airways or catheters	☐	☐	☐	☐

	S A T I S F A C T O R Y	U N S A T I S F A C T O R Y	N O T O B S E R V E D	N O T A P P L I C A B L E
18. States an overall impression of the film	☐	☐	☐	☐
19. Correlates the film with the clinical findings	☐	☐	☐	☐

Follow-up

20. Maintains/processes equipment	☐	☐	☐	☐
21. Disposes of infectious waste and washes hands	☐	☐	☐	☐
22. Records pertinent data in chart and departmental records	☐	☐	☐	☐
23. Notifies appropriate personnel and makes any necessary recommendations or modifications to the patient care plan	☐	☐	☐	☐

_____

Signature of Evaluator

_____

Signature of Student

PERFORMANCE RATING SCALE

5 EXCELLENT—FAR EXCEEDS EXPECTED LEVEL, FLAWLESS PERFORMANCE
4 ABOVE AVERAGE—NO PROMPTING REQUIRED, ABLE TO SELF-CORRECT
3 AVERAGE—THE MINIMUM COMPETENCY LEVEL, NO CRITICAL ERRORS
2 IMPROVEMENT NEEDED—PROBLEM AREAS EXIST; CRITICAL ERRORS, CORRECTIONS NEEDED
1 POOR AND UNACCEPTABLE PERFORMANCE—GROSS INACCURACIES, POTENTIALLY HARMFUL

PERFORMANCE CRITERIA	SCALE				
1. DISPLAYS KNOWLEDGE OF ESSENTIAL CONCEPTS	5	4	3	2	1
2. DEMONSTRATES THE RELATIONSHIP BETWEEN THEORY AND CLINICAL PRACTICE	5	4	3	2	1
3. FOLLOWS DIRECTIONS, EXHIBITS SOUND JUDGMENT, AND DEMONSTRATES ATTENTION TO SAFETY AND DETAIL	5	4	3	2	1
4. EXHIBITS THE REQUIRED MANUAL DEXTERITY	5	4	3	2	1
5. PERFORMS PROCEDURE IN A REASONABLE TIME FRAME	5	4	3	2	1
6. MAINTAINS STERILE OR ASEPTIC TECHNIQUE	5	4	3	2	1
7. INITIATES UNAMBIGUOUS GOAL-DIRECTED COMMUNICATION	5	4	3	2	1
8. PROVIDES FOR ADEQUATE CARE AND MAINTENANCE OF EQUIPMENT AND SUPPLIES	5	4	3	2	1
9. EXHIBITS COURTEOUS AND PLEASANT DEMEANOR	5	4	3	2	1
10. MAINTAINS CONCISE AND ACCURATE RECORDS	5	4	3	2	1

ADDITIONAL COMMENTS: INCLUDE ERRORS OF OMISSION OR COMMISSION, COMMUNICATIVE SKILLS, AND EFFECTIVENESS OF PATIENT INTERACTION:

SUMMARY PERFORMANCE EVALUATION AND RECOMMENDATIONS

SATISFACTORY PERFORMANCE—Performed without error or prompting, or able to self-correct, no critical errors.

_____ LABORATORY EVALUATION. SKILLS MAY BE APPLIED/OBSERVED IN THE CLINICAL SETTING.

_____ CLINICAL EVALUATION. STUDENT READY FOR MINIMALLY SUPERVISED APPLICATION AND REFINEMENT.

UNSATISFACTORY PERFORMANCE—Prompting required; performed with critical errors, potentially harmful.

_____ STUDENT REQUIRES ADDITIONAL LABORATORY PRACTICE.

_____ STUDENT REQUIRES ADDITIONAL SUPERVISED CLINICAL PRACTICE.

SIGNATURES

STUDENT: _____   EVALUATOR: _____

DATE: _____   DATE: _____

Arterial Blood Gas Sampling

Arterial blood gas sampling is a quick and reliable tool for patient assessment. Blood sampling from a peripheral artery or an indwelling **catheter** provides a specimen for the measurement of pH, carbon dioxide and oxygen pressures, total hemoglobin and hemoglobin saturation, and evaluation of abnormal hemoglobins. Analysis of these values helps evaluate the adequacy of ventilation and oxygenation. They are used to assess a patient's response to therapeutic interventions, for diagnostic evaluations, and to monitor the severity and progression of a disease process.[1]

Arterial blood sampling is an invasive procedure and is not without risk to both the patient and the respiratory care practitioner. It is essential that the skills required to perform these procedures be practiced until proficiency is achieved before performing these procedures in the clinical setting. Knowledge of anatomy and infection control practices is an integral part of the requirements for safe technique.

OBJECTIVES
Upon completion of this chapter, the student will be able to:

1. Practice communication skills needed to explain blood sampling procedures to patients.
2. Practice medical charting and documentation of performance of blood gas sampling procedures.
3. Apply infection control guidelines and standards associated with equipment and procedures, according to OSHA regulations and CDC guidelines.
4. Assemble and prepare the equipment necessary for performance of arterial puncture and arterial line sampling.
5. Review the medical record for information essential to the safe performance of arterial sampling.
6. Demonstrate the safe performance of arterial puncture and arterial line sampling.
7. Demonstrate safe postpuncture care.
8. Prepare an anaerobic blood gas sample for transport.
9. Identify the equipment and steps necessary to perform a capillary sample for blood gas analysis.

KEY TERMS

acid	calibration	embolism	laceration
anemia	catheter	erythema	lancet
anion	cation	exsanguination	latex
anticoagulant	coagulation	hematoma	Luer-Lok
base	coagulopathy	hemorrhage	polycythemia
bevel	collateral	intradermal	thrombus
buffer	dissociation	intraflow	valve stem
	ecchymosis	iodophor	wheal

EQUIPMENT REQUIRED

- Arterial arm simulators
- Sterile water
- Red dye
- Arterial blood gas kits or component parts:
  Preheparinized syringes, 1, 3, or 5 ml

1000-U/ml heparin vials
Various size needles: 20, 22, 23, and 25 gauge
Syringe caps and rubber stopper
Air bubble venting devices (optional)
Self-capping syringes (optional)
Sterile drape (optional)
Biohazard bags

Iodophor or alcohol-based disinfectant pads
Patient label
- Two-percent xylocaine solution
- Disposable **latex** and vinyl gloves, various sizes
- Gauze, 4 × 4 and 2 × 2
- Band-Aids
- Cloth tape
- Goggles
- Disposable gowns (optional)
- Sharps containers
- Arterial line setup:
  IV tubing
  Two 1000-ml IV solution bags
  Three-way stopcocks
  20-Gauge intracath needle
  Blood pressure cuff or pressure infuser
  Intraflow flush device
  Heparin 1-percent solution
- Towels
- Ice
- Sample blood gas analysis slips
- Heparinized capillary tubes
- Rubber capillary tube stoppers
- Metal mixing "fleas" and magnet
- **Lancets**

● E X E R C I S E S

EXERCISE 19.1 Preparation of Blood Gas Kit Components

1. Obtain an arterial blood gas kit. If preprepared kits are not available, gather the necessary items and identify the following components:
   a. Syringe. *Record the size syringe on your laboratory report.*
   b. Needles, various sizes. *Record the needle gauges available in your kit on your laboratory report.*
   c. Iodophor or alcohol prep pads.
   d. Band-Aids.
   e. Label.
   f. Biohazard transport bag.
   g. Syringe cap and rubber stoppers.
   h. Self-capping device (optional).
   i. Sterile drape (optional).
   j. Gauze.   *or dry Heparine*
   k. Liquid heparin vial (optional). Syringes may already be preheparinized with liquid sodium heparin or dry litholized lithium heparin. *Record the type of heparin used in your blood gas kit.*
   l. Air bubble removal device (optional). This may be available with kits that contain self-capping needle protection devices (Fig. 19.1).

   is the diameter of the bigger the gage the smaller The Needle indiameter

   Pprevent blood from clotting

2. Wash your hands and apply latex or vinyl gloves.

   NOTE: Some people have or may develop severe latex allergies.[2] Vinyl gloves are recommended in this case.

3. Select the smallest needle available in your kit for performing a radial puncture. *Record the gauge selected on your laboratory report.*

4. Secure the needle on the syringe by twisting it onto the **Luer-Lok** (see Fig. 19.1).

5. If a preheparinized dry heparin syringe is used, draw back the plunger to preset the desired sample amount to be obtained. In most modern blood gas analyzers, as little as

0.5 ml is needed, but it is advisable to draw some extra blood in case repeat analysis is required.

6. If a liquid heparin preheparinized plastic syringe is used, pull back the barrel of the syringe about halfway. Then turn the syringe so that the needle is pointing straight up (Fig. 19.2). To eject any excess air, slowly push the barrel back up to the point at which the heparin enters the needle. Turn the needle and syringe downward and discard any excess safely. Leave only the amount of heparin needed to fill the hub of the syringe and the needle.

   If a glass syringe is used, the barrel of the syringe must be lubricated with the heparin before ejecting the excess. This can be accomplished by sliding the barrel of the syringe up and down until it slides freely on its own.

7. Gently loosen the needle cap, but do not remove it.

8. Your instructor will give you a patient scenario. Fill out the patient label, charge slip, or both. Include the patient name and identification number.

EXERCISE 19.2 Modified Allen's Test

An arterial puncture can be performed via the radial, brachial, or femoral artery (Fig. 19.3). The radial artery is the most common site chosen. It is the most accessible, is easiest to stabilize, and has the best **collateral** circulation. A modified Allen's test is used to determine the presence of collateral circulation via the ulnar artery.

Perform the following steps on your laboratory partner:

1. Identify your "patient." Introduce yourself and your department. Explain to your partner in nonmedical terms that you are going to perform an arterial blood gas and what is involved. Confirm your partner's understanding, and answer any questions or concerns. The partner should simulate a patient's concern and fears about having this invasive procedure performed and about the fact that laboratory personnel were just here drawing blood. You should respond appropriately.

2. Determine which hand is the patient's dominant hand. Palpate both radial arteries and select the one with the strongest pulse. The nondominant hand is the preferred choice. The radial artery pulse can be found by placing your index finger, middle finger, or both on the lateral aspect of the wrist on the thumb side between the second and third wrist folds, then sliding your fingers into the groove between the bones and tendons.

3. Palpate the ulnar artery if possible. It is located on the lateral side of the wrist (closest to the little finger) in the groove between the tendons and the ulnar bone.

4. Have your partner hold his or her hand palm up. Using two hands, occlude both the radial and ulnar arteries as shown in Figure 19.4.

5. Instruct your partner to open and close his or her fist at least three times until you observe the palm of the hand blanching (turning pale).

6. Release the ulnar artery only (pinky side of partner's hand). The palm should flush within 3 to 5 sec (10 to 15 sec maximum).[3] If not, repeat the test on the other arm.

7. *Record the results of the Allen's test on your laboratory report.*

8. Practice the technique for performing a modified Allen's test on an unconscious patient. Hold the radial and ulnar arteries with one hand and raise the patient's arm. Keep the arm raised until the palm blanches. Lower the arm. Release the ulnar artery and look for the palm flushing as in the preceding steps.

You need
more → R.R. & FIO₂ before analysing the bloodgas.

A.

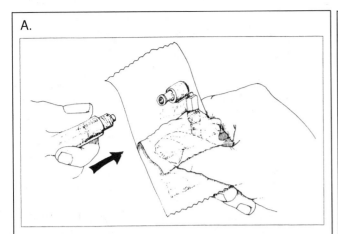

- Peel blister pouch open half way. (Do not touch Needle-Pro.) Grasp sheath using the plastic peel pouch. To prevent contamination, be careful not to touch Needle-Pro's locking end.

- With an easy twisting motion, attach syringe to the luer connection of Needle-Pro.

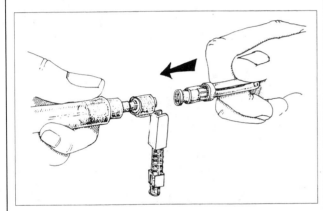

- Place a needle into the male fitting on the base of Needle-Pro.

- Remove the sheath from the needle and begin the procedure.

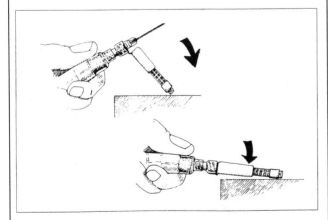

- After the procedure is completed, press the needle into the sheath using a one-handed technique. Perform the one-handed technique by gently pressing the sheath against a hard surface such as a bedside table. As the sheath is pressed, the needle is firmly snapped into the sheath.

FIGURE 19.1   Needle protection devices. (Courtesy of *[A and B]* Smiths Industries Medical Systems, Inc., Keene, NH; *[C]* Marquest Medical Products, Inc., Englewood, CO.)

B.

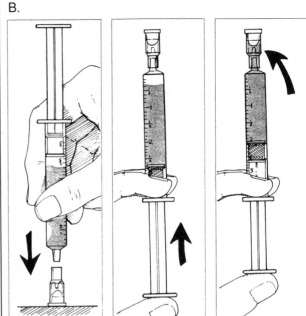

- Remove needle from arterial blood gas syringe (if attached) and dispose of properly.

- To remove air bubbles from sample, firmly push the Filter-Pro onto the syringe luer.

- Holding the luer end up, tap the syringe to position air bubbles at the tip.

- Gently push the plunger forward to expel air from the sample.

- Stop pushing plunger when sample wets filter. Too much pressure may release Filter-Pro from syringe.

- Transport syringe with Filter-Pro attached to laboratory for analysis.

C.

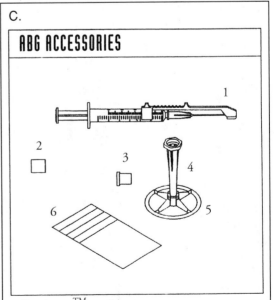

ABG ACCESSORIES

1. Peachcapp™ needle protector
2. Cubic needle stopper
3. L'uer tip caps
4. Silicone-filled sheath
5. Needle sheath holder
6. Three-part patient label

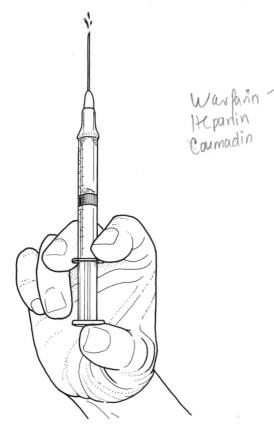

Warfarin
Heparin
Coumadin

FIGURE 19.2 Ejecting heparin from liquid heparin syringe.

EXERCISE 19.3 Performance of Arterial Puncture

An arterial arm simulator should be used for this procedure. Under no circumstances should students draw blood on each other. Iodophor preparations will stain the simulator and should be avoided during laboratory practice.

Perform or simulate the following steps:

1. Verify the physician's order or protocol. Check for time, special instructions (on or off O_2 or special position).

2. Scan the chart and note diagnosis, order, **coagulopathies, anticoagulant** therapy, oxygen concentration, and modality. Allergies to xylocaine should be checked if a local anesthetic will be used.

3. Gather and prepare the required equipment as in Exercise 19.1. Fill the bag with ice and water. Obtain a towel to use as a support for the patient's wrist.

4. Wash your hands and apply standard precautions and transmission-based isolation procedures as appropriate.

5. Introduce yourself and your department, and explain the procedure. Confirm the patient's understanding. Reassure as needed.

6. Verify the patient's identity by checking the identification band.

7. Verify the oxygen concentration or ventilator settings by double-checking in the room.

8. Fill in the patient information label, charge slip, or other appropriate documentation. In some situations this information may be input directly into a computer system. Include the following information:
   Date
   Time
   Patient name and identification
   Physician
   Puncture site (left or right radial artery, arterial line, brachial artery, etc.)
   Allen's test results
   F_IO_2: percent and modality
   Ventilatory status: spontaneous respiratory frequency or ventilator settings, if applicable, including machine tidal volume, machine frequency, mode of ventilation, any spontaneous tidal volume, and frequency noted
   Technician or therapist signature

Record this information on your laboratory report. In a clinical situation, the label may be filled out after the

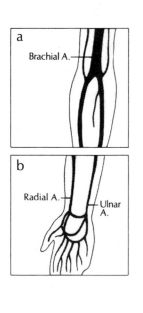

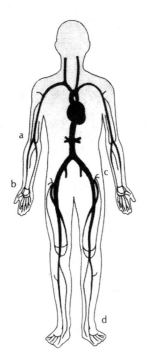

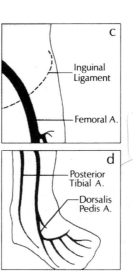

PaO_2 =	SpO_2
40	70
50	80
60	90

PaO_2 = 80-100

mild = 60-80
moderate = 50-70
severe = 40-50

FIGURE 19.3 Sites available for arterial puncture. (From Shapiro, BA, Peruzzi, WT and Templin, R: Clinical Application of Blood Gases, ed 5. Mosby-Year Book, St. Louis, 1994, p. 302, with permission.)

(a)

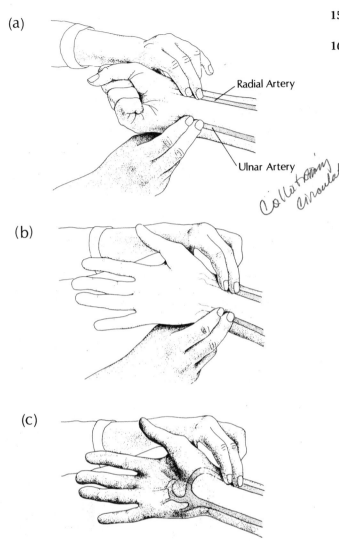

Radial Artery

Ulnar Artery

Collateral circulation

(b)

(c)

FIGURE 19.4 Performing the modified Allen's test. (From Shapiro, BA, Peruzzi, WT and Templin, R: Clinical Application of Blood Gases, ed 5. Mosby-Year Book, St. Louis, 1994, p. 304, with permission.)

15. Repalpate the puncture site, and determine the path of the artery.
16. Correctly perform the puncture.
    a. Place your hand in the palm of the patient's hand to stabilize it.
    b. With the **bevel** of the needle facing upward, enter the artery with the syringe at a 45-degree angle (Fig. 19.6). The puncture should be performed within 2 to 3 cm of the wrist skin folds (Fig. 19.7). Insert the tip of the needle quickly just through the skin, and then pause to verify the needle angle.
    c. *Slowly* advance the needle until a flash of blood is seen in the hub, indicating that the artery has been entered. Once the flash is seen and blood begins to fill the syringe, maintain your position until blood fills the syringe to the desired amount. The amount needed will vary with the size of the syringe and the type of blood gas analyzer being used. For most automated blood gas analyzers, 0.5 to 1 ml of blood is sufficient. More may be obtained if more than one analysis will be performed on the sample. If need be, slowly withdraw the needle to just below the surface of the skin. Do not completely withdraw it. Redirect the needle angle until the blood is obtained. *Do not* reangle the syringe while it is in the wrist. There is no set rule as to how many times repositioning the needle is acceptable. However, patient comfort and the availability of another competent person to attempt the puncture should be considered. If more than two or three repositions are needed, a beginning student should terminate the procedure and seek assistance.

NOTE: Arterial blood can be recognized by color, pulsation into syringe, self-filling, and data results as compared with clinical condition.

    d. Remove the syringe and immediately compress the artery with the gauze.
    e. Using the rubber stopper or self-capping needle protection device, plug the needle.

NOTE: *Never recap the needle manually using two hands.*

17. Continue to apply firm pressure to the site for 3 to 5 min or at least 10 min if the patient has any bleeding disorders or is receiving anticoagulant therapy.

puncture procedure. However, ventilatory status and F_IO_2 should be verified before the puncture.

9. Select the appropriate size needle and secure it to the syringe Luer-Lok.
10. Heparinize the syringe or set the barrel on the preheparinized syringe as in Exercise 19.1.
11. Palpate both radial arteries. Choose the best site.
12. Perform the modified Allen's test for the presence of collateral circulation as in Exercise 19.2.
13. Position the patient's arm so that it is extended and supported on a firm surface, palm up. Place a towel or similar item to support the wrist (Fig. 19.5). Place a sterile field under the wrist if available.
14. Prepare the intended puncture site by rubbing vigorously with antiseptic solution for at least 30 sec in a circular motion away from the puncture site. Allow it to dry. Disinfect the gloved fingers that you will be using to palpate the pulse.

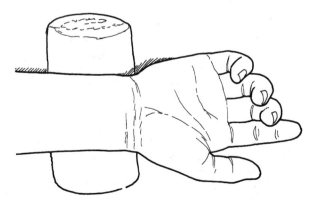

FIGURE 19.5 Positioning of wrist for radial artery puncture.

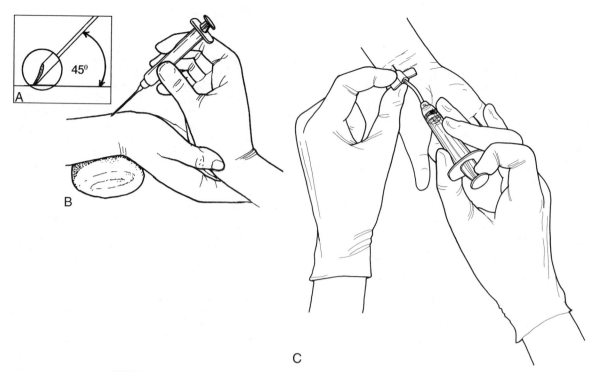

FIGURE 19.6 (*A*, *B*, and *C*)   Bevel position and needle angle for arterial puncture.

18. If a self-venting syringe is used, expel any air from the sample by pushing the barrel toward the plugged needle. Otherwise, remove the needle from the Luer-Lok and expel the air into a gauze pad. Venting devices may also be available. Once all air bubbles have been removed, cap the syringe and label it.

19. Mix blood and heparin by rolling the syringe in your palms.

20. Place the sample on ice if analysis will be delayed by more than 15 min.[1] Place the sample in a biohazard bag for transport.

21. Check the circulation distal to the puncture site. Continue to compress the artery until there is a return of pulses proximal and distal to the site and there is no evidence of bleeding, swelling, or discoloration.

22. Ensure patient safety and comfort.

23. Clean up. Discard needle in sharps container, and dispose of any infectious waste in the appropriate receptacle. Immediately clean any blood spills according to OSHA regulations with a sodium hypochlorite (bleach) solution.

24. Remove your gloves and wash your hands.

25. Transport the sample in the sealed container.

26. Record the procedure on the chart and on appropriate departmental records, as applicable. *"Chart" the procedure on your laboratory report. Indicate whether the blood sample was obtained and how many attempts were necessary.*

27. Repeat the exercise for brachial artery puncture.

28. Repeat the exercise simulating the use of local anesthetic.
    a. Attach a 25-gauge needle to a syringe.
    b. Using a 2-percent xylocaine solution, verify the medication vial contents.

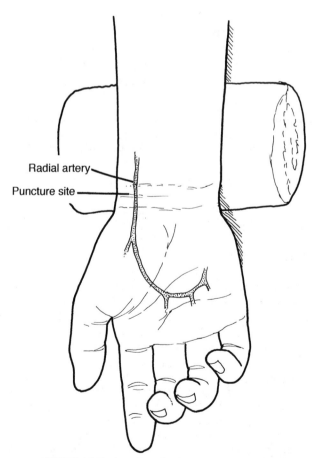

FIGURE 19.7   Location of radial artery puncture.

c. Wipe the rubber stopper of the vial with alcohol.
d. Verify vial contents again and aseptically draw about 0.5 to 1 ml into a syringe.
e. Remove any air bubbles from the syringe.
f. Disinfect the puncture site.
g. Palpate the artery to be punctured.
h. Verify one last time that the syringe was filled with the correct medication.
i. Insert the needle **intradermally** (the tip of the needle should be just below the surface of the skin).
j. Pull back on the barrel of the syringe to ensure that no blood vessel has been punctured.
k. Slowly inject the xylocaine into the skin until a small **wheal** is created.
l. Wait 5 to 10 min before performing arterial puncture.

EXERCISE 19.4 Arterial Line Sampling

EXERCISE 19.4.1 Arterial Line Setup

In unstable or critically ill patients who may require frequent blood gases or continuous blood pressure monitoring, the placement of an arterial line can facilitate sampling and be more comfortable for the patient than frequent arterial punctures.

Identify the components of the arterial line setup shown in Figure 19.8, and *record the corresponding letters on your laboratory report.*

Proximal three-way stopcock
Luer-Lok
Intraflow flush device
Monitor
Pressure tubing
Arterial catheter
Pressure infuser
IV bag with heparinized solution
Transducer
Valve stem

EXERCISE 19.4.2 Arterial Line Sampling

An arterial arm simulator should be used for this procedure. Perform or simulate the following steps:

1. Verify the physician's order. Check for time, special instructions (on or off O_2, special positioning).

2. Scan the chart and note the diagnosis, anticoagulant therapy, oxygen concentration and modality, and ventilator settings.

3. Gather and prepare the required equipment:
   Discard or waste syringe, 5-ml, nonheparinized
   Heparinized syringe, 1, 3, or 5 ml
   Syringe cap
   4 × 4 gauze
   Sterile field or towel
   Alcohol prep pads
   Patient label
   Biohazard transport bag filled with ice and water

4. Wash your hands and apply standard precautions and transmission-based isolation procedures as appropriate.

5. Introduce yourself and your department, and explain the procedure. Confirm the patient's understanding if possible and reassure.

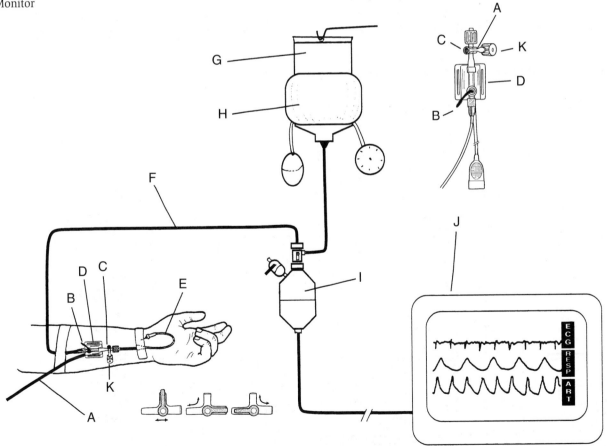

FIGURE 19.8   Identification of arterial line components.

6. Verify the patient's identity by checking the identification band.

7. Verify the oxygen concentration or ventilator settings by double-checking in the room.

8. Heparinize one syringe, or set the barrel on the preheparinized syringe as in Exercise 19.1.

9. Place a sterile field or towel under the sampling site to prevent soiling.

10. Check waveform and pressure readings on the monitor to verify line function.

11. Remove the Luer-Lok cap from the three-way stopcock closest to the catheter insertion site. Place it aseptically on the sterile field or on a sterile gauze pad.

12. Wipe the Luer-Lok of the three-way stopcock with an alcohol prep pad.

13. Attach the nonheparinized discard syringe on the Luer-Lok of the three-way stopcock, and twist to secure (Fig. 19.9).

14. Turn the **valve stem** of the stopcock toward the intraflow flush device (Fig. 19.10).

15. Fill the discard syringe until all flush solution has been removed from the catheter and whole blood begins to appear in the syringe.

16. Turn the valve stem of the stopcock back toward the Luer-Lok, as shown in Figure 19.11, and then remove the discard syringe.

17. Attach the heparinized sample syringe on the Luer-Lok of the three-way stopcock, and twist to secure. Turn the stopcock toward the intraflow flush device (Fig. 19.12). Fill it with the desired amount of blood for the sample.

18. Turn the valve stem of the stopcock back toward the Luer-Lok, and then remove the sample syringe.

19. If a self-venting syringe is used, expel any air from the sample by pushing the barrel toward the plugged needle. Otherwise, remove the needle from the Luer-Lok and expel the air into a gauze pad. Venting devices may also be available. Cap the syringe.

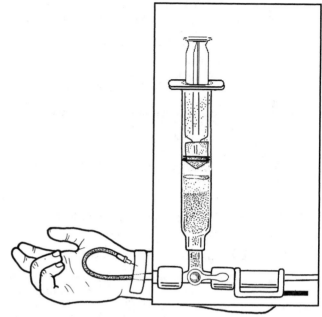

FIGURE 19.10 Draw waste solution into syringe until blood is obtained.

20. Activate the intraflow flush device, and flush the arterial line catheter until no blood is seen in the catheter (Fig. 19.13).

21. Turn the valve stem of the stopcock toward the catheter (off to the patient). Place a 4 × 4 gauze pad under the Luer-Lok, and activate the intraflow flush device to flush the Luer-Lok clean (Fig. 19.14). Wipe the Luer-Lok and cap with alcohol, and then recap the Luer-Lok (Fig. 19.15).

22. Mix blood and heparin in the syringe by rolling the syringe in your palms.

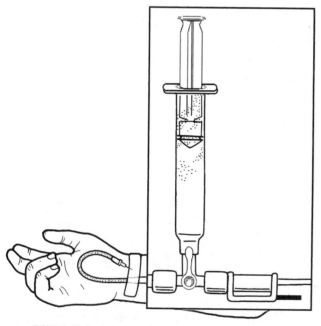

FIGURE 19.9 Attachment of waste syringe to stopcock.

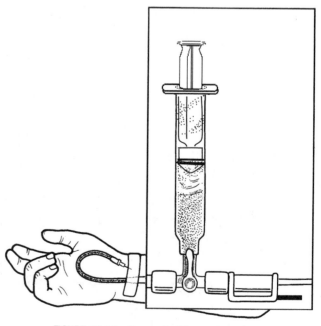

FIGURE 19.11 Removal of the waste syringe.

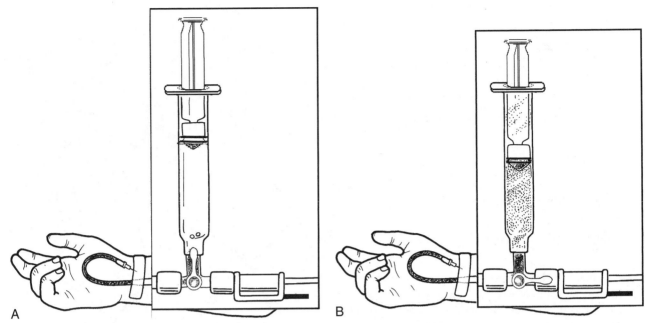

FIGURE 19.12 Attachment of sampling syringe to arterial line. Draw the blood sample into the syringe until the desired amount is obtained.

23. Label the syringe. Place the sample on ice if analysis will be delayed by more than 15 min.[3]

24. Ensure patient safety and comfort.

25. Clean up. Dispose of any infectious waste in the appropriate receptacle. Dispose of the discard syringe in a sharps container. Immediately clean any blood spills according to OSHA regulations with a bleach solution.

26. Fill in the patient information label, charge slip, and other appropriate documentation. In some situations this information may be input directly into a computer system. Include the following information:

    Date
    Time
    Patient name and identification
    Sample site (left or right radial, brachial or femoral line)
    F_IO_2: percent and modality
    Ventilatory status: spontaneous respiratory frequency or ventilator settings, if applicable, including machine tidal volume, machine frequency, mode of ventilation, any spontaneous tidal volume, and frequency noted
    Technician or therapist signature

27. Check waveform and pressure readings to verify line function.

28. Remove your gloves and wash your hands.

29. Transport the sample in a sealed biohazard container.

30. Record the procedure on the chart and on appropriate departmental records as applicable.

EXERCISE 19.5 Capillary Sampling

Capillary sticks may be used in infants and children to approximate pH and PCO_2 values. The sample may be taken from areas with large capillary surface area such as the fingertip, earlobe, or most commonly on the lateral aspect of the heel of the foot in infants only. Values obtained for PO_2 are generally less reliable. For acid-base balance and carbon dioxide tension to be reliable, the heel must be "arterialized" by warming before capillary sampling. The procedure is difficult to simulate in the laboratory setting. Students should identify the equipment needed for capillary heel sampling and review the procedure. Practice of the procedure will be reserved for the clinical setting.

1. Gather the necessary equipment:

    Disposable latex and vinyl gloves, various sizes
    2 × 2 gauze
    Iodophor or alcohol prep pads
    Band-Aids

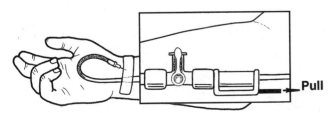

FIGURE 19.13 Flushing the arterial catheter by pulling the intraflow control device.

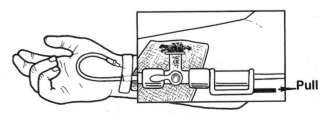

FIGURE 19.14 Flushing the Luer-Lok.

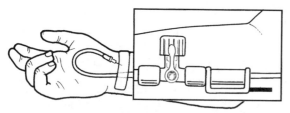

FIGURE 19.15   Recapped flushed line.

Cloth tape
Biohazard bag
Sharps containers
Towels or warm packs
Ice
Heparinized capillary tubes
Rubber capillary tube stoppers
Metal mixing "fleas" and magnet
Lancets
Sample blood gas analysis slips

2. Wash your hands and apply standard precautions and transmission-based isolation procedures as appropriate.

3. Warm the heel area for 5 to 10 min before the procedure to arterialize by wrapping the heel in a warm soak. The heel should turn pink or red before you obtain the sample.

4. Prep the site by vigorously rubbing with Betadine or an alcohol prep pad to disinfect it before puncture.

5. The acceptable locations for heel sticks are shown in Figure 19.16. Quickly puncture the lateral or medial aspect

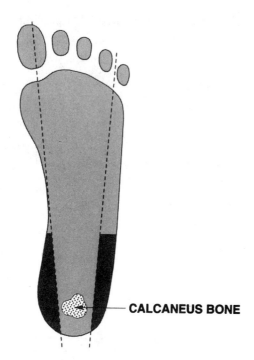

CALCANEUS BONE

■ **PUNCTURE ZONE**

FIGURE 19.16   Acceptable heel puncture sites. (From Strasinger, SK and DiLorenzo, MA: Phlebotomy Workbook for the Multiskilled Health Care Professional. FA Davis, Philadelphia, 1996, p. 268, with permission.)

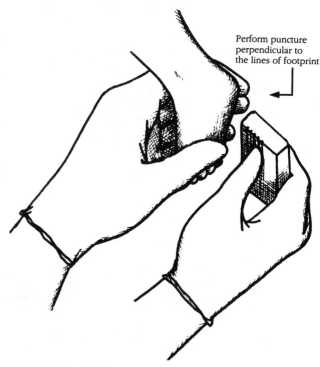

Perform puncture perpendicular to the lines of footprint

FIGURE 19.17   Capillary stick of the heel. (From Strasinger, SK and DiLorenzo, MA: Phlebotomy Workbook for the Multiskilled Health Care Professional. FA Davis, Philadelphia, 1996, p. 270, with permission.)

of the heel with the lancet (Fig. 19.17). The lancet should penetrate approximately 3 mm to ensure adequate blood flow.

6. Do not squeeze the heel. The result will be less accurate because of venous and interstitial fluid contaminating the sample. Blood should be flowing freely.

7. The initial drop of blood should be wiped away with gauze and discarded. Using the heparinized capillary tube, draw the sample into the tube up to the red line, making sure that no air bubbles are introduced.

8. Compress the puncture site with gauze until bleeding has stopped. A Band-Aid may then be applied.

9. Seal one end of the capillary tube with a rubber stopper. Introduce the metal flea into the tube, and place the circular magnet over the tube. Cap the other end of the tube as shown in Figure 19.18.

10. Mix the blood and heparin by sliding the magnet up and down the tube, thereby moving the metal flea.

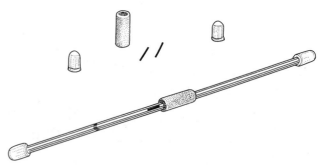

FIGURE 19.18   Capillary tube with metal flea and magnet.

11. Label the sample as in previous exercises.

12. Ice the sample if analysis will be delayed. Place the sample in a biohazard bag or container for transport.

13. Remove your gloves and wash your hands.

14. Make sure to remove the metal flea before analysis of the sample.

References

1. American Association for Respiratory Care: AARC clinical practice guideline: Sampling for arterial blood gas analysis. Respir Care 37:913–917, 1992.

2. Yassin, MS et al: Latex allergy in hospital employees. Ann Allergy 72:245–249, 1994.

3. Shapiro, B et al: Clinical Application of Blood Gases, ed 5. Year Book Medical Publishers, Chicago, 1994.

Related Readings

Eubanks, DH and Bone, RC: Principles and Applications of Cardiorespiratory Care Equipment. Mosby, St Louis, 1994.

Madama, V: Pulmonary Function Testing and Cardiopulmonary Stress Testing. Delmar Publishers, Albany, 1993.

McPherson, S: Respiratory Care Equipment, ed 5. Mosby, St Louis, 1995.

Scanlan, C et al (eds): Egan's Fundamentals of Respiratory Care, ed 6. Mosby, St Louis, 1995.

Shapiro, B et al: Clinical Application of Blood Gases, ed 5. Year Book Medical Publishers, Chicago, 1994.

Wilkins, R, Sheldon, R and Krider, S: Clinical Assessment in Respiratory Care, ed 3. Mosby, St Louis, 1995.

Selected Journal Articles

American Association for Respiratory Care: AARC clinical practice guideline: Sampling for arterial blood gas analysis. Respir Care 37:913–917, 1992.

American Association for Respiratory Care: AARC clinical practice guideline: Capillary blood gas sampling for neonatal and pediatric patients. Respir Care 39:1180–1183, 1994.

Barnes LP: Needle recapping: Do we practice what we preach? MCN Am J Matern Child Nurs 16:331, 1991.

Branson, RD and MacIntyre, N (eds): Blood gas measurements. Respiratory Care Clinics of North America 1:1–162, 1995.

Centers for Disease Control: Guideline for handwashing and hospital environmental control, 1985. U.S. Department of Health and Human Services, Atlanta, 99–1117, pp. 1–20, 1985.

Centers for Disease Control and Prevention: Guidelines for preventing the transmission of *Mycobacterium tuberculosis* in health-care facilities, 1994. U.S. Department of Health and Human Services, Atlanta, 43:RR-13, pp. 33–34.

HIV related infection precautions for personnel providing ABG analysis. Respir Care 34:734–740, 1989.

Liss, H and Payne, C: Stability of blood gases in ice and at room temperature. Chest 103:1120–1122, 1993.

OSHA: Regulations for bloodborne pathogens. Federal Register 31:41–47, 1992.

Shapiro, B: In-vivo monitoring of arterial blood gases and pH. Respir Care 37:165–169, 1992.

Tokars, JI et al: Surveillance of HIV infection and zidovudine use among health care workers after occupational exposure to HIV infected blood. Ann Intern Med 118:913–919, 1993.

Watson, ME: Median nerve damage from brachial artery puncture: A case report. Respir Care 40:1141–1143, 1995.

Yassin, MS et al: Latex allergy in hospital employees. Ann Allergy 72:245–249, 1994.

LABORATORY REPORT

CHAPTER 19: ARTERIAL BLOOD GAS SAMPLING

Name _____ Date _____

Course/Section _____ Instructor _____

Data Collection

EXERCISE 19.1   Preparation of Blood Gas Kit Components

Syringe size used: _____

Needle sizes available: _____

Type of heparin: _____

Needle gauge selected for radial puncture: _____

EXERCISE 19.2   Modified Allen's Test

Allen's test result: _____

EXERCISE 19.3   Performance of Arterial Puncture

Patient label/charge slip information:

_____

_____

_____

_____

Chart the arterial puncture:

_____

_____

_____

_____

EXERCISE 19.4   Arterial Line Sampling

EXERCISE 19.4.1   Arterial Line Setup

A. _____

B. _____

C. _____

D. _____

E. _____

F. _____

G. _____

H. _____

I. _____

J. _____

K. _____

CRITICAL THINKING QUESTIONS

1. Identify three conditions that would require compression of the artery for longer than 10 min during postpuncture care. Identify one condition that would require compression of the artery for less than 5 min.

2. Identify at least four complications of arterial line sampling, and state how each can be prevented.

3. You are performing a modified Allen's test to the right arm on Ms. Gordon, a 22-year-old African American woman. You notice that her fingertips are cold to the touch. After release of the ulnar artery, it takes 12 sec for color to return to the palm. What actions should you take at this time? What are the possible causes of a negative Allen's test in this patient?

4. While performing an arterial puncture on Ms. Gordon, the patient in Critical Thinking Question 3, you encounter the following difficulties. Describe all possible solutions for each problem.
   a. The tip of the needle touches the bedside table before insertion into the patient.

   b. The artery seems to roll away from the needle each time you approach it.

   c. You observe a blood flash in the hub of the needle, and then blood flow stops.

   d. The patient attempts to jerk her arm away as you are inserting the needle.

   e. You have reangled the needle three times and are still unable to get the blood sample.

   f. You notice swelling under the puncture site when you remove the needle.

   g. As you are corking the needle, you puncture your fingertip.

5. Why does the IV bag in an arterial line setup need to be pressurized?

Predicted respiratory flow

$$\% \text{ predicted} = \frac{actual}{predicted} \times 100$$

$$\% \text{ change} = \frac{post + pre}{pre} \times 100$$

6. Identify at least five complications of arterial puncture, and state how each can be prevented.

7. You are attempting to obtain a sample from an arterial line and encounter the following difficulties. Identify the probable cause(s), if applicable, and describe all possible solutions to the problems.
   a. You observe a blood backup halfway between the point of entrance of the catheter into the patient's arm and the sampling port.

   b. You drop the Luer-Lok cap on the floor.

   c. After removing the discard syringe from the Luer-Lok, blood continues to flow onto the bedsheets.

   d. As you are withdrawing the blood sample, the patient is moving her arm and blood is filling the syringe intermittently.

   e. After removal of the sample, you are unable to flush the catheter.

Anticoagulant Therapy

1. Warfarin
2. Heparin
3. Coumadin

high CO_2 produce acidosis
low CO_2 produce alcalosis

PH - 7.35 - 7.45

HCO_3^- 22-26

$B\bar{E}$ - -2 or +2

PaO_2 - 80-100

CO_2 = 35-45

pH
$PaCO_2$ > Ventilation

HCO_3
$B\bar{E}$ > metabolic

PaO_2 → oxygenation

PRODUCT INFORMATION

... of 0.7 days in the median time to complete healing, reduction of 0.7 days in the median time to complete relief. After 4 days of treatment there was a significant increase in both percent of patients with complete healing ... (37% vs. 27%) and percent of patients with complete resolution of pain (60% vs. 49%).

Relief occurred in conjunction with healing of the ulcer. Amlexanox oral paste, 5%, by itself, was not shown to be analgesic medication. The safety and effectiveness of product in immunocompromised individuals has not been assessed.

Cumulative % of Patients with Healed Ulcers

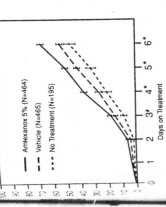

- Amlexanox 5% (N=464)
- Vehicle (N=465)
- No Treatment (N=195)

Days on Treatment

Results for amlexanox, 5%, vs. vehicle are based on three clinical trials. Results for amlexanox, 5%, vs. no treatment are based on ... clinical trials.
* ... was statistically significant superiority of amlexanox, 5%, vs. vehicle and no treatment.
... a ... proves statistically significant superiority of amlexanox, 5%, vs. ... to vehicle ... treatment.
Bars represent Standard Error of the Mean.

INDICATIONS AND USAGE

Amlexanox oral paste, 5%, is indicated for the treatment of aphthous ulcers in people with normal immune systems.

CONTRAINDICATIONS

Amlexanox oral paste, 5%, is contraindicated in patients with known hypersensitivity to amlexanox or other ingredients of the formulation.

PRECAUTIONS

Information for Patients: Wash hands immediately after applying amlexanox oral paste, 5%, directly to ulcers with the finger tips. In the event that a rash or contact mucositis occurs, discontinue ... Apply the paste as soon as possible after noticing the ...

dosing range, reflecting the greater frequency of decreased hepatic, renal, or cardiac function, and of concomitant disease or other drug therapy.

ADVERSE REACTIONS

Adverse reactions considered related or possibly related to amlexanox oral paste, 5%, were not reported by more than 5% of patients. Adverse reactions reported by 1–2% of patients were transient pain, stinging and/or burning at the site of application. Infrequent (< 1%) adverse reactions in the clinical studies were contact mucositis, nausea, and diarrhea.

OVERDOSAGE

There are no reports of human ingestion overdosage. Ingestion of a full tube of 5 grams of paste would result in systemic exposure well below the maximum nontoxic dose of amlexanox in animals. Gastrointestinal upset such as diarrhea and vomiting could result from an overdose.

DOSAGE AND ADMINISTRATION

The paste should be applied as soon as possible after noticing the symptoms of an aphthous ulcer and should be used four times daily, preferably following oral hygiene after breakfast, lunch, dinner, and at bedtime. Squeeze a dab of paste approximately 1/4 inch (0.5 cm) onto a finger tip. With gentle pressure, dab the paste onto each ulcer in the mouth. Use of the medication should be continued until the ulcer heals. If significant healing or pain reduction has not occurred in 10 days, consult your dentist or physician.

HOW SUPPLIED

Amlexanox oral paste, 5%, is supplied in 5 gram tubes (NDC 10158-059-01). Amlexanox oral paste, 5%, should be stored at controlled room temperature, 15°–30°C (59°–86°F).

Manufactured for:

Oral Health Care Division
Block Drug Company, Inc.
Jersey City, NJ 07302

By Reedco, Inc.
Humacao, Puerto Rico 00791

Aphthasol® is a registered trademark of Block Drug Company, Inc.
© 1999 Block Drug Company, Inc.
March 1999   APH-PI-01

Boehringer Ingelheim Pharmaceuticals, Inc.
A subsidiary of Boehringer Ingelheim Corporation
900 RIDGEBURY ROAD
POST OFFICE BOX 368
RIDGEFIELD, CT 06877-0368

BOEHRINGER INGELHEIM/787

Chemically, Alupent is 1-(3,5 dihydroxyphenyl)-2-isopropylaminoethanol sulfate, a white crystalline, racemic mixture of two optically active isomers.

metaproterenol sulfate (Alupent)
$(C_{11}H_{17}NO_3)_2 \cdot H_2SO_4$
Mol. Wt: 520.59

CLINICAL PHARMACOLOGY

Alupent® (metaproterenol sulfate USP) is a potent beta-adrenergic stimulator. Alupent Inhalation Solutions have a rapid onset of action. It is postulated that beta-adrenergic stimulants produce many of their pharmacological effects by activation of adenyl cyclase, the enzyme which catalyzes the conversion of adenosine triphosphate to cyclic adenosine monophosphate.

In vitro studies and in vivo pharmacologic studies have demonstrated that Alupent® (metaproterenol sulfate USP) has a preferential effect on beta-2 adrenergic receptors compared with isoproterenol. While it is recognized that beta-2 adrenergic receptors are the predominant receptors in bronchial smooth muscle, recent data indicate that there is a population of beta-2 receptors in the human heart existing in a concentration between 10–50%. The precise function of these, however, is not yet established (see WARNINGS section).

The pharmacologic effects of beta adrenergic agonist drugs, including Alupent, are at least in part attributable to stimulation through beta adrenergic receptors of intracellular adenyl cyclase, the enzyme which catalyzes the conversion of adenosine triphosphate (ATP) to cyclic-3',5'-adenosine monophosphate (c-AMP). Increased c-AMP levels are associated with relaxation of bronchial smooth muscle and inhibition of release of mediators of immediate hypersensitivity from cells, especially from mast cells.

Pharmacokinetics: Absorption, biotransformation and excretion studies in humans following administration by inhalation have shown that approximately 3 percent of the actuated dose is absorbed intact through the lungs.

Absorption, biotransformation and excretion studies in humans following oral administration indicate that an average of less than 10% of the drug is absorbed intact; it is not metabolized by catechol-O-methyl-transferase nor converted to glucuronide conjugates but is excreted primarily as the sulfate conjugate formed in the gut.

When administered orally or by inhalation, Alupent decreases reversible bronchospasm. Pulmonary function tests performed concomitantly usually show improvement follow-

formed with pulmonary function monitoring. The duration of effect of a single dose of Alupent Tablets 20 mg or Alupent Syrup (that is, the period of time during which there is a 15% or greater increase in FEV_1) was up to 4 hours. Controlled single- and multiple-dose studies have been performed with pulmonary function monitoring. The duration of effect of a single dose of two to three inhalations of Alupent Inhalation Aerosol (that is, the period of time during which there is a 20% or greater increase in FEV_1) has varied from 1 to 5 hours.

In repetitive-dosing studies (up to q.i.d.) the duration of effect for a similar dose of Alupent Inhalation Aerosol has ranged from about 1 to 2.5 hours. Present studies are inadequate to explain the divergence in duration of the FEV_1 effect between single- and repetitive-dosing studies, respectively.

Following controlled single dose studies with Alupent Inhalation Solution by an intermittent positive pressure breathing apparatus (IPPB) and by hand-bulb nebulizers, significant improvement (15% or greater increase in FEV_1) occurred within 5 to 30 minutes and persisted for periods varying from 2 to 6 hours.

In these studies, the longer duration of effect occurred in the studies in which the drug was administered by IPPB, i.e., 6 hours, versus 2 to 3 hours when administered by hand-bulb nebulizer. In these studies, the doses used were 0.3 ml by IPPB and 10 inhalations by hand-bulb nebulizer.

In controlled repetitive-dosing studies with Alupent Inhalation Solution by IPPB and by hand-bulb nebulizer the onset of effect occurred within 5 to 30 minutes and duration ranged from 4 to 6 hours. In these studies, the doses used were 0.3 ml b.i.d. or t.i.d. when given by IPPB, and 10 inhalations q.i.d. (no more often than q4h) when given by hand-bulb nebulizer. As in the single dose studies, effectiveness was measured as a sustained increase in FEV_1 of 15% or greater. In these repetitive-dosing studies there was no apparent difference in duration between the two methods of delivery.

Continued on next page

ALUPENT

[al 'u-pent]

(metaproterenol sulfate USP)

Bronchodilator		
Tablets 10 mg		BI-CODE 74
Tablets 20 mg		BI-CODE 72
Inhalation Aerosol 10 ml		BI-CODE 70
Syrup 10 mg/5 ml		BI-CODE 73
Inhalation Solution 5%		BI-CODE 71
Inhalation Solution	0.6%	BI-CODE 69
Unit-dose Vials	0.4%	BI-CODE 78

Prescribing Information

DESCRIPTION

Alupent® (metaproterenol sulfate USP) Inhalation Aerosol is a bronchodilator administered by oral inhalation. The Alupent Inhalation Aerosol containing 150 mg of metaproterenol sulfate as micronized powder is sufficient medication for 200 inhalations. Each metered dose delivers through the mouthpiece 0.65 mg of metaproterenol sulfate (each ml contains 15 mg). The inert ingredients are dichlorodifluoromethane, dichlorotetrafluoroethane and trichloromonofluoromethane as propellants, and sorbitan trioleate.

Alupent Inhalation Solution is administered by oral inhalation with the aid of a nebulizer or an intermittent positive pressure breathing apparatus (IPPB). It contains Alupent 5% in a pH-adjusted aqueous solution containing benzalkonium chloride and edetate disodium as preservatives.

Alupent Inhalation Solution Unit-dose Vial is administered by oral inhalation with the aid of an IPPB. It contains Alupent 0.4% or 0.6% in a sterile pH-adjusted aqueous solution with edetate disodium and sodium chloride.

Alupent Syrup is an oral bronchodilator. Each teaspoonful (5 ml) of syrup contains 10 mg of metaproterenol sulfate. The inactive ingredients are edetate disodium, FD&C Red No. 40, hydroxyethylcellulose, imitation black cherry flavor, methylparaben, propylparaben, saccharin, sorbitol solution.

Alupent Tablets are administered orally. Each tablet contains metaproterenol sulfate 10 mg or 20 mg. The inactive ingredients are colloidal silicon dioxide, corn starch, dibasic calcium phosphate, lactose, magnesium stearate.

... finger tip.

... dab the Aphthasol on to the ulcer. Repeat the procedure ... have more than one ulcer.

... your hands when you are done applying Aphthasol. ... eyes promptly if they should come in contact with ...

... the paste until the ulcer heals. If significant healing ... relief has not occurred in 10 days, consult your dentist/physician.

... out of the reach of children.

Mutagenesis, Impairment of Fertility: ... was not carcinogenic when administered ... rats for two years and to mice for 18 months. In ... and in vitro (mouse micronucleus) mutagenicity ... of amlexanox were negative. Amlexanox at doses up to ... times the projected human daily dose, on a ... respectively, the projected human daily ... basis did not significantly affect fertility or general ... performance in rats.

Category B: Teratology studies were performed ... rabbits at doses up to two hundred and six ... times the projected human daily ... on a mg/m² basis. No adverse fetal effects were observed ... up to two hundred times the projected human ... on a mg/m² basis, amlexanox did not have ... effect on peri- and postnatal development of rat ... There are no adequate and well-controlled studies ... Because animal reproduction studies ... predictive of human response, this drug ... during pregnancy only if clearly needed.

... Amlexanox was found in the milk of lac... therefore, caution should be exercised when administered ... to a nursing woman.

... Safety and effectiveness of amlexanox oral ... paste, 5%, to a nursing woman.

... in pediatric patients have not been established. ... Clinical studies of Aphthasol did not include ... of subjects aged 65 and over to determine ... they respond differently from younger subjects. ... clinical experience has not identified ... between the elderly and younger patient ... dose selection for an elderly patient ... starting at the low end of the

2. Scans chart for anticoagulant therapy

Oxygen conc. Ventilator settings & allergies y using local anesthetic

3. Select, necessary equipment

4. Wash & applies stort. prec. + Isol.

5. Ident. pt. sel. a dept.

6. Explain purpose of proc. & confirms pt. understanding.

7. Palpate pulse on 2 arms to determine best puncture site w/o non-dominant hand.

8. Performs Allen's test, if Negative repeats on other arm.

9. Prepares puncture site by rubbing in circular motion for at least 30 sec.
   disinfect gloved finger used for palp.

10. administer anesthetic if ordered.

Never
puncti site
wher 20 min.

[boxed notes on left:]
Includes data:
Sample time
pt name
w/l
F₁O₂

allow pt to talk.
Vent. setting.
tech or therap.
signature
physician order

puncture site

PROCEDURAL COMPETENCY EVALUATION

Name _____   Date _____

Arterial Puncture

Setting: ☐ Lab ☐ Clinical   Evaluator: ☐ Peer ☐ Instructor

Conditions (describe): _____

_____

Equipment Used

_____

_____

	S A T I S F A C T O R Y	U N S A T I S F A C T O R Y	N O T O B S E R V E D	N O T A P P L I C A B L E
Equipment and Patient Preparation				
NOTE: *Never recap needle.* Any needle stick *must* be reported.				
1. Verifies, interprets, and evaluates physician's order or protocol *Warfarin / Heparin / Coumadin*	☐	☐	☐	☐
2. Scans the chart for diagnosis, anticoagulant therapy, oxygen concentration, ventilator settings, and allergies if using local anesthetic	☐	☐	☐	☐
3. Selects, gathers, and assembles the necessary equipment	☐	☐	☐	☐
4. Washes hands and applies standard precautions and transmission-based isolation procedures as appropriate	☐	☐	☐	☐
5. Identifies patient, introduces self and department	☐	☐	☐	☐
6. Explains purpose of the procedure and confirms patient understanding	☐	☐	☐	☐
Assessment and Implementation				
7. Palpates pulse on both arms to determine best puncture site; uses nondominant hand, if possible	☐	☐	☐	☐
8. Performs modified Allen's test; if negative, repeats on other arm	☐	☐	☐	☐
9. Prepares the puncture site by rubbing vigorously in circular motion away from puncture site with an antiseptic solution for at least 30 sec; disinfects gloved fingers used for palpation	☐	☐	☐	☐
10. Administers anesthetic if ordered	☐	☐	☐	☐
11. Repalpates and positions puncture site by extending wrist; places self and patient in comfortable position	☐	☐	☐	☐
12. Correctly performs the puncture:				
a. Sets the plunger on a self-venting syringe to obtain the desired amount of blood (enough for repeated analysis)	☐	☐	☐	☐
b. Holds the syringe at 45-degree angle, needle bevel up	☐	☐	☐	☐
c. Slowly inserts needle between second and third skin fold on wrist; safely reangles needle if necessary	☐	☐	☐	☐
13. Obtains sample; removes needle and immediately applies pressure with sterile gauze	☐	☐	☐	☐
14. Corks needle with rubber stopper or automatic capping device	☐	☐	☐	☐
15. Maintains pressure on the puncture site for a minimum of 3 to 5 min; 10 min or longer if patient has bleeding disorder or uses anticoagulants	☐	☐	☐	☐
16. Checks puncture site for bleeding, swelling, discoloration, return of pulse proximal and distal to puncture site; ensures patient safety and comfort	☐	☐	☐	☐
17. Expels any air from sample following OSHA guidelines, using gauze pad or automatic venting cap	☐	☐	☐	☐

	S A T I S F A C T O R Y	U N S A T I S F A C T O R Y	N O T O B S E R V E D	N O T A P P L I C A B L E

Follow-up

18. Labels sample and charge ticket appropriately with date, time, patient identification, F_IO_2, puncture site, Allen's test results, ventilatory settings (if applicable), and technician or therapist signature; places in iced, sealed container for transport

	☐	☐	☐	☐

19. Cleans any blood spills with sodium hypochlorite solution

	☐	☐	☐	☐

20. Disposes of infectious waste and washes hands; changes gloves before transport of sample

	☐	☐	☐	☐

21. Records pertinent data in chart and departmental records

	☐	☐	☐	☐

22. Notifies appropriate personnel and makes any necessary recommendations or modifications to the respiratory care plan

	☐	☐	☐	☐

23. Rechecks puncture site after 20 min if pressure bandage used

	☐	☐	☐	☐

_____
Signature of Evaluator

_____
Signature of Student

PERFORMANCE RATING SCALE

5 EXCELLENT—FAR EXCEEDS EXPECTED LEVEL, FLAWLESS PERFORMANCE
4 ABOVE AVERAGE—NO PROMPTING REQUIRED, ABLE TO SELF-CORRECT
3 AVERAGE—THE MINIMUM COMPETENCY LEVEL, NO CRITICAL ERRORS
2 IMPROVEMENT NEEDED—PROBLEM AREAS EXIST; CRITICAL ERRORS, CORRECTIONS NEEDED
1 POOR AND UNACCEPTABLE PERFORMANCE—GROSS INACCURACIES, POTENTIALLY HARMFUL

PERFORMANCE CRITERIA	SCALE				
1. DISPLAYS KNOWLEDGE OF ESSENTIAL CONCEPTS	5	4	3	2	1
2. DEMONSTRATES THE RELATIONSHIP BETWEEN THEORY AND CLINICAL PRACTICE	5	4	3	2	1
3. FOLLOWS DIRECTIONS, EXHIBITS SOUND JUDGMENT, AND DEMONSTRATES ATTENTION TO SAFETY AND DETAIL	5	4	3	2	1
4. EXHIBITS THE REQUIRED MANUAL DEXTERITY	5	4	3	2	1
5. PERFORMS PROCEDURE IN A REASONABLE TIME FRAME	5	4	3	2	1
6. MAINTAINS STERILE OR ASEPTIC TECHNIQUE	5	4	3	2	1
7. INITIATES UNAMBIGUOUS GOAL-DIRECTED COMMUNICATION	5	4	3	2	1
8. PROVIDES FOR ADEQUATE CARE AND MAINTENANCE OF EQUIPMENT AND SUPPLIES	5	4	3	2	1
9. EXHIBITS COURTEOUS AND PLEASANT DEMEANOR	5	4	3	2	1
10. MAINTAINS CONCISE AND ACCURATE RECORDS	5	4	3	2	1

ADDITIONAL COMMENTS: INCLUDE ERRORS OF OMISSION OR COMMISSION, COMMUNICATIVE SKILLS, AND EFFECTIVENESS OF PATIENT INTERACTION:

SUMMARY PERFORMANCE EVALUATION AND RECOMMENDATIONS

SATISFACTORY PERFORMANCE—Performed without error or prompting, or able to self-correct, no critical errors.

_____ LABORATORY EVALUATION. SKILLS MAY BE APPLIED/OBSERVED IN THE CLINICAL SETTING.

_____ CLINICAL EVALUATION. STUDENT READY FOR MINIMALLY SUPERVISED APPLICATION AND REFINEMENT.

UNSATISFACTORY PERFORMANCE—Prompting required; performed with critical errors, potentially harmful.

_____ STUDENT REQUIRES ADDITIONAL LABORATORY PRACTICE.

_____ STUDENT REQUIRES ADDITIONAL SUPERVISED CLINICAL PRACTICE.

SIGNATURES

STUDENT: _____   EVALUATOR: _____

DATE: _____   DATE: _____

PROCEDURAL COMPETENCY EVALUATION

Name _____ Date _____

Arterial Line Sampling

Setting: ☐ Lab ☐ Clinical   Evaluator: ☐ Peer ☐ Instructor

Conditions (describe): _____

_____

Equipment Used

_____

_____

	SATISFACTORY	UNSATISFACTORY	NOT OBSERVED	NOT APPLICABLE
Equipment and Patient Preparation				
1. Verifies, interprets, and evaluates physician's order or protocol and F_IO_2 and ventilator settings	☐	☐	☐	☐
2. Scans chart for any other pertinent data and notes, including diagnosis	☐	☐	☐	☐
3. Selects, gathers, and assembles the necessary equipment	☐	☐	☐	☐
4. Washes hands and applies standard precautions and transmission-based isolation procedures as appropriate	☐	☐	☐	☐
5. Identifies patient, introduces self and department	☐	☐	☐	☐
6. Explains purpose of the procedure and confirms patient understanding	☐	☐	☐	☐
Assessment and Implementation				
7. Observes cardiac monitor for shape and height of arterial waveform	☐	☐	☐	☐
8. Identifies line/intraflow device	☐	☐	☐	☐
9. Removes cap from stopcock hub; aspirates flush into waste syringe				
a. Wipes hub with alcohol	☐	☐	☐	☐
b. Places cap aseptically on drape or gauze	☐	☐	☐	☐
c. Attaches unheparinized syringe and turns stopcock off to intraflow	☐	☐	☐	☐
d. Places gauze under the stopcock while aspirating approximately until flush solution removed and whole blood appears in syringe from the patient line	☐	☐	☐	☐
e. Turns stopcock off to syringe	☐	☐	☐	☐
f. Removes syringe and discards in sharps container	☐	☐	☐	☐
10. Aspirates sample				
a. Sets plunger of self-venting syringe for desired amount of blood (enough for repeated analysis)	☐	☐	☐	☐
b. Secures heparinized syringe on Luer-Lok hub	☐	☐	☐	☐
c. Reopens stopcock; collects sample	☐	☐	☐	☐
d. Turns stopcock off to syringe and removes syringe	☐	☐	☐	☐
11. Caps syringe, removes air bubbles following OSHA guidelines	☐	☐	☐	☐
12. Labels sample, places in sealed container	☐	☐	☐	☐
13. Maintains line: using intraflo, with stopcock turned toward Luer-Lok, flushes the line to the patient for one pass of the screen	☐	☐	☐	☐

	SATISFACTORY	UNSATISFACTORY	NOT OBSERVED	NOT APPLICABLE
14. Turns stopcock off to the patient; places gauze under hub; pulls the intraflow to flush the stopcock hub	☐	☐	☐	☐
15. Turns the stopcock off to the Luer-Lok; wipes hub with alcohol; replaces cap on hub; checks waveform	☐	☐	☐	☐

Follow-up

16. Ensures patient comfort and safety	☐	☐	☐	☐
17. Maintains/processes equipment: discards all disposables; disposes of sharps in puncture-proof container; sends blood to be analyzed after filling in date, time, F_IO_2, site, ventilation, setting on charge tickets, technician signature	☐	☐	☐	☐
18. Disposes of infectious waste and washes hands	☐	☐	☐	☐
19. Records pertinent data in chart and departmental records	☐	☐	☐	☐
20. Notifies appropriate personnel and makes any necessary recommendations or modifications to the patient care plan	☐	☐	☐	☐

_____
Signature of Evaluator

_____
Signature of Student

PERFORMANCE RATING SCALE

5 EXCELLENT—FAR EXCEEDS EXPECTED LEVEL, FLAWLESS PERFORMANCE
4 ABOVE AVERAGE—NO PROMPTING REQUIRED, ABLE TO SELF-CORRECT
3 AVERAGE—THE MINIMUM COMPETENCY LEVEL, NO CRITICAL ERRORS
2 IMPROVEMENT NEEDED—PROBLEM AREAS EXIST; CRITICAL ERRORS, CORRECTIONS NEEDED
1 POOR AND UNACCEPTABLE PERFORMANCE—GROSS INACCURACIES, POTENTIALLY HARMFUL

PERFORMANCE CRITERIA		SCALE			
1. DISPLAYS KNOWLEDGE OF ESSENTIAL CONCEPTS	5	4	3	2	1
2. DEMONSTRATES THE RELATIONSHIP BETWEEN THEORY AND CLINICAL PRACTICE	5	4	3	2	1
3. FOLLOWS DIRECTIONS, EXHIBITS SOUND JUDGMENT, AND DEMONSTRATES ATTENTION TO SAFETY AND DETAIL	5	4	3	2	1
4. EXHIBITS THE REQUIRED MANUAL DEXTERITY	5	4	3	2	1
5. PERFORMS PROCEDURE IN A REASONABLE TIME FRAME	5	4	3	2	1
6. MAINTAINS STERILE OR ASEPTIC TECHNIQUE	5	4	3	2	1
7. INITIATES UNAMBIGUOUS GOAL-DIRECTED COMMUNICATION	5	4	3	2	1
8. PROVIDES FOR ADEQUATE CARE AND MAINTENANCE OF EQUIPMENT AND SUPPLIES	5	4	3	2	1
9. EXHIBITS COURTEOUS AND PLEASANT DEMEANOR	5	4	3	2	1
10. MAINTAINS CONCISE AND ACCURATE RECORDS	5	4	3	2	1

ADDITIONAL COMMENTS: INCLUDE ERRORS OF OMISSION OR COMMISSION, COMMUNICATIVE SKILLS, AND EFFECTIVENESS OF PATIENT INTERACTION:

SUMMARY PERFORMANCE EVALUATION AND RECOMMENDATIONS

SATISFACTORY PERFORMANCE—Performed without error or prompting, or able to self-correct, no critical errors.

_____ LABORATORY EVALUATION. SKILLS MAY BE APPLIED/OBSERVED IN THE CLINICAL SETTING.

_____ CLINICAL EVALUATION. STUDENT READY FOR MINIMALLY SUPERVISED APPLICATION AND REFINEMENT.

UNSATISFACTORY PERFORMANCE—Prompting required; performed with critical errors, potentially harmful.

_____ STUDENT REQUIRES ADDITIONAL LABORATORY PRACTICE.

_____ STUDENT REQUIRES ADDITIONAL SUPERVISED CLINICAL PRACTICE.

SIGNATURES

STUDENT: _____   EVALUATOR: _____

DATE: _____   DATE: _____

Noninvasive Blood Gas Monitoring

INTRODUCTION

Monitoring devices are used to observe or record physiologic phenomena and to provide information on an ongoing basis without the need for removal of body fluids or tissue.[1] The use of noninvasive technology to monitor blood gases and trends has increased exponentially over the last decade. Devices such as pulse oximeters, **transcutaneous** monitors, and capnometers and capnographs can provide useful data for clinical decisions with less risk to the practitioner from infectious hazards and fewer risks to the patient than invasive techniques.

However, the data provided do not replace invasive blood gas measurements. A baseline arterial blood gas should still be obtained to correlate with the noninvasive data. Noninvasive devices have significant limitations that must be thoroughly understood. False-negative or false-positive findings may lead to inappropriate treatment of the patient.[2] When used appropriately, noninvasive monitors can be cost-effective and time-saving additions to patient ... t.

... e communication skills needed to explain noninvasive monitoring procedures to the ... t and confirm understanding.

... infection control guidelines and standards associated with equipment and proce- ... according to OSHA regulations and CDC guidelines.

... assemble, operate, and maintain the appropriate monitoring device for a given ... l situation.

... and correct malfunctions of noninvasive monitoring equipment.

... fy limitations of noninvasive monitoring devices and differentiate false-negative and ... ositive readings from reliable clinical data.

... ret data obtained from noninvasive monitors and correlate the results to the pa- ... condition.

... ce medical charting of noninvasive monitoring procedures and data obtained.

... ce verbal communication skills needed to report results of data collection and make ... mendations or modifications to the patient care plan.

KEY TERMS	erythema	oxidation	tourniquet
capnography	hydrolysis	phlebotomy	transcutaneous
capnometry	infrared absorption	sensor	transducer
colorimetric	monitoring	spectrophotometry	

EQUIPMENT REQUIRED

- Pulse oximeter
- Finger Phantoms (pulse oximeter accuracy-checking devices)
- Disposable and nondisposable oximeter probes
- Nail polish: red, black, and green
- Nail polish remover
- Cotton balls
- 4 × 4 gauze
- Oxygen gas source and regulator
- Nonrebreathing masks

- Bucket or large basin
- Ice water
- Elastic **phlebotomy tourniquet** or blood pressure cuff
- Barometer (mercury or aneroid)
- Capnograph
- Mainstream or sidestream **sensor** and connectors
- Calibration gas source for capnograph
- Disposable **colorimetric** capnometer (Easy Cap)
- Disposable cannula probe
- Alcohol prep pads
- Intubated airway management trainer
- Swivel ventilator adaptor and 50-ml corrugated tubing

- Transcutaneous oxygen/carbon dioxide monitor
- Zero solution
- Transcutaneous electrodes
- Calibration gas source for transcutaneous monitor
- Adhesive tape
- Intubated airway management trainer

⬤ EXERCISES

EXERCISE 20.1 Pulse Oximetry

EXERCISE 20.1.1 Measurement of Saturation and Pulse

1. Gather the necessary equipment:
   Pulse oximeter
   Probe
   Electrical power cord
   Alcohol prep pads
   Finger Phantoms (pulse oximeter accuracy-checking devices)

2. Visually inspect the power cord (if applicable) and probe cable for any frayed or exposed wires.

3. Plug the power cord into a three-prong electrical outlet, if applicable. If a battery-operated oximeter is used, continuous monitoring could run down the battery and render the unit inoperative.

4. Determine the accuracy of the pulse oximeter by using Finger Phantom pulse oximeter accuracy-checking devices, if available, as shown in Figure 20.1. These come preset with three levels of saturation (97 percent, 90 percent, and 80 percent). Place the Finger Phantom in the holder, and insert it into the pulse oximeter probe. *Record the saturation reading on the pulse oximeter for each level on your laboratory report.*

5. Using your laboratory partner as the patient, introduce yourself to your patient, explain the procedure, and confirm understanding.

6. With the patient seated comfortably, measure the patient's pulse rate manually. *Record it on your laboratory report.*

7. Select a site for the probe application. Clean it with an alcohol prep pad. Possible application sites are shown in Figure 20.2.

8. Turn on the oximeter.

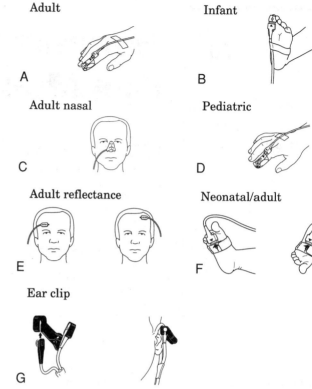

FIGURE 20.2 Oximeter probe application sites. (Reprinted by permission of Nellcor Puritan Bennett, Pleasanton, CA.)

9. Disinfect the probe if a nondisposable probe is used. Attach the probe to the selected site. If a digit is selected, place the probe so that the light source is over the nail bed as shown in Figure 20.3.

10. Measure the time required for equilibration, and *record it on your laboratory report.*

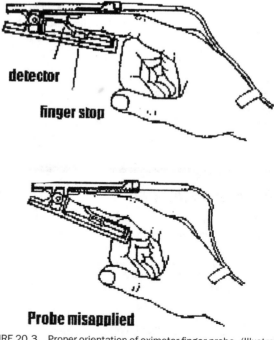

FIGURE 20.3 Proper orientation of oximeter finger probe. (Illustration courtesy of Ohmeda, Inc., Louisville, CO.)

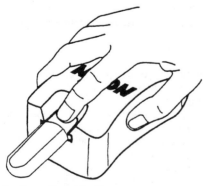

FIGURE 20.1 Finger Phantoms® pulse oximeter accuracy checking device. (Courtesy of Nonin Medical, Inc., Plymouth, MN.)

11. (
12.
13.
14.
15.
16.
results obtained and explain what they mean.

17. Using your laboratory partner as the physician, report the results obtained and make any necessary recommendations or modifications to the patient care plan.

EXERCISE 20.1.2 Effect of Nail Polish on Saturation

1. Polish three fingernails, each with two coats of each of the following colors:
   Black
   Red
   Green
2. Allow the nail polish to dry thoroughly.
3. Using the procedure outlined in Exercise 20.1.1, *record the manual pulse, oximeter pulse, and saturation level for each color on your laboratory report.*
4. Remove and disinfect the probe.
5. Remove the nail polish if desired.

EXERCISE 20.1.3 Effects of Perfusion Changes on Pulse Oximetry

Before performing these exercises, perform a modified Allen's test, as performed in Chapter 19, on your laboratory partner. *Note the result on your laboratory report.*

1. Place ice water in a basin. Soak your hand in the ice water for several minutes.
2. Using the procedure outlined in Exercise 20.1.1, *record which hand was used, the manual pulse, oximeter pulse, and saturation level obtained on your laboratory report.*
3. Using the opposite hand from that used in step 2, place an elastic phlebotomy tourniquet or blood pressure cuff snugly around the biceps of the upper arm. If a cuff is used, inflate the bladder until a radial pulse cannot be felt.
4. Using the procedure outlined in Exercise 20.1.1, *record which hand was used, the manual pulse, oximeter pulse, and saturation level obtained on your laboratory report.*
5. Deflate the cuff or remove the elastic phlebotomy tourniquet as soon as you complete the measurements.
6. Remove and disinfect the probe.

EXERCISE 20.1.4 Metabolic Effects on Pulse Oximetry

1. With the pulse oximeter probe attached, hold your breath as long as possible. *Record the time of the breath hold, manual pulse, oximeter pulse, and saturation level obtained on your laboratory report.*
2. Apply oxygen via a nonrebreathing mask for 5 to 10 min. *Record the manual pulse, oximeter pulse, and saturation level obtained on your laboratory report.*

3. Remove the oxygen mask. Run in place for several minutes. *Record the time of the exercise, manual pulse, oximeter pulse, and saturation level obtained on your laboratory report.*
4. Remove and disinfect the probe.

EXERCISE 20.2 Capnography

EXERCISE 20.2.1 Disposable Capnometer (Easy Cap)™

1. Obtain a disposable colorimetric capnometer and remove it from the wrapper.
2. Observe the face of the capnometer and note the ranges indicated, as shown in Figure 20.4. *Record the color of the capnometer on your laboratory report.*
3. Have your laboratory partner place the adaptor in his or her mouth and breathe normally through the device. Note the change in color. *Record the color changes and the range observed on your laboratory report.*
4. Identify the amount of deadspace of the device. *Record on your laboratory report.*

EXERCISE 20.2.2 Continuous Capnographic Monitoring

1. Obtain the manual for the specific capnograph available in your laboratory.
2. Follow the instructions for the setup and calibration of the device. This usually requires a zero-point calibration on room air and a high-point (slope) calibration gas of 5-percent carbon dioxide (CO_2). The calibration is usually performed every 12 to 24 hours, and the accuracy should be within 12 percent or 4 mm Hg.[3] *Record the following on your laboratory report:*
   Barometric pressure
   Percent CO_2 used
   Calculation of slope calibration point (show your work!)

   Adjust the readings to the calibration points calculated.
3. Note the location of the sensor placement relative to the patient's airway. Is this a mainstream or sidestream sampling system? Examples of these two types of setups

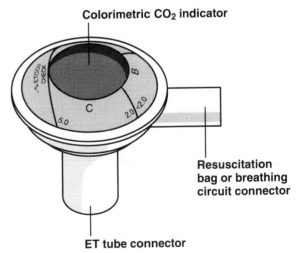

Colorimetric CO₂ indicator

Resuscitation bag or breathing circuit connector

ET tube connector

FIGURE 20.4 Colorimetric capnometer. (Reprinted by permission of Nellcor Puritan Bennett, Pleasanton, CA.)

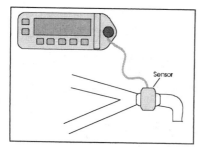

FIGURE 20.5 Mainstream capnography. (Courtesy of Novametrix Medical Systems Inc., Wallingford, CT.)

are shown in Figures 20.5 and 20.6. *Record your answer on your laboratory report.*

4. Attach a cannula sensing device to the capnograph (Fig. 20.7).

5. Using your laboratory partner as the patient, explain the procedure and confirm understanding.

6. Place the cannula on your patient.

7. Instruct the patient to breathe normally through the nose. Observe the time required for the reading to stabilize. If the device has printer capabilities, *obtain a capnogram and attach it to your laboratory report.* If the unit does not have a printer, *observe the shape of the capnograph wave and draw a facsimile of the observed tracing on your laboratory report.*

8. Instruct your partner to breathe through the mouth. Observe the reading, and *record any changes in the reading on your laboratory report.*

9. Instruct your partner to breathe slowly and shallowly. *Obtain a capnogram and attach it to your laboratory report.* If the unit does not have a printer, *observe the shape of the capnograph wave and draw a facsimile of the observed tracing on your laboratory report.*

10. Instruct your partner to breathe quickly and deeply. *Obtain a capnogram and attach it to your laboratory report.* If the unit does not have a printer, *observe the shape of the capnograph wave and draw a facsimile of the observed tracing on your laboratory report.*

11. Instruct your partner to hold his or her breath. Record the length of the breath hold and the CO_2 level once the breath is released. *Obtain a capnogram and attach it to your laboratory report.* If the unit does not have a printer, *observe the shape of the capnograph wave and draw a facsimile of the observed tracing on your laboratory report.*

12. Dispose of the cannula in the proper receptacle.

13. Set up the device on an intubated mannequin (Fig. 20.8).

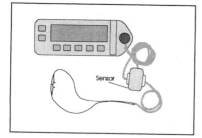

FIGURE 20.6 Sidestream capnography. (Courtesy of Novametrix Medical Systems Inc., Wallingford, CT.)

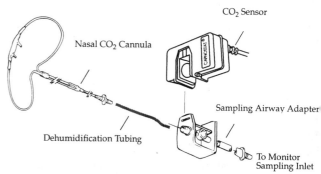

FIGURE 20.7 Cannula for capnography monitoring electrodes. (Courtesy of Novametrix Medical Systems Inc., Wallingford, CT.)

EXERCISE 20.3 Transcutaneous Monitors

1. Obtain a transcutaneous monitor and electrodes (Fig. 20.9).

2. Read the manual and determine whether the monitor is a $P_{TC}CO_2$, $P_{TC}O_2$, or combined unit. *Record the type of unit on your laboratory report.*

3. Following the manufacturer's instructions, calibrate the unit using the appropriate zero solution and slope gas.

4. Select an electrode site that is away from flat, boney areas, large veins, or thick skin. Possible site selections are shown in Figure 20.10.

5. Cleanse the selected site with an alcohol prep pad and dry it.

6. Using your laboratory partner as the patient, explain the procedure and confirm understanding.

7. Attach the electrode as directed in the manual. *Record the location on your laboratory report.*

8. Adjust the temperature to 44 to 45°C.

9. Observe the length of time required for equilibration.

10. *Record the $P_{TC}CO_2$ and $P_{TC}O_2$ readings on your laboratory report.*

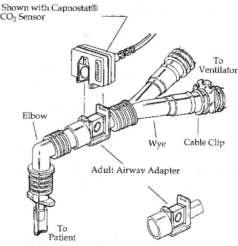

FIGURE 20.8 Application of a capnograph sensor to an artificial airway. (Reprinted by permission of Nellcor Puritan Bennett, Pleasanton, CA.)

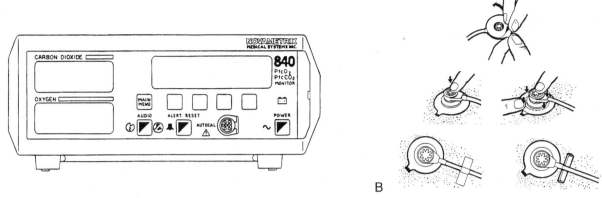

FIGURE 20.9 *(A)* Transcutaneous monitor and *(B)* electrodes. (Courtesy of Novametrix Medical Systems Inc., Wallingford, CT.)

11. With the electrode still in place, place your laboratory partner on a nonrebreathing mask, and *record the $P_{TC}CO_2$ and $P_{TC}O_2$ readings on your laboratory report.*

12. With the electrode still in place, instruct your laboratory partner to hold his or her breath. *Record the $P_{TC}CO_2$ and $P_{TC}O_2$ readings on your laboratory report.*

13. Repeat the exercise, placing the electrode in one of the following locations:
    Palm of the hand
    Sole of the foot
    Underside of the forearm
    Clavicle

    Record the site selected on your laboratory report. Observe the length of time required for equilibration and any differences in readings. *Record the $P_{TC}CO_2$ and $P_{TC}O_2$ readings on your laboratory report.*

14. Detach the electrode and clean it as instructed in the manufacturer's manual.

15. Shut off the unit and clean it as required.

References

1. Peruzzi, WT and Shapiro, BA: Blood gas monitors. Respir Care Clin North Am 1:143, 1995.
2. American Association for Respiratory Care: AARC clinical practice guideline: Pulse oximetry. Respir Care 36:1406–1409, 1991.
3. Eubanks, DH and Bone, RC: Principles and Applications of Cardiorespiratory Care Equipment. Mosby, St Louis, 1994, p 312.

Related Readings

Eubanks, DH and Bone, RC: Principles and Applications of Cardiorespiratory Care Equipment. Mosby, St Louis, 1994.
McPherson, S: Respiratory Care Equipment, ed 5. Mosby, St Louis, 1995.
Scanlan, C et al (eds): Egan's Fundamentals of Respiratory Care. Mosby, St Louis, 1995.

Selected Journal Articles

American Association for Respiratory Care: AARC clinical practice guideline: Pulse oximetry. Respir Care 36:1406–1409, 1991.
American Association for Respiratory Care: AARC clinical practice guideline: Transcutaneous blood gas monitoring for neonatal and pediatric patients. Respir Care 39:1176–1179, 1994.
Blanchette, T, Dziodzio, J and Harris, K: Pulse oximetry and normoxemia in the neonatal intensive care unit. Respir Care 1:25–32, 1991.
Branson, RD and MacIntyre, N (eds): Blood gas measurements. Respir Care Clin North Am 1:1–162, 1995.
Harris, K: Noninvasive monitoring of gas exchange. Respir Care 32:544–557.
Special issue: Noninvasive monitoring part I. Respir Care 35:449–608, 1990.
Special issue: Noninvasive monitoring part II. Respir Care 35:609–768, 1990.

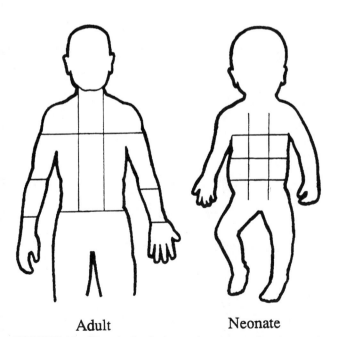

Adult   Neonate

FIGURE 20.10 Site selection for transcutaneous monitor placement. (Courtesy of Novametrix Medical Systems Inc., Wallingford, CT.)

LABORATORY REPORT

CHAPTER 20: NONINVASIVE BLOOD GAS MONITORING

Name _____   Date _____

Course/Section _____   Instructor _____

Data Collection

EXERCISE 20.1   Pulse Oximetry

EXERCISE 20.1.1   Measurement of Saturation and Pulse

Pulse Oximetry Accuracy Check

97% Phantom reading: _____

90% Phantom reading: _____

80% Phantom reading: _____

Resting pulse rate: _____

Oximeter equilibration time: _____

Pulse difference: _____

SpO_2: _____

Capillary refill: _____

Charting: _____

_____

_____

_____

EXERCISE 20.1.2   Effect of Nail Polish on Saturation

Black Nail Polish

SpO_2: _____

Pulse: _____

Manual pulse measurement: _____

Red Nail Polish

SpO_2: _____

Pulse: _____

Manual pulse measurement: _____

Green Nail Polish

SpO_2: _____

Pulse: _____

Manual pulse measurement: _____

EXERCISE 20.1.3   Effects of Perfusion Changes on Pulse Oximetry

Modified Allen's test result: _____

Iced Hand

Hand used: _____

SpO$_2$: _____

Pulse: _____

Manual pulse measurement: _____

Tourniquet or Blood Pressure Cuff:

Hand used: _____

SpO$_2$: _____

Pulse: _____

Manual pulse measurement: _____

EXERCISE 20.1.4   Metabolic Effects on Pulse Oximetry

Pulse Oximeter Readings with Breath Hold

Time of breath hold: _____

SpO$_2$: _____

Pulse: _____

Manual pulse measurement: _____

Pulse Oximeter Readings with 100% Oxygen

SpO$_2$: _____

Pulse: _____

Manual pulse measurement: _____

Pulse Oximeter Reading after Exercise

Duration of exercise: _____

SpO$_2$: _____

Pulse: _____

Manual pulse measurement: _____

EXERCISE 20.2   Capnography

EXERCISE 20.2.1   Disposable Capnometer (Easy Cap)™

Initial color: _____

Ranges available: _____

Color change: _____

Range measured: _____

Deadspace: _____

EXERCISE 20.2.2   Continuous Capnographic Monitoring

Barometric pressure: _____

Percent CO_2 used: _____

Calculation of slope calibration point: _____

Mainstream or sidestream? _____

Tracing of tidal breathing:

Observed differences between nose and mouth breathing: _____

_____

_____

Tracing of hypoventilation: CO_2 level = _____

Tracing of hyperventilation: CO_2 level = _____

Tracing of breath hold: CO_2 level = _____

EXERCISE 20.3   Transcutaneous Monitors

Type of device used: _____

Electrode placement site: _____

$P_{TC}CO_2$: _____

$P_{TC}O_2$: _____

Nonrebreather

$P_{TC}CO_2$: _____

$P_{TC}O_2$: _____

Breath Hold

$P_{TC}CO_2$: _____

$P_{TC}O_2$: _____

New electrode placement site: _____

$P_{TC}CO_2$: _____

$P_{TC}O_2$: _____

Differences observed: _____

_____

CRITICAL THINKING QUESTIONS

1. Explain the principle of operation of a pulse oximeter.

2. Identify four limitations to the use of a pulse oximeter compared with a co-oximeter, and explain how each would affect the accuracy or reliability of the reading.

3. Describe how a pulse oximeter could be used to wean a patient from oxygen.

4. What complications are associated with the use of pulse oximetry?

5. Explain the use of capnography for trending in mechanically ventilated patients. What factors might affect the trends, related to false-negative or false-positive findings?

6. Identify three conditions in which the capnography reading is lower than the $PaCO_2$.

7. In what conditions would the capnography reading be most comparable with the $PaCO_2$ in a mechanically ventilated patient?

8. Calculate the V_D/V_T ratio and the deadspace in milliliters for the following:
   a. A COPD patient
      $P_ECO_2 = 30$ mm Hg
      $PaCO_2 = 60$ mm Hg
      $V_T = 400$ ml
   b. A drug overdose patient
      $P_ECO_2 = 55$ mm Hg
      $PaCO_2 = 60$ mm Hg
      $V_T = 500$ ml
   c. A head injury patient
      $P_ECO_2 = 28$ mm Hg
      $PaCO_2 = 30$ mm Hg
      $V_T = 800$ ml
   d. A patient with pulmonary emboli
      $P_ECO_2 = 20$ mm Hg
      $PaCO_2 = 45$ mm Hg
      $V_T = 600$ ml

9. What are the complications of capnography?

10. Identify four factors that would make the reading for $P_{TC}O_2$ monitoring unreliable.

11. What complications are associated with transcutaneous monitoring?

12. How often and when should calibration of a transcutaneous monitor be performed?

PROCEDURAL COMPETENCY EVALUATION

ne _Celeca Ayala_   Date _6/25/00_

Pulse Oximetry ~(95 +/- 4)~

ing: ☑ Lab ☐ Clinical   Evaluator: ☐ Peer ☑ Instructor

nditions (describe): _____

_____

Equipment Used

_____

_____

	S A T I S F A C T O R Y	U N S A T I S F A C T O R Y	N O T O B S E R V E D	N O T A P P L I C A B L E

Equipment and Patient Preparation

1. Verifies, interprets, and evaluates physician's order or protocol; determines F_IO_2 ☑ ☐ ☐ ☐

2. Scans chart for diagnosis and any other pertinent data and notes   ☑ ☐ ☐ ☐

3. Selects, gathers, and assembles the necessary equipment   ☑ ☐ ☐ ☐

4. Visually inspects the power cord (if applicable) and probe cable for any frayed or exposed wires   ☑ ☐ ☐ ☐

5. Washes hands and applies standard precautions and transmission-based isolation procedures as appropriate   ☑ ☐ ☐ ☐

6. Identifies patient, introduces self and department   ☑ ☐ ☐ ☐

7. Explains purpose of the procedure and confirms patient understanding   ☑ ☐ ☐ ☐

Assessment and Implementation

8. Assesses patient by measuring the patient's pulse rate manually or verifying the heart rate displayed on ECG monitor (if applicable)   ☑ ☐ ☐ ☐

9. Confirms the F_IO_2 in the patient's ~room~   ☑ ☐ ☐ ☐

10. Turns on the oximeter and allows for appropriate warm-up _ex ear, finger, flute_   ☑ ☐ ☐ ☐

11. Selects a site for the probe application and checks for adequate perfusion; removes nail polish if necessary _because they have different sites_   ☑ ☐ ☐ ☐

12. Cleans site with alcohol prep pad   ☑ ☐ ☐ ☐

13. Attaches probe to the selected site   ☑ ☐ ☐ ☐

14. Allows for proper stabilization   ☑ ☐ ☐ ☐

15. Observes the pulse rate on the oximeter; correlates it with the manually measured rate or ECG rate   ☑ ☐ ☐ ☐

16. Records the pulse rate and saturation & FIO_2 ☑ ☐ ☐ ☐

Follow-up

17. Disconnects and turns unit off if not a continuous monitoring situation   ☑ ☐ ☐ ☐

18. Disinfects probe if nondisposable   ☑ ☐ ☐ ☐

19. Washes hands and disposes of any infectious waste   ☑ ☐ ☐ ☐

20. Records pertinent data in chart and departmental records   ☑ ☐ ☐ ☐

21. Notifies appropriate personnel and makes any necessary recommendations or modifications to the patient care plan   ☑ ☐ ☐ ☐

_____   _____
Signature of Evaluator   Signature of Student

PERFORMANCE RATING SCALE

5 EXCELLENT—FAR EXCEEDS EXPECTED LEVEL, FLAWLESS PERFORMANCE
4 ABOVE AVERAGE—NO PROMPTING REQUIRED, ABLE TO SELF-CORRECT
3 AVERAGE—THE MINIMUM COMPETENCY LEVEL, NO CRITICAL ERRORS
2 IMPROVEMENT NEEDED—PROBLEM AREAS EXIST; CRITICAL ERRORS, CORRECTIONS NEEDED
1 POOR AND UNACCEPTABLE PERFORMANCE—GROSS INACCURACIES, POTENTIALLY HARMFUL

PERFORMANCE CRITERIA	SCALE				
1. DISPLAYS KNOWLEDGE OF ESSENTIAL CONCEPTS	5	4	3	2	1
2. DEMONSTRATES THE RELATIONSHIP BETWEEN THEORY AND CLINICAL PRACTICE	5	4	3	2	1
3. FOLLOWS DIRECTIONS, EXHIBITS SOUND JUDGMENT, AND DEMONSTRATES ATTENTION TO SAFETY AND DETAIL	5	4	3	2	1
4. EXHIBITS THE REQUIRED MANUAL DEXTERITY	5	4	3	2	1
5. PERFORMS PROCEDURE IN A REASONABLE TIME FRAME	5	4	3	2	1
6. MAINTAINS STERILE OR ASEPTIC TECHNIQUE	5	4	3	2	1
7. INITIATES UNAMBIGUOUS GOAL-DIRECTED COMMUNICATION	5	4	3	2	1
8. PROVIDES FOR ADEQUATE CARE AND MAINTENANCE OF EQUIPMENT AND SUPPLIES	5	4	3	2	1
9. EXHIBITS COURTEOUS AND PLEASANT DEMEANOR	5	4	3	2	1
10. MAINTAINS CONCISE AND ACCURATE RECORDS	5	4	3	2	1

ADDITIONAL COMMENTS: INCLUDE ERRORS OF OMISSION OR COMMISSION, COMMUNICATIVE SKILLS, AND EFFECTIVENESS OF PATIENT INTERACTION:

SUMMARY PERFORMANCE EVALUATION AND RECOMMENDATIONS

SATISFACTORY PERFORMANCE—Performed without error or prompting, or able to self-correct, no critical errors.

_____ LABORATORY EVALUATION. SKILLS MAY BE APPLIED/OBSERVED IN THE CLINICAL SETTING.

_____ CLINICAL EVALUATION. STUDENT READY FOR MINIMALLY SUPERVISED APPLICATION AND REFINEMENT.

UNSATISFACTORY PERFORMANCE—Prompting required; performed with critical errors, potentially harmful.

_____ STUDENT REQUIRES ADDITIONAL LABORATORY PRACTICE.

_____ STUDENT REQUIRES ADDITIONAL SUPERVISED CLINICAL PRACTICE.

SIGNATURES

STUDENT: _____   EVALUATOR: _____

DATE: _____   DATE: _____

PROCEDURAL COMPETENCY EVALUATION

Name _____ Date _____

Capnography

Setting: ☐ Lab ☐ Clinical   Evaluator: ☐ Peer ☐ Instructor

Conditions (describe): _____

_____

Equipment Used

_____

_____

	SATISFACTORY	UNSATISFACTORY	NOT OBSERVED	NOT APPLICABLE
Equipment and Patient Preparation				
1. Verifies, interprets, and evaluates physician's order or protocol; determines F_IO_2 and ventilator settings	☐	☐	☐	☐
2. Scans chart for diagnosis and any other pertinent data and notes	☐	☐	☐	☐
3. Selects, gathers, and assembles the necessary equipment	☐	☐	☐	☐
4. Tests equipment and verifies calibration	☐	☐	☐	☐
5. Washes hands and applies standard precautions and transmission-based isolation procedures as appropriate	☐	☐	☐	☐
6. Identifies patient, introduces self and department	☐	☐	☐	☐
7. Explains purpose of the procedure and confirms patient understanding	☐	☐	☐	☐
Assessment and Implementation				
8. Assesses patient and confirms F_IO_2 and ventilator settings	☐	☐	☐	☐
9. Turns unit on and allows warm-up time	☐	☐	☐	☐
10. Connects sampling tube to patient's nose or in-line to ventilator circuit with proper adaptor	☐	☐	☐	☐
11. Ensures that there is no excess pull on airway	☐	☐	☐	☐
12. Records highest P_ECO_2 after 3 min	☐	☐	☐	☐
13. Prints capnograph wave if applicable and determines ventilatory status	☐	☐	☐	☐
Follow-up				
14. Maintains/processes equipment as necessary; if continuous monitoring performed, checks line and water trap for moisture, debris	☐	☐	☐	☐
15. Disposes of infectious waste and washes hands	☐	☐	☐	☐
16. Records pertinent data in chart and departmental records	☐	☐	☐	☐
17. Notifies appropriate personnel and makes any necessary recommendations or modifications to the patient care plan	☐	☐	☐	☐

_____   _____
Signature of Evaluator   Signature of Student

PERFORMANCE RATING SCALE

5 EXCELLENT—FAR EXCEEDS EXPECTED LEVEL, FLAWLESS PERFORMANCE
4 ABOVE AVERAGE—NO PROMPTING REQUIRED, ABLE TO SELF-CORRECT
3 AVERAGE—THE MINIMUM COMPETENCY LEVEL, NO CRITICAL ERRORS
2 IMPROVEMENT NEEDED—PROBLEM AREAS EXIST; CRITICAL ERRORS, CORRECTIONS NEEDED
1 POOR AND UNACCEPTABLE PERFORMANCE—GROSS INACCURACIES, POTENTIALLY HARMFUL

PERFORMANCE CRITERIA	SCALE				
1. DISPLAYS KNOWLEDGE OF ESSENTIAL CONCEPTS	5	4	3	2	1
2. DEMONSTRATES THE RELATIONSHIP BETWEEN THEORY AND CLINICAL PRACTICE	5	4	3	2	1
3. FOLLOWS DIRECTIONS, EXHIBITS SOUND JUDGMENT, AND DEMONSTRATES ATTENTION TO SAFETY AND DETAIL	5	4	3	2	1
4. EXHIBITS THE REQUIRED MANUAL DEXTERITY	5	4	3	2	1
5. PERFORMS PROCEDURE IN A REASONABLE TIME FRAME	5	4	3	2	1
6. MAINTAINS STERILE OR ASEPTIC TECHNIQUE	5	4	3	2	1
7. INITIATES UNAMBIGUOUS GOAL-DIRECTED COMMUNICATION	5	4	3	2	1
8. PROVIDES FOR ADEQUATE CARE AND MAINTENANCE OF EQUIPMENT AND SUPPLIES	5	4	3	2	1
9. EXHIBITS COURTEOUS AND PLEASANT DEMEANOR	5	4	3	2	1
10. MAINTAINS CONCISE AND ACCURATE RECORDS	5	4	3	2	1

ADDITIONAL COMMENTS: INCLUDE ERRORS OF OMISSION OR COMMISSION, COMMUNICATIVE SKILLS, AND EFFECTIVENESS OF PATIENT INTERACTION:

SUMMARY PERFORMANCE EVALUATION AND RECOMMENDATIONS

SATISFACTORY PERFORMANCE—Performed without error or prompting, or able to self-correct, no critical errors.

_____ LABORATORY EVALUATION. SKILLS MAY BE APPLIED/OBSERVED IN THE CLINICAL SETTING.

_____ CLINICAL EVALUATION. STUDENT READY FOR MINIMALLY SUPERVISED APPLICATION AND REFINEMENT.

UNSATISFACTORY PERFORMANCE—Prompting required; performed with critical errors, potentially harmful.

_____ STUDENT REQUIRES ADDITIONAL LABORATORY PRACTICE.

_____ STUDENT REQUIRES ADDITIONAL SUPERVISED CLINICAL PRACTICE.

SIGNATURES

STUDENT: _____   EVALUATOR: _____

DATE: _____   DATE: _____

PROCEDURAL COMPETENCY EVALUATION

Name _____ Date _____

Transcutaneous Monitoring

Setting: ☐ Lab ☐ Clinical

Evaluator: ☐ Peer ☐ Instructor

Conditions (describe): _____

_____

Equipment Used

_____

_____

	SATISFACTORY	UNSATISFACTORY	NOT OBSERVED	NOT APPLICABLE
Equipment and Patient Preparation				
1. Verifies, interprets, and evaluates physician's order or protocol; determines F_IO_2 and ventilator settings	☐	☐	☐	☐
2. Scans chart for diagnosis and any other pertinent data and notes	☐	☐	☐	☐
3. Selects, gathers, and assembles the necessary equipment	☐	☐	☐	☐
4. Calibrates the unit using the appropriate zero solution and slope gas	☐	☐	☐	☐
5. Washes hands and applies standard precautions and transmission-based isolation procedures as appropriate	☐	☐	☐	☐
6. Identifies patient, introduces self and department	☐	☐	☐	☐
7. Explains purpose of the procedure and confirms patient or family's understanding	☐	☐	☐	☐
Assessment and Implementation				
8. Assesses patient and confirms F_IO_2 and ventilator settings	☐	☐	☐	☐
9. Selects an electrode site away from flat, boney areas, large veins, or thick skin	☐	☐	☐	☐
10. Cleanses the selected site with an alcohol prep pad and dries it	☐	☐	☐	☐
11. Adjusts the temperature to 43 to 45°C as appropriate for patient's age	☐	☐	☐	☐
12. Allows for equilibration	☐	☐	☐	☐
13. Records the $P_{TC}CO_2$ and $P_{TC}O_2$ readings as applicable	☐	☐	☐	☐
14. Reassesses patient and electrode site periodically; changes electrode placement at least every 4 hours	☐	☐	☐	☐
Follow-up				
15. Maintains/processes equipment	☐	☐	☐	☐
16. Disposes of infectious waste and washes hands	☐	☐	☐	☐
17. Records pertinent data in chart and departmental records	☐	☐	☐	☐
18. Notifies appropriate personnel and makes any necessary recommendations or modifications to the patient care plan	☐	☐	☐	☐

_____

Signature of Evaluator

_____

Signature of Student

PERFORMANCE RATING SCALE

5 EXCELLENT—FAR EXCEEDS EXPECTED LEVEL, FLAWLESS PERFORMANCE
4 ABOVE AVERAGE—NO PROMPTING REQUIRED, ABLE TO SELF-CORRECT
3 AVERAGE—THE MINIMUM COMPETENCY LEVEL, NO CRITICAL ERRORS
2 IMPROVEMENT NEEDED—PROBLEM AREAS EXIST; CRITICAL ERRORS, CORRECTIONS NEEDED
1 POOR AND UNACCEPTABLE PERFORMANCE—GROSS INACCURACIES, POTENTIALLY HARMFUL

PERFORMANCE CRITERIA		SCALE			
1. DISPLAYS KNOWLEDGE OF ESSENTIAL CONCEPTS	5	4	3	2	1
2. DEMONSTRATES THE RELATIONSHIP BETWEEN THEORY AND CLINICAL PRACTICE	5	4	3	2	1
3. FOLLOWS DIRECTIONS, EXHIBITS SOUND JUDGMENT, AND DEMONSTRATES ATTENTION TO SAFETY AND DETAIL	5	4	3	2	1
4. EXHIBITS THE REQUIRED MANUAL DEXTERITY	5	4	3	2	1
5. PERFORMS PROCEDURE IN A REASONABLE TIME FRAME	5	4	3	2	1
6. MAINTAINS STERILE OR ASEPTIC TECHNIQUE	5	4	3	2	1
7. INITIATES UNAMBIGUOUS GOAL-DIRECTED COMMUNICATION	5	4	3	2	1
8. PROVIDES FOR ADEQUATE CARE AND MAINTENANCE OF EQUIPMENT AND SUPPLIES	5	4	3	2	1
9. EXHIBITS COURTEOUS AND PLEASANT DEMEANOR	5	4	3	2	1
10. MAINTAINS CONCISE AND ACCURATE RECORDS	5	4	3	2	1

ADDITIONAL COMMENTS: INCLUDE ERRORS OF OMISSION OR COMMISSION, COMMUNICATIVE SKILLS, AND EFFECTIVENESS OF PATIENT INTERACTION:

SUMMARY PERFORMANCE EVALUATION AND RECOMMENDATIONS

SATISFACTORY PERFORMANCE—Performed without error or prompting, or able to self-correct, no critical errors.

_____ LABORATORY EVALUATION. SKILLS MAY BE APPLIED/OBSERVED IN THE CLINICAL SETTING.

_____ CLINICAL EVALUATION. STUDENT READY FOR MINIMALLY SUPERVISED APPLICATION AND REFINEMENT.

UNSATISFACTORY PERFORMANCE—Prompting required; performed with critical errors, potentially harmful.

_____ STUDENT REQUIRES ADDITIONAL LABORATORY PRACTICE.

_____ STUDENT REQUIRES ADDITIONAL SUPERVISED CLINICAL PRACTICE.

SIGNATURES

STUDENT: _____   EVALUATOR: _____

DATE: _____   DATE: _____

Blood Gas Interpretation and Calculations

INTRODUCTION

The respiratory care practitioner must not only be proficient in obtaining blood gas samples but also must be able to interpret the results in order to make recommendations and modify therapeutic interventions related to acid-base, ventilation, and oxygenation status. Many calculations and formulas assist in estimating the adequacy of physiologic indexes or approximating needed changes in oxygen or ventilator parameters. Calculations also are helpful in verifying the accuracy of derived values from blood gas sampling measurements.

OBJECTIVES

Upon completion of this chapter, the student will be able to:

1. Identify and correct **preanalytical** errors affecting blood gas results, including inadvertent venous sampling, air bubbles in sample, excess heparinization, and delayed analysis.

2. Interpret arterial blood gas analysis results and make recommendations for oxygen therapy based on the interpretations.

3. Calculate P_AO_2, $P(A - a)DO_2$, arterial/alveolar oxygen tension (a/A) ratio, CaO_2, CvO_2 and $C(a - v)O_2$, VO_2 and cardiac output using the Fick equation, acid/base ratios, pH, Hco_3^- and total carbon dioxide.

4. Estimate the F_IO_2 needed to obtain a desired PaO_2.

5. Using a graphic representation of the oxyhemoglobin dissociation curve, determine SaO_2, CaO_2, PaO_2, and P-50.

KEY TERMS

acidosis	alkalosis	hyperoxia	preanalytical
	exacerbation	logarithm	superimposed

EQUIPMENT REQUIRED

- Arterial blood gas results:
  - Logs
  - Computer runs
  - Computer tutorials
- **Logarithm** table or calculator with log function
- Metric ruler

● EXERCISES

EXERCISE 21.1 Interpretation of Arterial Blood Gas Values

Review normal arterial and venous values (Table 21.1). Perform the following steps to interpret arterial blood gas sample results:

1. Obtain blood gas analysis results to interpret. Your instructor will provide you with one or more of the following:

   Blood gas log records
   Computer runs of blood gas results
   Blood gas record slips
   Computerized practice and drill tutorials

2. Consider the following abnormalities:

   pH
   　<7.35: acidotic
   　>7.45: alkalotic
   PCO₂—Respiratory Component
   　>45 mm Hg: acidotic (hypoventilation)
   　<35 mm Hg: alkalotic (hyperventilation)
   HCO₃⁻—Metabolic Component
   　<22 mEq/L: acidotic
   　>26 mEq/L: alkalotic
   BE—Metabolic Component
   　<−2: acidotic
   　>+2: alkalotic
   PO₂
   　<80 mm Hg mild hypoxemia
   　<60 mm Hg moderate hypoxemia
   　<40 mm Hg severe hypoxemia
   　>100 mm Hg **hyperoxia**
   a. Must consider correlation with oxygen therapy (uncorrected, corrected, or overcorrected).

Arterial	Venous
pH: 7.40 (7.35-7.45)	pH: 7.34-7.36
$PaCO_2$: 40 (35-45) mm Hg	$PvCO_2$: 46-48 mm Hg
PaO_2: 100 (80-100) mm Hg	PvO_2: 40 (37-43) mm Hg
SaO_2: 97%	SvO_2: 70%-75%
HCO_3^-: 22-26 mEq/L	
BE: ±2	

b. Must consider age of patient:
   (1) Newborn normal PaO_2 is 40 to 70 mm Hg.
   (2) Over 60 years old, PaO_2 may decrease approximately 1 mm Hg per year.
   (3) Any PaO_2 below 60 mm Hg is abnormal.

3. Interpret acid/base status:
   a. Look at the pH and decide whether it is acidotic, alkalotic, or normal. If normal, is it on the acidotic or alkalotic side of 7.40? Mark your decision next to the pH value.
   b. Look at the $PaCO_2$ and determine whether it is normal, acidotic, or alkalotic.
   c. Look at HCO_3^-/BE. Determine whether it is normal, acidotic, or alkalotic.
   d. Determine whether the primary condition is respiratory or metabolic. See which component (CO_2 or base) matches the pH (same direction, alkalotic, or acidotic).
   e. Determine how much compensation is occurring.
      (1) Look at the nonprimary component to see if it is normal. If normal, this is an *acute uncompensated* condition.
      (2) If the nonprimary component is abnormal, determine in which direction it is occurring. If it is in the opposite direction of the primary problem, *compensation* has begun. This is a *chronic, partially compensated* condition.
      (3) If the pH is normal, compensation is *complete*.
      (4) If the nonprimary component is abnormal in the same direction as the primary component, it is a *mixed* condition.

4. You *must* consider the patient history, diagnosis, and treatment, if known, to fully interpret. There may be an acute problem **superimposed** on a chronic problem—for example, a COPD patient with chronic hypercarbia placed on a mechanical ventilator or having an acute exacerbation. The following series of blood gases are given as an illustration:

	"Normal state"	On admission	After ventilation
pH	7.37	7.25	7.47
PCO_2	55	70	45
HCO_3^-	31	30	32
BE	+4	+5	+3

5. Oxygenation status:
   a. Look at the PO_2 and determine whether it is normal, hypoxemic, or hyperoxic.
   b. Look at the oxygen therapy being given, if any, and determine whether the PO_2 is uncorrected, corrected, or overcorrected.
   c. Remember to consider the age of the patient.
   d. Look at the hemoglobin, SO_2, oxygen content, and vital signs to determine whether there are any indications of tissue hypoxia.

6. Compare the results with the patient's previous results, if available, and the clinical condition.

7. Consider any possible sources of error, such as excess heparin, air bubbles, inadvertent venous sample, improperly iced sample or delayed analysis, or analyzer temperature not at 37°C.

NOTE: There is a lack of a scientific basis for correction of blood gases for changes in patient body temperature. Appropriate clinical interpretation is better accomplished when temperature correction is avoided.[1]

EXERCISE 21.2 Calculation of Oxygenation Parameters

EXERCISE 21.2.1 Oxygen Dissociation Curve

The following problems should be answered using the oxygen dissociation curve in Figure 21.1. Do not "calculate" answers.

Use your ruler to line up the y and x axes on the graph to determine the following parameters. *Record your answers on your laboratory report.*

1. With the curve in a normal position, for the following values of PO_2, determine the SaO_2.
   a. 60 mm Hg
   b. 50 mm Hg
   c. 90 mm Hg
   d. 40 mm Hg

2. With the curve in the normal position, for the following values of PO_2, determine the CaO_2.
   a. 60 mm Hg
   b. 20 mm Hg
   c. 90 mm Hg
   d. 40 mm Hg

3. For the following P-50 values, determine whether the curve has shifted left or right.
   a. 20 mm Hg
   b. 30 mm Hg

4. For the shifted curves shown in Figure 21.2, determine the P-50 value by lining up your ruler with an SO_2 value of 50 percent, intersecting the curve, and then drawing a perpendicular line down to the corresponding PO_2 value. For the curves shifted to the left and to the right, *record your answers on your laboratory report.*

EXERCISE 21.2.2 Calculation of Alveolar Air Equation, Alveolar Arterial Oxygen Gradient, and Arterial/Alveolar Oxygen Ratio

The following equation can be used to determine the PaO_2. Because PaO_2 should approximate PaO_2, the formula is helpful in determining the maximum possible PaO_2 for a given F_IO_2. This is useful in evaluating possible preanalytical error from air bubble inclusion.

$$PAO_2 = [F_IO_2 (P_B - 47)] - (PaCO_2 \times 1.25)$$

From this calculation, the $P(A - a)DO_2$ can then be determined by using the following formula:

$$PAO_2 - PaO_2 = P(A - a)DO_2$$

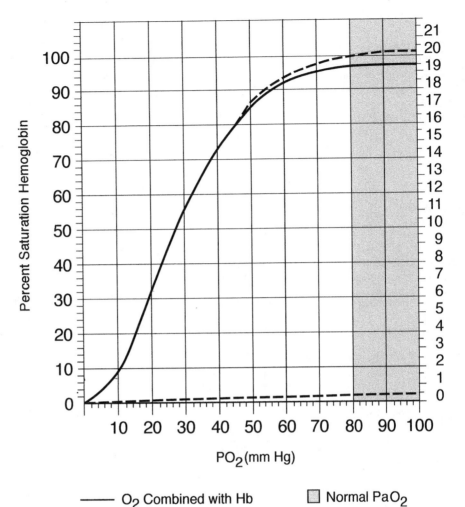

FIGURE 21.1 The oxyhemoglobin dissociation curve.

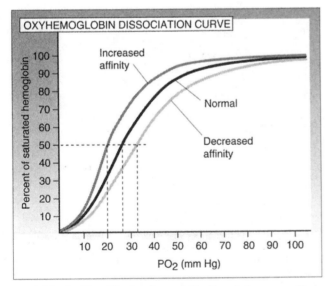

FIGURE 21.2 The shifted oxyhemoglobin dissociation curve. (From Persing, G: Entry-Level Respiratory Care Review: Study Guide and Workbook, ed 2. WB Saunders, Philadelphia, 1996, p. 79, with permission.)

This formula can be used to estimate the degree of hypoxemia or the degree of physiologic shunt.[2]

The arterial/alveolar oxygen ratio is an indicator of the efficiency of oxygen diffusion. A low a/A ratio reflects ventilation perfusion (V/Q) mismatches, diffusion defects, or shunts.[3] The a/A ratio is determined by the following formula:

$$\frac{PaO_2}{PAO_2} = a/A \text{ ratio}$$

For each of the following, calculate the PAO_2, the $P(A - a)DO_2$, and the a/A ratio. *Show your work and record your answers on your laboratory report.*

1. $F_IO_2 = 0.21$
   $PB = 760 \text{ mm Hg}$
   $PaCO_2 = 40 \text{ mm Hg}$
   $PaO_2 = 100 \text{ mm Hg}$

2. $F_IO_2 = 1.00$
   $PB = 760 \text{ mm Hg}$
   $PaCO_2 = 40 \text{ mm Hg}$
   $PaO_2 = 650 \text{ mm Hg}$

3. $F_IO_2 = 0.50$
   $PB = 750 \text{ mm Hg}$
   $PaCO_2 = 50 \text{ mm Hg}$
   $PaO_2 = 60 \text{ mm Hg}$

4. $F_IO_2 = 0.21$
   $P_B = 755$ mm Hg
   $PaCO_2 = 20$ mm Hg
   $PaO_2 = 110$ mm Hg

5. Calculate the highest possible values of PaO_2 for the following values of $PaCO_2$ for patients breathing room air at sea level.
   a. $PaCO_2 = 25$ mm Hg
   b. $PaCO_2 = 15$ mm Hg
   c. $PaCO_2 = 30$ mm Hg
   d. $PaCO_2 = 50$ mm Hg
   e. $PaCO_2 = 70$ mm Hg

EXERCISE 21.2.3 F_IO_2 Needed for a Desired PaO_2

This calculation is useful to estimate the F_IO_2 needed for a desired PaO_2 in a patient with hypoxemia caused by V/Q mismatch or hypoventilation. It is less reliable in severe intrapulmonary shunts.[4]

Step 1: Calculate the P_AO_2 as in the preceding exercises.

Step 2: Calculate the a/A ratio as in the preceding exercises.

Step 3: Calculate the P_AO_2 needed.

$$P_AO_2 \text{ needed} = \frac{PaO_2 \text{ desired}}{\text{a/A ratio}}$$

Step 4: Calculate the F_IO_2 needed.

$$F_IO_2 \text{ needed} = \frac{P_AO_2 \text{ needed} + (PaCO_2 \times 1.25)}{P_B - 47}$$

For the following blood gas examples, calculate the F_IO_2 needed. *Show your work and record your answers on your laboratory report.*

1. $PaO_2 = 40$ mm Hg
   $PaCO_2 = 30$ mm Hg
   $F_IO_2 = 0.21$
   $P_B = 760$ mm Hg
   Desired $PaO_2 = 80$ mm Hg

2. $PaO_2 = 50$ mm Hg
   $PaCO_2 = 60$ mm Hg
   $F_IO_2 = 0.25$
   $P_B = 750$
   Desired $PaO_2 = 60$ mm Hg

3. $PaO_2 = 500$ mm Hg
   $PaCO_2 = 40$ mm Hg
   $F_IO_2 = 1.0$
   $P_B = 765$
   Desired $PaO_2 = 90$ mm Hg

EXERCISE 21.2.4 Arterial Oxygen Content, Venous Oxygen Content, Arterial Venous Oxygen Difference, Oxygen Consumption, and Cardiac Output Using the Fick Equation

$$CaO_2 = (PaO_2 \times 0.003) + (Hb \times 1.39) \, SaO_2$$
$$CvO_2 = (PvO_2 \times 0.003) + (Hb \times 1.39) \, SvO_2$$
$$C(a-v)O_2 = CaO_2 - CvO_2$$
$$VO_2 = C(a-v)O_2 \times (\text{cardiac output}) \times 10$$

For each of the following, perform the above calculations. *Show your work and record your answers on your laboratory report.*

1.

	Arterial	Mixed venous
pH	7.25	7.22
PCO_2	55 mm Hg	62 mm Hg
PaO_2	60 mm Hg	30 mm Hg
SaO_2	88%	65%
Hb	18 g/100 ml	
Cardiac output	4.0 L/min	
F_IO_2	0.21	

2.

	Arterial	Mixed venous
pH	7.35	7.32
PCO_2	65 mm Hg	72 mm Hg
PaO_2	50 mm Hg	20 mm Hg
SaO_2	85%	60%
Hb	10 g/100 ml	
VO_2	180 ml/min	
F_IO_2	0.24	

EXERCISE 21.3 Acid-Base Calculations

The following formulas are used to calculate acid-base parameters:

$$\text{Base:acid ratio} = \frac{HCO_3^-}{PaCO_2 \times 0.03}$$

$$pH = 6.1 + \log\left[\frac{HCO_3^-}{PaCO_2 \times 0.03}\right]$$

$$\text{Total } CO_2 \text{ mM/L} = (PaCO_2 \times 0.03) + HCO_3^-$$

For each of the following, calculate the base:acid ratio, pH, and total CO_2. *Show your work and record your answers on your laboratory report.*

1. $HCO_3^- = 20$ mEq/L
   $PCO_2 = 37$ mm Hg

2. $HCO_3^- = 32$ mEq/L
   $PCO_2 = 42$ mm Hg

3. $HCO_3^- = 35$ mEq/L
   $PCO_2 = 55$ mm Hg

4. $HCO_3^- = 17$ mEq/L
   $PCO_2 = 28$ mm Hg

For the following, calculate the HCO_3^-. *Show all work and record your answers on your laboratory report.*

5. pH = 7.35
   $PCO_2 = 60$

6. pH = 7.45
   $PCO_2 = 45$

7. pH = 7.15
   $PCO_2 = 20$

8. pH = 7.55
   $PCO_2 = 20$

References

1. Shapiro, BA, Peruzzi, WT and Kozelowski-Templin, R: Clinical Application of Blood Gases. Mosby, St Louis, 1994, p 231.
2. Chang, DW: Respiratory Care Calculations. Delmar, Albany, 1994, p 10.
3. Chang, DW: Respiratory Care Calculations. Delmar, Albany, 1994, p 14.
4. Chang, DW: Respiratory Care Calculations. Delmar, Albany, 1994, p 48.

Related Readings

Chang, DW: Respiratory Care Calculations. Delmar, Albany, 1994.

Eubanks, DH and Bone, RC: Principles and Applications of Cardiorespiratory Care Equipment. Mosby, St Louis, 1994.

Madama, V: Pulmonary Function Testing and Cardiopulmonary Stress Testing. Delmar, Albany, 1993.

Scanlan, C et al (eds): Egan's Fundamentals of Respiratory Care, ed 6. Mosby, St Louis, 1995.

Shapiro, B et al: Clinical Application of Blood Gases, ed 5. Year Book Medical Publishers, Chicago, 1994.

West, J: Respiratory Physiology: The Essentials, ed 5. Williams & Wilkins, Baltimore, 1995.

Wilkins, R, Sheldon, R and Krider, S: Clinical Assessment in Respiratory Care, ed 3. Mosby, St Louis, 1995.

Selected Journal Articles

American Association for Respiratory Care: AARC clinical practice guideline: In-vitro pH and blood gas analysis and hemoximetry. Respir Care 38:505–510, 1993.

American Association for Respiratory Care: AARC clinical practice guideline: Pulse oximetry. Respir Care 36:1406–1409, 1991.

American Association for Respiratory Care: AARC clinical practice guideline: Sampling for arterial blood gas analysis. Respir Care 37:913–917, 1992.

Branson, RD and MacIntyre, N (eds): Blood gas measurements. Respir Care Clin North Am 1:1–162, 1995.

Martin, L: Abbreviating the alveolar gas equation: An argument for simplicity. Respir Care 31:40–44, 1986.

Nelson, L and Rutherford, E: Monitoring mixed venous oxygen. Respir Care 37:154, 1992.

LABORATORY REPORT

CHAPTER 21: BLOOD GAS INTERPRETATION AND CALCULATIONS

Name _____   Date _____

Course/Section _____   Instructor _____

Data Collection

EXERCISE 21.2   Calculation of Oxygen Parameters

EXERCISE 21.2.1   Oxygen Dissociation Curve

1. a. 60 mm Hg = _____

    b. 50 mm Hg = _____

    c. 90 mm Hg = _____

    d. 40 mm Hg = _____

2. a. 60 mm Hg = _____

    b. 20 mm Hg = _____

    c. 90 mm Hg = _____

    d. 40 mm Hg = _____

3. For the following P-50 values, determine whether the curve has shifted left or right:

    a. 20 mm Hg _____

    b. 30 mm Hg _____

4. For the curve shifted to the left, P-50 = _____

    For the curve shifted to the right, P-50 = _____

EXERCISE 21.2.2   Calculation of P_AO_2, $P(A - a)DO_2$, a/A Ratio

Show your work on the laboratory report!

1. P_AO_2 = _____

    $P(A - a)DO_2$ = _____

    a/A Ratio = _____

2. P_AO_2 = _____

    $P(A - a)DO_2$ = _____

    a/A Ratio = _____

3. P_AO_2 = _____

    $P(A - a)DO_2$ = _____

    a/A Ratio = _____

4. P_AO_2 = _____

    $P(A - a)DO_2$ = _____

    a/A Ratio = _____

5. Calculation of PaO_2 (see text):

    a. $PaO_2 = $ _____

    b. $PaO_2 = $ _____

    c. $PaO_2 = $ _____

    d. $PaO_2 = $ _____

    e. $PaO_2 = $ _____

EXERCISE 21.2.3 F_IO_2 Needed for a Desired PaO_2

Show all work for all steps!

1. $P_AO_2 = $ _____

    a/A Ratio = _____

    P_AO_2 needed = _____

    F_IO_2 needed = _____

2. $P_AO_2 = $ _____

    a/A Ratio = _____

    P_AO_2 needed = _____

    F_IO_2 needed = _____

3. $P_AO_2 = $ _____

    a/A Ratio = _____

    P_AO_2 needed = _____

    F_IO_2 needed = _____

EXERCISE 21.2.4 CaO_2, CvO_2, $C(a-v)O_2$, VO_2, Cardiac Output (C. O.) Using the Fick Equation

Show all work for all steps!

1. $CaO_2 = $ _____

    $CvO_2 = $ _____

    $C(a-v)O_2 = $ _____

    $VO_2 = $ _____

2. $CaO_2 = $ _____

    $CvO_2 = $ _____

    $C(a-v)O_2 = $ _____

    C. O. = _____

EXERCISE 21.3 Acid-Base Calculations

Show all work for all steps!

1. Base : acid ratio = _____

    pH = _____

    Total $CO_2 = $ _____

2. Base : acid ratio = _____

    pH = _____

    Total CO_2 = _____

3. Base : acid ratio = _____

    pH = _____

    Total CO_2 = _____

4. Base : acid ratio = _____

    pH = _____

    Total CO_2 = _____

5. HCO_3^- = _____

6. HCO_3^- = _____

7. HCO_3^- = _____

8. HCO_3^- = _____

CRITICAL THINKING QUESTIONS

Mr. Sample is a 33-year-old nonsmoking healthy man who has volunteered to serve as a control in a research study. An arterial blood gas sample is drawn on room air as part of the study. The blood gas kit used did not contain a preheparinized syringe. Liquid heparin was used to heparinize the syringe before sampling.

1. If the following blood gas result was obtained, what type of preanalytical error would you suspect, if any? What action would you take at this time, if any?
   pH 7.35
   $PaCO_2$ 46 mm Hg
   PaO_2 45 mm Hg
   SaO_2 77%
   HCO_3^- 23 mEq/L

2. If the following blood gas result was obtained, what type of preanalytical error would you suspect, if any? What action would you take at this time, if any?
   pH 7.50
   $PaCO_2$ 25 mm Hg
   PaO_2 150 mm Hg
   SaO_2 100%
   HCO_3^- 26 mEq/L

3. If excess heparin remained in the syringe during sampling, how would it affect the pH and $PaCO_2$ values obtained?

4. If analysis of the sample was delayed by 1 hour without icing the sample, how would the pH, $PaCO_2$, and PaO_2 be changed? Why?

Mr. Khan is a 65-year-old with a history of atrial fibrillation. He takes Coumadin. He complained of increasing shortness of breath and was transported to the ER by the paramedics with a nonrebreathing mask in place. The patient is lethargic. You are called to draw an arterial blood gas.

5. What factors might you consider while performing the puncture?

6. Interpret and explain the following results:
   pH = 7.30
   $PaCO_2$ = 68 mm Hg
   PaO_2 = 122 mm Hg
   HCO_3^- = 32 mEq/L

7. What recommendations would you make concerning an appropriate oxygen delivery device?

8. After successful cardiopulmonary resuscitation, the following blood gas results were obtained while the patient was still being manually ventilated with an F_IO_2 of 0.50:
   pH = 7.10
   $PaCO_2$ = 50 mm Hg
   PaO_2 = 55 mm Hg
   HCO_3^- = 15 mEq/L
   a. Interpret the results.
   b. Explain the cause(s) for these results.
   c. What specific recommendations would you make at this time?

CHAPTER 22

Arterial Blood Gas Analysis and Maintenance

INTRODUCTION

Clinical decisions based on blood gas data may have serious implications for the well-being of the patient. It is imperative that these decisions be based on reliable data from a well-maintained blood gas laboratory.

A total quality assurance program for a blood gas laboratory should include documented policies and procedures for the analysis of samples and machine maintenance, verifiable technician competence, scheduled preventive maintenance of the analyzers, performance of calibrations, quality control sampling, **proficiency** testing, and documentation of sample analysis results. Review of patient data would include the statistical analysis of sampling done and identifying whether procedures were indicated.

This chapter introduces students to the procedures involved in maintaining a blood gas laboratory. Because of the significant expense of equipment and **reagents** and the lack of real blood samples for programs that are not hospital based, some of the procedures described may be performed only in the clinical setting.

OBJECTIVES
Upon completion of this chapter, the student will be able to:

1. Apply infection control guidelines and standards associated with equipment and procedures, according to OSHA regulations and CDC guidelines.
2. Analyze an arterial blood gas sample for pH, $PaCO_2$, and PaO_2 via a standard blood gas analyzer.
3. Analyze an arterial blood gas sample for total hemoglobin, oxyhemoglobin saturation, and dyshemoglobins via a co-oximeter.
4. Perform one- and two-point calibrations of blood gas analyzers.
5. Perform daily and weekly maintenance according to manufacturer's specifications.
6. Remembrane a pH, PCO_2, and PO_2 electrode.
7. Analyze quality control test samples and document the results.

KEY TERMS

diluent	proficiency	reagents	slope

EQUIPMENT REQUIRED

- Blood gas analyzer
- Co-oximeter
- Reagents: pH buffers, PO_2 and PCO_2 electrolytes, flush solution, KCl solution or KCl donuts
- Electrode cleaning solution
- Deproteinizing solution
- Calibration gases
- Barometer, mercury or anaeroid
- **Diluent**
- Zeroing solution
- Quality control test samples for analyzer and co-oximeter
- Blank blood gas report forms or equivalent
- Electrode membrane changing kits for pH, PCO_2, and PO_2
- Electrode membrane changing tools and holder
- 4×4 gauze
- Arterial blood gas syringes
- 3-ml syringes with 22- or 23-gauge needles
- Plastic specimen containers or equivalent
- Heparinized capillary sample tubes
- Magnet and metal rods ("fleas")
- Disposable waste containers
- Sharps containers
- 5.25-percent sodium hypochlorite (bleach) (1:10) solution
- Disposable latex and vinyl gloves, various sizes
- Goggles, disposable gowns (optional)
- Cotton swabs
- Stopwatch or watch with second hand
- Calculator (optional)

⬤ EXERCISES

EXERCISE 22.1 Blood Gas Analysis

EXERCISE 22.1.1 Identification of Components of Blood Gas Analyzers

1. Identify the brand of blood gas analyzer being used for this exercise, and *record it on your laboratory report*. Some commonly used analyzers are depicted in Figure 22.1.
2. Identify the controls located on the control panel, and *record them on your laboratory report*. Draw a schematic representation of the location of these controls. Be sure to include the location of the sampling ports and electrodes.

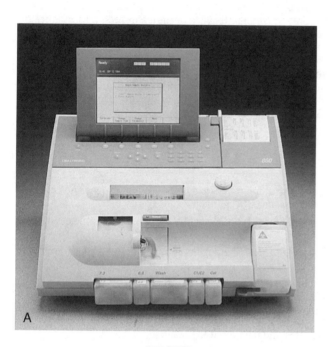

ABL™500
Blood Gas System

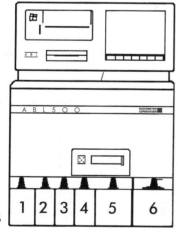

FIGURE 22.1   Commonly used blood gas analyzers. (*[A]* Courtesy of Chiron Diagnostics Corporation, East Walpole, MA 02032; *[B]* drawing courtesy of Radiometer, Radiometer America, Westlake, OH.)

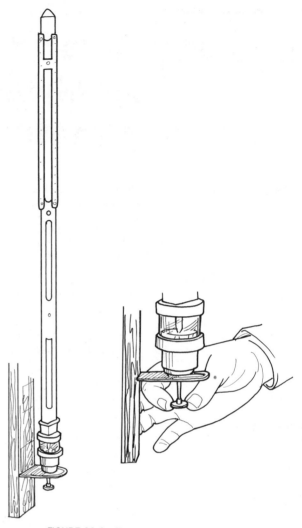

FIGURE 22.2   Zeroing a mercury barometer.

3. Locate the reagents and the waste receptacle. *Record the pH of the buffers for the analyzer on your laboratory report.*
4. Locate the calibration gases. Note the pressures on the gauges, and *record them on your laboratory report*. Note the concentrations of gases in the tanks, and *record them on your laboratory report*.
5. Locate the water bath (if applicable). *Record the temperature on your laboratory report*. Count the rate of gases bubbling through the water bath for 15 sec, and *record it on your laboratory report*.
6. Locate the barometer in your laboratory. If a mercury barometer is used, make sure it is zeroed by adjusting the needle tip so that it just touches the surface of the mercury pool (Fig. 22.2).
7. Determine the barometric pressure in your laboratory, and *record it on your laboratory report*.
8. Calculate the calibration point for **slope** and balance based on your recorded barometric pressure using the following formula:

$$P = (\text{Barometric pressure} - 47 \text{ mm Hg}) \times F_I$$

where P is the partial pressure of calibration gas and F_I is the fractional decimal expression of the gas concentration. *Show your work and calculations on your laboratory report.*

EXERCISE 22.1.2 Calibration of Blood Gas Analyzers

Performance of this exercise and the specific sequence of steps will vary depending on the brand and level of automation of the analyzer used. Consult the operator's manual for the analyzer you are using.

Two-Point Calibration

Initiate the two-point calibration sequence for your analyzer. Using a stopwatch or a watch with a second hand, time how long the two-point calibration takes for your analyzer. *Record the time on your laboratory report.* Pay attention to the sequence in which the reagents and gases are introduced into the analyzer. *Record the sequence of reagents and gases on your laboratory report.*

The following steps are usually involved in a two-point calibration:

1. Flush the pH electrode.
2. Introduce the low-pH buffer into the pH electrode.
3. Allow sufficient time for the reading to stabilize.
4. Adjust the pH balance control.
5. Flush the pH electrode.
6. Introduce the high-pH buffer into the pH electrode.
7. Allow sufficient time for the reading to stabilize.
8. Adjust the pH slope control.
9. Calculate the balance and slope gas calibration points.
10. Introduce low-calibration gases into the PaO_2 and $PaCO_2$ electrodes.
11. Allow sufficient time for the readings to stabilize.
12. Adjust the PO_2 and PCO_2 balance controls.
13. Flush the electrodes.
14. Introduce high-calibration gases into the PO_2 and PCO_2 electrodes.
15. Allow sufficient time for the readings to stabilize.
16. Adjust the PO_2 and PCO_2 slope controls.
17. Flush the sampling chamber.
18. Determine from the analyzer manual or observation how often the machine performs a two-point calibration. *Record this information on your laboratory report.*

One-Point Calibration

Initiate the one-point calibration sequence for your analyzer. Using a stopwatch or a watch with a second hand, time how long the one-point calibration takes for your analyzer. *Record the time on your laboratory report.* Pay attention to the sequence in which the reagents and gases are introduced into the analyzer. *Record the sequence of reagents and gases on your laboratory report.*

The following steps are usually involved in a one-point calibration:

1. Flush the pH electrode.
2. Expose the pH electrode to the high-pH buffer.
3. Allow sufficient time for the readings to stabilize.
4. Adjust the balance control.
5. Flush the sampling chamber.
6. Introduce the low-calibration gases.
7. Allow sufficient time for the readings to stabilize.
8. Adjust the PCO_2 and PO_2 balance controls.

9. Determine how often the machine performs a one-point calibration. *Record the frequency on your laboratory report.*

EXERCISE 22.1.3 Analysis of Quality Control Test Media

Three levels of controls must be analyzed every 8 hours and appropriately documented. Depending on the medium used, the medium may need to be anaerobically drawn up into sampling syringes before insertion into the blood gas analyzer. The following instructions are for media that come in small glass vials. If a different medium is used, follow the manufacturer's directions.

1. Apply latex or vinyl gloves and other standard precautions and transmission-based isolation procedures as applicable.
2. Perform a one-point calibration before analysis.
3. Verify the quality control medium expiration data and lot number.
4. Mix the quality control medium gently by swirling the vial. Break open the vial carefully, and draw up an anaerobic sample of the level I medium into a syringe using a 22- or 23-gauge needle, or aspirate directly into the analyzer's sampling tube. A glass ampule protection device may be used (Fig. 22.3).
5. Initiate the sampling sequence on your analyzer.
6. Insert the syringe into the sampling port. (On some analyzers this may require inserting the analyzer sampling tube into the syringe.)
7. Slowly inject the sample into the analyzer until a continuous line of the sample can be seen past the electrode block or until the machine indicates that enough blood has been introduced. Be certain that no air bubbles are introduced. In most modern machines less than 0.5 ml of sample is needed. In older machines 1 to 2 ml may be needed.
8. Allow sufficient time for the readings to stabilize.
9. *Record the results on your laboratory report.* Print out the results if a printer and blood gas recording slips are available.
10. Flush the sampling chamber. (This will be done automatically on most machines.)

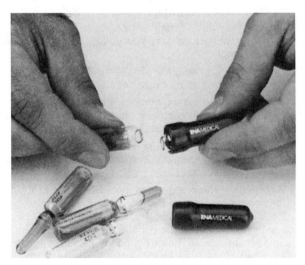

FIGURE 22.3 Glass ampule protection device. (Courtesy of RNA Medical, Division of Bionostics, Inc., Acton, MA.)

11. Discard the syringe in a sharps container.

12. Repeat the preceding steps with level II and level III and *record the results on your laboratory report.*

13. If the control levels are out of range, take corrective actions. *Record the actions taken on your laboratory report.*

14. Remove your gloves and discard them in an infectious waste container. Wash your hands.

EXERCISE 22.1.4 Trending of Quality Control Data: Levy-Jennings Plots

For the following exercise, you will need to obtain quality control data for a period of time and do statistical analysis.

1. Determine what method or methods of recording and analyzing quality control data are performed at your clinical site (manual or computerized). *Record this information on your laboratory report.*

2. Collect at least 2 days worth of quality control data for all shifts and levels. *Attach this information to your laboratory report.*

3. Obtain the lot number of the quality control medium and the acceptable ranges for quality control data for each level. *Record this information on your laboratory report.*

4. Obtain a printout or copy of a Levy-Jennings plot, as shown in Figure 22.4, from your clinical site for the time period in which you collected your data. *Attach it to your laboratory report. Identify any values that indicate random error, trending, or out-of-control data.*

EXERCISE 22.1.5 Blood Gas Analysis

Blood samples may not be readily available in a school laboratory setting. *Do not* introduce the red dye "blood" solution used in the arterial arm simulators into the blood gas analyzers. A saline or water solution or quality control medium may be used as a substitute for blood samples. *Record the type of specimen used on your lab report.*

1. Apply latex or vinyl gloves and other standard precautions and transmission-based isolation procedures as applicable. Gowns and goggles may be worn when dealing with human blood samples.

2. Perform a one-point calibration before blood analysis.

3. Remove the sample from the ice bath, and mix the blood sample by rolling it between your palms. Verify that it is an air-free sample.

4. Remove the cap from the sample syringe. Eject a small amount of blood into a gauze pad.

5. Initiate the sampling sequence on your analyzer. Analyzers interfaced with computers may require that patient data and other information be entered.

6. Insert the syringe into the sampling port. (On some analyzers this may require inserting the analyzer sampling tube into the syringe.)

7. Slowly inject the blood sample into the analyzer until a continuous line of blood can be seen past the electrode block or until the machine indicates that enough blood has been introduced. Be certain that no air bubbles or clots are introduced. In most modern machines less than 0.5 ml of blood is needed. In older machines 1 to 2 ml may be needed. In some newer models, the blood sample may be aspirated into the machine automatically.

8. Allow sufficient time for the readings to stabilize.

9. *Record the results on your laboratory report.* Print out the results if a printer and blood gas recording slips are available.

10. Flush the sampling chamber. (This will be done automatically on most machines.)

11. Discard the syringe in a sharps container.

12. Clean up any blood spills with a 1:10 solution of sodium hypochlorite (bleach) solution.

13. Remove your gloves and discard them in an infectious waste container. Wash your hands.

EXERCISE 22.1.6 Maintenance of a Blood Gas Analyzer

The steps required for daily and weekly preventive maintenance will vary depending on the type of analyzer and the level of automation. Refer to the operator's manual for specific sequences. All activities should be performed with appropriate standard precautions, including gloves, gowns, and goggles if blood splashing may occur.

Daily Maintenance

1. Empty or change the waste container. Modern analyzers may have disposable waste bottles. Remove the container and replace it with a new one. If a disposable container is not available, discard the waste in an infectious waste container, followed by a small amount of bleach. Rinse the container with hot water, pour a small amount of bleach into the container, and place it back onto the analyzer.

2. Check the calibration gas tank pressures.

3. Check the fluid and reagent levels.

4. Check the barometric pressure. Zero the base of the manometer if needed.

5. Verify that the water bath temperature is 37°C.

6. Check the water level in the humidifier (if applicable). Refill it if needed with sterile water.

7. Clean the sample port with a cotton swab and bleach solution or alcohol.

8. Debubble and dry the electrode chambers if disposable electrodes are not being used. Newer electrodes are maintenance free.

Weekly or Biweekly Maintenance

1. Insert a syringe with cleaning solution once per week. Allow it to sit in sampling chamber. Flush when complete.

2. Insert a sample of deproteinizing solution. Allow it to sit in the sampling chamber. Flush when complete.

3. Change the membranes. Newer electrodes on some brands of analyzers are maintenance free. The entire electrode block is replaced about once a year. Other brands have snap on membrane kits that are easier to remembrane. Figure 22.5 depicts a reference pH, PCO_2, and PO_2 electrode. The following steps are usually involved in membrane changing:
   a. Remove the electrode from the machine.
   b. Remove the old membrane, O-ring, and electrolyte solution.
   c. Rinse with sterile water.

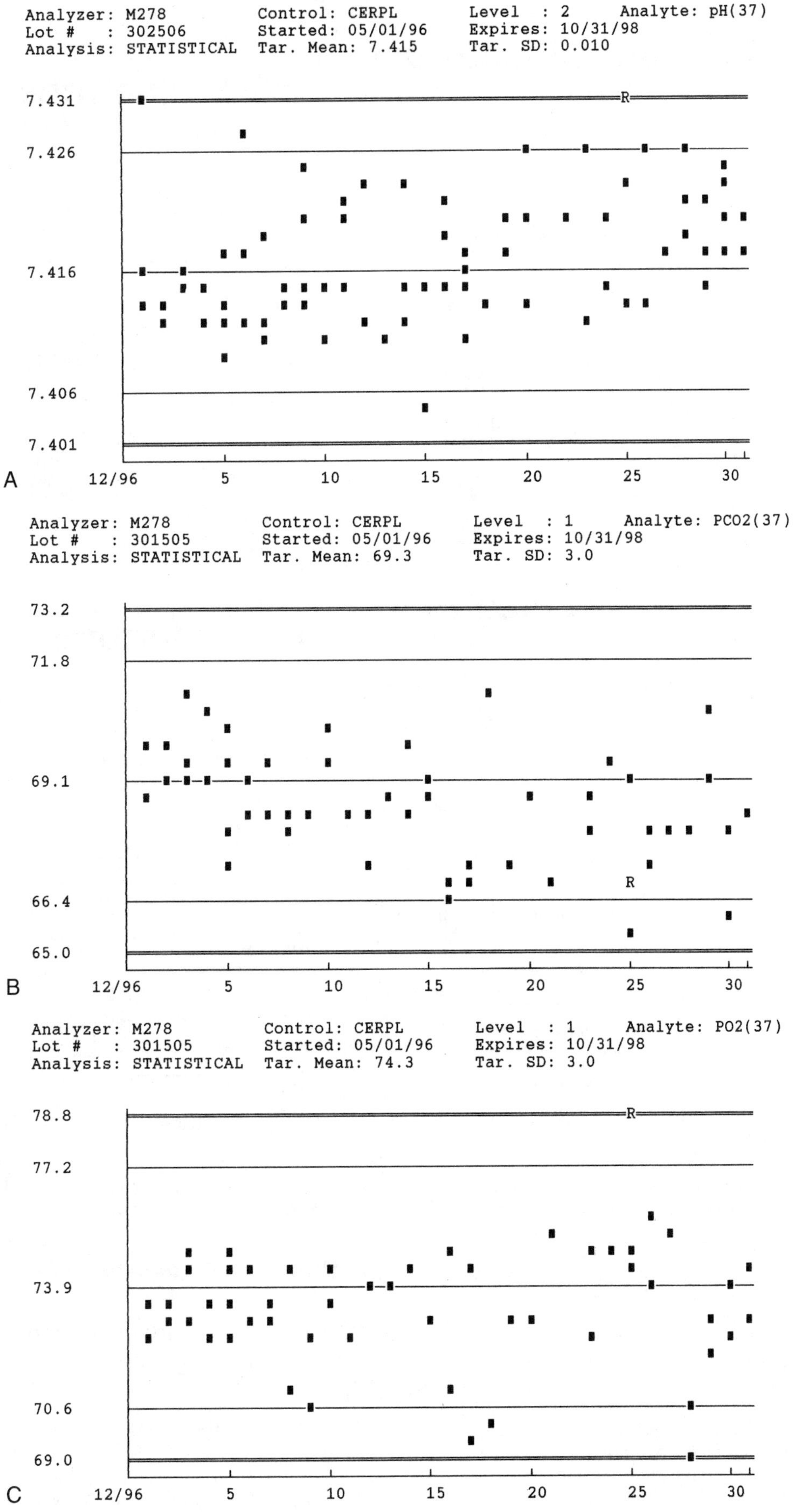

FIGURE 22.4   Sample Levy-Jennings plot. (Courtesy of Helen Hayes Hospital, W. Haverstraw, NY.)

Reference Electrodes

*p*CO$_2$ Electrode

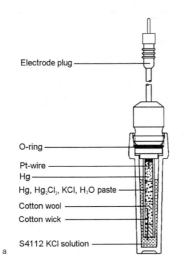

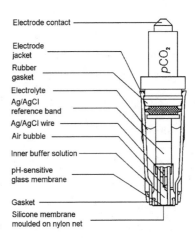

pH Electrode

*p*O$_2$ Electrode

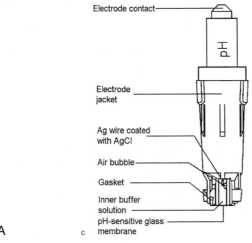

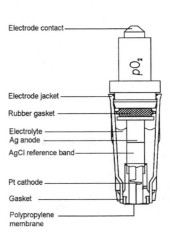

FIGURE 22.5   Schematic of pH, PCO$_2$, and PO$_2$ electrodes. (Courtesy of Radiometer America, Westlake, OH.)

d. The PO$_2$ electrode tip may be polished with a small amount of pumice on a gauze pad and then rinsed with sterile water.

e. Soak the electrode in the appropriate solution.

f. Place a new O-ring on the appropriate membrane changing tool and insert it into the holder.

g. Place a new membrane over the tool, letters down.

h. Place a drop of electrolyte on the membrane.

i. For the CO$_2$ electrode, place a nylon spacer over the tip of the electrode.

j. Insert the tip of the electrode into the tool and push down until the O-ring snaps into place.

k. Inspect the membrane and remove any wrinkles. Trim if necessary and remove the cardboard holder.

l. Fill the electrode with fresh electrolyte solution, leaving a 1-mm air bubble in the chamber.

m. Dry the outside of the electrode, and check for leaks. Place the "boot" over the tip of the membrane.

EXERCISE 22.2 Co-oximetry

EXERCISE 22.2.1 Identification of Controls for a Co-oximeter

1. Identify the brand of co-oximeter being used for this exercise, and *record it on your laboratory report.* Some brands of co-oximeters are depicted in Figure 22.6.

2. Identify the controls located on the control panel. *Record them on your laboratory report.* Draw a schematic representation of the location of these controls.

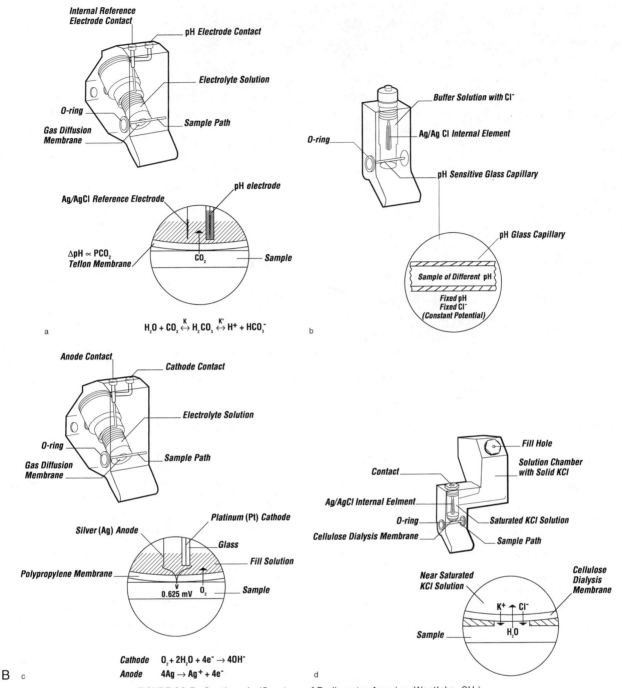

FIGURE 22.5, *Continued* (Courtesy of Radiometer America, Westlake, OH.)

3. Locate the reagents and waste receptacle. *Record which reagents are used for the co-oximeter on your laboratory report.*

EXERCISE 22.2.2 Calibration and Quality Controls for a Co-oximeter

The steps required for calibration and quality control media sampling will vary depending on the type of analyzer and the level of automation. Refer to the operator's manual for specific sequences. All activities should be performed with appropriate standard precautions and transmission-based isolation procedures, including gloves, gowns, and goggles if blood splashing may occur.

The following steps are usually involved for calibration and quality control for a co-oximeter:

1. Activate the flush.

2. Aspirate the sample chamber.

3. Alternate between flush and aspirate until all bubbles are removed from the fluidics.

4. Push the start button.

5. Insert the calibration sample into the sample port.

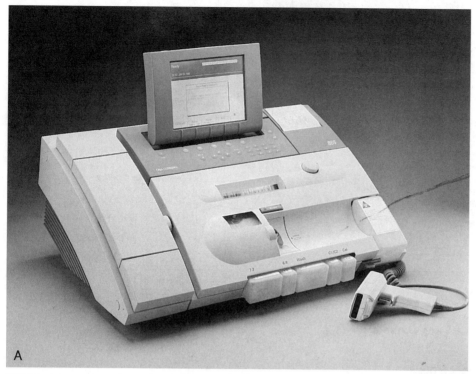

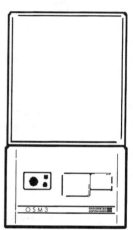

OSM™3 Hemoximeter™

FIGURE 22.6   Commonly used co-oximeters. (*[A]* Courtesy of Chiron Diagnostics Corporation, East Walpole, MA 02032; *[B]* drawing courtesy of Radiometer, Radiometer America, Westlake, OH.)

6. Once the readings stabilize, adjust the calibration value if necessary.

7. Repeat the procedure for the quality control media.

Related Readings

Eubanks, DH and Bone, RC: Principles and Applications of Cardiorespiratory Care Equipment. Mosby, St Louis, 1994.

Madama, V: Pulmonary Function Testing and Cardiopulmonary Stress Testing. Delmar, Albany, 1993.

McPherson, S: Respiratory Care Equipment, ed 5. Mosby, St Louis, 1995.

Scanlan, C et al (eds): Egan's Fundamentals of Respiratory Care, ed 6. Mosby, St Louis, 1995.

Shapiro, B et al: Clinical Application of Blood Gases, ed 5. Mosby–Year Book Medical Publishers, Chicago, 1993.

Wilkins, R, Sheldon, R and Krider, S: Clinical Assessment in Respiratory Care, ed 3. Mosby, St Louis, 1995.

Selected Journal Articles

American Association for Respiratory Care: AARC clinical practice guideline: In-vitro pH and blood gas analysis and hemoximetry. Respir Care 38:505–510, 1993.

American Association for Respiratory Care: AARC clinical practice guideline: Sampling for arterial blood gas analysis. Respir Care 37:913–917, 1992.

American Association for Respiratory Care: HIV related infection precautions for personnel providing ABG analysis. Respir Care 34:734, 1989.

Beasley, KE, Darrin, JM and Durbin, CG Jr: The effect of respiratory care department management of a blood gas analyzer on the appropriateness of arterial blood gas utilization. Respir Care 37:343–347, 1992.

CLIA '88 update: HCFA clarifies several issues. AARC Times 19:42–43, 1995.

Yost, JA: Questions and answers: Understanding CLIA '88 provisions. Lab Med 20:105, 1995.

LABORATORY REPORT

CHAPTER 22: ARTERIAL BLOOD GAS ANALYSIS AND MAINTENANCE

Name _____   Date _____

Course/Section _____   Instructor _____

Data Collection

EXERCISE 22.1   Blood Gas Analysis

EXERCISE 22.1.1   Identification of Components of Blood Gas Analyzers

1. Analyzer brand: _____

2. Control panel:

_____   _____

_____   _____

_____   _____

_____   _____

_____   _____

_____   _____

_____   _____

_____   _____

_____   _____

_____   _____

Schematic:

3. pH of the buffers:

_____

_____

4. Calibration gas pressures: _____

   Concentration of gases: _____

5. Water bath temperature: _____

   Bubbling rate: _____ /15 sec

6. Type of barometer: _____

7. Barometric pressure: _____

8. Calculation of calibration points: *Show your work!*

   P_B = _____

   Slope gases: CO_2 = _____ O_2 = _____

   Balance gases: CO_2 = _____ O_2 = _____

EXERCISE 22.1.2   Calibration of Blood Gas Analyzers

Duration (time) of two-point calibration: _____

Sequence for reagents in two-point calibration: _____

_____

_____

Frequency (time) between two-point calibrations:

_____

Duration of one-point calibration: _____

Sequence for reagents in one-point calibration: _____

_____

_____

Frequency of one-point calibration: _____

EXERCISE 22.1.3   Analysis of Quality Control Test Media

Type of quality control media used: _____

Level I	*Level II*	*Level III*
EXPECTED RANGES	EXPECTED RANGES	EXPECTED RANGES
pH: _____	pH: _____	pH: _____
PCO_2: _____	PCO_2: _____	PCO_2: _____
PO_2: _____	PO_2: _____	PO_2: _____
ACTUAL RESULTS	ACTUAL RESULTS	ACTUAL RESULTS
pH: _____	pH: _____	pH: _____
PCO_2: _____	PCO_2: _____	PCO_2: _____
PO_2: _____	PO_2: _____	PO_2: _____

Describe corrective actions (if applicable) if out of range:

_____

_____

EXERCISE 22.1.4   Trending of Quality Control Data: Levy-Jennings Plots

1. Method(s) of recording and analyzing quality control data

    Clinical site: _____

    Method(s) used: _____

2. Quality control data: _____

3. Lot number: _____

Acceptable ranges for quality control data

Level I	*Level II*	*Level III*
pH: _____	pH: _____	pH: _____
PCO_2: _____	PCO_2: _____	PCO_2: _____
PO_2: _____	PO_2: _____	PO_2: _____

4. Attach the Levy-Jennings plot. Identify any values on the attached plot that indicate
   a. Random error
   b. Trending
   c. Out of control

EXERCISE 22.1.5   Blood Gas Analysis

Type of specimen used: _____ Fio_2 _____

pH: _____

$PaCO_2$: _____

PaO_2: _____

HCO_3^-: _____

SaO_2: _____

EXERCISE 22.2   Co-oximetry

EXERCISE 22.2.1   Identification of Controls for a Co-oximeter

1. Brand of co-oximeter: _____

2. Control panel:

_____   _____

_____   _____

_____   _____

_____   _____

_____   _____

_____   _____

_____   _____

_____   _____

_____   _____

_____   _____

Schematic:

3. Reagents used for the cooximeter: _____

CRITICAL THINKING QUESTIONS

1. For each of the following, *identify* what it measures, *describe* the components of the device, and *explain* its principle of operation.
   a. Sanz electrode
   b. Severinghaus electrode
   c. Clark electrode
   d. Co-oximeter

2. What effect will a water bath temperature of less than 37°C have on the measured pH, $PaCO_2$, and PaO_2? What effect will a water bath temperature of greater than 37°C have on the measured pH, $PaCO_2$, and PaO_2? Whose gas law explains this?

3. Why is it important to eject a small amount of blood from the syringe sample onto a gauze pad before injecting the sample into the machine?

4. Under what circumstances and how often should a two-point calibration be performed on a blood gas analyzer? A one-point calibration?

5. Given a barometric pressure of 750 mm Hg, calculate the calibration points for the following *(show your work!)*:
   a. 10% CO_2 and 0% oxygen
   b. 5% CO_2 and 12% oxygen
   c. 20% oxygen and 12% CO_2

6. List five common causes of inaccurate results obtained from blood gas sampling and analysis.

7. A patient is being treated for smoke inhalation and third-degree burns. Silvadene has been applied to large portions of the patient's body surface. How might the patient's condition affect the analysis of blood for co-oximetry?

8. Identify three factors that would make the reading of a co-oximeter unreliable.

PROCEDURAL COMPETENCY EVALUATION

Name _____   Date _____

Arterial Blood Gas Calibration, Maintenance, and Quality Assurance

Setting: ☐ Lab ☐ Clinical   Evaluator: ☐ Peer ☐ Instructor

Conditions (describe): _____

_____

Equipment Used

_____

_____

	SATISFACTORY	UNSATISFACTORY	NOT OBSERVED	NOT APPLICABLE
Preparation				
1. Applies personal protective equipment and performs daily maintenance				
a. Checks fluid level of pH and flush	☐	☐	☐	☐
b. Checks cal and slope tanks and gas flow	☐	☐	☐	☐
c. Checks levels of humidifiers	☐	☐	☐	☐
d. Empties waste bottle	☐	☐	☐	☐
e. Inserts daily cleaner	☐	☐	☐	☐
2. Calibrates blood gas analyzer				
a. Obtains correct barometric pressure	☐	☐	☐	☐
b. Performs a two-point calibration going from low-high buffer (pH), then from low gas–high gas (PCO_2 and PO_2); using the following formula, calculates correct gas values: $(BP - 47) \times \%\text{gas in tank} = \text{mm Hg}$ to be calibrated	☐	☐	☐	☐
3. Inserts three levels of quality control (acidosis, normal, alkalosis); ensures proper calibration of ABG analyzer	☐	☐	☐	☐
4. Electrode maintenance				
a. Replaces the pH reference PCO_2 and PO_2 membranes every 2 weeks	☐	☐	☐	☐
b. Obtains equipment	☐	☐	☐	☐
c. Remembranes following procedure manual; fills with electrolyte solution; cleans out chamber and puts electrode back	☐	☐	☐	☐
(1) PCO_2: removes from machine, empties solution, and removes membrane; cleans and remembranes following procedure manual for the machine; fills with electrolyte solution; cleans out electrode chamber and puts electrode back	☐	☐	☐	☐
(2) PO_2 electrodes: removes from machine, empties solution, and removes membrane; cleans and remembranes according to procedure manual for machine; fills with electrolyte solution; cleans out electrode chamber and puts electrode back	☐	☐	☐	☐
5. Calibrates the machine	☐	☐	☐	☐
6. Performs quality control	☐	☐	☐	☐
7. Documents results according to departmental policy	☐	☐	☐	☐

_____   _____
Signature of Evaluator   Signature of Student

PERFORMANCE RATING SCALE

5 EXCELLENT—FAR EXCEEDS EXPECTED LEVEL, FLAWLESS PERFORMANCE
4 ABOVE AVERAGE—NO PROMPTING REQUIRED, ABLE TO SELF-CORRECT
3 AVERAGE—THE MINIMUM COMPETENCY LEVEL, NO CRITICAL ERRORS
2 IMPROVEMENT NEEDED—PROBLEM AREAS EXIST; CRITICAL ERRORS, CORRECTIONS NEEDED
1 POOR AND UNACCEPTABLE PERFORMANCE—GROSS INACCURACIES, POTENTIALLY HARMFUL

PERFORMANCE CRITERIA	SCALE				
1. DISPLAYS KNOWLEDGE OF ESSENTIAL CONCEPTS	5	4	3	2	1
2. DEMONSTRATES THE RELATIONSHIP BETWEEN THEORY AND CLINICAL PRACTICE	5	4	3	2	1
3. FOLLOWS DIRECTIONS, EXHIBITS SOUND JUDGMENT, AND DEMONSTRATES ATTENTION TO SAFETY AND DETAIL	5	4	3	2	1
4. EXHIBITS THE REQUIRED MANUAL DEXTERITY	5	4	3	2	1
5. PERFORMS PROCEDURE IN A REASONABLE TIME FRAME	5	4	3	2	1
6. MAINTAINS STERILE OR ASEPTIC TECHNIQUE	5	4	3	2	1
7. INITIATES UNAMBIGUOUS GOAL-DIRECTED COMMUNICATION	5	4	3	2	1
8. PROVIDES FOR ADEQUATE CARE AND MAINTENANCE OF EQUIPMENT AND SUPPLIES	5	4	3	2	1
9. EXHIBITS COURTEOUS AND PLEASANT DEMEANOR	5	4	3	2	1
10. MAINTAINS CONCISE AND ACCURATE RECORDS	5	4	3	2	1

ADDITIONAL COMMENTS: INCLUDE ERRORS OF OMISSION OR COMMISSION, COMMUNICATIVE SKILLS, AND EFFECTIVENESS OF PATIENT INTERACTION:

SUMMARY PERFORMANCE EVALUATION AND RECOMMENDATIONS

SATISFACTORY PERFORMANCE—Performed without error or prompting, or able to self-correct, no critical errors.

_____ LABORATORY EVALUATION. SKILLS MAY BE APPLIED/OBSERVED IN THE CLINICAL SETTING.

_____ CLINICAL EVALUATION. STUDENT READY FOR MINIMALLY SUPERVISED APPLICATION AND REFINEMENT.

UNSATISFACTORY PERFORMANCE—Prompting required; performed with critical errors, potentially harmful.

_____ STUDENT REQUIRES ADDITIONAL LABORATORY PRACTICE.

_____ STUDENT REQUIRES ADDITIONAL SUPERVISED CLINICAL PRACTICE.

SIGNATURES

STUDENT: _____   EVALUATOR: _____

DATE: _____   DATE: _____

Pulmonary Function Testing

The development and use of advanced medical techniques have allowed people to live longer, particularly patients with lung disease and victims of major trauma. Because of these medical advances, more people with severe respiratory disease, and other diseases with respiratory complications, are accessing medical care. It therefore became necessary to develop sophisticated methods to objectively measure the function of the respiratory system in order to better evaluate these individuals.

Many lung diseases develop insidiously over time. The pulmonary system has a significant amount of functional reserve so that a large degree of dysfunction can occur through illness or injury[1] before outward signs and symptoms are noted. Detection of lung dysfunction is important for the diagnosis, prevention, treatment, and rehabilitation of patients with lung disease.

Pulmonary function testing (PFT) is a series of diagnostic tests devised to evaluate all aspects of respiratory system function, including,[1] but not limited to, the following:

1. Ventilatory volumes and capacities
2. Airway integrity through measurement of flows and resistance
3. Respiratory muscle strength
4. Mechanical properties of lungs and thoracic cage
5. Efficiency of gas exchange and function of A/C membrane
6. Exercise response
7. Response to irritants and bronchoactive drugs

The goals of pulmonary function testing include the following[2,3]:

1. Determine absence or presence of pulmonary disease abnormalities
2. Allow for earlier detection and intervention
3. Measure the severity of the disorder (degree of impairment and extent of disability—how it affects daily activities)
4. Characterize the type of pathophysiology
5. Follow the course of disease and progression
6. Measure response to therapy regimens and rehabilitation efforts
7. Preoperative evaluation—determine surgical risk for postoperative pulmonary complications

Pulmonary function testing has some limitations. One cannot identify specific diseases entirely without other correlating information such as the patient's history and physical examination and other diagnostic tests. The variable sensitivity of pulmonary function tests and the large **variability** of what is considered normal make early detection difficult.

Four factors that play an important role in determining the **validity** and **reliability** of pulmonary function testing are equipment use, technician competence, level of patient cooperation and effort, and **reproducibility** of the results. Standards for equipment and test performance help minimize variability and improve the reliability and validity of the test results.

Many different testing protocols, including bedside assessment, screening, complete testing, and specialized testing, are performed for various indications. This chapter focuses on simple spirometry, screening, protocols, flow-volume loops, and postbronchodilator studies.

1. Practice communication skills needed for the active forceful coaching instruction of subjects performing a forced vital capacity (FVC) maneuver.
2. Practice medical charting for maintaining legal records of pulmonary function results.
3. Apply infection control guidelines and standards associated with equipment and procedures, according to OSHA regulations and CDC guidelines.

4. Calibrate and maintain volume displacement and flow sensing spirometry equipment.

5. Perform valid and reliable pulmonary function testing of a slow vital capacity (SVC) and FVC maneuver, postbronchodilator study, and maximum voluntary ventilation (MVV) according to American Thoracic Society (ATS) guidelines for spirometry.

6. Interpret graphic representations of volume-time and flow-volume tracings of FVC maneuvers.

7. Manually calculate the FVC, FEV_1, $FEF_{25\%-75\%}$, predicted values, and percent predicted values for a valid spirogram.

8. Interpret pulmonary function testing results.

9. Define the four lung volumes and four lung capacities and analyze their interrelationships.

KEY TERMS

accuracy	extrathoracic	precision	specificity
calibration	intersection	regression equation	standard deviation
discrimination	kymograph	reliability	transducer
displacement	nomogram	reproducibility	validity
extrapolation	plateau	resolution	variability
	pneumotachometer	sensitivity	

EQUIPMENT REQUIRED

- Volume **displacement** spirometers
- Disposable mouthpieces
- Main large-bore tubing
- Flow sensing spirometers
- Disposable flow sensors or in-line filters
- Disposable noseclips
- Calibrated graph paper
- Marking pens
- Chair
- Centigrade thermometer
- 3-L calibration syringe and adaptors
- Unit-dose bronchodilators
- Small volume nebulizer, connecting tubing, and gas source
- Metric rulers
- Tissues
- Medical waste receptacles
- Pencils
- Calculators
- Stopwatch
- BTPS conversion charts
- Predicted values tables or **nomograms**

● E X E R C I S E S

EXERCISE 23.1 Equipment Identification

EXERCISE 23.1.1 Identification of Volume Displacement Spirometers

Identify the types of volume displacement spirometers shown in Figure 23.1, and *record them on your laboratory report.*

EXERCISE 23.1.2 Identification of Flow Sensing Spirometers (Pneumotachometers)

Identify the types of flow sensing spirometers (**pneumotachometers**) shown in Figure 23.2, and *record them on your laboratory report.*

EXERCISE 23.2 Calibration and Maintenance of Spirometric Equipment

1. Identify the type of spirometer and brand used, and *record it on your laboratory report.*

2. Check to make sure you have an adequate paper supply. Note the paper speed of the machine used (**calibration** in mm/sec), and *record it on your laboratory report.*

3. Check to make sure the recording pen (if applicable) is functional and that spares are available.

4. Plug the unit in, if applicable. If a computerized device is used, follow the manufacturer's instructions to enter the date and time.

5. If a volume displacement spirometer is used, check the unit for leaks by occluding the main inlet and attempting to move the piston/bell/bellows connection where the recording pen attaches. No movement should be observed if no leaks are present.

6. Attach the main tubing and repeat step 5. If a leak is detected, check the tubing for holes or tears and replace as necessary.

7. If possible, turn on the recording device and make sure the pen is recording on the baseline.

8. Check the room temperature. Enter it into your computerized spirometer as applicable. *Record the temperature in both Fahrenheit and Celsius on your laboratory report.*

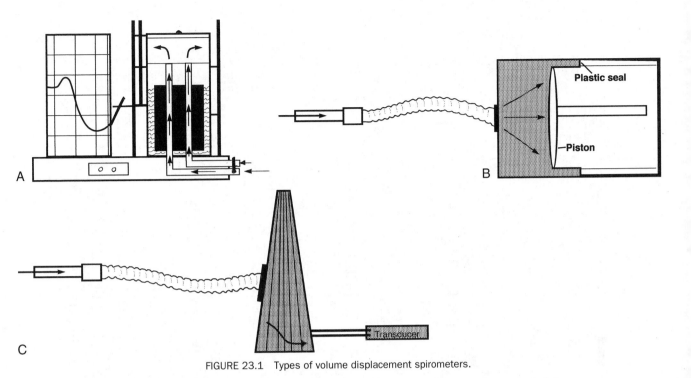

FIGURE 23.1   Types of volume displacement spirometers.

FIGURE 23.2   Types of flow sensing spirometers. (Courtesy of *[A]* Nellcor Puritan Bennett Corporation, Carlsbad, CA.)

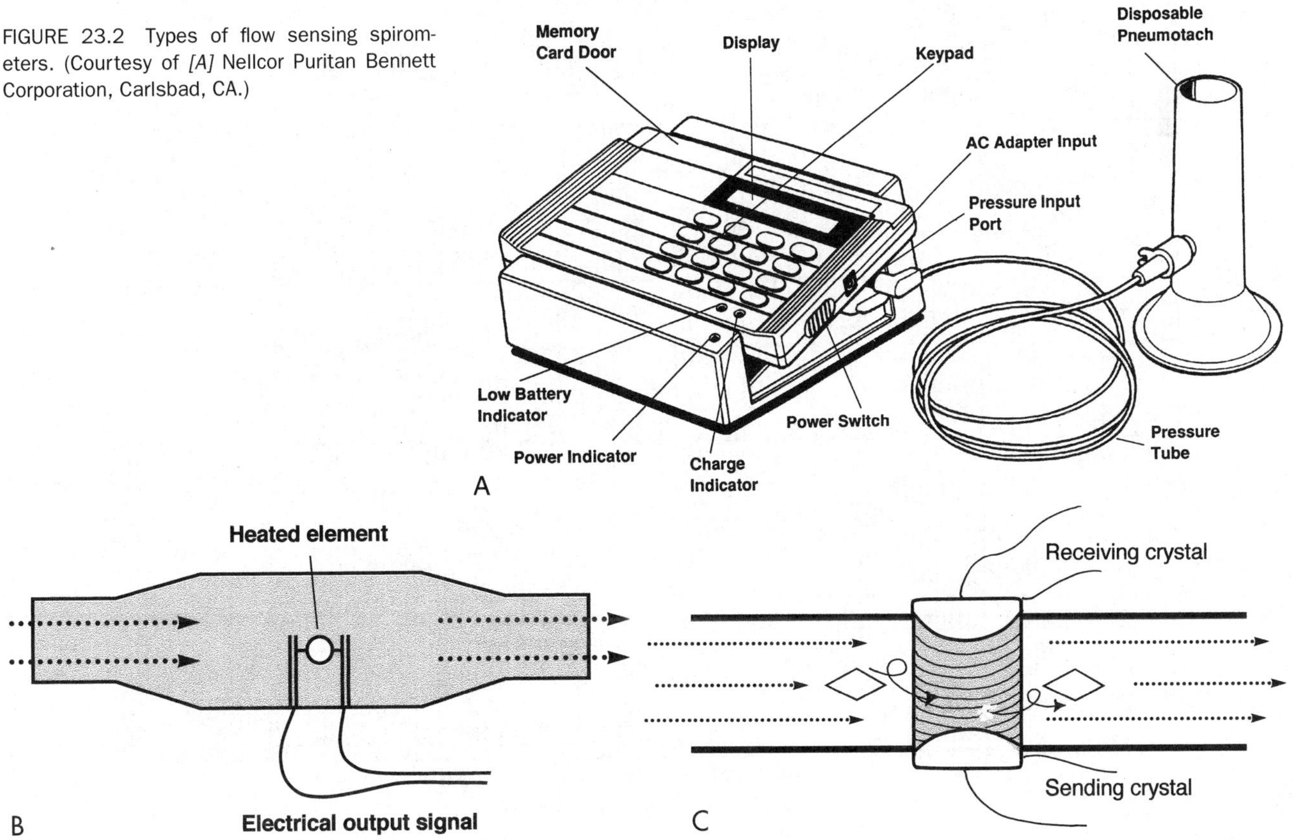

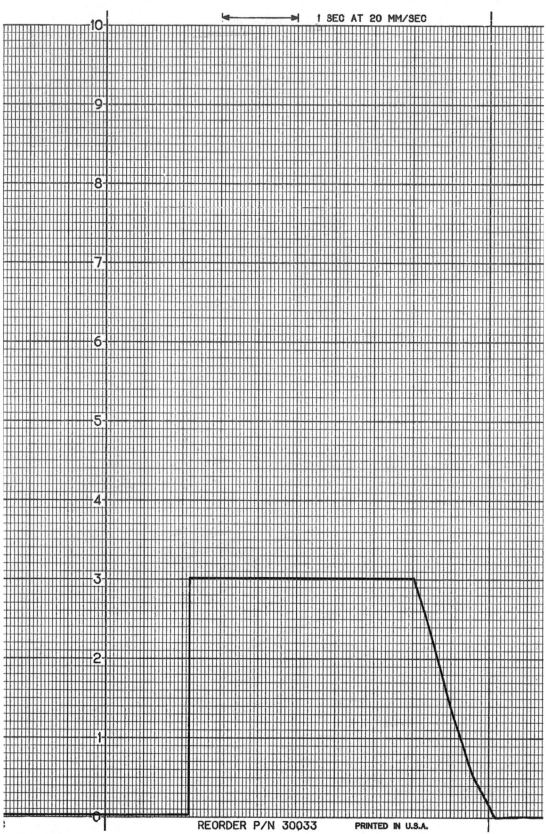

FIGURE 23.3   Calibration tracing.

9. Using a 3-L calibration syringe, check the spirometer for **accuracy.**
   a. Turn the machine on and enter the calibration mode, if applicable, on a computerized machine.
   b. Pull ‘back the plunger to set the syringe to the 3-L volume.
   c. Attach the syringe (an adaptor may be required) securely to the main tubing or flow sensing device.
   d. Start the recording device or activate the machine according to manufacturer's directions, and push the entire 3-L volume into the device. The calibration tracing will appear as shown in Figure 23.3.
   e. *Record the measured volume on your laboratory report.* According to ATS standards, the spirometer must be accurate to 3 percent of the calibrating volume or ±50 ml, whichever is greater.[4]
   f. Calculate the percent accuracy of your measurement by the following formula, and *record it on your laboratory report:*

   $$\frac{\text{Measured volume} - 3\ \text{L}}{3\ \text{L}} \times 100 = \text{Percent accuracy}$$

   g. Repeat the calibration while varying the speed at which the calibration volume is injected. *Record your observations of how fast or slow the volume is injected and the effects on the calibration volume on your laboratory report.*

h. For volume displacement spirometers using a kymograph recording device, verify the time calibration by checking the paper speed using a stopwatch. Make a mark on your recording paper. Simultaneously start the recording device and activate the stopwatch. At exactly 10 sec, simultaneously stop the recording and the stopwatch. Verify that 10 sec of recording paper have been used.

EXERCISE 23.3 Respiratory History

Using your lab partner as the patient, obtain a baseline spirometry screening test. This involves obtaining three valid, reproducible FVC maneuvers that meet all ATS standards for spirometry. A screening should not be performed on anyone with an acute illness.

1. Introduce yourself and your department to your subject.
2. Briefly explain the purpose of the test and confirm your subject's understanding by having the subject repeat the instructions back to you.
3. *Have your subject record his or her information on his or her own laboratory report. Record your information on your laboratory report.* Although you will be performing testing on your laboratory partner, for purposes of student confi-

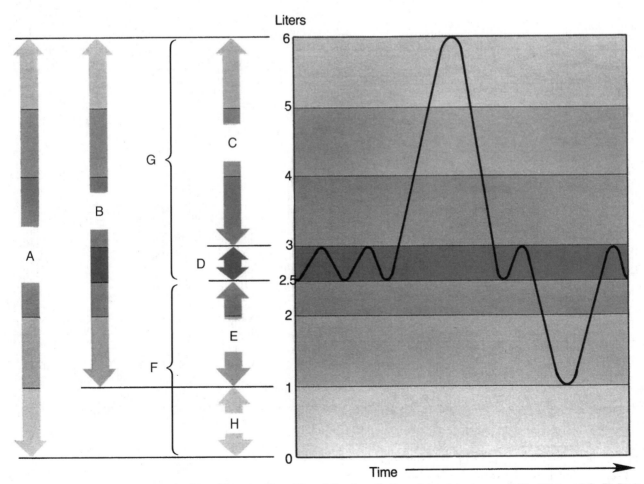

FIGURE 23.4 Lung volumes and capacities. (From Scanlon, VC and Sanders, T: Essentials of Anatomy and Physiology, ed 2. FA Davis, Philadelphia, 1991, p. 349, with permission.)

dentiality, *use only your own information and test results for your laboratory report.*

a. Name and identification number
b. Age on day of testing
c. Height in stocking feet
d. Gender
e. Race (indicate white or nonwhite for purposes of race correction according to NIOSH and OSHA regulations for spirometry)

4. Determine whether previous testing has ever been done and whether it was done sitting or standing. *Record the information on your laboratory report.*

5. Elicit a respiratory history by asking your subject the following questions. *Record the information on your laboratory report.*

   a. Do you usually have a cough first thing in the morning? Do you cough up any secretions? If so, how much and what color is it usually?

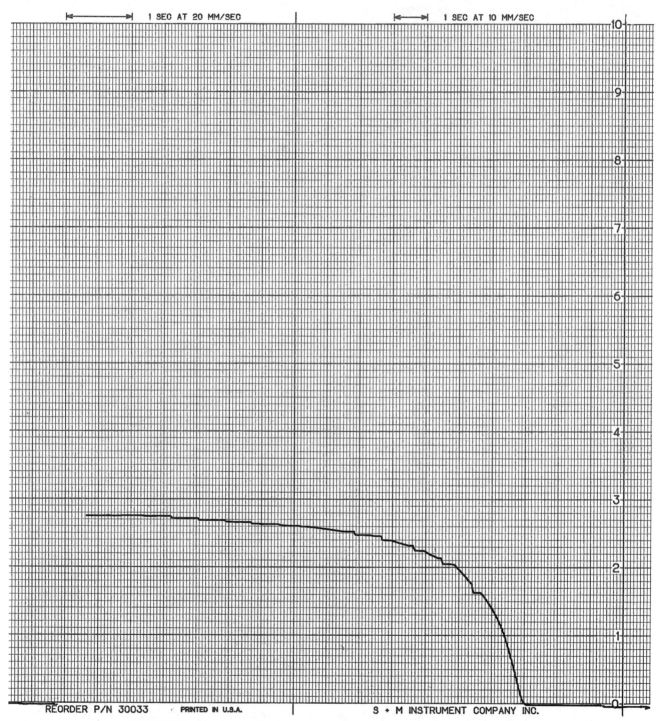

FIGURE 23.5 Cough or glottic closure on a volume-time tracing. Shown at reduced size.

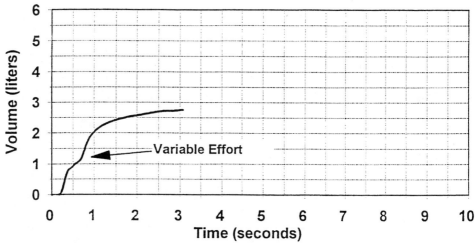

FIGURE 23.6 Variable effort on a volume-time tracing.

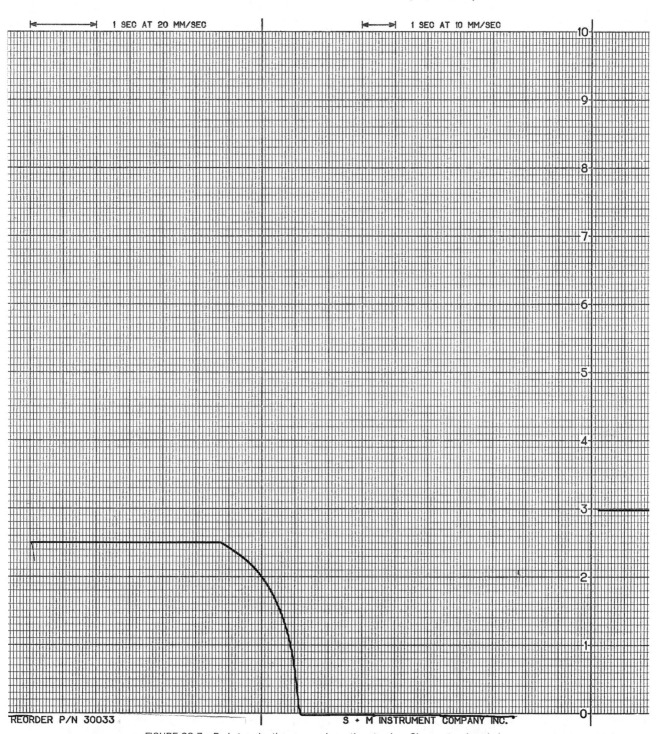

FIGURE 23.7 Early termination on a volume-time tracing. Shown at reduced size.

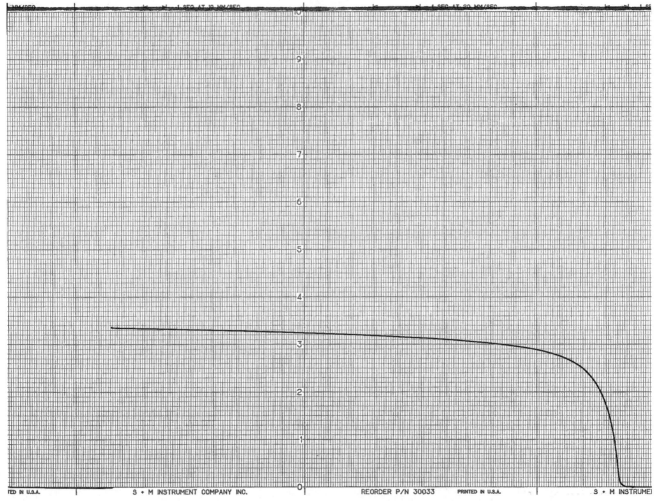

FIGURE 23.8 Failure to plateau on a volume-time tracing. Shown at reduced size.

b. Do you cough for as much as 3 months a year?
c. Do you ever experience chest tightness, wheezing, shortness of breath on exertion or at rest, or chest pain? Describe quality and location. Are you having any chest pain now?
d. Have you ever had or been told you have asthma, allergies, pneumonia, chronic bronchitis, emphysema, or tuberculosis?
e. Do you have a heart condition for which you are under a doctor's care?
f. Do you take or have you ever taken prescription medicine for a respiratory or cardiac illness? If so, what medications?
g. Do you take nonprescription medicine for a respiratory illness?
h. Smoking history:
   (1) Have you ever smoked?
   (2) Do you smoke now?
   (3) How many packs of cigarettes do/did you smoke per day?
   (4) How old were you when you started smoking?
   (5) How long ago did you quit smoking?
   (6) How many years/months have you been smoking?
   (7) Calculate the subject's pack/year history: [(Age now − Age started smoking) − years since stopped smoking] × packs per day = pack/years. *Show your work and answer on your laboratory report.*

i. Occupational history:
   (1) What type of work do you presently do?
   (2) What other types of work have you done in the past?
   (3) Have you ever worked in mining, construction, or with insulation? Have you ever been exposed to dusts, fumes, or mists at work?
j. Family history: list ages, state of health, age at death, and cause of death for mother, father, and siblings.

EXERCISE 23.4 Spirometry Screening

NOTE: The following exercises should be done with a volume displacement spirometer if available so that hand calculation of the results can be practiced as part of the laboratory exercises. It should then be repeated with a flow sensing spirometer as well so students gain experience with both types of equipment. Also, each student must practice being both tester and subject in order to have appropriate data to complete the laboratory report.

EXERCISE 23.4.1 Identification of Lung Volumes and Capacities

Identify the lung volumes and capacities labeled in Figure 23.4. *Record them on your laboratory report.*

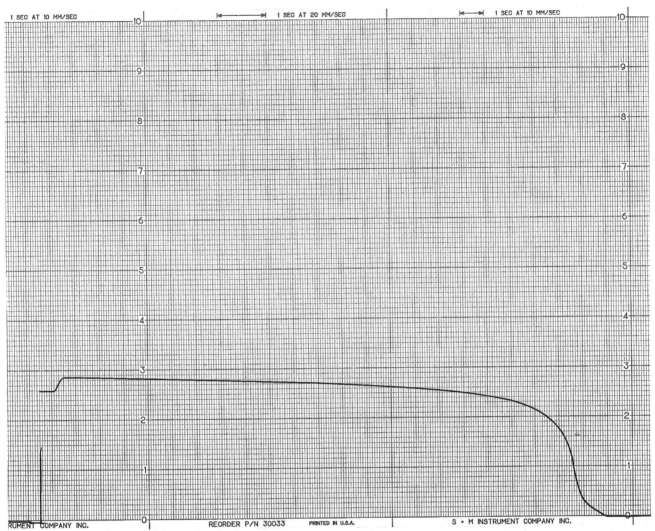

FIGURE 23.9   Hesitation at the start of the test on a volume-time tracing. Shown at reduced size.

EXERCISE 23.4.2 Measuring Spirometric Lung Volumes and Capacities

1. Wash your hands and apply standard precautions and transmission-based isolation procedures as applicable.

2. Aseptically take a clean disposable mouthpiece or flow sensing device and attach it to the main tubing. If disposable pneumotachometers are used, each one should be calibrated before use in testing.

3. Instruct the subject in the performance of a simple spirogram. Instruct the subject, when indicated, to place

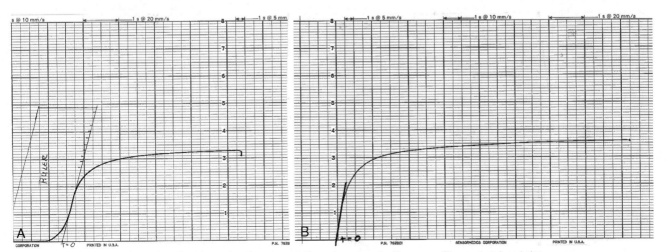

FIGURE 23.10   Measuring the extrapolation volumes under the curve. Shown at reduced size.

the mouthpiece tightly between the teeth with the lips sealed, without the tongue blocking the opening and without biting down, and to relax and breathe normally in and out for five or six breaths. Observe for consistency of tidal volume and breathing pattern. Instruct the subject to take the deepest breath possible and then blow it out *slowly* until you say to stop. Confirm your subject's understanding by having the subject repeat the instructions back to you.

4. Place the noseclips on the subject and verify that there are no leaks. If the subject refuses to use the noseclips, have the subject hold his or her nose if possible.

5. Have the subject sit or stand straight, chin slightly elevated. If the subject is obese, pregnant, or a child, the test should be performed standing. A chair without wheels should be placed behind the subject under these circumstances for safety.

6. Have the subject begin tidal breathing until a relaxed pattern is noted, and then activate the machine and the recording device. Reinforce instructions throughout the test. Record five or six tidal breaths.

7. Actively coach the subject throughout inspiration and expiration to perform the SVC maneuver. At the end of a normal exhalation, instruct the subject to take a maximal inspiration until the lungs are completely full and then exhale slowly until the lungs are completely empty. Remind the subject to continue exhaling until instructed to stop.

8. Observe the subject for adequate effort and proper performance during the maneuver. Reinstruct as necessary.

9. Remove the noseclips and allow the subject to be seated if needed between tests.

10. *Have the subject sign the tracing. Record the room temperature on your laboratory report. Attach the spirogram tracing to the subject's laboratory report. From the spirogram, calculate the values listed on the laboratory report.*

EXERCISE 23.4.3 Performance of Slow Vital Capacity and Forced Vital Capacity Maneuvers

1. Determine whether there are any contraindications to the performance of a baseline spirometry screening at this time by asking the subject the following questions (the mnemonic "FRED'S SAFE" may help you remember them):
   a. (F) Have you had upper respiratory tract illness, in*f*luenza, or bronchitis within the last 3 weeks?
   b. (R) Are you wearing any tight or *r*estrictive clothing that may interfere with the performance of the test?
   c. (E) Have you *e*aten a heavy meal within the last 2 hours?
   d. (D) Do you have any *d*ental appliances, loose teeth, caps, gum, or candy in your mouth? Note that dentures should usually be left in place to allow for an adequate seal around the mouthpiece unless they are so loose that they may come out during the test.
   e. (S) Have you *s*moked within the last hour?
   f. (S) Have you had any recent *s*urgeries?
   g. (A) Have you used an *a*erosolized bronchodilator within the last 4 to 6 hours?
   h. (F) How are you *f*eeling today? Do you have any acute illness at the present time?
   i. (E) Have you had any *e*ar infections in the last 3 weeks?

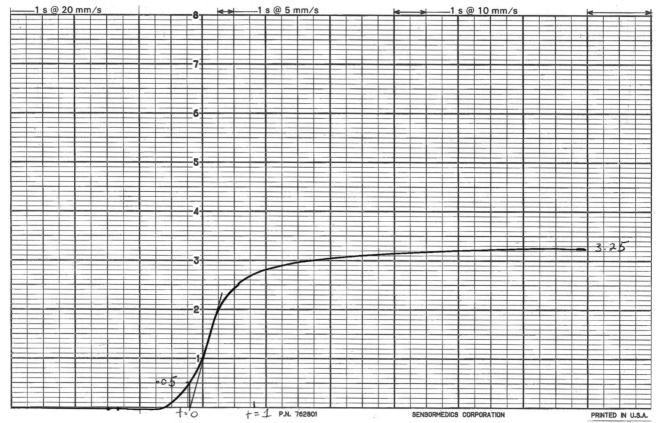

FIGURE 23.11   Measuring the FEV$_1$ by measuring the 1-sec distance from the zero point. Shown at reduced size.

2. If a positive response is obtained to any of the preceding questions, the problem should be corrected or screening spirometry should be postponed for the appropriate length of time. The subject must be free from any acute illness for at least 3 weeks before screening.[5]

3. Wash your hands and apply standard precautions and transmission-based isolation procedures as applicable.

4. Aseptically take a clean disposable mouthpiece or flow sensing device and attach it to the main tubing. If disposable pneumotachometers are used, each one should be calibrated before use in testing.

5. Instruct the subject in the performance of the SVC maneuver. Explain (and demonstrate, if necessary) the following:
   a. When you indicate, the subject should take as deep a breath as possible, completely filling his or her lungs.

b. The subject should place the mouthpiece tightly between the teeth with the lips sealed, without the tongue blocking the opening and without biting down.

c. Without hesitation, the subject should then *slowly* blow the air out until the lungs are as completely empty as possible, until you say to stop.

6. Confirm your subject's understanding by having the subject repeat the instructions back to you.

7. Place the noseclips on the subject and verify that there are no leaks. If the subject refuses to use the noseclips, have the subject hold his or her nose if possible.

8. Have the subject sit or stand straight, chin slightly elevated. If the subject is obese, pregnant, or a child, the test should be performed standing. A chair without wheels should be placed behind the subject under these circumstances for safety.

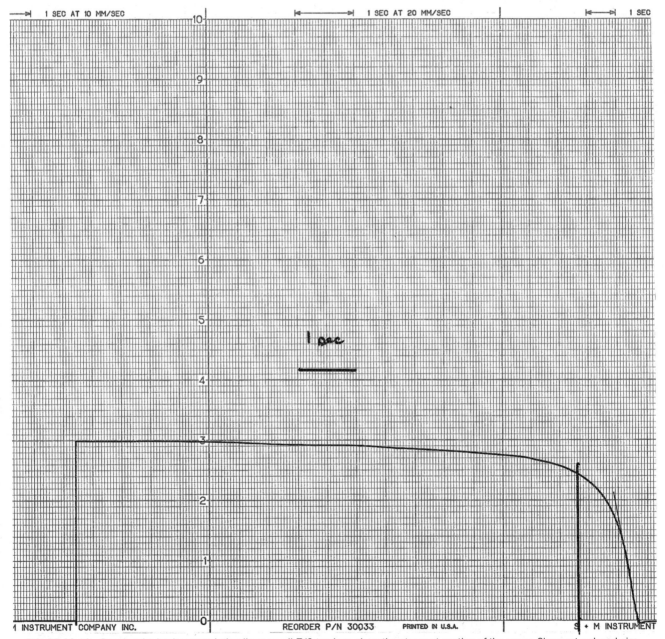

FIGURE 23.12   Drawing the back extrapolation lines on all FVC tracings along the steepest portion of the curve. Shown at reduced size.

9. Activate the machine and the recording device. Actively coach the subject throughout inspiration and expiration, and perform the SVC.

10. Observe the subject for adequate effort and proper performance during the maneuver. Reinstruct as necessary.

11. Note the volume obtained and *record it on your laboratory report.*

12. Allow for adequate recovery of the subject. Remove the noseclips and allow the subject to be seated if needed between tests.

13. Replace the noseclips, reinstruct the subject, and repeat the SVC maneuver with active, forceful coaching until three tracings of consistent volume are observed. The two best volumes should be within 200 ml or 5 percent.

14. Instruct the subject in the performance of the FVC maneuver. Explain (and demonstrate, if necessary) the following:
    a. When you indicate, the subject should take as deep a breath as possible, completely filling his or her lungs.
    b. The subject should place the mouthpiece tightly between the teeth with the lips sealed, without the tongue blocking the opening and without biting down.
    c. Without hesitation, the subject should then blow the air out as hard, fast, and completely as possible, until you say to stop.

15. Confirm your subject's understanding by having the subject repeat the instructions back to you.

16. Place the noseclips on the subject and verify that there are no leaks. If the subject refuses to use the noseclips, have the subject hold his or her nose if possible.

17. Have the subject sit or stand straight, chin slightly elevated. If the subject is obese, pregnant, or a child, the test should be performed standing. A chair without wheels should be placed behind the subject under these circumstances for safety.

18. Activate the machine and the recording device. Actively coach the subject throughout inspiration and expiration, and perform the FVC.

19. Observe the subject for adequate effort and proper performance during the maneuver. Reinstruct as necessary.

20. Note the volume obtained, the shape, and the appearance of the graphic representation, if available.

21. Allow for adequate recovery of the subject. Remove the noseclips and allow the subject to be seated if needed between tests.

22. Verify that the results meet ATS standards for acceptability. The FVC tracings should be free from the following[6]:
    a. Cough or glottic closure (Fig. 23.5).
    b. Variable effort (Fig. 23.6).
    c. Early termination (Fig. 23.7). A **plateau** should be achieved and is defined as no change in volume in the last 1 sec of the tracing. The test should be at least 6 sec in duration. In subjects with severe chronic obstructive lung disease, the spirometer should be capable of recording for at least 15 sec. Failure to plateau is shown in Figure 23.8.
    d. Hesitation at the start of the test (Fig. 23.9). Extrapolated volume must be less than 5 percent of the FVC or 150 ml, whichever is greater.
    e. Baseline error or leaks.
    f. Excessive variability. There should be less than 5 percent or 200 ml difference between the two best FVC and FEV_1 results. The 1994 ATS standards require less

than 200 ml; however, this variability may be excessive with smaller lung volumes.[5,6]

23. It is advisable to have the subject sign and date the spirometric tracing, due to the often litigious nature of pulmonary disability or workers' compensation cases. *Attach it to his or her laboratory report.*

24. Repeat spirometry with a flow sensing computerized spirometer. *Attach the subject's results to his or her laboratory report for comparison.*

25. Discard any disposable noseclips, mouthpieces, or flow sensors in an infectious waste container when testing is completed. Disinfect any nondisposable mouthpieces and tubings when finished with the laboratory.

EXERCISE 23.5 Calculation of Spirometric Results

Using your own graph obtained from a volume displacement spirometer, calculate the following. *Show your work and record the results on your laboratory report.*

1. Determine validity as indicated by three acceptable FVC tracings free from the following:
   Cough or glottic closure
   Early termination of expiration
   Variable effort
   Baseline error
   Excessive hesitation at start of test

2. Measure the SVC at the highest point of the plateau.

3. Measure the FVC in each tracing at the highest point of the plateau.
   a. No excessive variability: two best curves within 5 percent or 100 ml, whichever is greater.

$$\frac{\text{Volume A (largest)} - \text{Volume B}}{\text{Volume A (largest)}} \times 100 = \text{Percent}$$

   b. Select the largest FVC.

TABLE 23.1 **BTPS Conversion Factors**

Gas Temperature °C (ATPS)	Conversion Factor
18	1.114
19	1.111
20	1.102
21	1.096
22	1.091
23	1.085
24	1.080
25	1.075
26	1.068
27	1.063
28	1.057
29	1.051
30	1.045
31	1.039
32	1.032
33	1.026
34	1.020
35	1.014
36	1.007
37	1.000

$$°C = 5 \frac{(°F - 32)}{9}$$

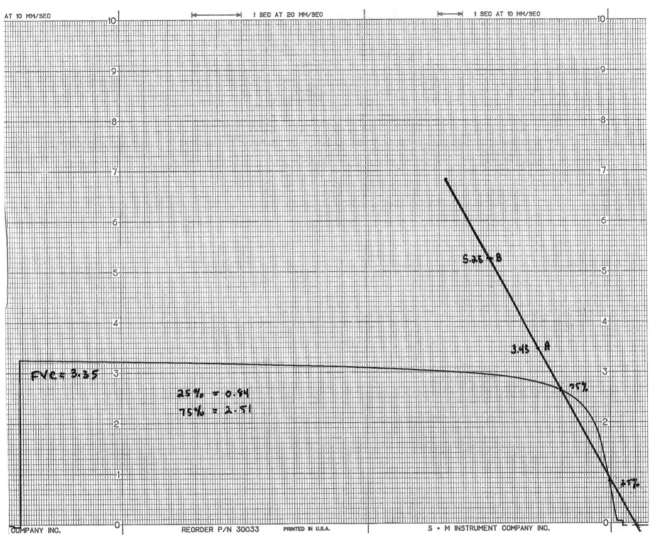

FIGURE 23.13   FEF$_{25\%-75\%}$ calculation. Shown at reduced size.

4. Calculate the variability between the SVC and FVC:

$$\frac{SVC - FVC}{SVC} \times 100 = Percent$$

5. Using a metric ruler placed on the volume-time tracing, draw back-extrapolation lines on all FVC tracings on the steepest portion of the curve, as shown in Figure 23.10.
   a. The tracing is valid if the extrapolation volume is less than 5 percent or 150 ml of the FVC on that curve (volume inside triangle as shown in Fig. 23.11).
   b. Use the point at which the back-extrapolation line intersects the baseline (x axis) as the zero point determination.

6. Measure the FEV$_1$ on all three tracings by measuring the 1-sec distance from the zero point determined in step 3 (Fig. 23.12). Choose the best FEV$_1$ regardless of which curve it is from, even if it is not the same curve as the best FVC.

7. Calculate the FEV$_1$/FVC% ratio.

$$\frac{FEV_1}{FVC} \times 100 = FEV_1/FVC\% \ (FEV_1\%)$$

8. Determine the BTPS correction factor from Table 23.1 using ambient temperature. Correct all volumes and flow rates to BTPS. *Do not* correct the FEV$_1$% ratio.

SVC × BTPS correction factor = SVC actual BTPS corrected

FVC × BTPS correction factor = FVC actual BTPS corrected

FEV$_1$ × BTPS correction factor = FEV$_1$ actual BTPS corrected

FEF$_{25\%-75\%}$ × BTPS correction factor
$$= FEF_{25\%-75\%} \ actual \ BTPS \ corrected$$

9. Determine predicted values from tables or nomograms. Correct for race if necessary.

Predicted value × .85 = Race-corrected value

10. Calculate the percent predicted.

$$\frac{Actual \ (BTPS)}{\substack{Predicted \ (race \ corrected \\ if \ necessary}} \times 100 = Percent \ predicted$$

NOTE: Round all volumes to two decimal places and all percentages to one decimal place. Label all results correctly.

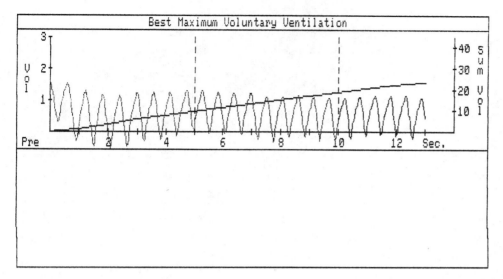

FIGURE 23.14   MVV tracing.

11. $FEF_{25\%-75\%}$ (Fig. 23.13):
   a. Choose the "best" curve, that is, the one with best sum of FEV_1 and FVC.
   b. Calculate 25 percent of FVC. Calculate 75 percent of FVC. Mark 25- and 75-percent points on the curve.
   c. Draw a line connecting the 25- and 75-percent points.
   d. Find any two points *A* and *B* that are 1 sec apart on the FEF line.
   e. Measure the volumes at points *A* and *B* (note that these are *not* the 25- and 75-percent points).
   f. Subtract the difference in volume (point $B - A$).
   g. Correct for BTPS. Answer in liters per second.
   h. Obtain a predicted value for the $FEF_{25\%-75\%}$.

EXERCISE 23.6 Postbronchodilator Study

If any students presently have a prescription for bronchodilators, a prebronchodilator-postbronchodilator comparison may be done with the student's consent.

1. Have the subject administer the bronchodilator via MDI or SVN as previously instructed (Chapter 9).
2. Repeat Exercise 23.4.3.
3. Calculate the percent change in FEV_1 as follows, and *record on your laboratory report:*

$$\frac{FE\overset{\bullet}{V}_1 \text{ prebronchodilator} - FEV_1 \text{ postbronchodilator}}{FEV_1 \text{ postbronchodilator}} \times 100$$

4. Calculate the percent change in FEV_1/FVC ratio ($FEV_1\%$) as follows, *and record on your laboratory report:*

$$FEV_1\% \text{ pre} - FEV_1\% \text{ post} = \text{percent change}$$

EXERCISE 23.7 Maximum Voluntary Ventilation

1. Introduce yourself and your department to your subject.
2. Briefly explain the purpose of the test. Confirm your subject's understanding by having the subject repeat the instructions back to you.

3. Wash your hands and apply standard precautions and transmission-based isolation procedures as applicable.
4. Aseptically attach the mouthpiece to the main tubing.
5. Instruct the subject in the performance of the test. Explain that he or she will be breathing as rapidly and deeply as possible for 12 to 15 sec (depending on the device used).
6. With the subject seated, actively coach him or her to begin breathing as rapidly and deeply as possible. Activate the machine and obtain a tracing (Fig. 23.14). *Record the result on your laboratory report and attach the tracing.*
7. Multiply the volume achieved by 5 (for a 12-sec observation) or 4 (for a 15-sec observation) to obtain the volume per minute. *Record the duration of the test on your laboratory report. Record the result on your laboratory report.*

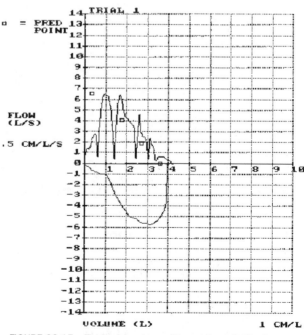

FIGURE 23.15   Flow volume loop with cough or glottic closure.

EXERCISE 23.8 Flow Volume Loops

If the spirometer you are using is capable of performing a flow volume loop, follow the manufacturer's directions and complete the following:

1. Introduce yourself and your department to the subject.
2. Explain the purpose of the test. Confirm understanding by having the subject repeat the instructions back to you.
3. Obtain subject information (age, gender, height, weight, and race) and enter the data into the spirometer.
4. Wash your hands and apply standard precautions and transmission-based isolation procedures as applicable.
5. Aseptically take a clean disposable mouthpiece or flow sensing device and attach it to the main tubing. If disposable pneumotachometers are used, each one should be calibrated before use in testing.
6. Instruct the subject in the performance of the flow volume loop maneuver. Explain (and demonstrate, if necessary) the following:
   a. The subject should place the mouthpiece tightly between the teeth with the lips sealed, without the tongue blocking the opening and without biting down.
   b. When you indicate, the subject should take as deep a breath as possible, completely filling the lungs.
   c. Without hesitation, the subject should then blow the air out as hard, fast, and completely as possible, until you say to stop. As soon as the subject's lungs are empty, the subject should take a maximum deep breath without removing the mouthpiece.
7. Confirm your subject's understanding by having the subject repeat the instructions back to you.
8. Place the noseclips on the subject and verify that there are no leaks. If the subject refuses to use the noseclips, have the subject hold his or her nose if possible.

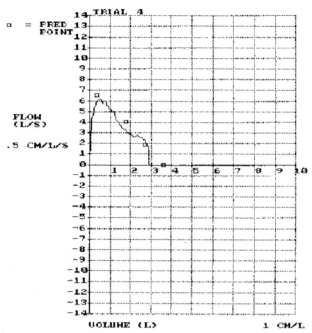

FIGURE 23.17   Flow volume loop with early termination.

9. Have the subject sit or stand straight, chin slightly elevated. If the subject is obese, pregnant, or a child, the test should be performed standing. A chair without wheels should be placed behind the subject under these circumstances for safety.
10. Activate the machine and the recording device. Actively coach the subject throughout inspiration and expiration, and perform the flow volume loop.
11. Observe the subject for adequate effort and proper performance during the maneuver. Reinstruct as necessary.

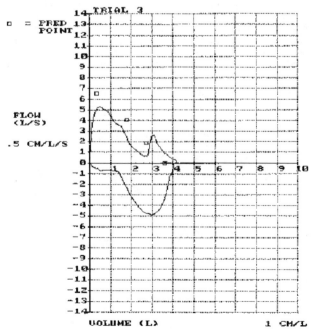

FIGURE 23.16   Flow volume loop with variable effort.

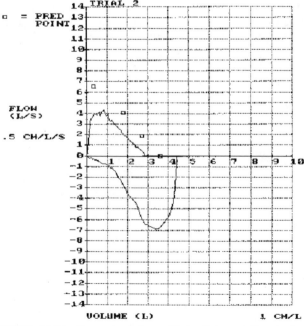

FIGURE 23.18   Flow volume loop with hesitation at the start of the test.

12. Note the volume obtained on the first effort and the shape and appearance of the graphic representation if available.

13. Allow for adequate recovery of the subject. Remove the noseclips and allow the subject to be seated if needed between tests.

14. Replace the noseclips, reinstruct the subject, and repeat the maneuver with active, forceful coaching until three acceptable tracings are obtained according to ATS standards. The three tracings should be free from the following:
    a. Cough or glottic closure (Fig. 23.15).
    b. Variable effort (Fig. 23.16).
    c. Early termination (Fig. 23.17).
    d. Hesitation at the start of the test (Fig. 23.18). The extrapolated volume must be less than 5 percent of the FVC or 150 ml, whichever is greater.
    e. Baseline error.
    f. Excessive variability. There should be no more than 5 percent or 200 ml difference between the two best FVC and FEV_1 results.

15. Have the subject sign and date the spirometric tracing. *Attach it to his or her laboratory report.*

References

1. Madama, V: Pulmonary Function Testing and Cardiopulmonary Stress Testing. Delmar Publishers, Albany, 1993.
2. Ruppel, G: Manual of Pulmonary Function Testing, ed 6. Mosby, St Louis, 1994.
3. American Association for Respiratory Care: AARC clinical practice guideline: Spirometry. Respir Care 36:1414–1417, 1991.
4. American Thoracic Society: Standardization of spirometry: 1987 update. Am Rev Respir Dis 136:1285–1298, 1987.
5. NIOSH Spirometry Training Guide. Universities Occupational Safety and Health Educational Resource Center Continuing Education and Outreach Program and Centers for Disease Control and Prevention National Institute for Occupational Safety and Health. Morgantown, West Virginia, 1997.
6. American Thoracic Society: Standardization of spirometry: 1994 update. Am J Respir Crit Care Med 152:1107–1136, 1995.

Related Readings

Eubanks, DH and Bone, RC: Principles and Applications of Cardiorespiratory Care Equipment. Mosby, St Louis, 1994.
Madama, V: Pulmonary Function Testing and Cardiopulmonary Stress Testing. Delmar Publishers, Albany, 1993.
McPherson, S: Respiratory Care Equipment, ed 5. Mosby, St Louis, 1995.
Ruppel, G: Manual of Pulmonary Function Testing, ed 6. Mosby, St Louis, 1994.
Scanlan, C et al (eds): Egan's Fundamentals of Respiratory Care, ed 6. Mosby, St Louis, 1995.
Wanger, J: Pulmonary Function Testing. Williams & Wilkins, Baltimore, 1992.
Wilkins, R, Sheldon, R and Krider, S: Clinical Assessment in Respiratory Care, ed 3. Mosby, St Louis, 1995.

Selected Journal Articles

American Association for Respiratory Care: AARC clinical practice guideline: Spirometry. Respir Care 36:1414–1417, 1991.
American Association for Respiratory Care: AARC clinical practice guideline: Spirometry, 1996 update. Respir Care 41:629–636, 1996.
American Thoracic Society: Standardization of spirometry: 1987 update. Am Rev Respir Dis 136:1285–1298, 1987.
American Thoracic Society: Standardization of spirometry: 1994 update. Am J Respir Crit Care Med 152:1107–1136, 1995.
Bosse, CG and Criner, GJ: Using spirometry in the primary care office: A guide to technique and interpretation of results. Postgrad Med 93:122–124, 1993.
Fluck, R and MacIntyre, N: Special issue: Pulmonary function testing. Part I. Respir Care 34:393–544, 1989.
Fluck, R and MacIntyre, N: Special issue: Pulmonary function testing. Part II. Respir Care 34:545–696, 1989.
Gardner, RM: Pulmonary function laboratory standards. 34:651–660, 1989.
Gardner, RM: Quality assurance in spirometry. Choices Respir Manage 19:88, 94, 96–97, 1989.
Gleadhill, I et al: Upper airway collapsibility in snorers and in patients with obstructive hypopnea and apnea. Am Rev Respir Dis 143: 1300–1303, 1991.
Glindmeyer, H et al: Blue-collar normative spirometric values for Caucasian and African American men and women aged 18 to 65. Am J Respir Crit Care Med 151:412–422, 1995.
Hankinson, J: Quality control in pulmonary function laboratories. Respir Care 27:830–833, 1982.
Hankinson, J and Wagner, GR: Medical screening using periodic spirometry for detection of chronic lung disease. Occup Med 8:353–361, 1993.
Lareau, SC et al: Development and testing of the pulmonary functional status and dyspnea questionnaire. Heart Lung 23:242–250, 1994.
Mahler, DA and Loke, J: The pulmonary function laboratory. Clin Chest Med 10:129–134, 1989.
Nelson, S et al: Performance evaluation of contemporary spirometers. Chest 97:288–297, 1990.
Tablan, OC, Williams, WW and Martone, WJ: Infection control in pulmonary function laboratories. Infect Control 6:442–444, 1985.
White, NW et al: Review and analysis of variation between spirometric values reported in 29 studies of healthy African adults. Am J Respir Crit Care Med 150:348–355, 1995.

LABORATORY REPORT

CHAPTER 23: PULMONARY FUNCTION TESTING

Name _____ Date _____

Course/Section _____ Instructor _____

Data Collection

EXERCISE 23.1   Equipment Identification

EXERCISE 23.1.1   Identification of Volume Displacement Spirometers

A. _____

B. _____

C. _____

EXERCISE 23.1.2   Identification of Flow Sensing Spirometers (Pneumotachometers)

A. _____

B. _____

C. _____

EXERCISE 23.2   Calibration and Maintenance of Spirometric Equipment

1. Type: _____

   Brand: _____

2. Paper speed (calibration mm/sec): _____

3. Room temperature: _____ °F (_____ °C)

4. Calibration volume: _____

   Percent accuracy: _____ *(show your work!)*

   Calibration injection speed observations: _____

   _____

   _____

EXERCISE 23.3   Respiratory History

1. Name and identification number: _____

2. Age on day of testing: _____

3. Height in stocking feet: _____

4. Gender: _____

5. Race: _____

6. Previous testing: _____

7. Sitting or standing: _____

8. Respiratory history

a. Do you usually have a cough first thing in the morning? _____

b. Do you cough up any secretions? If so, how much and what color is it usually? _____

c. Do you cough for as much as 3 months a year? _____

d. Do you ever experience chest tightness, wheezing, shortness of breath (on exertion or at rest), or chest

pain (quality and duration)? _____

e. Have you ever had or been told you have asthma, allergies, pneumonia, chronic bronchitis, emphysema,

or tuberculosis? _____

f. Do you have a heart condition for which you are under a doctor's care? Do you have any chest

pain now? _____

g. Do you take or have you ever taken prescription medicine for a respiratory or cardiac illness? If so,

what medications? _____

h. Do you take nonprescription medicine for a respiratory illness? _____

9. Smoking history

a. Have you ever smoked? _____

b. Do you smoke now? _____

c. How many packs of cigarettes do/did you smoke per day? _____

d. How old were you when you started smoking? _____

e. How long ago did you quit smoking? _____

f. How many years/months have you been smoking? _____

g. Calculate the subject's pack/year history

(show your work): _____

_____

_____

10. Occupational history

a. What type of work do you presently do? _____

b. What other types of work have you done in the past? _____

c. Have you ever worked in mining, in construction, or with insulation? Have you ever been exposed to

dusts, fumes, or mists at work? _____

11. Family history

a. Mother: _____

b. Father: _____

c. Siblings: _____

EXERCISE 23.4 Spirometry Screening

EXERCISE 23.4.1 Identification of Lung Volumes and Capacities

A. _____

B. _____

C. _____

D. _____

E. _____

F. _____

G. _____

H. _____

EXERCISE 23.4.2   Measuring Spirometric Lung Volumes and Capacities

From the attached spirogram, calculate the following:

Room temperature: _____

Measure all tidal breaths recorded: _____

Average the V_T *(show your work)*: _____

_____

Correct for BTPS: $V_T \times$ BTPS correction factor: _____
Measure the following from the spirometric tracing:

   IC (BTPS) = _____

   IRV (BTPS) = _____

   VC (BTPS) = _____

   ERV (BTPS) = _____

EXERCISE 23.4.3   Performance of Slow Vital Capacity and Forced Vital Capacity Maneuvers

Recorded SVC: _____

Attach results from volume displacement and flow sensing spirometer.

EXERCISE 23.5   Calculation of Spirometric Results

Attach the spirometric volume-time tracing obtained with your measurements and calculate the following *(show your work)*:

Date: _____

Time: _____

Temperature: _____

FVC results

   A: _____

   B: _____

   C: _____

Percent variability for FVC: _____

SVC results: _____

Percent variability between SVC and FVC: _____

FEV_1 results

   A: _____

   B: _____

   C: _____

Whose predicted values used: _____

Best FEV_1 (BTPS): _____

FEV_1 predicted: _____

FEV_1 percent predicted: _____

Best FVC (BTPS): _____

FVC predicted: _____

FVC percent predicted: _____

$FEV_1/FVC\%$: _____

$FEF_{25\%-75\%}$: _____

Compare your hand-calculated results with the computerized spirometric results: _____

_____

_____

EXERCISE 23.6 Postbronchodilator Study

Attach results of postbronchodilator study, if applicable. Compare prebronchodilator and postbronchodilator results:

Percent change FEV_1: _____

Percent change $FEV_1/FVC\%$: _____

EXERCISE 23.7 Maximum Voluntary Ventilation

Duration (sec) of test: _____

MVV: _____ L/min

EXERCISE 23.8 Flow Volume Loops

Attach the results of the flow volume loop, if available.

CRITICAL THINKING QUESTIONS

1. What lung volumes and capacities cannot be measured difrectly by spirometry?

2. Identify three methods to measure the volumes and capacities listed in Critical Thinking Question 1.

3. What is considered a significant change in preshift to postshift or prebronchodilator or postbronchodilator spirometric results? What factors might account for a change in spirometric values from preshift to postshift workers?

4. What is considered a significant change in annual spirometric results? What factors might account for changes in annual spirometry?

5. Calculate the following *(show all work)*:
   V_T = 500 ml
   IRV = 3000 ml
   ERV = 1000 ml
   RV = 1500 ml

   a. TLC = _____

   b. VC = _____

   c. IC = _____

   d. FRC = _____

6. Calculate the following *(show all work)*:
  V_T = 400 ml
  IC = 1000 ml
  FRC = 3000 ml
  ERV = 600 ml

  a. VC = _____

  b. TLC = _____

  c. RV = _____

  d. IRV: _____

7. Calculate the following *(show all work)*:
  TLC = 6000 ml
  FRC = 3500 ml
  ERV = 1500 ml
  V_T = 500 ml

  a. VC = _____

  b. IC = _____

8. For the flow volume loop shown in Figure 23.19, calculate the FVC, FIVC, PEF_{max} (peak expiratory flow), PIF_{max} (peak inspiratory flow), and ratio of $PEF_{50\%}/PIF_{50\%}$.

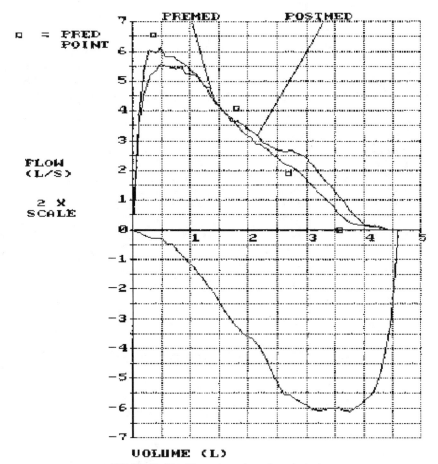

FIGURE 23.19   Flow volume loop for calculation.

9. What would sawtoothing on the inspiratory loop of a flow volume tracing most likely represent?

10. Interpret the following pulmonary function tests:

a. A 39-year-old man has a chief complaint of shortness of breath on exertion. Results of the spirometry screening are as follows:

	Prebronchodilator	Predicted	Percent predicted	Postbronchodilator	Percent predicted
FVC	4.09 L	4.64 L	88.1%	4.00 L	86.2%
FEV_1	1.94 L	3.73 L	52.0%	1.98 L	53.1%
$FEV_1/FVC\%$	47.4%	80.4%	—	49.5%	—

b. A slightly dyspneic coal miner who is a heavy smoker has a respiratory rate of 25/min with the following PFT results:

pH   7.43
$PaCO_2$ 50
HCO_3^- 32
PaO_2 55

	Predicted	Actual
VC	4.4 L	3.0 L
FEV_1	3.4	1.8 L
$FEF_{25\%-75\%}$	3.8 L/sec	2.0 L/sec
D_LCO	26	24
MVV	150 lpm	85 lpm
FRC	6.0 L	4.0 L

c. John Bart, 40 years of age, 72 inches tall, and 165 pounds, has been working in the steel mill since he was 17 years old. During the past 6 months, he has been experiencing worsening of his shortness of breath. He is now not able to work. He quit smoking 1 week ago. He had been smoking one pack a day since he was 16. Results are as follows:

Spirometry	Prebronchodilator	Predicted	Percent predicted	Postbronchodilator	Percent predicted
FVC	3.25 L	5.42	60.0%	3.22 L	59.4%
FEV_1	2.30 L	4.08 L	56.4%	2.35 L	57.6%
$FEV_1/FVC\%$	70.8	75.3	—	73.0	—
$FEF_{25\%-75\%}$	1.59 L/sec	4.55 L/sec	35.0%	1.77 L/sec	38.9%
MVV	88 lpm	147 lpm	60.0%	95 lpm	64.6%
FRC	2.98 L	4.20 L	71.0%		
RV	1.52 L	2.20 L	69.0%		
TLC	4.77 L	7.62 L	63.0%		
RV/TLC%	31.9%	28.9%			
D_LCO	8.4	30.9	27.2%		

PROCEDURAL COMPETENCY EVALUATION

Name _____ Date _____

Spirometry Screening

Setting: ☐ Lab ☐ Clinical   Evaluator: ☐ Peer ☐ Instructor

Conditions (describe): _____

_____

Equipment Used

_____

_____

	SATISFACTORY	UNSATISFACTORY	NOT OBSERVED	NOT APPLICABLE
Equipment and Patient Preparation				
1. Verifies, interprets, and evaluates physician's order or protocol	☐	☐	☐	☐
2. Selects, gathers, and assembles the necessary equipment	☐	☐	☐	☐
3. Checks for adequate paper supply	☐	☐	☐	☐
4. Checks for functional recording pens (if applicable)	☐	☐	☐	☐
5. Plugs the unit in if applicable; enters the date and time	☐	☐	☐	☐
6. If a volume displacement spirometer is used, checks the unit for leaks	☐	☐	☐	☐
7. If possible, turns on the recording device and makes sure the pen is recording on the baseline	☐	☐	☐	☐
8. Checks and enters the room temperature	☐	☐	☐	☐
9. Using a 3-L calibration syringe, checks the spirometer for accuracy; calculates or records the percent accuracy; repeats the calibration while varying the speed of volume injection	☐	☐	☐	☐
10. Washes hands and applies standard precautions and transmission-based isolation procedures as appropriate	☐	☐	☐	☐
11. Identifies subject; introduces self and department	☐	☐	☐	☐
12. Explains purpose of the procedure and confirms subject's understanding	☐	☐	☐	☐
Assessment and Implementation				
13. Assesses subject by obtaining the following information:				
a. Name and identification number	☐	☐	☐	☐
b. Age on day of testing	☐	☐	☐	☐
c. Height in stocking feet (or arm span)	☐	☐	☐	☐
d. Gender	☐	☐	☐	☐
e. Race (indicate white or nonwhite for purposes of race correction according to NIOSH and OSHA regulations for spirometry)	☐	☐	☐	☐
14. Determines whether previous testing has ever been done and whether it was done sitting or standing	☐	☐	☐	☐
15. Elicits a respiratory history, including cough/sputum production, smoking history, dyspnea at rest and on exertion, medications, employment history, and previous illnesses	☐	☐	☐	☐
16. Determines whether there are any contraindications to the performance of a baseline spirometry screening at this time by asking the subject the following questions:				
a. Upper respiratory tract illness, influenza, or bronchitis within the last 3 weeks?	☐	☐	☐	☐
b. Any tight or restrictive clothing that may interfere with the performance of the test?	☐	☐	☐	☐

	S A T I S F A C T O R Y	U N S A T I S F A C T O R Y	N O T O B S E R V E D	N O T A P P L I C A B L E
c. Eaten a heavy meal within the last 2 hours?	☐	☐	☐	☐
d. Any dental appliances, loose teeth, caps, gum or candy in mouth? Remove as appropriate	☐	☐	☐	☐
e. Smoked within the last hour?	☐	☐	☐	☐
f. Recent surgeries?	☐	☐	☐	☐
g. Used an aerosolized bronchodilator within the last 4 to 6 hours?	☐	☐	☐	☐
h. How are you feeling today? Any acute illness at the present time?	☐	☐	☐	☐
i. Ear infections in the last 3 weeks?	☐	☐	☐	☐
17. If a positive response is obtained to any of the preceding questions, corrects problems or postpones test for the appropriate time period	☐	☐	☐	☐
18. Aseptically attaches clean disposable mouthpiece or flow sensing device to the main tubing; calibrates as needed	☐	☐	☐	☐
19. Instructs the subject in the performance of the SVC maneuver and confirms subject's understanding	☐	☐	☐	☐
20. Places the noseclips on the subject and verifies that there are no leaks	☐	☐	☐	☐
21. Positions the subject by instructing him or her to sit or stand straight, as appropriate, with chin slightly elevated; places a chair without wheels behind the subject if standing	☐	☐	☐	☐
22. Activates the machine and recording device; actively coaches the subject throughout inspiration and expiration and performs the SVC	☐	☐	☐	☐
23. Observes the subject for adequate effort and proper performance during the maneuver; reinstructs as necessary	☐	☐	☐	☐
24. Notes the volume obtained	☐	☐	☐	☐
25. Allows for adequate recovery of the subject	☐	☐	☐	☐
26. Repeats the SVC maneuver with active, forceful coaching until three tracings within 200 ml or 5 percent of each other are obtained	☐	☐	☐	☐
27. Instructs the subject in the performance of the FVC maneuver and confirms understanding	☐	☐	☐	☐
28. Places the noseclips on the subject and verifies that there are no leaks	☐	☐	☐	☐
29. Repositions subject	☐	☐	☐	☐
30. Activates machine and performs the FVC with active forceful coaching throughout inspiration and expiration	☐	☐	☐	☐
31. Observes the subject for adequate effort and proper performance during the maneuver; reinstructs as necessary	☐	☐	☐	☐
32. Notes the volume obtained and the shape and appearance of the graphic representation, if available	☐	☐	☐	☐
33. Allows for adequate recovery of the subject	☐	☐	☐	☐
34. Determines validity of the test				
a. Three acceptable tracings free from cough or glottic closure, early termination of expiration, variable effort, leaks, and baseline error	☐	☐	☐	☐

	SATISFACTORY	UNSATISFACTORY	NOT OBSERVED	NOT APPLICABLE
b. Excessive hesitation at start of test: extrapolated volume must be less than 5 percent of the FVC or 150 ml, whichever is greater	☐	☐	☐	☐
c. Plateau defined as no change in volume in the last 1 sec of the tracing; test should be at least 6 sec in duration	☐	☐	☐	☐
d. Excessive variability: should be less than 5 percent or 200 ml difference between the two best FVC and FEV_1 results	☐	☐	☐	☐
35. Has the subject sign and date the spirometric tracing	☐	☐	☐	☐
36. Compares the SVC and FVC volumes and explains any discrepancies	☐	☐	☐	☐
37. If a postbronchodilator test is ordered, administers the medication, waits an appropriate length of time, and repeats the FVC	☐	☐	☐	☐
38. Calculates the percent change in FEV_1	☐	☐	☐	☐
39. Calculates the percent change in FEV_1/FVC ratio (FEV_1%)	☐	☐	☐	☐
40. Instructs the subject in the MVV maneuver, if appropriate, and confirms understanding	☐	☐	☐	☐
41. With the subject seated, has subject begin breathing as rapidly and deeply as possible; activates the machine and actively coaches test performance for 12 to 15 sec	☐	☐	☐	☐
42. Allows for adequate recovery of subject	☐	☐	☐	☐
43. Multiplies the volume achieved by 6 or 4 to obtain the volume per minute; records the results	☐	☐	☐	☐

Follow-up

	SATISFACTORY	UNSATISFACTORY	NOT OBSERVED	NOT APPLICABLE
44. Discards any disposable noseclips, mouthpieces, or flow sensors in an infectious waste container; disinfects any nondisposable mouthpieces and tubings	☐	☐	☐	☐
45. Washes hands	☐	☐	☐	☐
46. Records pertinent data in chart and departmental records	☐	☐	☐	☐
47. Notifies appropriate personnel and makes any necessary recommendations or modifications to the patient care plan	☐	☐	☐	☐

_____
Signature of Evaluator

_____
Signature of Student

PERFORMANCE RATING SCALE

5 EXCELLENT—FAR EXCEEDS EXPECTED LEVEL, FLAWLESS PERFORMANCE
4 ABOVE AVERAGE—NO PROMPTING REQUIRED, ABLE TO SELF-CORRECT
3 AVERAGE—THE MINIMUM COMPETENCY LEVEL, NO CRITICAL ERRORS
2 IMPROVEMENT NEEDED—PROBLEM AREAS EXIST; CRITICAL ERRORS, CORRECTIONS NEEDED
1 POOR AND UNACCEPTABLE PERFORMANCE—GROSS INACCURACIES, POTENTIALLY HARMFUL

PERFORMANCE CRITERIA	SCALE				
1. DISPLAYS KNOWLEDGE OF ESSENTIAL CONCEPTS	5	4	3	2	1
2. DEMONSTRATES THE RELATIONSHIP BETWEEN THEORY AND CLINICAL PRACTICE	5	4	3	2	1
3. FOLLOWS DIRECTIONS, EXHIBITS SOUND JUDGMENT, AND DEMONSTRATES ATTENTION TO SAFETY AND DETAIL	5	4	3	2	1
4. EXHIBITS THE REQUIRED MANUAL DEXTERITY	5	4	3	2	1
5. PERFORMS PROCEDURE IN A REASONABLE TIME FRAME	5	4	3	2	1
6. MAINTAINS STERILE OR ASEPTIC TECHNIQUE	5	4	3	2	1
7. INITIATES UNAMBIGUOUS GOAL-DIRECTED COMMUNICATION	5	4	3	2	1
8. PROVIDES FOR ADEQUATE CARE AND MAINTENANCE OF EQUIPMENT AND SUPPLIES	5	4	3	2	1
9. EXHIBITS COURTEOUS AND PLEASANT DEMEANOR	5	4	3	2	1
10. MAINTAINS CONCISE AND ACCURATE RECORDS	5	4	3	2	1

ADDITIONAL COMMENTS: INCLUDE ERRORS OF OMISSION OR COMMISSION, COMMUNICATIVE SKILLS, AND EFFECTIVENESS OF PATIENT INTERACTION:

SUMMARY PERFORMANCE EVALUATION AND RECOMMENDATIONS

SATISFACTORY PERFORMANCE—Performed without error or prompting, or able to self-correct, no critical errors.

_____ LABORATORY EVALUATION. SKILLS MAY BE APPLIED/OBSERVED IN THE CLINICAL SETTING.

_____ CLINICAL EVALUATION. STUDENT READY FOR MINIMALLY SUPERVISED APPLICATION AND REFINEMENT.

UNSATISFACTORY PERFORMANCE—Prompting required; performed with critical errors, potentially harmful.

_____ STUDENT REQUIRES ADDITIONAL LABORATORY PRACTICE.

_____ STUDENT REQUIRES ADDITIONAL SUPERVISED CLINICAL PRACTICE.

SIGNATURES

STUDENT: _____   EVALUATOR: _____

DATE: _____   DATE: _____

Noninvasive Ventilation

Some of the most common complications associated with mechanical ventilation arise from the use of artificial airways. Besides trauma to the airway and the potential for obstruction, endotracheal tubes and tracheostomy tubes provide a route for infection and serve as a barrier to communication. During the polio epidemic in the 1950s in the United States, negative pressure ventilators were designed to provide long-term ventilatory assistance to patients with this neuromuscular disease. Although more physiologic than positive pressure ventilation, they proved awkward and made routine care difficult. Today, the **cuirass** and the **poncho** types provide an alternative to positive pressure ventilation.

Other alternative methods to positive pressure ventilation have been employed with varying degrees of success. Rocking beds, pneumobelts, and phrenic nerve stimulators (diaphragmatic pacemakers) are used primarily for a select group of quadriplegic patients in rehabilitation facilities. Hands-on practice with these devices is beyond the scope of the laboratory setting.

Microprocessor-controlled positive pressure devices are now capable of providing another noninvasive alternative in the forms of continuous positive airway pressure (CPAP), bi-level positive airway pressure (BiPAP™), and, most recently, demand positive airway pressure (DPAP). These devices are now common in the acute care and home care environments. The respiratory care practitioner must be familiar with the capabilities and limitations of these devices.

OBJECTIVES

Upon completion of this chapter, the student will be able to:

1. Practice communication skills needed for the instruction of patients or their families in noninvasive ventilator initiation.
2. Identify the components of negative pressure, CPAP, BiPAP™, and DPAP units.
3. Assess patient for indications requiring noninvasive ventilation.
4. Apply infection control guidelines and standards associated with noninvasive ventilation equipment and procedures, according to OSHA regulations and CDC guidelines.
5. Select the equipment needed and assess the patient for proper fit of masks, cuirass shell, or poncho, as appropriate.
6. Initiate noninvasive ventilation.
7. Troubleshoot and solve common problems associated with noninvasive ventilators.
8. Assess the patient for tolerance and response to noninvasive ventilation.
9. Titrate oxygen in conjunction with noninvasive ventilators to vary F_IO_2.
10. Make recommendations or modifications to ventilation techniques or equipment as needed.
11. Practice medical charting for application of noninvasive ventilation procedures.

KEY TERMS

barotrauma
cuirass
poncho
volutrauma

EQUIPMENT REQUIRED

- Negative pressure ventilators
- Cuirass shells or ponchos, various sizes if available
- CPAP unit
- BiPAP unit
- DPAP unit
- Mask sizing gauge
- Nasal masks, various sizes
- Head straps
- Spacers
- Oxygen supply tubing

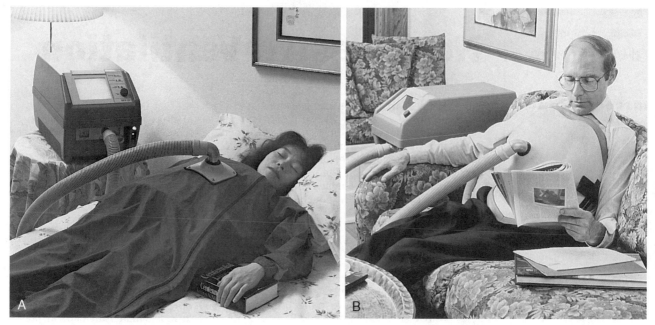

FIGURE 24.1   Negative pressure ventilators. (Courtesy of LIFECARE International, Inc., Westminster, CO.)

- Oxygen analyzer
- Adaptors
- Oxygen enrichment adaptor
- Oxygen source or concentrator
- Watch with second hand
- Respirometer
- One-way valves
- Blood pressure cuffs and sphygmomanometer
- Pulse oximeter

● EXERCISES

EXERCISE 24.1 Negative Pressure Ventilator

1. Select a negative pressure ventilator as shown in Figure 24.1. *Record the type used on your laboratory report.*

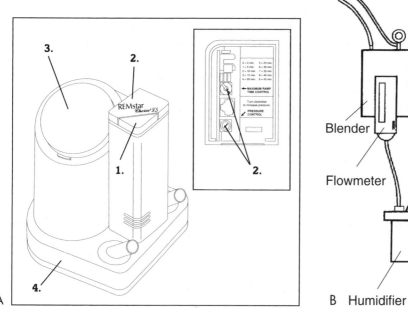

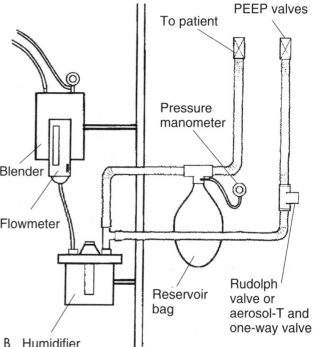

FIGURE 24.2   Continuous positive airway pressure (CPAP) systems: *(A)* Commercial CPAP system: *1.* ramp start button, *2.* pressure control and maximum ramp time control, *3.* filter cap, *4.* humidifier; *(B)* Assembly of a CPAP system from component parts.

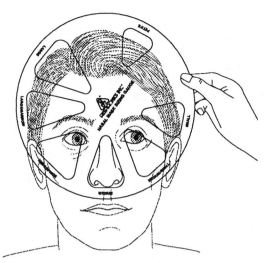

FIGURE 24.3 Fitting a CPAP mask. (Courtesy of Respironics, Murrysville, PA.)

2. Identify the controls. *Record the available controls on your laboratory report.*

3. Use your laboratory partner as the patient.

4. Wash your hands and apply standard precautions and transmission-based isolation procedures as appropriate.

5. Identify your "patient." Introduce yourself and your department. Explain to your partner in nonmedical terms that you are going to place the patient in the noninvasive ventilator device and what is involved. Confirm your partner's understanding and answer any questions or concerns. The partner should simulate a patient's concern and fears about having this procedure performed. You should respond appropriately.

6. Assess the patient for vital signs, SpO$_2$, breath sounds, and ventilatory status. *Record your findings on your laboratory report.*

7. Prepare the patient for noninvasive ventilation. Select the correct size cuirass shell or poncho.

8. Place the cuirass or poncho on the patient and check for proper fit and patient comfort.

9. Adjust the negative pressure to –10 cm H$_2$O.

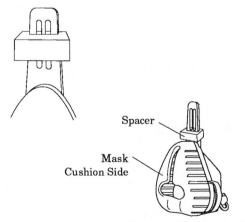

FIGURE 24.4 CPAP mask spacers. (Courtesy of Respironics, Murrysville, PA.)

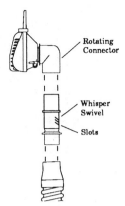

FIGURE 24.5 Hose attachment. (Courtesy of Respironics, Murrysville, PA.)

10. Adjust the rate to 12/min. Have your partner count 1 to 10 as the ventilator cycles. *Record your observations on your laboratory report.*

11. Using the spirometer and one-way valve, measure the exhaled tidal volume. *Record the volume on your laboratory report.*

12. Reassess your patient's vital signs, SpO$_2$, breath sounds, and ventilatory status. *Record your findings on your laboratory report.*

13. *"Chart" the application of noninvasive ventilation on your laboratory report.*

14. Loosen the cuirass or the poncho.

15. Measure the exhaled tidal volume. *Record the volume on your laboratory report.*

EXERCISE 24.2 Continuous Positive Airway Pressure Setup

1. Select a CPAP unit and identify the controls. *Record the type of unit used and the available controls on your laboratory*

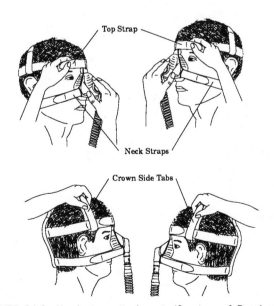

FIGURE 24.6 Head strap attachment. (Courtesy of Respironics, Murrysville, PA.)

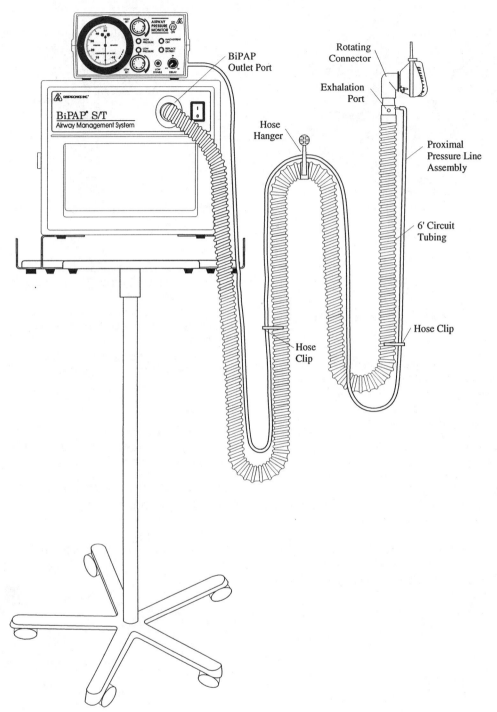

FIGURE 24.7 BiPAP™ S/T ventilatory support system on a mobile stand with an airway pressure monitor. (Courtesy of Respironics, Murrysville, PA.)

report. If a commercial CPAP unit is not available, a system can be assembled as shown in Figure 24.2.

2. Wash your hands and apply standard precautions and transmission-based isolation procedures as appropriate.

3. Use your laboratory partner as the patient. Identify your patient. Introduce yourself and your department. Explain to your partner in nonmedical terms that you are going to apply a mask CPAP device and what is involved. Confirm your partner's understanding and answer any questions or concerns. The partner should simulate a patient's concern and fears about having this procedure performed. You should respond appropriately.

4. Assess the patient's vital signs, SpO_2, breath sounds, and ventilatory status. *Record your findings on your laboratory report.*

5. Take the mask sizing gauge and measure your lab partner. Select the smallest mask possible that will come close to, but not contact, the nasal bone, external nares, and upper

lip, as shown in Figure 24.3. *Record the mask size on your laboratory report.* Remember to explain everything to your partner.

6. Use spacers to fill any gaps, as shown in Figure 24.4.

7. Attach the mask to the hose, as shown in Figure 24.5.

8. Turn the CPAP unit or system on.

9. Attach the head straps to your partner's head as shown in Figure 24.6. Confirm proper fit and comfort.

10. Adjust the CPAP pressure to 5 cm H_2O.

11. Reassess vital signs, SpO_2, breath sounds, and ventilatory status. *Record your findings on your laboratory report.*

12. Ask your partner how he or she is tolerating the pressure. Have your partner try to mouth breathe and talk. *Record your observations on your laboratory report.*

13. *"Chart" the initiation of CPAP on your laboratory report.*

EXERCISE 24.3 BiPAP™ Setup

1. Select a BiPAP™ unit, as shown in Figure 24.7. Note the various connections and air filter locations and identify the controls. *Record the type of unit and the available controls on your laboratory report.*

2. Wash your hands and apply standard precautions and transmission-based isolation procedures as appropriate.

3. Use your laboratory partner as the patient. Identify your patient. Introduce yourself and your department. Explain to your partner in nonmedical terms that you are going to apply a mask BiPAP™ device and what is involved. Confirm your partner's understanding, and answer any questions or concerns.

4. Assess the patient's vital signs, SpO_2, breath sounds, and ventilatory status. *Record your findings on your laboratory report.*

5. Using the same steps as in the CPAP exercise, measure your partner for the correct size mask and attach your partner to the unit using the following settings:

   Mode: spontaneous
   IPAP: 10 cm H_2O
   EPAP: 6 cm H_2O
   Percent IPAP: 20 percent
   Low pressure alarm: 4 cm H_2O
   High pressure alarm: 15 cm H_2O

6. Observe the pressure manometer for several breathing cycles. Determine the I:E ratio. (See Chapter 1.) Elicit from your partner any differences between breathing on a CPAP unit versus BiPAP™. *Record your observations on your laboratory report.*

7. Adjust the low pressure alarm to 8 cm H_2O. Note any pressure changes and other occurrences. *Record your observations on your laboratory report.* Correct any malfunctions or alarms. *Record what adjustments were made on your laboratory report.*

8. Loosen the mask from your lab partner. Note any pressure changes and other occurrences. *Record your observations on your laboratory report.* Resecure the mask in place.

9. Change the mode to spontaneous/timed and set the rate to 14/min.

10. Ask your partner if any appreciable difference is felt. *Record your observations on your laboratory report.*

11. Obtain an oxygen enrichment adaptor and oxygen analyzer. Place in-line as shown in Figure 24.8.

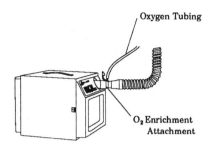
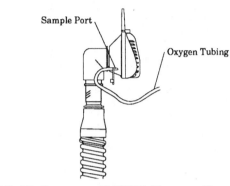

FIGURE 24.8 Titrating oxygen with BiPAP™. (Courtesy of Respironics, Murrysville, PA.)

12. Titrate low flow oxygen until an F_IO_2 of 0.28 is achieved. *Record the liter flow required on your laboratory report.*

    NOTE: Supplemental oxygen may also be directly titrated into the mask via the oxygen bleed-in port.

13. Adjust the unit to the following settings:
    Mode: spontaneous
    IPAP: 2 cm H_2O
    EPAP: 10 cm H_2O
    Percent IPAP: 20 percent
    Low pressure alarm: 0 cm H_2O

14. Ask your partner if any appreciable difference is felt. Note any pressure changes and other occurrences. *Record your observations on your laboratory report.*

15. Adjust the settings to correct any malfunctions or alarms. *Record what adjustments were made on your laboratory report.*

16. Obtain a DPAP unit. Set it up according to the manufacturer's instructions and apply it to your laboratory partner.

17. Ask your partner if any appreciable difference is felt between DPAP and BiPAP™. Note any pressure changes and other occurrences. *Record your observations on your laboratory report.*

Related Readings

Eubanks, DH and Bone, RC: Principles and Applications of Cardiorespiratory Care Equipment. Mosby, St Louis, 1994.

Hodgkin, JE, Connors, GL and Bell, CW: Pulmonary Rehabilitation: Guidelines to Success, ed 2. JB Lippincott, Philadelphia, 1993.

Kacmarek, RM, Mack, CW and Dimas, S: The Essentials of Respiratory Care, ed 3. Mosby, St Louis, 1990.

McPherson, S: Respiratory Care Equipment, ed 5. Mosby, St Louis, 1995.

Scanlan, C et al (eds): Egan's Fundamentals of Respiratory Care, ed 6. Mosby, St Louis, 1995.

Selected Journal Articles

Bach, JR and Saporito, LR: Indications and criteria for decannulation and transition from invasive to non-invasive long-term ventilatory support. Respir Care 39:515–531, 1994.

Brochard, L: Non-invasive ventilation: Practical issues. Intensive Care Med 19:431–432, 1993.

Brochard, L et al: Reversal of acute exacerbations of chronic obstructive lung disease by inspiratory assistance with a face mask. N Engl J Med 323:1523–1530, 1990.

Campbell, DA et al: Phrenic nerve pacing in two young quadriplegic ventilator dependent patients. Aust N Z J Med 22:463–468, 1992.

Elliott, MW et al: A comparison of different modes of noninvasive ventilatory support: Effects on ventilation and inspiratory muscle effort. Anesthesia 49:279–283, 1994.

Fredrick, C: Non-invasive mechanical ventilation with the iron lung. Crit Care Nurs Clin North Am 6:831–840, 1994.

Hill, N et al: Efficacy of nocturnal nasal ventilation in patients with restrictive thoracic disease. Am Rev Respir Dis 145:365–371, 1992.

Hill, NS and Bach, JR: Noninvasive mechanical ventilation. Clinics of North America 2:161–352, 1996.

Khan, Y et al: Effects of nasal ventilation on nocturnal hypoxemia in neuromuscular patients. Am Rev Respir Dis 145:A563, 1992.

Kovach, GM and Henry, S: Phrenic nerve pacing—an alternative to positive pressure ventilation: The required nursing care. AACN Clinical Issues in Critical Care Nursing 4:573–577, 1993.

Marino, W: Intermittent volume cycled mechanical ventilation via nasal mask in patient with respiratory failure due to COPD. Chest 99:681–684, 1991.

Meyer, TJ and Hill, NS: Noninvasive positive pressure ventilation to treat respiratory failure. Ann Intern Med 120:760–770, 1994.

Miller, JH, Thomas, E and Wilmont, CB: Pneumobelt use among high quadriplegic population. Arch Phys Med Rehabil 69:369, 1988.

Padman, R et al: Use of independently adjusted inspiratory and exhalatory positive airway pressure via nasal mask in acute and chronic respiratory insufficiency in pediatric patients. Am Rev Respir Dis 145:A555, 1992.

Padman, R, Lawless, S and Von Nessen, S: Use of BiPAP™ by nasal mask in the treatment of respiratory insufficiency in pediatric patients: Preliminary investigation. Pediatr Pulmonol 17:119–123, 1994.

Parisi, R, England, S and Santiago, T: Treatment of central sleep apnea with respiratory-cycled variable nasal positive pressure (BiPAP™). Am Rev Respir Dis 143:A586, 1991.

Piper, A et al. Nocturnal nasal IPPV stabilizes patients with cystic fibrosis and hypercapneic respiratory failure. Chest 102:846–850, 1992.

Renston, J, DiMarco, A and Supinski, G: Respiratory muscle rest using nasal BiPAP™ ventilation in patients with stable severe COPD. Chest 145:4, 1994.

Sanders, M and Kern, N: Obstructive sleep apnea treated by independently adjusted inspiratory pressure via nasal mask. Chest 98:317–324, 1990.

Spessert, CK, Weilitz, PB, and Goodenberger, DM: A protocol for initiation of positive pressure nasal ventilation. Am J Crit Care 2:54–60, 1993.

Strumpf, D et al: An evaluation of the Respironics BiPAP™ bi-level CPAP device for delivery of assisted ventilation. Respir Care 35:415–422, 1990.

Teague, W et al: Nasal bi-level positive airway pressure acutely improves ventilation and oxygen saturation in children with upper airway obstruction. Am Rev Respir Dis 143:A505, 1991.

Vitacca, M et al: Non-invasive modalities of positive pressure ventilation improve the outcome of acute exacerbations in COLD patients. Eur Respir J 5:433s, 1992.

Waldhorn, R: Nocturnal intermittent positive pressure ventilation with bi-level positive airway pressure (BiPAP™) in respiratory failure. Chest 101:516–521, 1992.

LABORATORY REPORT

CHAPTER 24: NONINVASIVE VENTILATION

Name _____   Date _____

Course/Section _____   Instructor _____

Data Collection

EXERCISE 24.1   Negative Pressure Ventilator

Type of ventilator used: _____

Controls available: _____

_____

_____

Patient assessment: _____

_____

Observations: _____

_____

_____

_____

Exhaled tidal volume: _____

Patient assessment: _____

_____

Chart the initiation of noninvasive ventilation as you would on a legal medical record:

_____

_____

_____

_____

_____

_____

_____

Exhaled tidal volume with loosened cuirass: _____

EXERCISE 24.2   Continuous Positive Airway Pressure Setup

Type of ventilator used: _____

Controls available: _____

Mask size: _____

Patient assessment: _____

_____

Observations: _____

_____

_____

_____

_____

_____

Chart the initiation of CPAP as you would on a legal medical record:

_____

_____

_____

_____

_____

_____

_____

_____

_____

EXERCISE 24.3   BiPAP Setup

Type of ventilator used: _____

Controls available: _____

_____

Patient assessment: _____

_____

I:E ratio: _____
(Show your work for any calculations!)

IPAP = 10 cm H_2O; EPAP = 6 cm H_2O; pressure alarm = 4 cm H_2O.

Observations: _____

_____

_____

_____

Pressure alarm = 8 cm H_2O.

Observations: _____

_____

_____

_____

Adjustments made: _____

Observation with loose mask: _____

_____

_____

Observations in the timed mode: _____

_____

_____

Liter flow: _____

Observations with IPAP = 2, EPAP = 10: _____

_____

_____

_____

Adjustments made: _____

DPAP observations: _____

_____

_____

_____

CRITICAL THINKING QUESTIONS

1. What types of patients would not be candidates for noninvasive ventilation?

2. Based on the exercises, what limitations of noninvasive ventilation did you observe?

Mr. Pickwick has obstructive sleep apnea, and the doctor has ordered him placed on BiPAP™ at the following settings: mode, S/T; rate, 12/min; IPAP, 12 cm H_2O; EPAP, 6 cm H_2O. You enter his room, identify yourself, and explain everything to him. You also perform a complete assessment. After applying BiPAP™ you note a drop in blood pressure and oxygen saturation.

3. What changes or modifications would you recommend?

4. What would you recommend to Mr. Pickwick for infection control in the home?

You are a newly employed home care therapist and are visiting Mr. Pickwick for the first time. While checking his BiPAP™ setup you observe that 2 lpm of oxygen from an oxygen concentrator is being titrated directly into the mask.

5. How would you determine the F_IO_2 being delivered? Explain your answer.

6. How can you assess the adequacy of the oxygen therapy being provided?

PROCEDURAL COMPETENCY EVALUATION

Name _____ Date _____

Mask CPAP/BiPAP™ Initiation

Setting: ☐ Lab ☐ Clinical   Evaluator: ☐ Peer ☐ Instructor

Conditions (describe): _____
_____

Equipment Used

_____
_____

	SATISFACTORY	UNSATISFACTORY	NOT OBSERVED	NOT APPLICABLE
Equipment and Patient Preparation				
1. Verifies, interprets, and evaluates physician's order or protocol for appropriate modality	☐	☐	☐	☐
2. Scans chart for diagnosis and any other pertinent data and notes	☐	☐	☐	☐
3. Selects, gathers, and assembles the necessary equipment	☐	☐	☐	☐
4. Washes hands and applies standard precautions and transmission-based isolation procedures as appropriate	☐	☐	☐	☐
5. Identifies patient, introduces self and department	☐	☐	☐	☐
6. Explains in nonmedical terms that a mask CPAP/BiPAP™ device is going to be applied and what is involved; confirms the patient's understanding and answers any questions or concerns	☐	☐	☐	☐
Assessment and Implementation				
7. Assesses the patient's vital signs, SpO$_2$, breath sounds, and ventilatory status	☐	☐	☐	☐
8. Positions patient and measures the patient for the appropriate mask size	☐	☐	☐	☐
9. Uses spacers to fill any gaps	☐	☐	☐	☐
10. Attaches the mask to the hose	☐	☐	☐	☐
11. Turns the unit or system on and selects proper mode	☐	☐	☐	☐
12. Attaches the head straps to the patient's head; confirms proper fit and comfort	☐	☐	☐	☐
13. Adjusts the pressure to conform with the physician's order	☐	☐	☐	☐
14. Reassess vital signs, SpO$_2$, breath sounds, and ventilatory status	☐	☐	☐	☐
15. Asks the patient how he or she is tolerating the pressure; readjusts mask if necessary	☐	☐	☐	☐
Follow-up				
16. Maintains/processes equipment	☐	☐	☐	☐
17. Disposes of infectious waste	☐	☐	☐	☐
18. Washes hands	☐	☐	☐	☐
19. Records pertinent data in chart and departmental records	☐	☐	☐	☐
20. Notifies appropriate personnel and makes any necessary recommendations or modifications to the patient care plan	☐	☐	☐	☐

_____   _____
Signature of Evaluator   Signature of Student

PERFORMANCE RATING SCALE

5 EXCELLENT—FAR EXCEEDS EXPECTED LEVEL, FLAWLESS PERFORMANCE
4 ABOVE AVERAGE—NO PROMPTING REQUIRED, ABLE TO SELF-CORRECT
3 AVERAGE—THE MINIMUM COMPETENCY LEVEL, NO CRITICAL ERRORS
2 IMPROVEMENT NEEDED—PROBLEM AREAS EXIST; CRITICAL ERRORS, CORRECTIONS NEEDED
1 POOR AND UNACCEPTABLE PERFORMANCE—GROSS INACCURACIES, POTENTIALLY HARMFUL

PERFORMANCE CRITERIA		SCALE			
1. DISPLAYS KNOWLEDGE OF ESSENTIAL CONCEPTS	5	4	3	2	1
2. DEMONSTRATES THE RELATIONSHIP BETWEEN THEORY AND CLINICAL PRACTICE	5	4	3	2	1
3. FOLLOWS DIRECTIONS, EXHIBITS SOUND JUDGMENT, AND DEMONSTRATES ATTENTION TO SAFETY AND DETAIL	5	4	3	2	1
4. EXHIBITS THE REQUIRED MANUAL DEXTERITY	5	4	3	2	1
5. PERFORMS PROCEDURE IN A REASONABLE TIME FRAME	5	4	3	2	1
6. MAINTAINS STERILE OR ASEPTIC TECHNIQUE	5	4	3	2	1
7. INITIATES UNAMBIGUOUS GOAL-DIRECTED COMMUNICATION	5	4	3	2	1
8. PROVIDES FOR ADEQUATE CARE AND MAINTENANCE OF EQUIPMENT AND SUPPLIES	5	4	3	2	1
9. EXHIBITS COURTEOUS AND PLEASANT DEMEANOR	5	4	3	2	1
10. MAINTAINS CONCISE AND ACCURATE RECORDS	5	4	3	2	1

ADDITIONAL COMMENTS: INCLUDE ERRORS OF OMISSION OR COMMISSION, COMMUNICATIVE SKILLS, AND EFFECTIVENESS OF PATIENT INTERACTION:

SUMMARY PERFORMANCE EVALUATION AND RECOMMENDATIONS

SATISFACTORY PERFORMANCE—Performed without error or prompting, or able to self-correct, no critical errors.

_____ LABORATORY EVALUATION. SKILLS MAY BE APPLIED/OBSERVED IN THE CLINICAL SETTING.

_____ CLINICAL EVALUATION. STUDENT READY FOR MINIMALLY SUPERVISED APPLICATION AND REFINEMENT.

UNSATISFACTORY PERFORMANCE—Prompting required; performed with critical errors, potentially harmful.

_____ STUDENT REQUIRES ADDITIONAL LABORATORY PRACTICE.

_____ STUDENT REQUIRES ADDITIONAL SUPERVISED CLINICAL PRACTICE.

SIGNATURES

STUDENT: _____ EVALUATOR: _____

DATE: _____ DATE: _____

Pressure Ventilators

Although pressure limited–volume variable ventilation is not used as the primary ventilatory mode in the adult intensive care setting, it is increasingly used as an alternative modality. Understanding the relationships between pressure, flow, volume, and time will help the student grasp the complexities of mechanical ventilation. The student must be able to apply these concepts in order to initiate ventilation and monitor patients using the more advanced modes available on current highly sophisticated equipment.

This chapter is intended to introduce the student to the relationships between pressure, flow, volume, and time in preparation for more in-depth exploration of mechanical ventilation in later chapters. In preparation for these exercises, the student should review the IPPB exercises in Chapter 10.

OBJECTIVES
Upon completion of this chapter, the student will be able to:

1. Identify the components of an adult breathing circuit.
2. Test the circuit for leaks.
3. Identify and operate the controls of a pressure limited ventilator.
4. Initiate and monitor pressure limited ventilation.
5. Compare the interrelationships between pressure, volume, flow, and time.
6. Relate the changes that might occur in the parameters of pressure, volume, flow, and time with changes in compliance and resistance.
7. Chart data related to pressure limited ventilation in the medical record.

KEY TERMS
See Chapters 10 and 24.

EQUIPMENT REQUIRED

- Pressure ventilator (Bird series or Bennett PR II)
- Respirometer and adaptor
- Lung simulator or test lungs
- Adult breathing circuits
- Corrugated tubing
- Watch with second hand
- 50-psi gas source
- High-pressure hose

● EXERCISES

EXERCISE 25.1 Identification of an Adult Breathing Circuit and Leak Testing

1. Select an adult breathing circuit for a pressure limited ventilator.
2. Examine the components shown in Figure 25.1.
3. Connect the circuit to the unit as practiced in Chapter 10.
4. Using the same technique as in Chapter 10, Exercise 10.3, step 3, test the circuit for leaks. Observe for leaks and correct if necessary. *Record the ventilator used, your observations, and any corrective actions on your laboratory report.*

EXERCISE 25.2 Controls

1. Attach the ventilator circuit to a lung simulator or test lung as shown in Figure 25.2. Adjust the lung simulator to normal compliance and resistance values.
2. Adjust the pressure to 10 cm H_2O.
3. Adjust the flow rate to 15 if using a Bird.
4. If using a PR II, turn the peak flow to the minimum setting and the terminal flow to maximum.
5. Adjust the apnea control or rate control to achieve a breath rate of 12.
6. Attach a respirometer to the exhalation port. *Record the tidal volume achieved on your laboratory report.*
7. Measure the inspiratory and expiratory times and *record them on your laboratory report. Calculate the I:E ratio and record it on your laboratory report.*
8. Increase the pressure to 15 cm H_2O. *Record the tidal volume achieved on your laboratory report.*
9. Measure the inspiratory and expiratory times and *record them on your laboratory report. Calculate the I:E ratio and record it on your laboratory report.*

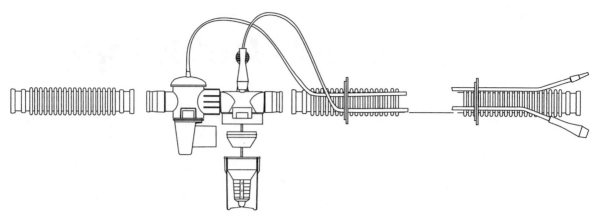

FIGURE 25.1   Adult breathing circuit for pressure ventilators. (Courtesy of Hudson RCI, Temecula, CA.)

10. Return the pressure to 10 cm H_2O.

11. Increase the flow rate to 20 (Bird) or maximum peak flow (PR II). *Record the tidal volume achieved on your laboratory report.*

12. Measure the inspiratory and expiratory times and *record them on your laboratory report. Calculate the I:E ratio and record it on your laboratory report.*

13. Decrease the flow rate to 10 (Bird). *Record the volume achieved on your laboratory report.*

14. Measure the inspiratory and expiratory times and *record them on your laboratory report. Calculate the I:E ratio on your laboratory report.*

15. Increase the pressure to 20 cm H_2O and the flow to 20. *Record the tidal volume achieved on your laboratory report.*

16. Measure the inspiratory and expiratory times and *record them on your laboratory report. Calculate the I:E ratio and record it on your laboratory report.*

EXERCISE 25.3 Initiation and Monitoring

Given the following information, complete the exercise as directed. Use the lung simulator as your patient. Your instructor will show you how to operate the simulator. Depending on the brand of simulator, you might have to change adaptors or settings in order to vary compliance and resistance. Use the

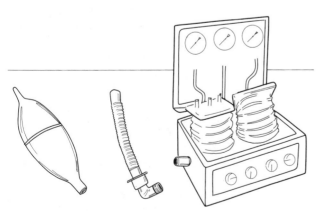

FIGURE 25.2   Attaching the circuit to a test lung.

settings on your simulator that correspond to the compliance and resistance settings in the exercises. Initially use the R5 resistance adaptors (normal resistance) and set the compliance of both lungs at 0.10 L/cm H_2O (normal resistance and compliance settings).

Mrs. Gandhi is a 45-year-old nonsmoker with a history of asthma. She is in the recovery room following a colon resection. She is not yet reactive and is not breathing spontaneously. She is 150 lb. You have been called to place her on a pressure ventilator until she becomes reactive.

1. Using the formula of 10 to 15 mL/kg, set the ventilator to give the patient an appropriate tidal volume and respiratory rate of 12/min. *Record your settings for pressure and flow on your laboratory report.*

2. Measure the tidal volume, inspiratory time, and expiratory time, and *record them on your laboratory report. Calculate the I:E ratio on your laboratory report.*

3. Change the resistance adaptor to R20 (high resistance). Measure the tidal volume, and observe any changes in volume and I:E ratio. *Record them on your laboratory report.*

4. Increase the pressure until you have achieved the tidal volume in step 1. *Record it on your laboratory report.*

5. Using the flow control, adjust the inspiratory time until the I:E ratio returns to original value. *Record the settings and your observations on your laboratory report.*

6. Return the resistance to R5 (normal resistance). Set the compliance setting for the right lung to 0.08 L/cm H_2O (low compliance). Measure the tidal volume, inspiratory time, and expiratory time, and *record them on your laboratory report. Calculate the I:E ratio on your laboratory report.*

7. Set the left lung to the same compliance setting as in step 6. Measure the tidal volume, inspiratory time, and expiratory time, and *record them on your laboratory report. Calculate the I:E ratio on your laboratory report.*

8. Increase the pressure until you have achieved the tidal volume in step 1. *Record it on your laboratory report.*

9. Using the flow control, set an appropriate I:E ratio. *Record the settings and your observations on your laboratory report.*

10. Set the compliance to 0.01 L/cm H_2O and the resistance to R20. Measure the tidal volume, inspiratory time, and expiratory time, and *record them on your laboratory report. Calculate the I:E ratio on your laboratory report.*

Related Readings

Eubanks, DH and Bone, RC: Principles and Applications of Cardiorespiratory Care Equipment. Mosby, St Louis, 1994.

McPherson, S: Respiratory Care Equipment, ed 5. Mosby, St Louis, 1995.

Scanlan, C et al (eds): Egan's Fundamentals of Respiratory Care, ed 6. Mosby, St Louis, 1995.

Selected Journal Articles

Bellman, MJ et al: Efficacy of positive versus negative pressure ventilation in unloading the respiratory muscles. Chest 98:850–856, 1990.

Leger, P: Non-invasive positive pressure ventilation at home. Respir Care 39:501–514, 1994.

LABORATORY REPORT

CHAPTER 25: PRESSURE VENTILATORS

Name _____ Date _____

Course/Section _____ Instructor _____

Data Collection

EXERCISE 25.1   Identification of an Adult Breathing Circuit and Leak Testing

Ventilator used: _____

Observations: _____

_____

_____

_____

_____

EXERCISE 25.2   Controls

Normal Resistance and Compliance
PRESSURE 10 cm H_2O, FLOW 15

Tidal volume: _____

Inspiratory time: _____

Expiratory time: _____

I:E ratio (show your work): _____
PRESSURE 15 cm H_2O, FLOW 15

Tidal volume: _____

Inspiratory time: _____

Expiratory time: _____

I:E ratio (show your work!): _____
PRESSURE 10 cm H_2O, FLOW 20

Tidal volume: _____

Inspiratory time: _____

Expiratory time: _____

I:E ratio (show your work!) _____
PRESSURE 10 cm H_2O, FLOW 10

Tidal volume: _____

Inspiratory time: _____

Expiratory time: _____

I:E ratio (show your work!) _____

PRESSURE 20 CM H_2O, FLOW 20

Tidal volume: _____

Inspiratory time: _____

Expiratory time: _____

I:E ratio (show your work!) _____

EXERCISE 25.3   Initiation and Monitoring

Peak pressure: _____

Respiratory rate: _____

Peak flow: _____

Tidal volume: _____

Inspiratory time: _____

Expiratory time: _____

I:E ratio: _____

Tidal volume with high resistance (R20): _____

Inspiratory time: _____

Expiratory time: _____

I:E ratio: _____

Pressure setting: _____

Flow setting: _____

Tidal volume with decreased compliance right lung (C_L.08 L/cm H_2O): _____

Inspiratory time: _____

Expiratory time: _____

I:E ratio: _____

Pressure setting: _____

Flow setting: _____

Tidal volume with decreased compliance both lungs (C_L.08 L/cm H_2O): _____

Inspiratory time: _____

Expiratory time: _____

I:E ratio: _____

Pressure setting: _____

Flow setting: _____

Tidal volume with low compliance and high resistance (C_L.01 and R20): _____

Inspiratory time: _____

Expiratory time: _____

I:E ratio: _____

Pressure setting: _____

Flow setting: _____

CRITICAL THINKING QUESTIONS

1. Given the scenario with Mrs. Gandhi, answer the following:
   a. What clinical situations were simulated by increasing the airway resistance?

   b. What clinical situations were simulated by decreasing the compliance in the right lung? In both lungs?

2. What patient assessment techniques would you use to evaluate the ventilatory status of Mrs. Gandhi?

3. Construct a sample charting note using the initial settings and data obtained in Exercise 25.3. Be sure to include all assessment information.

4. Based on your observations and measurements:
   a. What effect did increasing resistance have on the exhaled tidal volume and I:E ratio?

   b. What parameter(s) would you change to maintain adequate ventilation and I:E ratio?

   c. What effect did decreasing compliance have on the exhaled tidal volume and I:E ratio?

   d. What parameter(s) would you change to maintain adequate ventilation and I:E ratio?

Volume Ventilators

The selection, assembly, verification of function, initiation, and maintenance of mechanical ventilators has long been the responsibility of the respiratory care practitioner. Increasingly sophisticated technology has made volume ventilators more and more complex. It is essential to safe and effective patient care that these devices be properly set up before use. Nothing is more embarrassing and damaging to the image of the profession or dangerous to the patient than a respiratory care practitioner trying to initiate mechanical ventilation in a critical care setting when the machine is not assembled and functioning properly.

OBJECTIVES
Upon completion of this chapter, the student will be able to:

1. Identify the components of an adult breathing circuit.
2. Differentiate between ventilator breathing circuit variations.
3. Locate, identify, and use the basic controls on a volume ventilator for volume and rate (or minute ventilation), F_IO_2, flow rate, or inspiratory:expiratory ratio.
4. Test the circuit for leaks.
5. Determine the tubing compliance factor.
6. Calculate **compressible volume.**

KEY TERMS
chronometer

compressibility factor
compressible volume

proximal

wye

EQUIPMENT REQUIRED

- Adult breathing circuits, with and without exhalation valve
- HEPA bacteria filter
- Manufacturer's operation and maintenance manuals (videos if available)
- Water traps
- Humidifiers (HME, cascade, and wick)
- Sterile water
- Volume ventilators
- 50 psi oxygen source
- 50 psig regulator
- High-pressure hoses
- Air compressor
- Blender
- Wrench
- Test lung or lung simulator

● EXERCISES

EXERCISE 26.1 Adult Breathing Circuit

1. Select an adult breathing circuit with an external exhalation valve. Identify the components as illustrated in Figure 26.1, and *record them on your laboratory report.*

Inspiratory limb
Expiratory limb
Nebulizer
Wye
Patient connection adaptor
Proximal temperature port
Proximal pressure port
Exhalation valve
Exhalation drive line
Connection to humidifier
Connection to spirometer

2. Select an adult breathing circuit for use with ventilators using an internal exhalation valve as shown in Figure 26.2. Compare the circuit components with the circuit in step 1. *Record your observations regarding the variations between the circuits on your laboratory report.*

EXERCISE 26.2 Ventilator Assembly

1. Select a volume ventilator, water traps, bacteria filters, humidifier, and test lung. *Record the ventilator brand and model on your laboratory report.*
2. Obtain the maintenance manual for the ventilator selected. In the manual, find the manufacturer's recommendations for changing and cleaning of bacteria filters, fan filters, sterilization or disinfection instructions for internal and external parts and surfaces, and requirements for routine

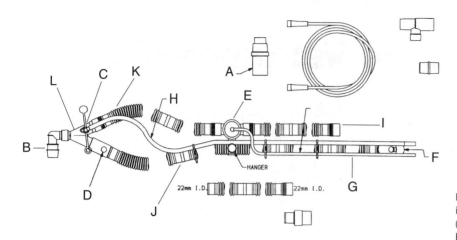

FIGURE 26.1   Components of an adult breathing circuit with an external exhalation valve. (Courtesy of Marquest Medical Products, Inc., Englewood, CO.)

maintenance. *Record this information on your laboratory report.*

3. Locate the **chronometer** and *record the number of hours of use on your laboratory report.*

4. Assemble the ventilator as shown in Figure 26.3, with humidifier, and Figure 26.4, with HME. Note any difficulties encountered while assembling the ventilator, and *record them on your laboratory report.*

5. Repeat this exercise for each ventilator provided.

EXERCISE 26.3 Identification of Controls

1. On the same ventilator used in Exercise 26.2, identify the following controls. It is important to note that not all ventilators have the same controls, but they have several controls in common. Several ventilator panels are shown in Figure 26.5. *Record the controls identified on your laboratory report.*

    Tidal volume or minute volume
    Rate
    F_IO_2
    Flow or percent inspiratory time
    Sigh volume
    Sigh rate
    High-pressure limit
    Low-pressure limit
    F_IO_2 alarms
    Low exhaled volume alarm

2. Repeat this exercise for each ventilator provided.

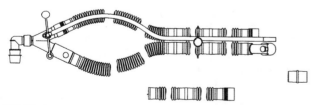

FIGURE 26.2   Components of an adult breathing circuit without an external exhalation valve. (Courtesy of Marquest Medical Products, Inc., Englewood, CO.)

EXERCISE 26.4 Leak Testing

Using the same equipment from Exercises 26.2 and 26.3, perform the following steps.

> NOTE: When initially turning on the ventilator, the Puritan Bennett 7200 ventilator will provide an option for an extended self-test (EST) procedure. Follow your instructor's directions to complete the EST before starting the exercise.

1. Turn all settings to the minimum or off setting.

2. Increase the tidal volume to 400 ml.

3. Increase the high-pressure limit to 80 cm H_2O or to the maximum setting.

4. Occlude the patient adaptor at the wye.

5. Cycle the ventilator. *Record your observations and the pressure achieved on your laboratory report.*

6. Loosen the water trap on the inspiratory limb.

7. Occlude the patient adaptor at the wye.

8. Cycle the ventilator. *Record your observations and the pressure achieved on your laboratory report.*

9. Return the water trap to its previous status.

10. Disconnect the inspiratory limb from the ventilator or humidifier outlet.

11. Occlude the patient adaptor at the wye.

12. Cycle the ventilator. *Record your observations and the pressure achieved on your laboratory report.*

13. Reconnect all tubes.

14. Repeat this exercise for each ventilator provided.

EXERCISE 26.5 Determination of Tubing Compliance Factor and Calculation of Lost Volume

Utilizing the same ventilator, perform the following:

1. Set the flow to the minimum setting.

2. Set the tidal volume to 300 ml.

3. Ensure that the high-pressure limit is set at the maximum.

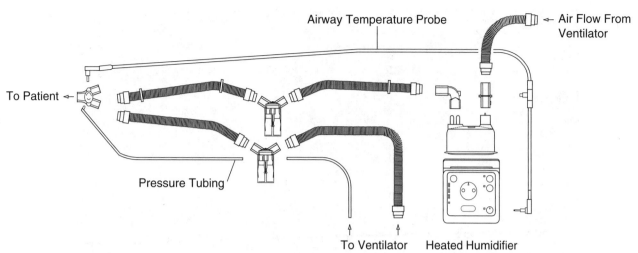

FIGURE 26.3   Ventilator circuit assembly with humidifier and water traps. (Courtesy of Fisher & Paykel Healthcare, Auckland, New Zealand.)

4. Occlude the patient adaptor at the wye.

5. Cycle the ventilator. *Record your observations and the pressure achieved on your laboratory report.*

6. Determine the **compressibility factor** (CF) using the following formula:

$$\frac{\text{Set } V_T - \text{Observed exhaled } V_T}{\text{Pressure}} = \text{Compressibility factor}$$

Record the compressibility factor on your laboratory report.

Related Readings

Chang, D: Clinical Application of Mechanical Ventilation. Delmar, Albany, 1997.

Eubanks, DH and Bone, RC: Principles and Applications of Cardiorespiratory Care Equipment. Mosby, St Louis, 1994.

McPherson, S: Respiratory Care Equipment, ed 5. Mosby, St Louis, 1995.

Scanlan, C et al (eds): Egan's Fundamentals of Respiratory Care, ed 6. Mosby, St Louis, 1995.

Selected Journal Articles

AARC: Special Issue. Conference on Mechanical Ventilation Part I. Respir Care 32:385–496, 1986.

AARC: Special Issue. Conference on Mechanical Ventilation Part II. Respir Care 32:497–640, 1986.

Bach, JR: A comparison of long-term ventilatory support alternatives from the perspective of the patient and caregiver. Chest 104:1702–1706, 1993.

Branson, RD and Davis, K: Work of breathing imposed by five ventilators used for long-term support: The effects of PEEP and simulated patient demand. Respir Care 40:1270–1278, 1995.

Consensus statement on mechanical ventilators. Respir Care 37:1000–1008, 1992.

Gammon et al: Mechanical ventilation: A review for the internist. Am J Med 99:533–562, 1995.

Kacmarek, RM and Venneger, JV: Mechanical ventilatory rates and tidal volumes. Respir Care 32:466–474, 1987.

Marini, JJ: Patient-ventilator interaction: Rational strategies for acute ventilatory management. Respir Care 38:482–493, 1993.

Slutski, AS: Consensus conference. Chest 104:1833–1859, 1993.

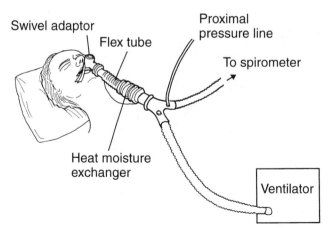

FIGURE 26.4   Ventilator circuit assembly with a heat and moisture exchanger (HME).

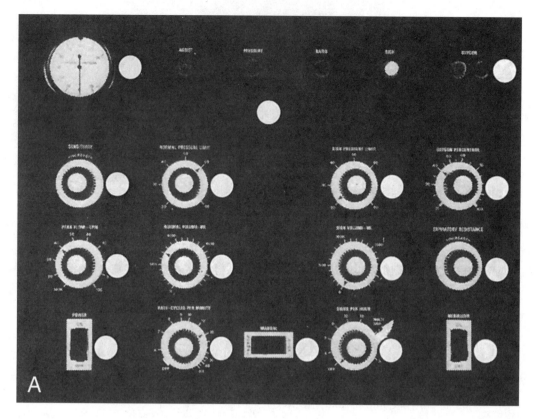

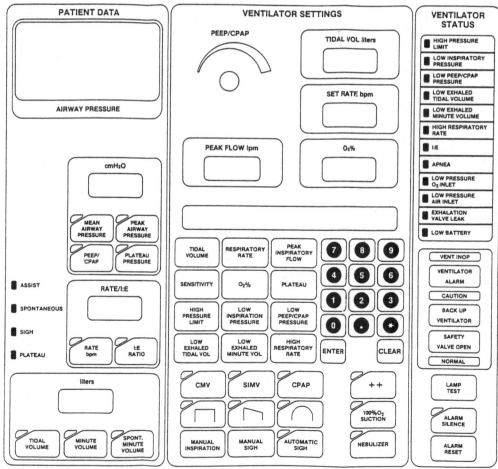

FIGURE 26.5   Control panels of common volume ventilators: *(A)* Puritan Bennett MA-1. *(B)* Puritan Bennett 7200. (Courtesy of Nellcor Puritan Bennett Inc., Carlsbad, CA.)

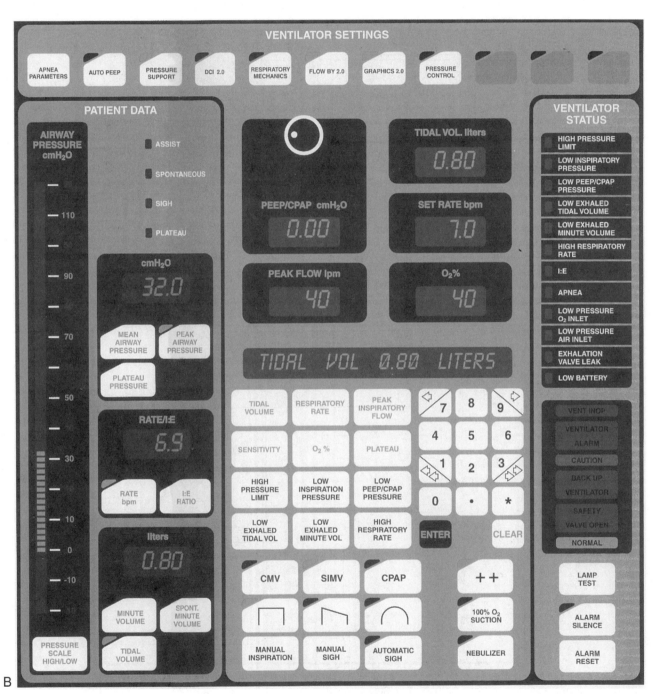

FIGURE 26.5   *(B, continued)* Puritan Bennett 7200. (Courtesy of Nellcor Puritan Bennett Inc., Carlsbad, CA.)

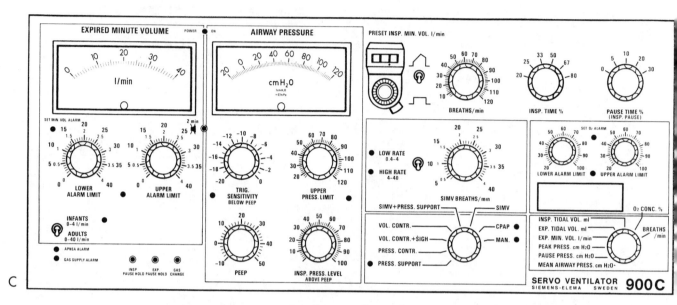

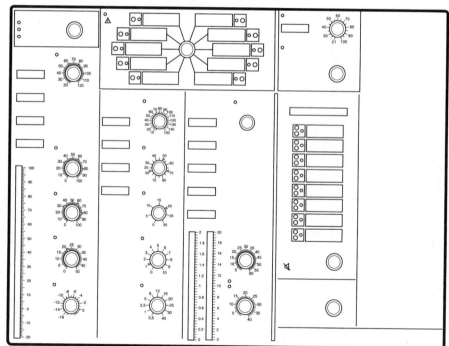

FIGURE 26.5 *Continued* *(C)* Servo 900C. (Courtesy of Siemens Medical Systems, Electromedical Group, Danvers, MA.) *(D)* Siemens 300E. (Courtesy of Siemens Medical Systems, Electromedical Group, Danvers, MA.)

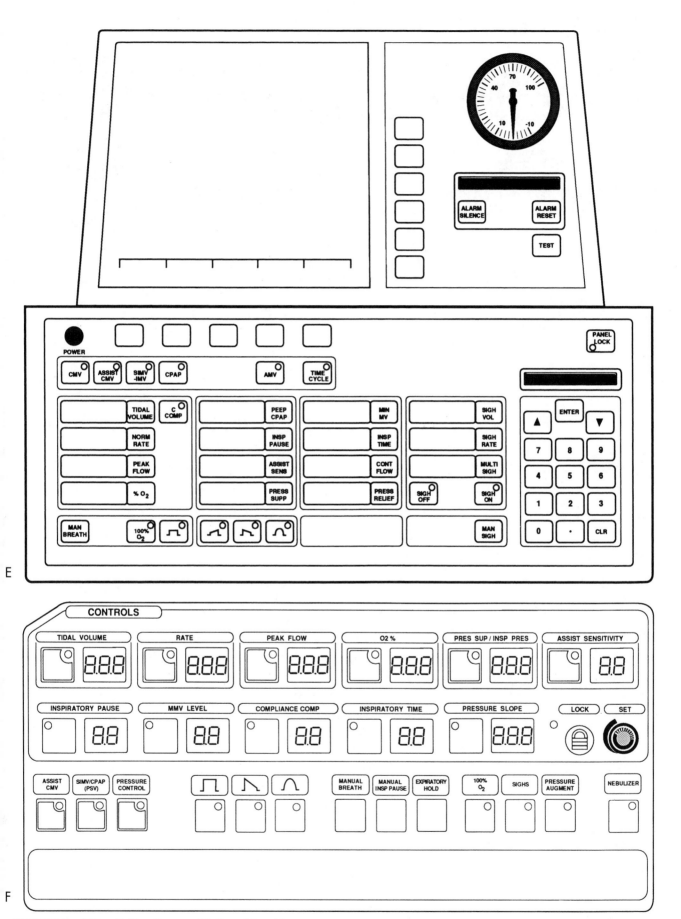

FIGURE 26.5 *(E)* Bear 5. (From Branson, RD, Hess, DR and Chatburn, RL: Respiratory Care Equipment. JB Lippincott, Philadelphia, 1995, p. 314, with permission.) *(F)* Bear 1000. (Courtesy of Bear Medical Systems, Riverside, CA.)

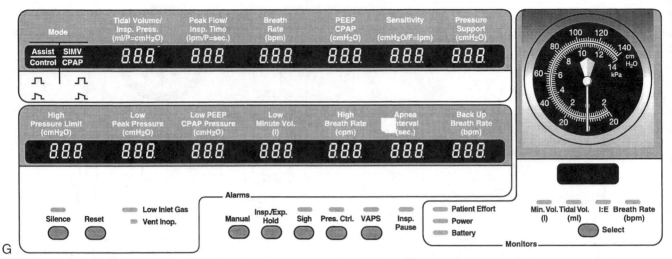

FIGURE 26.5 *Continued* *(G)* Bird 8400ST. (Courtesy of Bird Products Corporation, Palm Springs, CA.)

LABORATORY REPORT

CHAPTER 26: VOLUME VENTILATORS

Name _____   Date _____

Course/Section _____   Instructor _____

Data Collection

EXERCISE 26.1   Adult Breathing Circuit

A. _____

B. _____

C. _____

D. _____

E. _____

F. _____

G. _____

H. _____

I. _____

J. _____

K. _____

L. _____

Comparison of ventilator circuit types: _____

_____

_____

_____

EXERCISE 26.2   Ventilator Assembly   (attach separate sheet for additional ventilators used)

Ventilator brand and model: _____

Manufacturer's Recommendations

Changing and cleaning of bacteria filters: _____

_____

Fan filters: _____

_____

Sterilization or disinfection instructions for internal and external parts and surfaces: _____

_____

_____

Requirements for routine maintenance: _____

_____

Hours of use: _____

What difficulties, if any, did you encounter when assembling the ventilator? _____

_____

EXERCISE 26.3 Identification of Controls (attach separate sheet for each ventilator used)

List the controls identified: _____

_____

_____

_____

_____

_____

EXERCISE 26.4 Leak Testing (attach separate sheet for each ventilator provided)

Pressure reading and observations after setup: _____

_____

_____

Pressure reading and observations with a loose water trap: _____

_____

_____

Pressure reading and observations with a large disconnect: _____

_____

_____

EXERCISE 26.5 Determination of Tubing Compliance Factor (CF) and Calculation of Lost Volume

Set tidal volume: _____

Observed exhaled tidal volume: _____

Pressure reading: _____

Observations: _____

Calculated compressibility factor (CF) (show your work!):

CRITICAL THINKING QUESTIONS

1. Compare and contrast the assembly of a volume ventilator with the following:
   a. Internal exhalation valve vs. external exhalation valve
   b. HME vs. cascade or wick humidifier

2. You have just assembled a volume ventilator and performed a leak test. The cycling pressure achieved when the wye was occluded was only 55 cm H_2O. Describe the step-by-step procedure you would use to rectify the problem.

3. You have successfully rectified the problem in Critical Thinking Question 2. How would you communicate to the incoming shift that this ventilator is ready for patient use?

4. Given the following data, calculate the compressible volume loss and actual V_T. Show your work!
   a. V_T = 500 ml
      CF = 4 ml/cm H_2O
      Peak pressure = 20 cm H_2O

      Lost volume = _____ ml

      Actual V_T = _____ ml
   b. V_T = 800 ml
      CF = 2 ml/cm H_2O
      Peak pressure = 30 cm H_2O

      Lost volume = _____ ml

      Actual V_T = _____ ml
   c. V_T = 700 ml
      CF = 3.5 ml/cm H_2O
      Peak pressure = 40 cm H_2O

      Lost volume = _____ ml

      Actual V_T = _____ ml
   d. V_T = 200 ml
      CF = 2 ml/cm H_2O
      Peak pressure = 50 cm H_2O

      Lost volume = _____ ml

      Actual V_T = _____ ml

Ventilator Modes

INTRODUCTION

Technological advances have increased the variety of ways that one can mechanically ventilate a patient. Each method has a different goal. Is the goal to rest the patient's respiratory muscles, or do we allow the patient to do some work? Will we allow the patient to breathe spontaneously as a supplement to machine breaths or as the sole method of ventilation? Do we need to **augment** the patient's spontaneous breaths or increase the FRC? Does the patient have difficulty primarily with oxygenation, ventilation, or both? What is the condition of the patient's airways and lung-thorax relationship? Is the patient "fighting the ventilator" or ready to be weaned? The way in which the ventilator achieves these goals is by the mode selected. The ventilator mode will determine how the patient and machine function in harmony. The practitioner, therefore, must comprehend the capabilities of each machine in order to know if a specific mode is available and must also know the intricacies of each mode and how it may be best applied for each individual patient.

Once the appropriate mode is selected, the practitioner must, in concert with the physician or through the use of protocol, determine the most appropriate values for other ventilator parameters, including F_IO_2, tidal volume and respiratory rate (or minute ventilation), flow rate and pattern, inspiratory-to-expiratory ratios, inspiratory or expiratory pauses, sighs, and any pressure adjuncts.

This chapter explores the common modes of mechanical ventilation and ventilator capabilities. Guidelines for initiation of ventilation and parameter selection, alarm settings, monitoring, and discontinuance of mechanical ventilation are addressed in the next chapter.

OBJECTIVES
Upon completion of this chapter, the student will be able to:

1. Differentiate the various modes of mechanical ventilation: control, assist/control, synchronized intermittent **mandatory** ventilation (SIMV), pressure control and **inverse** I:E ratio ventilation, pressure support, PEEP, and CPAP.

2. Given any mechanical ventilator, locate and identify each mode and adjunct parameter available and determine how to use it.

3. Assess the limitations of each ventilator.

4. Evaluate the effects of manipulation of the various interdependent modes and adjunct parameters.

5. Compare and contrast the capabilities of critical care ventilators with home care ventilators.

KEY TERMS

augment	inverse	mandatory	synchrony

EQUIPMENT REQUIRED

- Adult breathing circuits for ventilators available (needed for critical care and home care ventilators)
- HEPA bacteria filters
- Manufacturer's operation and maintenance manuals (videos if available)
- Water traps
- Humidifiers (HME, cascade, and wick)
- Sterile water
- Volume ventilators
- Home care ventilators
- 50 psi oxygen source
- 50 psig regulator
- Bourdon gauge and Thorpe tube flowmeters
- High-pressure hoses
- Air compressor
- Blender
- Wrench
- T-adaptor with small-bore tubing connection and cap
- Test lungs and lung simulator (if available)
- Watch with a second hand
- Respirometer
- Oxygen analyzer and in-line adaptor

- Spring-loaded PEEP valve
- Self-contained (or sealed marine) 12-volt battery with connecting cables

⬤ E X E R C I S E S

It is suggested that the following exercises be performed with the ventilator alarms set on minimum/maximum settings so that students will not be intimidated by the noise and confusion during the initial learning experience (and so that instructors will not be unnerved). Once students gain comfort with the operation of the various ventilator controls, it would be valuable for the exercises to be repeated with the alarms set appropriately for clinical situations. Students can then observe the relationship between the machine settings, alarms, and patient care implications. The goals of the various modes of mechanical ventilation are outlined in Table 27.1. Most modern ventilators can achieve all of these modes. The student should perform all the exercises on a selected ventilator and then repeat the entire set of exercises on any other available brands, taking particular notice of the differences between the brands of ventilators used.

EXERCISE 27.1 Control and Assist/Control

1. Assemble a volume ventilator and verify its proper function as performed in Chapter 26. *Record the type/brand of ventilator used on your laboratory report.*

TABLE 27.1 **Goals of Mechanical Ventilation Modes**

Mode	Goal
Control	Precise $\dot{V}_E$; patient's ventilatory drive controlled with medication
Assist/control	Ventilator does almost all work; ventilatory muscles rested.
SIMV	Patient breathes spontaneously between mandatory ventilator breaths; ventilatory muscles used; also can be used as weaning technique or to help stabilize a patient fighting assist/control mode
Pressure support	Augments the V_T with a preselected amount of positive pressure; decreases work of breathing, including that superimposed by the artificial airway and circuitry
CPAP	Patient breathes spontaneously; continuous positive pressure gradient aids in oxygenation by increasing FRC
PEEP	Not a true mode but an adjunct to exhalation; aids oxygenation by increasing FRC
Pressure control	Used when one needs to reduce the mean airway pressure when high pressures are being used in volume ventilation
Inverse I:E	Aids in oxygenation
Airway pressure release ventilation (APRV)	Strategy for use with ARDS: improves oxygenation and lowers mean airway pressure; available only on Irisa ventilator

2. Adjust the settings to the following:
   $V_T = 600$ ml
   $f = 15$/min
   Peak flow = 30 lpm (or percent inspiratory time = 33 percent)
   $F_IO_2 = 0.21$
   Make sure that all the alarms are set to the minimum/maximum settings.

3. Adjust the sensitivity to -10 cm H_2O.

4. Attach the test lung to the patient wye connection.

5. Count the respiratory rate, and compare it with the rate set on the machine. *Record the result on your laboratory report.*

6. Observe the exhaled tidal volume, and *record the result on your laboratory report.*

7. Squeeze the test lung several times to simulate an inspiratory effort. Observe the manometer. Count the rate at which you are squeezing the test lung, and compare it with the displayed rate on the machine. *Record the results on your laboratory report. Explain why the ventilator responded in this manner on your laboratory report.*

8. Adjust the sensitivity to -2 cm H_2O.

9. Squeeze the test lung several times to simulate an inspiratory effort. Listen to the sound of the machine. Observe the manometer. Count the rate at which you are squeezing the test lung, and compare it with the displayed rate on the machine. *Record the results and observations on your laboratory report.*

10. Observe the exhaled tidal volume, and compare it with the displayed machine volume. *Record the result on your laboratory report.*

11. Adjust the rate to 4/min. Squeeze the test lung at a minimum rate of 15/min. Listen to the sound of the machine. Observe the manometer. Count the rate at which you are squeezing the test lung, and compare it with the displayed rate on the machine. *Record the results and observations on your laboratory report.*

12. Observe the exhaled tidal volume, and compare it with the displayed machine volume. *Record the result on your laboratory report.*

13. Stop squeezing the test lung. Wait 1 min and observe the ventilator response. Count the ventilator rate. *Record your results and observations on your laboratory report.*

14. Repeat the exercise with a second ventilator.

EXERCISE 27.2 Synchronized Intermittent Mandatory Ventilation

1. Using the same equipment, change the mode to IMV or SIMV. *Record the type/brand of ventilator on your laboratory report.*

2. Maintain the settings as follows:
   $V_T = 600$ ml
   $f = 15$/min
   Peak flow = 30 lpm (or percent inspiratory time = 33 percent)
   $F_IO_2 = 0.21$
   Make sure that all the alarms are set to the minimum/maximum settings.

3. Adjust the sensitivity to -2 cm H_2O.

4. Count the respiratory rate and observe the tidal volume, and *record on your laboratory report.*

5. Squeeze the test lung several times to simulate an inspiratory effort. Observe the manometer. Count the rate at which you are squeezing the test lung, and compare it with the displayed rate on the machine. *Record the results on your laboratory report.*

6. Continue to squeeze the lung. Listen to the sound of the machine, and compare it with the control/assist control mode. Observe the tidal volume for your manual squeezes and machine-delivered breaths. *Record the result and your observations on your laboratory report. Determine if the machine is using IMV or SIMV.*

7. Decrease the set respiratory rate to four breaths per minute.

8. Squeeze the test lung to simulate an inspiratory effort.

9. Continue to squeeze the lung, and count the rate at which you are squeezing. Listen to the sound of the machine, and compare it with step 6. Observe and compare the spontaneous rate with the machine rate displayed. Observe and compare the tidal volume for your manual squeezes and machine-delivered breaths. *Record the results on your laboratory report.*

10. Stop squeezing the test lung. Wait 1 min, listen to the sound of the machine, and observe the machine response. *Record your observations on the laboratory report.*

11. Reset any alarms if necessary. Resume squeezing the test lung. Observe the machine response, and *record your observations on the laboratory report.*

12. Compare the ventilator responses in the SIMV mode to the assist control mode. *Explain why these differences occur on your laboratory report.*

EXERCISE 27.3 Positive End-Expiratory Pressure/Continuous Positive Airway Pressure

1. Using the same equipment, set the mode to assist/control. *Record the type/brand of ventilator used on your laboratory report.*

2. Adjust the settings to the following:
   V_T = 500 ml
   f = 15/min
   Peak flow = 30 lpm (or percent inspiratory time = 25 percent)
   F_IO_2 = 0.21
   Make sure that all the alarms are set to the minimum/maximum settings.

3. Adjust the sensitivity to –3 cm H_2O.

4. Attach the test lung and turn on the ventilator.

5. Observe and compare the pressure manometer and the filling of the test lung at the end of inspiration and at the end of expiration. *Record the pressure readings at end inspiration and end expiration and your observations on your laboratory report.*

6. Adjust the PEEP to 5 cm H_2O.

7. Observe and compare the pressure manometer and the filling of the test lung at the end of inspiration and at the end of expiration. *Record the pressure readings at end inspiration and end expiration and your observations on your laboratory report. Did the sensitivity need to be adjusted?*

8. Adjust the PEEP to 8 cm H_2O.

9. Observe and compare the pressure manometer and the filling of the test lung at the end of inspiration and at the end of expiration. *Record the pressure readings at end inspiration and end expiration and your observations on your laboratory report. Did the sensitivity need to be adjusted?*

10. Decrease the PEEP setting to 0.

11. Change the mode to CPAP.

12. Adjust the CPAP pressure to 5 cm H_2O.

13. Squeeze the test lung to simulate a spontaneous breath.

14. Observe the pressure manometer and the filling of the test lung. *Record the pressure reading and your observations on your laboratory report.*

15. Adjust the CPAP to 10 cm H_2O.

16. Squeeze the test lung to simulate a spontaneous breath. Count the respiratory rate, and *record it on your laboratory report.*

17. Observe and compare the pressure manometer and the filling of the test lung at the end of inspiration and at the end of expiration. *Record the pressure readings at end inspiration and end expiration and your observations on your laboratory report.*

18. Stop squeezing the test lung. Wait 1 min, and observe the machine response, rate, and tidal volume. *Record your results and observations on your laboratory report. Explain why the ventilator responded as it did on your laboratory report.*

19. Repeat the exercise with a second ventilator.

EXERCISE 27.4 Pressure Support Mode

EXERCISE 27.4.1 Synchronized Intermittent Mandatory Ventilation with Pressure Support

1. Using the same equipment, modify the mode to activate pressure support with the SIMV mode. *Record the type/brand of ventilator used on your laboratory report.*

2. Maintain the settings as at the end of Exercise 27.3:
   V_T = 600 ml
   f = 4/min
   Peak flow = 30 lpm (or percent inspiratory time = 33 percent)
   F_IO_2 = 0.21
   Make sure that all the alarms are set to the minimum/maximum settings.

3. Adjust the sensitivity to –2 cm H_2O.

4. Adjust the pressure support level to 5 cm H_2O.

5. Squeeze the test lung to simulate an inspiratory effort.

6. Continue to squeeze the lung, and count the respiratory rate. Observe the tidal volume and manometer pressure readings for your manual squeezes and machine-delivered breaths. *Record the results on your laboratory report.*

7. While still squeezing the test lung, observe the pressure manometer. Listen to the sound of the machine. Compare the sound of the machine during a spontaneous breath in SIMV with pressure support with a spontaneous breath in SIMV without pressure support. *Record the pressure reading and your observations on your laboratory report.*

8. Increase the pressure support to 10 cm H_2O.

9. Squeeze the test lung to simulate an inspiratory effort.

10. Continue to squeeze the lung and count the respiratory rate. Listen to the sound of the machine, and compare it with step 7. Observe the tidal volume for your manual squeezes and machine-delivered breaths. *Record the results and your observations on your laboratory report.*

EXERCISE 27.4.2 Pressure Support

1. Using the same equipment, modify the mode to activate pressure support without SIMV. This may require you to consult the operation manual to determine how this is achieved on a given ventilator. It may require the use of the CPAP mode.

2. Adjust the pressure support level to 0 cm H_2O. If the CPAP mode is required, make sure that the CPAP or PEEP pressure is set at zero.

3. Squeeze the test lung to simulate an inspiratory effort.

4. Continue to squeeze the lung. Observe the rate and tidal volume for your manual squeezes and machine-delivered breaths. *Record the results and observations on your laboratory report.*

5. While still squeezing the test lung, observe the pressure manometer. Listen to the sound of the machine. *Record the pressure reading and your observations on your laboratory report.*

6. Increase the pressure support to 5 cm H_2O.

7. Squeeze the test lung to simulate an inspiratory effort.

8. Continue to squeeze the lung. Listen to the sound of the machine and compare it with step 6. Observe the rate and tidal volume for your manual squeezes. *Record the results and your observations on your laboratory report.*

9. Increase the pressure support to 10 cm H_2O.

10. Squeeze the test lung to simulate an inspiratory effort.

11. Continue to squeeze the lung. Listen to the sound of the machine and compare it with step 6. Observe the rate and tidal volume for your manual squeezes. *Record the results and your observations on your laboratory report.*

12. Stop squeezing the test lung. Wait 1 min, and observe the rate and tidal volume. Observe the machine response. *Record your results and observations on your laboratory report.*

13. Repeat the exercise with a second ventilator.

EXERCISE 27.4.3 Pressure Support with Continuous Positive Airway Pressure

1. Maintain the ventilator in the pressure support mode as in Exercise 27.4.2. Set the pressure support to 10 cm H_2O. *Record the type/brand of ventilator used on your laboratory report.*

2. Squeeze the test lung to simulate an inspiratory effort.

3. Continue to squeeze the lung. Listen to the sound of the machine. Observe the rate, tidal volume, and filling of the test lung for your manual squeezes. *Record the results and your observations on your laboratory report.*

4. Add CPAP of 5 cm H_2O.

5. Continue to squeeze the lung. Listen to the sound of the machine and compare it with step 3. Observe the rate, tidal volume, and filling of the test lung for your manual squeezes. *Record the results and your observations on your laboratory report.*

EXERCISE 27.5 Inverse I:E Ratio, Pressure Control Ventilation

EXERCISE 27.5.1 Pressure Control

1. Using the same ventilator, set the mode control to pressure control, if available.

2. Connect the test lung or lung simulator to the patient wye. If you are using a lung simulator, set the compliance at 0.15 L/cm H_2O, the most compliant setting.

3. Set the controls to the following:
   Inspiratory pressure = 10 cm H_2O
   f = 15/min
   Peak flow = 30 lpm (or percent inspiratory time = 33 percent)

4. Monitor the exhaled tidal volume, and *record it on your laboratory report.*

5. Measure the I:E ratio and *record it on your laboratory report.*

6. Adjust the compliance to 0.05 L/cm H_2O.

7. Observe the exhaled tidal volume, and *record it on your laboratory report.*

8. Measure the I:E ratio, and *record it on your laboratory report.*

9. Repeat the exercise with a second ventilator.

EXERCISE 27.5.2 Inverse I:E Ratio Ventilation

1. Using the same ventilator, set the mode control to pressure control, if available.

2. Connect the test lung or lung simulator to the patient wye.

3. Set the controls to the following:
   Inspiratory pressure = 15 cm H_2O
   f = 15/min
   Compliance = 0.05 L/cm H_2O (decreased compliance)

4. Adjust the ventilator to inverse I:E ratio of 2:1 (if using the Siemens Servo 900C, adjust the percent inspiratory time to 67 percent).

5. Observe the exhaled tidal volume, and *record it on your laboratory report.*

6. Measure the I:E ratio, and *record it on your laboratory report.*

7. Calculate or determine the peak flow rate, and *record it on your laboratory report.*

EXERCISE 27.6 Home Care Ventilators

EXERCISE 27.6.1 Home Care Ventilator Circuits and Maintenance

Obtain a home care ventilator and appropriate breathing circuit. Selected control panels for common home care ventilators are shown in Figure 27.1.

1. Select a breathing circuit for home care ventilator use as shown in Figure 27.2. Contrast the components to those

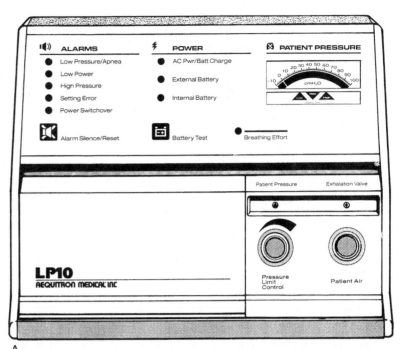

A

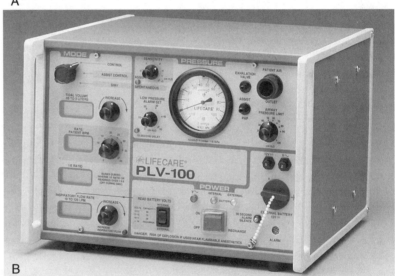

B

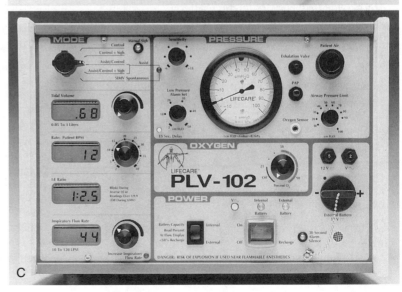

C

FIGURE 27.1 Ventilator control panels for *(A)* Life Products LP-10. (Courtesy of Aequitron Medical Inc., Minneapolis, MN.) *(B)* Lifecare PLV-100. (Courtesy of LIFECARE International, Inc., Westminster, CO.) *(C)* Lifecare PLV-102. (Courtesy of LIFECARE International, Inc., Westminster, CO.)

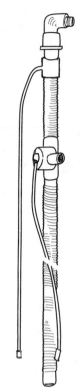

FIGURE 27.2   Home care ventilator circuit.

used on adult critical care ventilator circuits. *Record the major differences on your laboratory report.*

2. Select a home care ventilator, bacteria filters, humidifier or HME, and test lung. *Record the ventilator brand and model on your laboratory report.*

3. Obtain the maintenance manual for the ventilator selected. In the manual, find the manufacturer's recommendations for the following:
   Changing and cleaning of bacteria filters
   Fan filters
   Sterilization or disinfection instructions for internal and external parts and surfaces
   Requirements for routine maintenance
   Charging frequency for internal battery
   Locate the port where the external battery is connected. *Record this information on your laboratory report.*

4. Locate the chronometer, if available, and *record the number of hours of use on your laboratory report.*

5. Assemble the ventilator circuit as shown in Figure 27.2.

6. Repeat this exercise for each ventilator provided.

EXERCISE 27.6.2 Identification of Controls

1. On the same ventilator used in Exercise 27.6.1, identify the following controls. It is important to note that home care ventilators do not have the same controls as critical care ventilators, but they have several controls in common. Determine if the following parameters can be controlled:
   Tidal volume or minute volume
   Rate
   Mode
   Sensitivity
   F_IO_2
   Flow or I:E ratio
   Sigh volume and rate
   PEEP
   High-pressure limit
   Low-pressure limit
   Battery alarm
   Low exhaled volume alarm
   *Record the controls or alarms identified, and what controls are **not** available, on your laboratory report.*

2. Repeat this exercise for each ventilator provided.

3. Lift each ventilator carefully and compare their weights.

EXERCISE 27.6.3 Leak Testing

Using the same equipment from Exercise 27.6.1, perform the following steps. *Record the type/brand of ventilator used on your laboratory report.*

1. Turn all settings to the minimum or off setting.

2. Increase the tidal volume to 400 ml.

3. Increase the high-pressure limit to 80 cm H_2O or to the maximum setting.

4. Occlude the patient adaptor at the wye.

5. Cycle the ventilator, and *record your observations and the pressure achieved on your laboratory report.*

6. Loosen the medication cup (if available) on the inspiratory limb.

7. Occlude the patient adaptor at the wye.

8. Cycle the ventilator, and *record your observations and the pressure achieved on your laboratory report.*

9. Return the medication cup to its previous status.

10. Disconnect the inspiratory limb from the ventilator or humidifier outlet.

11. Occlude the patient adaptor at the wye.

12. Cycle the ventilator, and *record your observations and the pressure achieved on your laboratory report.*

13. Reconnect all tubes.

14. Repeat this exercise for each ventilator provided.

EXERCISE 27.6.4 F_IO_2 and Positive End-Expiratory Pressure on Home Care Ventilators

Using the same equipment from Exercise 27.6.1, perform the following steps.

1. Adjust the ventilator controls as follows:
   V_T: 500 ml
   f: 12/min
   Mode: assist/control
   Sensitivity: −2 cm H_2O

2. Obtain an oxygen T-adaptor with a small-bore tubing connection and cap, and insert it into the inspiratory limb of the circuit proximal to the humidifier as shown in Figure 27.3.

3. Connect the adaptor to an oxygen flowmeter at a liter flow of 2 lpm.

4. Insert a calibrated oxygen analyzer in-line distal to the humidifier.

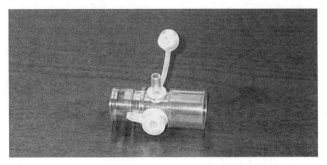

FIGURE 27.3   Oxygen T-adaptor.

5. Adjust the flow to obtain an F_IO_2 of 0.3. *Record the flow required on your laboratory report.*

6. Adjust the rate to 20/min. Allow at least 1 min for the F_IO_2 to stabilize. *Record any change in the F_IO_2 on your laboratory report.*

7. Readjust the liter flow to obtain an F_IO_2 of 0.3. *Record any changes required on your laboratory report.*

8. Observe the pressure manometer. *Record any back pressure reflected on your laboratory report.*

9. Squeeze the test lung to simulate spontaneous breathing effort at a rate of 25/min. *Record any change in the F_IO_2 on your laboratory report.*

10. Return the rate to 12/min.

11. Obtain a 5 cm H_2O spring-loaded PEEP valve. If adjustable, the pressure must be set after connection. Connect the valve to the exhalation port as shown in Figure 27.4.

12. Adjust the PEEP pressure to 5 cm H_2O if required.

13. Observe the PIP and PEEP pressure on the manometer and record the pressures on your laboratory report.

14. Squeeze the test lung to simulate spontaneous breathing at a rate of 20/min. Observe the manometer and breath rate, and *record your observations on your laboratory report.*

15. Select the appropriate control, and adjust it so that the machine cycles appropriately when spontaneous breathing is simulated. *Record the control selected and the adjustments required on your laboratory report.*

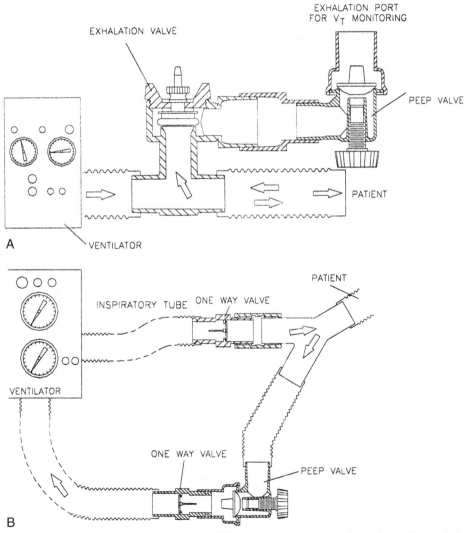

FIGURE 27.4   *(A)* PEEP valve connected to the exhalation port. *(B)* PEEP valve attachment to ventilator circuit without exhalation valve. (Courtesy of Instrumentation Industries, Inc., Bethel Park, PA.)

Related Readings

Chang, DW: Clinical Application of Mechanical Ventilation. Delmar, Albany, 1997.

Eubanks, DH and Bone, RC: Principles and Applications of Cardiorespiratory Care Equipment. Mosby, St Louis, 1994.

McPherson, SP: Respiratory Care Equipment, ed 5. Mosby, St Louis, 1995.

Pilbeam, S: Mechanical Ventilation: Physiological and Clinical Applications. Mosby, St Louis, 1992.

Scanlan, C et al (eds): Egan's Fundamentals of Respiratory Care, ed 6. Mosby, St Louis, 1995.

Selected Journal Articles

Bach, JR: A comparison of long-term ventilatory support alternatives from the perspective of the patient and the care giver. Chest 104:1702–1706, 1993.

Banner, M et al: Decreasing imposed work of the breathing apparatus to zero using pressure support ventilation. Crit Care Med 219:1333–1338, 1993.

Cane, RD, Peruzzi, WT and Shapiro, BA: Airway pressure release ventilation in severe acute respiratory failure. Chest 100:460–463, 1991.

Chiang, AA et al: Demand flow airway pressure release ventilation as a partial ventilatory support mode: Comparison with synchronized intermittent mandatory ventilation and pressure support ventilation. Crit Care Med 22:1431–1437, 1994.

Davis K, et al: Airway pressure release ventilation. Arch Surg 128: 1348–1352, 1993.

Gurevitch, M et al: Improved oxygenation and lower peak airway pressure in severe adult respiratory distress syndrome treatment with inverse I:E ratio ventilation. Chest 89:211–213, 1986.

Keilty, S et al: Effect of inspiratory pressure support on exercise tolerance and breathlessness in patients with severe stable obstructive pulmonary disease. Thorax 49:990–994, 1994.

Lessard, M et al: Effects of pressure controlled with different I:E ratio versus volume controlled ventilation on respiratory mechanics, gas exchange, and hemodynamics in patients with adult respiratory distress syndrome. Anesthesiology 80:983–991, 1994.

MacIntyre, N: Respiratory function during pressure support ventilation. Chest 89:677–683, 1986.

MacIntyre, N: Pressure support: Coming of age. Semin Respir Med 14:293–298, 1993.

Mancebo, J et al: Volume controlled ventilation and pressure controlled inverse ratio ventilation: A comparison of their effects in ARDS patients. Arch Chest Dis 49:201–207, 1994.

Marini, J: Recent advances in mechanical ventilation. Semin Respir Med 14:251–299, 1993.

Marini, J: Patient-ventilator interaction: Rational strategies for acute ventilatory management. Respir Care 38:482–493, 1993.

Morris, AH: Adult respiratory distress syndrome and new modes of mechanical ventilation: Reducing the complications of high volume and high pressure. New Horiz 2:19–33, 1994.

Stock, M: Conceptual basis for inverse ratio and airway pressure release ventilation. Semin Respir Med 14:270–274, 1993.

LABORATORY REPORT

CHAPTER 27: VENTILATOR MODES

Name _____   Date _____

Course/Section _____   Instructor _____

Data Collection

EXERCISE 27.1   Control and Assist/Control

Type/brand of ventilator 1: _____

Assist/Control Rate of 15

SENSITIVITY −10 cm H_2O

V_T = 600; f = 15/min; Peak flow = 30 lpm

Respiratory rate: _____

Exhaled V_T: _____

SIMULATED SPONTANEOUS BREATHING

Manometer observation and respiratory rate: _____

_____

_____

Exhaled V_T: _____

Explain why the ventilator responded in this manner: _____

_____

SENSITIVITY −2 cm H_2O

Manometer observation and respiratory rate: _____

_____

_____

Exhaled V_T: _____

Assist/Control Rate of 4 with Spontaneous Rate

Respiratory rate: _____

Exhaled V_T: _____

Manometer observation: _____

_____

_____

STOP SQUEEZING

Exhaled V_T: _____

Observations and rate: _____

_____

_____

Type/brand of ventilator 2: _____

Assist/Control Rate of 15

SENSITIVITY –10 cm H_2O

Respiratory rate: _____

Exhaled V_T: _____

SIMULATED SPONTANEOUS BREATHING

Manometer observation and respiratory rate: _____

_____

_____

Exhaled V_T: _____

SENSITIVITY –2 cm H_2O

Manometer observation and respiratory rate: _____

_____

_____

Exhaled V_T: _____

Assist/Control Rate of 4

Respiratory rate: _____

Exhaled V_T: _____

Manometer observation: _____

_____

_____

STOP SQUEEZING

Exhaled V_T: _____

Observations and rate: _____

_____

_____

Attach separate paper if additional ventilators are used.

EXERCISE 27.2   Synchronized Intermittent Mandatory Ventilation

Type/brand of ventilator 1: _____

With Sensitivity at –2 cm H_2O

Machine rate: _____

Machine exhaled V_T: _____

Spontaneous respiratory rate: _____

Spontaneous exhaled V_T: _____

SIMV Rate 4/min

Machine rate: _____

Machine V_T: _____

Spontaneous respiratory rate: _____

Spontaneous exhaled V_T: _____

Stop Squeezing

Observations: _____

_____

Resume Squeezing

Observations: _____

_____

Type/brand of ventilator 2: _____

With Sensitivity at −2 cm H₂O

Machine rate: _____

Machine exhaled V_T: _____

Spontaneous respiratory rate: _____

Spontaneous exhaled V_T: _____

SIMV Rate 4/min

Machine rate: _____

Machine V_T: _____

Spontaneous respiratory rate: _____

Spontaneous exhaled V_T: _____

Stop Squeezing

Observations: _____

_____

Resume Squeezing

Observations: _____

_____

Compare the ventilator response and your observations in the assist/control mode to the SIMV mode with spontaneous ventilations. Explain why these differences occur: _____

_____

_____

_____

Attach separate paper if additional ventilators are used.

EXERCISE 27.3   Positive End-Expiratory Pressure/Continuous Positive Airway Pressure

Type/brand of ventilator 1: _____

Initial pressure readings and observations: _____

_____

_____

5 cm H_2O pressure reading and observations: _____

_____

_____

Did the sensitivity need to be adjusted? _____

8 cm H_2O pressure reading and observations: _____

_____

_____

Did the sensitivity need to be adjusted? _____

CPAP 5 cm H_2O pressure reading and observations: _____

_____

_____

CPAP 10 cm H_2O pressure reading and observations: _____

_____

_____

Respiratory rate: _____

Stop Squeezing

Pressure reading and observations: _____

_____

_____

_____

Respiratory rate: _____ V_T: _____

Identify what clinical condition this exercise is supposed to simulate. Explain why the ventilator responded as it did: _____

_____

_____

_____

Type/brand of ventilator 2: _____

Initial pressure readings and observations: _____

_____

_____

5 cm H_2O pressure reading and observations: _____

_____

_____

Did the sensitivity need to be adjusted? _____

8 cm H_2O pressure reading and observations: _____

_____

_____

Did the sensitivity need to be adjusted? _____

CPAP 5 cm H_2O pressure reading and observations: _____

_____

_____

CPAP 10 cm H_2O pressure reading and observations: _____

_____

_____

Respiratory rate:

vations: _____

_____

_____

V_T: _____

)onse with that of ventilator 1: _____

_____

_____

mal ventilators are used.

pport Mode

ed Intermittent Mandatory Ventilation with

Type/brand of ventilator 1: _____

Pressure Support 5 cm H_2O

SIMV respiratory f: _____

Exhaled machine V_T: _____

Machine peak pressure: _____

Spontaneous respiratory f: _____

Spontaneous exhaled V_T: _____

Spontaneous peak pressure: _____

Observations: _____

_____

Pressure Support 10 cm H_2O

SIMV f: _____

Exhaled machine V_T: _____

Machine peak pressure: _____

Spontaneous f: _____

Spontaneous exhaled V_T: _____

Spontaneous peak pressure: _____

Observations: _____

_____

Type/brand of ventilator 2: _____

Pressure Support 5 cm H_2O

SIMV f: _____

Exhaled machine V_T: _____

Machine peak pressure: _____

Spontaneous f: _____

Spontaneous exhaled V_T: _____

Spontaneous peak pressure: _____

Observations: _____

_____

Pressure Support 10 cm H_2O

SIMV f: _____

Exhaled machine V_T: _____

Machine peak pressure: _____

Spontaneous f: _____

Spontaneous exhaled V_T: _____

Spontaneous peak pressure: _____

Observations: _____

_____

Attach separate paper if additional ventilators are used.

EXERCISE 27.4.2   Pressure Support

Type/brand of ventilator 1: _____

Pressure Support 0 cm H_2O

f: _____

V_T: _____

Pressure reading: _____

Observations: _____

Pressure Support 5 cm H_2O

f: _____

V_T: _____

Pressure reading: _____

Observations: _____

Pressure Support 10 cm H_2O

f: _____

V_T: _____

Pressure reading: _____

Observations: _____

Stop Squeezing

f: _____

V_T: _____

Observations: _____

Type/brand of ventilator 2: _____

Pressure Support 0 cm H_2O

f: _____

V_T: _____

Pressure reading: _____

Observations: _____

Pressure Support 5 cm H_2O

f: _____

V_T: _____

Pressure reading: _____

Observations: _____

Pressure Support 10 cm H_2O

f: _____

V_T: _____

Pressure reading: _____

Observations: _____

Stop Squeezing

f: _____

V_T: _____

Observations: _____

Attach separate paper if additional ventilators are used.

EXERCISE 27.4.3   Pressure Support with Continuous Positive Airway Pressure

Type/brand of ventilator 1: _____

CPAP 0 cm H₂O, Pressure Support 10 cm H₂O

f: _____

Observation of test lung: _____

_____

CPAP 5 cm H₂O, Pressure Support 10 cm H₂O

f: _____

V_T: _____

Observation of test lung: _____

_____

Type/brand of ventilator 2: _____

CPAP 0 cm H₂O, Pressure Support 10 cm H₂O

f: _____

V_T: _____

Observation of test lung: _____

_____

CPAP 5 cm H₂O, Pressure Support 10 cm H₂O

f: _____

V_T: _____

Observation of test lung: _____

_____

Attach separate paper if additional ventilators are used.

What is the effect of pressure support on the spontaneous exhaled volumes as compared with SIMV without

pressure support or CPAP without pressure support? _____

What is the best way to determine the ideal pressure support setting? _____

_____

_____

EXERCISE 27.5   Inverse I:E Ratio, Pressure Control Ventilation
EXERCISE 27.5.1   Pressure Control

Type/brand of ventilator 1: _____

Exhaled V_T (most compliant): _____

Exhaled V_T (least compliant): _____

I:E ratio: _____

Type/brand of ventilator 2: _____

Exhaled V_T (most compliant): _____

Exhaled V_T (least compliant): _____

I:E ratio: _____

Attach separate paper if additional ventilators are used.

What type of patient conditions would be simulated by the most compliant setting? _____

What type of patient conditions would be simulated by the least compliant settings? _____

How does the lung compliance affect the I:E ratio? Why?

_____

_____

EXERCISE 27.5.2   Inverse I:E Ratio Ventilation

Type/brand of ventilator 1: _____

Exhaled V_T: _____

I:E ratio: _____

Peak flow rate: _____

Type/brand of ventilator 2: _____

Exhaled V_T: _____

I:E ratio: _____

Peak flow rate: _____

Attach separate paper if additional ventilators are used.

What precautions must be taken when using this mode of ventilation? Why? _____

_____

_____

_____

EXERCISE 27.6   Home Care Ventilators
EXERCISE 27.6.1   Home Care Ventilator Circuits and Maintenance

Type/brand of ventilator 1: _____

Comparison of breathing circuits: _____

_____

_____

Maintenance procedures: _____

_____

_____

_____

_____

_____

_____

Chronometer hours: _____

Type/brand of ventilator 2: _____

Comparison of breathing circuits: _____

_____

_____

Maintenance procedures: _____

_____

_____

_____

_____

_____

_____

Chronometer hours: _____

Attach separate paper if additional ventilators are used.

EXERCISE 27.6.2   Identification of Controls

Type/brand of ventilator 1: _____

Comparison of available controls: _____

_____

_____

_____

Controls not available: _____

_____

_____

Type/brand of ventilator 2: _____

Comparison of available controls: _____

_____

_____

_____

Controls not available: _____

_____

_____

Attach separate paper if additional ventilators are used.

Explain the probable rationale for the differences between critical care and home care ventilators: _____

_____

_____

_____

EXERCISE 27.6.3　Leak Testing

Type/brand of ventilator 1: _____

Observations and pressure: _____

Loose medication cup observations and pressure: _____

_____

Disconnected inspiratory limb: _____

_____

Type/brand of ventilator 2: _____

Observations and pressure: _____

Loose medication cup observations and pressure: _____

_____

Disconnected inspiratory limb: _____

_____

EXERCISE 27.6.4　F_IO_2 and Positive End-Expiratory Pressure on Home Care Ventilators
V_T 500 ml; f 12/min; Assist/Control

F_IO_2 0.30; flow required: _____

f 20/min

Analyzed F_IO_2: _____

F_IO_2 0.30; flow required: _____

Back pressure: _____

Spontaneous f 25/min

Analyzed F_IO_2: _____

What effect will changes in the patient's spontaneous breathing pattern have on the F_IO_2? _____

_____

_____

f 12/min; PEEP 5 cm H_2O

PIP: _____

PEEP pressure achieved: _____

Spontaneous f 20/min

Observations and breath rate: _____

_____

Control selected: _____

Adjustments required: _____

Explain the rationale for these adjustments: _____

_____

_____

CRITICAL THINKING QUESTION

1. Based on the data you collected during the laboratory exercises, do the following:
   a. Contrast the major differences of each brand of ventilator.
   b. Discuss possible advantages and disadvantages of these differences. Relate these to effects on quality of patient care and patient comfort, ease of use for the practitioner, and cost-effectiveness (may require a literature search).

Ventilator Initiation

INTRODUCTION

Now that the student has a better understanding of the types of ventilators, available parameters, and their interrelationships, the art of ventilator initiation can be explored. Although guidelines have been established for initial settings, each patient must be assessed individually and the ventilator parameters selected to achieve the optimal patient outcomes. This requires a prerequisite and comprehensive understanding of anatomy, physiology, pathophysiology, and fundamentals of respiratory care such as gas administration and airway management.

Once the initial ventilator settings have been determined, the corresponding alarm parameters must be selected to ensure patient safety. It is extremely important that the student be able to set these parameters appropriately and understand the implications of the alarm limits. Although different ventilators have different alarm systems, there are certain alarms that are basic to any ventilator.[1] Some professionals consider that the new generation of ventilators may be over-alarmed, which can lead to an ignoring of nuisance or false alarms. "There are so many alarms, buzzers, beeps, tweets, and honks that you begin to ignore them after a while. Maybe we would be better off with fewer alarms."[2]

Mechanical ventilation has many hazards and complications. By appropriately adjusting ventilator settings and alarm parameters to meet individual patient needs, **iatrogenic** complications can be minimized.

OBJECTIVES

Upon completion of this chapter, the student will be able to:

1. Practice communication skills needed for the initiation of mechanical ventilation.
2. Determine the location and proper setting of available alarms on critical care and home care ventilators.
3. Given patient scenarios, determine the most appropriate mode of ventilation, tidal volume, respiratory rate, F_IO_2, peak flow rate or percent inspiratory time, I:E ratio, and pressure adjuncts and initiate ventilation using critical care and home care ventilators.
4. Given the parameters selected in the scenarios, appropriately set the alarms.
5. Make recommendations and modifications to the ventilator settings based on patient assessment and data collection.
6. Apply infection control guidelines and standards associated with equipment and procedures, according to OSHA regulations and CDC guidelines.
7. Change the ventilator circuit, ensuring physical integrity and proper function with minimal risk or harm to the patient and health care provider.[2]

KEY TERMS

iatrogenic	myelitis	quadriplegia	transverse

EQUIPMENT REQUIRED

- Adult breathing circuits for ventilators available (needed for critical care and home care ventilators)
- HEPA bacteria filters
- Manufacturer's operation and maintenance manuals (videos if available)
- Water traps
- Humidifiers (HME, cascade, and wick)
- Sterile water
- Volume ventilators
- Home care ventilators
- 50 psi oxygen source
- 50 psig regulator
- Bourdon gauge and Thorpe tube flowmeters
- High-pressure hoses
- Air compressor
- Blender
- Wrench
- T-adaptor with small-bore tubing connection and cap
- Test lungs and lung simulator (if available)
- Watch with a second hand
- Respirometer
- Oxygen analyzer and in-line adaptor
- Spring-loaded PEEP valve
- Self-contained (or sealed marine) 12-volt battery with connecting cables
- Intubated or tracheostomized airway management trainer
- Hospital bed

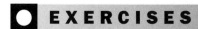

EXERCISE 28.1 Setting Alarm Parameters

Not all ventilators have the same number and types of alarms. *Record the manufacturer, model of the ventilator to be used, and the alarm parameters available on your laboratory report.*

EXERCISE 28.1.1 F_IO_2 or Gas Pressure Alarms

Obtain a critical care ventilator. Assemble the ventilator as in previous exercises. Be sure to check the unit for proper function, and correct any malfunctions before use.

1. Observe the ventilator panel and determine what type of ventilator F_IO_2 alarm or gas pressure alarm is present. You may have to consult the manufacturer's manual. *Record the available alarms on your laboratory report.*

2. Connect the high-pressure hose to a Bourdon gauge or Thorpe tube flowmeter instead of a 50 psig oxygen source. Adjust the flow rate to 8 lpm.

3. Set the ventilator parameters as follows:
   Mode = A/C
   f = 10/min
   V_T = 500 ml
   F_IO_2 = 0.50
   Peak flow = 40 lpm (or percent inspiratory time = 33 percent)

   Make sure that all alarm parameters are still set at minimum/maximum.

4. Turn on the ventilator and connect it to a test lung or lung simulator.

5. If the ventilator does not have a built-in oxygen analyzer, place one in-line.

6. Set the F_IO_2 alarm 5 percent lower than the F_IO_2 set on the ventilator.

7. Analyze the F_IO_2 and observe the ventilator for any activated alarms. *Record the F_IO_2 analyzed and observations of alarm status on your laboratory report.*

8. Adjust the flow rate to 15 lpm.

9. Set the ventilator parameters as follows:
   Mode = A/C
   f = 20/min
   V_T = 700 ml
   F_IO_2 = 1.0
   Peak flow = 70 lpm (or percent inspiratory time = 20 percent)

   Make sure that all alarm parameters are still set at minimum/maximum.

10. Analyze the F_IO_2 and observe the ventilator for any activated alarms. *Record the F_IO_2 analyzed and observations of alarm status on your laboratory report.*

11. Turn the ventilator off. Disconnect the high-pressure hose and connect it to a 50 psig gas source.

12. Turn the ventilator on. Analyze the F_IO_2 and observe the ventilator for any activated alarms. *Record the F_IO_2 analyzed and observations of alarm status on your laboratory report.*

EXERCISE 28.1.2 High-Pressure/Low-Pressure Alarms

1. Using the same ventilator as in Exercise 28.1.1, set the ventilator parameters as follows:
   Mode = A/C
   f = 12/min
   V_T = 700 ml
   F_IO_2 = 0.21
   Peak flow = 35 lpm (or percent inspiratory time = 25 percent)

2. Turn on the ventilator and connect it to a test lung or lung simulator.

3. Observe the system pressure on the manometer or digital display and the exhaled tidal volume, and *record the pressure and exhaled tidal volume on your laboratory report.*

4. Set the high-pressure limit 10 cm H_2O above the observed system pressure,[1] and *record the setting on your laboratory report.*

5. If available, set the low-pressure limit 10 cm H_2O below the observed system pressure,[1] and *record the setting on your laboratory report.*

6. Completely occlude the wye with your finger. Observe the pressure manometer and exhaled tidal volume, and *record your observations and the alarms activated on your laboratory report.*

7. Remove your finger and disconnect the test lung. Observe the pressure manometer and exhaled tidal volume, and *record your observations and the alarms activated on your laboratory report.*

8. Reconnect the ventilator.

EXERCISE 28.1.3 Low Exhaled Volume Alarms

1. Using the same ventilator, set the exhaled tidal volume alarm 100 to 150 ml lower than the exhaled tidal volume. If a low exhaled minute volume is available, set it by calculating a minute ventilation that has tidal volumes 100 to 150 ml less than the delivered tidal volume. *Record these settings on your laboratory report.*

2. Completely occlude the wye with your finger. Observe the pressure manometer and exhaled tidal volume, and *record your observations and the alarms activated on your laboratory report.*

3. Remove your finger and disconnect the test lung. Observe the pressure manometer and exhaled tidal volume, and *record your observations and the alarms activated on your laboratory report.*

4. Reconnect the ventilator.

5. Change the following parameters:
   Mode = SIMV
   f = 6/min

6. Squeeze the test lung to simulate spontaneous breathing at a rate of 6/min, for a total rate of 12/min.

7. Observe the ventilator, and *record your observations and the alarms activated on your laboratory report.*

8. Readjust the alarms appropriately, if needed, and *record the adjusted alarm settings on your laboratory report.*

EXERCISE 28.1.4 Other Ventilator Alarms

From the information gathered at the start of the exercises, set any of the other available alarm parameters, and *record them on your laboratory report*. Remember that some of these choices will depend on the patient's clinical condition. Be prepared to defend the rationale used to determine your selections.

EXERCISE 28.2 Ventilator Initiation

Given the following scenarios, select the mode and initial ventilator settings that you feel are appropriate. Be sure to set the alarms as well. Refer to Table 28.1 and Table 27.1 to aid in your selection. Each scenario should be performed on all critical care ventilators available in the laboratory.

Scenario 1

You have been called to the trauma room. Mr. Scott is a 20-year-old, 150-lb, unrestrained driver of an automobile involved in a motor vehicle accident (MVA). He is unconscious and apneic with multiple rib fractures. He is already intubated with an 8.0 mm ID endotracheal (ET) tube. The resident asks you to determine the initial ventilator settings.

1. Select the initial ventilator settings, and *record them on your laboratory report*.

2. Evaluate the patient by performing the following:
   Vital signs
   Physical assessment of the chest
   Auscultation
   Suctioning
   Record what you would expect to find for the above parameters on your laboratory report.

3. Set the alarm parameters, and *record them on your laboratory report*.

Scenario 2

Ms. Fumo is a 70-year-old, 100-lb, well-known COPD patient. She was admitted to the ER with fever, dyspnea, and productive cough. Over the past several hours her dyspnea has worsened and she has become lethargic. Her arterial blood gases (ABGs) on 2 L of nasal oxygen reveal the following:
   pH = 7.18
   $PaCO_2$ = 77 mm Hg
   PaO_2 = 52 mm Hg

   Her attending physician orders her intubated and asks for your recommendations for ventilator settings.

1. Select the initial ventilator settings, and *record them on your laboratory report*.

TABLE 28.1 **Guidelines for Initial Ventilator Setting Selection**

Patient Type	Rate	V_T
Adults		
Normal lungs	8–12	12–15 ml/kg
Obstructive	8–10	10–12 ml/kg
Chronic or acute restrictive	12–20	10 ml/kg or less
Children		
8–16 yr	20–30	8–10 ml/kg
0–8 yr	30–40	6–8 ml/kg

Adapted from Scanlan, C et al (eds): Egan's Fundamentals of Respiratory Care, ed 6. Mosby, St. Louis, 1995, pp. 898, 900.

2. Evaluate the patient by performing the following:
   Vital signs
   Physical assessment of the chest
   Auscultation
   Suctioning
   Record what you would expect to find for the above parameters on your laboratory report.

3. Set the alarm parameters, and *record them on your laboratory report*.

Scenario 3

Ms. Hoey is a 27-year-old, 90-lb, HIV-positive patient admitted with fever, dyspnea, and cough. A chest x-ray reveals bilateral pneumonia. Stat ABGs are drawn on a nonrebreather mask:
   pH = 7.48
   $PaCO_2$ = 32 mm Hg
   PaO_2 = 48 mm Hg

   Her vital signs are as follows:
   Pulse = 120/min
   Respiratory rate = 32/min and labored
   Blood pressure = 110/60

1. Select the initial ventilator settings, and *record them on your laboratory report*.

2. Evaluate the patient by performing the following:
   Vital signs
   Physical assessment of the chest
   Auscultation
   Suctioning
   Record what you would expect to find for the above parameters on your laboratory report.

3. Set the alarm parameters, and *record them on your laboratory report*.

Scenario 4

You are the only therapist on duty. There was a cardiac arrest in the ER, and the patient must be placed on a ventilator. Mrs. Raju is 65 years old, weighs 195 lb, and has an extensive cardiac history. She is intubated with an 8.0 mm ID ET tube. She is currently apneic. Her ABGs are as follows:
   pH = 7.32
   $PaCO_2$ = 33 mm Hg
   PaO_2 = 122 mm Hg

   These were drawn during the code while being manually ventilated with 1.0 F_IO_2.

1. Select the initial ventilator settings, and *record them on your laboratory report*.

2. Evaluate the patient by performing the following:
   Vital signs
   Physical assessment of the chest
   Auscultation
   Suctioning
   Record what you would expect to find for the above parameters on your laboratory report.

3. Set the alarm parameters, and *record them on your laboratory report*.

   Repeat the scenarios for each available critical care ventilator, and *record all parameters on your laboratory report*.

EXERCISE 28.3 Home Care Ventilators

EXERCISE 28.3.1 Alarms

1. Select a home care ventilator. Compare the alarms available on the home care ventilator with the alarms available on the

critical care ventilator. *Record the alarms available on the home care ventilator on your laboratory report.*

2. Plug the unit into an electrical outlet.

3. Set the following parameters:
   Mode = A/C
   V_T = 600 ml
   f = 12/min.

4. Turn the unit on.

5. After several breaths, unplug the power source. *Record your observations and the alarms activated on your laboratory report.*

6. Reset the alarm, and connect the ventilator to an external 12-volt power source according to the manufacturer's recommendations. *Record your observations and the alarms activated on your laboratory report.*

7. Reset the alarm.

8. Switch the power source back to the wall outlet.

EXERCISE 28.3.2 Ventilator Initiation Using a Home Care Ventilator

In the following scenario, initiate ventilation using the home care ventilator from the previous exercise. Be sure to set all alarms.

Scenario
You are working in a ventilator-dependent **quadriplegia** unit. You are called to initiate ventilation on the new admission, a 17-year-old with a **transverse myelitis** of C-2. Jean-Claude is alert but apprehensive. He is trached with a size 7 Portex tube with the cuff partially inflated to allow a large enough leak to permit phonation. The physician requests the following settings:
   Mode = A/C
   V_T = 1.0 L
   F_IO_2 = 0.30
   PEEP = 5 cm H_2O

1. Set the initial ventilator settings, select the additional parameters not ordered, and *record them on your laboratory report.*

2. Evaluate the patient by performing the following:
   Vital signs
   Physical assessment of the chest
   Auscultation
   Suctioning
   Record what you would expect to find for the above parameters on your laboratory report.

3. Set the alarm parameters, and *record them on your laboratory report.*

EXERCISE 28.4 Circuit Changes

To simulate the conditions in the clinical setting, an intubated or tracheostomized airway management trainer should be positioned in a hospital bed if available. Have your laboratory partner count how many breaths are missed during the circuit change.

1. Set the ventilator to the following parameters:
   Mode = Control
   f = 15
   V_T = 600 ml
   F_IO_2 = 0.40

2. Gather the necessary equipment to perform a complete ventilator circuit change.

3. Assemble the equipment as completely as possible.

4. Place the assembled circuit on the bed with the wye placed aseptically proximal to the patient. Place the other ends proximal to their corresponding connections on the ventilator as shown in Figure 28.1.

5. Silence the alarms.

6. Adjust the F_IO_2 on the ventilator to hyperoxygenate the patient before disconnection.

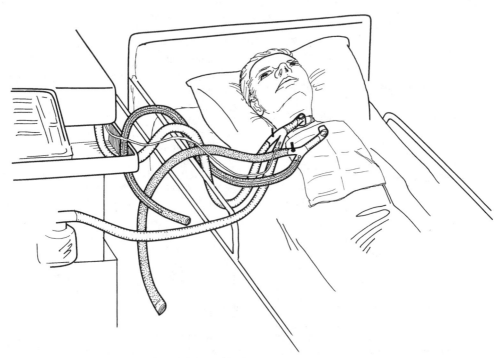

FIGURE 28.1 Changing a ventilator circuit.

7. Instruct your partner to hold his or her breath beginning simultaneously from the time of patient disconnection and to continue breath holding until the patient is reconnected.

8. Quickly disconnect the circuit from the patient wye.

9. Quickly disconnect the other circuit connections from the ventilator.

10. Quickly attach the ends of the new circuit to the corresponding connections on the ventilator.

11. Rapidly assess the circuit for leaks and ensure ventilator function.

12. Reconnect the patient to the ventilator circuit. *Instruct your partner to resume breathing.*

13. Observe the pressure manometer and exhaled volumes.

14. Readjust the F_IO_2 and reset the alarms.

15. Determine the number of breaths lost by the patient and the total time to complete the circuit change. *Record the number of breaths and time taken on your laboratory report. Record your partner's impressions of his or her breath-holding experience.*

16. Repeat this exercise using the home care ventilator.

References

1. Chang, DW: Clinical Application of Mechanical Ventilation. Delmar, Albany, 1997, p 132.
2. Pilbeam, S: Mechanical Ventilation: Physiological and Clinical Applications, ed 2. Mosby, St Louis, 1992, p 198.
3. American Association for Respiratory Care: The AARC clinical practice guideline: Ventilator circuit changes. Respir Care 39:797–802, 1994.
4. Scanlan, C, Spearman, C and Sheldon, R et al. (eds): Egan's Fundamentals of Respiratory Care, ed 6. Mosby, St Louis, 1995, pp 898, 900.

Related Readings

Chang, DW: Clinical Application of Mechanical Ventilation. Delmar, Albany, 1997.

Eubanks, DH and Bone, RC: Principles and Applications of Cardiorespiratory Care Equipment. Mosby, St Louis, 1994.

McPherson, SP: Respiratory Care Equipment, ed 5. Mosby, St Louis, 1995.

Pilbeam, S: Mechanical Ventilation: Physiological and Clinical Applications, ed 2. Mosby, St Louis, 1992.

Scanlan, C et al (eds): Egan's Fundamentals of Respiratory Care, ed 6. Mosby, St Louis, 1995.

Selected Journal Articles

American Association for Respiratory Care: The AARC clinical practice guideline: Patient-ventilator system checks. Respir Care 37:882–886, 1992.

Brown, BR: Understanding mechanical ventilation: Indications for and initiation of therapy. J Okla State Med Assoc 87:353–357, 1994.

Chiang, AA et al: Demand flow airway pressure release ventilation as a partial ventilatory support mode: Comparison with synchronized intermittent mandatory ventilation and pressure support ventilation. Crit Care Med 22:1431–1437, 1994.

Hess, D: Guideline for the prevention of nosocomial pneumonia and ventilator circuits: Time for change? Respir Care 39:1149–1153, 1994.

LABORATORY REPORT

CHAPTER 28: VENTILATOR INITIATION

Name _____   Date _____

Course/Section _____   Instructor _____

Data Collection

EXERCISE 28.1   Setting Alarm Parameters

Type/brand of ventilator 1: _____

Alarm parameters available: _____

_____

_____

_____

Type/brand of ventilator 2: _____

Alarm parameters available: _____

_____

_____

_____

EXERCISE 28.1.1 F_IO_2 or Gas Pressure Alarms

Type/brand of ventilator 1: _____

F_IO_2 or gas pressure alarms available: _____

_____

Type/brand of ventilator 2: _____

F_IO_2 or gas pressure alarms available: _____

_____

Connection to a Flowmeter

Type/brand of ventilator 1: _____

Flow 8 lpm; f 10; V_T 500 ml; F_IO_2 0.50; PEFR 40 lpm

F_IO_2 analyzed: _____

Observations: _____

_____

_____

Flow 15 lpm; f 20; V_T 700 ml; F_IO_2 1.0; PEFR 70 lpm

F_IO_2 analyzed: _____

Observations: _____

_____

_____

CONNECTION TO 50 PSIG SOURCE

F_IO_2 analyzed: _____

Observations: _____

_____

_____

_____

Type/brand of ventilator 2: _____

Flow 8 lpm; f 10; V_T 500 ml; F_IO_2 0.50; PEFR 40 lpm

F_IO_2 analyzed: _____

Observations: _____

_____

_____

Flow 15 lpm; f 20; V_T 700 ml; F_IO_2 1.0; PEFR 70 lpm

F_IO_2 analyzed: _____

Observations: _____

_____

_____

CONNECTION TO 50 PSIG SOURCE

F_IO_2 analyzed: _____

Observations: _____

_____

Explain why the observations made in this exercise occurred.

_____

_____

What can you conclude regarding the relationships between pressures, flows, and F_IO_2? _____

_____

_____

How does this affect the ventilator setup? _____

_____

_____

EXERCISE 28.1.2   High-Pressure/Low-Pressure Alarms

Type/brand of ventilator 1: _____

f 12; V_T 700 ml; F_IO_2 0.21; PEFR 35 lpm

Initial pressure observed: _____

Initial exhaled tidal volume: _____

High-pressure limit setting: _____

Low-pressure limit setting: _____

Wye Occluded

Pressure observed: _____

Exhaled tidal volume: _____

Alarms activated: _____

Test Lung Disconnected

Pressure observed: _____

Exhaled tidal volume: _____

Alarms activated: _____

Type/brand of ventilator 2: _____

f 12; V_T 700 ml; F_IO_2 0.21; PEFR 35 lpm

Initial pressure observed: _____

Initial exhaled tidal volume: _____

High-pressure limit setting: _____

Low-pressure limit setting: _____

Wye Occluded

Pressure observed: _____

Exhaled tidal volume: _____

Alarms activated: _____

Test Lung Disconnected

Pressure observed: _____

Exhaled tidal volume: _____

Alarms activated: _____

EXERCISE 28.1.3   Low Exhaled Volume Alarms

Type/brand of ventilator 1: _____

Low exhaled tidal volume alarm setting: _____

Low exhaled minute volume setting: _____

Wye Occluded

Pressure observed: _____

Exhaled tidal volume: _____

Alarms activated: _____

Test Lung Disconnected

Pressure observed: _____

Exhaled tidal volume: _____

Alarms activated: _____

SIMV 6/Spontaneous Rate 6

Alarms activated: _____

Alarm readjustment: _____

Type/brand of ventilator 2: _____

Low exhaled tidal volume alarm setting: _____

Low exhaled minute volume setting: _____

Wye Occluded

Pressure observed: _____

Exhaled tidal volume: _____

Alarms activated: _____

Test Lung Disconnected

Pressure observed: _____

Exhaled tidal volume: _____

Alarms activated: _____

SIMV 6/Spontaneous Rate 6

Alarms activated: _____

Alarm readjustment: _____

EXERCISE 28.1.4   Other Ventilator Alarms

Type/brand of ventilator 1: _____

Alarms available	*Setting determination*	*Rationale*
_____	_____	_____
_____	_____	_____
_____	_____	_____
_____	_____	_____
_____	_____	_____
_____	_____	_____
_____	_____	_____

Type/brand of ventilator 2: _____

Alarms available	*Setting determination*	*Rationale*
_____	_____	_____
_____	_____	_____
_____	_____	_____
_____	_____	_____
_____	_____	_____
_____	_____	_____

EXERCISE 28.2 Ventilator Initiation

Scenario 1

Type/brand of ventilator 1: _____

Mode: _____

V_T: _____

f: _____

Flow or percent inspiratory time: _____

F_IO_2: _____

Patient assessment:

Vital signs: _____

Physical assessment of the chest: _____

Auscultation: _____

Suctioning: _____

Alarm settings: _____

_____

_____

Type/brand of ventilator 2: _____

Mode: _____

V_T: _____

f: _____

Flow or percent inspiratory time: _____

F_IO_2: _____

Patient assessment:

Vital signs: _____

Physical assessment of the chest: _____

Auscultation: _____

Suctioning: _____

Alarm settings: _____

_____

_____

Scenario 2

Type/brand of ventilator 1: _____

Mode: _____

V_T: _____

f: _____

Flow or percent inspiratory time: _____

F_IO_2: _____

Patient assessment:

Vital signs: _____

Physical assessment of the chest: _____

Auscultation: _____

Suctioning: _____

Alarm settings: _____

_____

_____

Type/brand of ventilator 2: _____

Mode: _____

V_T: _____

f: _____

Flow or percent inspiratory time: _____

F_IO_2: _____

Patient assessment:

Vital signs: _____

Physical assessment of the chest: _____

Auscultation: _____

Suctioning: _____

Alarm settings: _____

_____

_____

Scenario 3

Type/brand of ventilator 1: _____

Mode: _____

V_T: _____

f: _____

Flow or percent inspiratory time: _____

F_IO_2: _____

Patient assessment:

Vital signs: _____

Physical assessment of the chest: _____

Auscultation: _____

Suctioning: _____

Alarm settings: _____
_____
_____

Type/brand of ventilator 2: _____

Mode: _____

V_T: _____

f: _____

Flow or percent inspiratory time: _____

F_IO_2: _____

Patient assessment:

Vital signs: _____

Physical assessment of the chest: _____

Auscultation: _____

Suctioning: _____

Alarm settings: _____
_____
_____

Scenario 4

Type/brand of ventilator 1: _____

Mode: _____

V_T: _____

f: _____

Flow or percent inspiratory time: _____

F_IO_2: _____

Patient assessment:

Vital signs: _____

Physical assessment of the chest: _____

Auscultation: _____

Suctioning: _____

Alarm settings: _____
_____
_____

Type/brand of ventilator 2: _____

Mode: _____

V_T: _____

f: _____

Flow or percent inspiratory time: _____

F_1O_2: _____

Patient assessment: _____

Vital signs: _____

Physical assessment of the chest: _____

Auscultation: _____

Suctioning: _____

Alarm settings: _____

_____

_____

EXERCISE 28.3 Home Care Ventilators
EXERCISE 28.3.1 Alarms

Type/brand of ventilator 1: _____

Available alarms: _____

_____

_____

_____

_____

Power disconnection—alarm activated and observations: _____

_____

_____

External battery—alarm activated and observations: _____

_____

_____

Type/brand of ventilator 2: _____

Available alarms: _____

_____

_____

_____

_____

Power disconnection—alarm activated and observations: _____

_____

_____

External battery—alarm activated and observations: _____

_____

_____

EXERCISE 28.3.2   Ventilator Initiation Using a Home Care Ventilator

Type/brand of ventilator 1: _____

Mode: _____

V_T: _____

f: _____

Flow: _____

F_IO_2: _____

PEEP: _____

Patient assessment:

Vital signs: _____

Physical assessment of the chest: _____

Auscultation: _____

Suctioning: _____

Alarm settings: _____

_____

_____

_____

Type/brand of ventilator 2: _____

Mode: _____

V_T: _____

f: _____

Flow: _____

F_IO_2: _____

PEEP: _____

Patient assessment:

Vital signs: _____

Physical assessment of the chest: _____

Auscultation: _____

Suctioning: _____

Alarm settings: _____

_____

_____

EXERCISE 28.4   Circuit Changes

Type/brand of ventilator 1: _____

Breaths lost: _____

Time taken: _____

Breath-holding impressions: _____

Type/brand of ventilator 2: _____

Breaths lost: _____

Time taken: _____

Breath-holding impressions: _____

_____

CRITICAL THINKING QUESTIONS

1. What are the purposes of alarms?

2. How can nuisance alarms be avoided?

3. The physicians in the scenarios want you to justify your initial ventilator settings in scenarios 1, 2, 3, and 4. How would you respond? Remember to include your rationale for machine and mode selection. (This question can also be done as an oral exercise with a fellow student or lab instructor acting as the physician.)
Scenario 1:

Scenario 2:

Scenario 3:

Scenario 4:

4. What differences in initiation and setting modification did you observe when using the home care ventilator?

5. The patient Jean-Claude from Exercise 28.3.2 is being discharged to home. You are asked to do an inspection of the home before his discharge. What specifics about the home environment must you check to ensure safety and access for Jean-Claude and all the equipment he will require?

6. What safety precautions should be taken when performing a ventilator circuit change?

PROCEDURAL COMPETENCY EVALUATION

Name _____ Date _____

Ventilator Initiation

Setting: ☐ Lab ☐ Clinical   Evaluator: ☐ Peer ☐ Instructor

Conditions (describe): _____

_____

Equipment Used

_____

_____

	SATISFACTORY	UNSATISFACTORY	NOT OBSERVED	NOT APPLICABLE
Equipment and Patient Preparation				
1. Verifies, interprets, and evaluates physician's order or protocol	☐	☐	☐	☐
2. Reviews any pertinent information (history and interview, lab data, x-rays) in the patient's chart as the acuity of the circumstances permits	☐	☐	☐	☐
3. Selects, gathers, and assembles the necessary equipment	☐	☐	☐	☐
4. Washes hands and applies standard precautions and transmission-based isolation procedures as appropriate	☐	☐	☐	☐
5. Identifies patient, introduces self and department	☐	☐	☐	☐
6. Explains purpose of the procedure and confirms patient understanding	☐	☐	☐	☐
7. Connects the ventilator to the appropriate emergency electrical outlets	☐	☐	☐	☐
8. Connects the high-pressure hoses to the appropriate 50 psi gas source outlets	☐	☐	☐	☐
9. Turns on the ventilator and performs any required tests	☐	☐	☐	☐
10. Performs any additional leak tests and verifies ventilator function	☐	☐	☐	☐
Assessment and Implementation				
11. Evaluates the patient by performing	☐	☐	☐	☐
a. Vital signs	☐	☐	☐	☐
b. Physical assessment of the chest	☐	☐	☐	☐
c. Auscultation	☐	☐	☐	☐
d. ECG, blood gas, or noninvasive monitoring of CO_2 and SpO_2	☐	☐	☐	☐
e. Suctioning	☐	☐	☐	☐
12. Selects the initial ventilator settings	☐	☐	☐	☐
13. Sets the alarm parameters	☐	☐	☐	☐
14. Analyzes the F_IO_2	☐	☐	☐	☐
15. Reassesses the patient, including blood gas or noninvasive monitoring and ECG	☐	☐	☐	☐
Follow-up				
16. Maintains/processes equipment	☐	☐	☐	☐
17. Disposes of infectious waste and washes hands	☐	☐	☐	☐
18. Records pertinent data in chart and departmental records	☐	☐	☐	☐
19. Notifies appropriate personnel and makes any necessary recommendations or modifications to the patient care plan	☐	☐	☐	☐

_____   _____
Signature of Evaluator   Signature of Student

PERFORMANCE RATING SCALE

5 EXCELLENT—FAR EXCEEDS EXPECTED LEVEL, FLAWLESS PERFORMANCE
4 ABOVE AVERAGE—NO PROMPTING REQUIRED, ABLE TO SELF-CORRECT
3 AVERAGE—THE MINIMUM COMPETENCY LEVEL, NO CRITICAL ERRORS
2 IMPROVEMENT NEEDED—PROBLEM AREAS EXIST; CRITICAL ERRORS, CORRECTIONS NEEDED
1 POOR AND UNACCEPTABLE PERFORMANCE—GROSS INACCURACIES, POTENTIALLY HARMFUL

PERFORMANCE CRITERIA   SCALE

1. DISPLAYS KNOWLEDGE OF ESSENTIAL CONCEPTS	5	4	3	2	1
2. DEMONSTRATES THE RELATIONSHIP BETWEEN THEORY AND CLINICAL PRACTICE	5	4	3	2	1
3. FOLLOWS DIRECTIONS, EXHIBITS SOUND JUDGMENT, AND DEMONSTRATES ATTENTION TO SAFETY AND DETAIL	5	4	3	2	1
4. EXHIBITS THE REQUIRED MANUAL DEXTERITY	5	4	3	2	1
5. PERFORMS PROCEDURE IN A REASONABLE TIME FRAME	5	4	3	2	1
6. MAINTAINS STERILE OR ASEPTIC TECHNIQUE	5	4	3	2	1
7. INITIATES UNAMBIGUOUS GOAL-DIRECTED COMMUNICATION	5	4	3	2	1
8. PROVIDES FOR ADEQUATE CARE AND MAINTENANCE OF EQUIPMENT AND SUPPLIES	5	4	3	2	1
9. EXHIBITS COURTEOUS AND PLEASANT DEMEANOR	5	4	3	2	1
10. MAINTAINS CONCISE AND ACCURATE RECORDS	5	4	3	2	1

ADDITIONAL COMMENTS: INCLUDE ERRORS OF OMISSION OR COMMISSION, COMMUNICATIVE SKILLS, AND EFFECTIVENESS OF PATIENT INTERACTION:

SUMMARY PERFORMANCE EVALUATION AND RECOMMENDATIONS

SATISFACTORY PERFORMANCE—Performed without error or prompting, or able to self-correct, no critical errors.

_____ LABORATORY EVALUATION. SKILLS MAY BE APPLIED/OBSERVED IN THE CLINICAL SETTING.

_____ CLINICAL EVALUATION. STUDENT READY FOR MINIMALLY SUPERVISED APPLICATION AND REFINEMENT.

UNSATISFACTORY PERFORMANCE—Prompting required; performed with critical errors, potentially harmful.

_____ STUDENT REQUIRES ADDITIONAL LABORATORY PRACTICE.

_____ STUDENT REQUIRES ADDITIONAL SUPERVISED CLINICAL PRACTICE.

SIGNATURES

STUDENT: _____   EVALUATOR: _____

DATE: _____   DATE: _____

PROCEDURAL COMPETENCY EVALUATION

Name _____ Date _____

Ventilator Circuit Change

Setting: ☐ Lab ☐ Clinical   Evaluator: ☐ Peer ☐ Instructor

Conditions (describe): _____

_____

Equipment Used

_____

_____

	SATISFACTORY	UNSATISFACTORY	NOT OBSERVED	NOT APPLICABLE
Equipment and Patient Preparation				
1. Verifies, interprets, and evaluates physician's orders or protocol	☐	☐	☐	☐
2. Selects, gathers, and assembles the necessary equipment	☐	☐	☐	☐
3. Washes hands and applies standard precautions and transmission-based isolation procedures as appropriate	☐	☐	☐	☐
4. Identifies patient, introduces self and department	☐	☐	☐	☐
5. Explains purpose of the procedure and confirms patient understanding	☐	☐	☐	☐
Assessment and Implementation				
6. Assesses the patient and ventilator system before performing the circuit change	☐	☐	☐	☐
7. Assembles the equipment as completely as possible	☐	☐	☐	☐
8. Places the assembled circuit on the bed with the wye positioned aseptically proximal to the patient	☐	☐	☐	☐
9. Places the other ends proximal to their corresponding connections on the ventilator	☐	☐	☐	☐
10. Silences the alarms	☐	☐	☐	☐
11. Ensures emergency equipment is available	☐	☐	☐	☐
12. Adjusts the F_IO_2 on the ventilator to hyperoxygenate the patient before disconnection (or manually hyperinflates as appropriate)	☐	☐	☐	☐
13. Quickly disconnects the circuit from the patient wye	☐	☐	☐	☐
14. Quickly disconnects the other circuit connections from the ventilator	☐	☐	☐	☐
15. Quickly attaches the ends of the new circuit to the corresponding connections on the ventilator	☐	☐	☐	☐
16. Rapidly assesses the circuit for leaks and ensures ventilator function	☐	☐	☐	☐
17. Reconnects the patient to the ventilator circuit	☐	☐	☐	☐
18. Observes the pressure manometer and exhaled volumes	☐	☐	☐	☐
19. Readjusts the F_IO_2 and resets the alarms	☐	☐	☐	☐
20. Reassesses the patient	☐	☐	☐	☐
Follow-up				
21. Maintains/processes equipment	☐	☐	☐	☐
22. Disposes of infectious waste and washes hands	☐	☐	☐	☐
23. Records pertinent data in chart and departmental records	☐	☐	☐	☐
24. Notifies appropriate personnel and makes any necessary recommendations or modifications to the patient care plan	☐	☐	☐	☐

_____   _____
Signature of Evaluator   Signature of Student

PERFORMANCE RATING SCALE

5 EXCELLENT—FAR EXCEEDS EXPECTED LEVEL, FLAWLESS PERFORMANCE
4 ABOVE AVERAGE—NO PROMPTING REQUIRED, ABLE TO SELF-CORRECT
3 AVERAGE—THE MINIMUM COMPETENCY LEVEL, NO CRITICAL ERRORS
2 IMPROVEMENT NEEDED—PROBLEM AREAS EXIST; CRITICAL ERRORS, CORRECTIONS NEEDED
1 POOR AND UNACCEPTABLE PERFORMANCE—GROSS INACCURACIES, POTENTIALLY HARMFUL

PERFORMANCE CRITERIA		SCALE			
1. DISPLAYS KNOWLEDGE OF ESSENTIAL CONCEPTS	5	4	3	2	1
2. DEMONSTRATES THE RELATIONSHIP BETWEEN THEORY AND CLINICAL PRACTICE	5	4	3	2	1
3. FOLLOWS DIRECTIONS, EXHIBITS SOUND JUDGMENT, AND DEMONSTRATES ATTENTION TO SAFETY AND DETAIL	5	4	3	2	1
4. EXHIBITS THE REQUIRED MANUAL DEXTERITY	5	4	3	2	1
5. PERFORMS PROCEDURE IN A REASONABLE TIME FRAME	5	4	3	2	1
6. MAINTAINS STERILE OR ASEPTIC TECHNIQUE	5	4	3	2	1
7. INITIATES UNAMBIGUOUS GOAL-DIRECTED COMMUNICATION	5	4	3	2	1
8. PROVIDES FOR ADEQUATE CARE AND MAINTENANCE OF EQUIPMENT AND SUPPLIES	5	4	3	2	1
9. EXHIBITS COURTEOUS AND PLEASANT DEMEANOR	5	4	3	2	1
10. MAINTAINS CONCISE AND ACCURATE RECORDS	5	4	3	2	1

ADDITIONAL COMMENTS: INCLUDE ERRORS OF OMISSION OR COMMISSION, COMMUNICATIVE SKILLS, AND EFFECTIVENESS OF PATIENT INTERACTION:

SUMMARY PERFORMANCE EVALUATION AND RECOMMENDATIONS

SATISFACTORY PERFORMANCE—Performed without error or prompting, or able to self-correct, no critical errors.

_____ LABORATORY EVALUATION. SKILLS MAY BE APPLIED/OBSERVED IN THE CLINICAL SETTING.

_____ CLINICAL EVALUATION. STUDENT READY FOR MINIMALLY SUPERVISED APPLICATION AND REFINEMENT.

UNSATISFACTORY PERFORMANCE—Prompting required; performed with critical errors, potentially harmful.

_____ STUDENT REQUIRES ADDITIONAL LABORATORY PRACTICE.

_____ STUDENT REQUIRES ADDITIONAL SUPERVISED CLINICAL PRACTICE.

SIGNATURES

STUDENT: _____   EVALUATOR: _____

DATE: _____   DATE: _____

CHAPTER 29

Patient-Ventilator System Care

INTRODUCTION

From the initial application to the discontinuance of mechanical ventilation, respiratory care practitioners must be able to assess the integrity and effectiveness of the patient-ventilator system in order to make appropriate modifications to the care plan. The AARC clinical practice guideline is specific in defining the patient-ventilator system check. It is the documented *evaluation* of a mechanical ventilator's function *and* of the patient's response to ventilatory support.[1] It is therefore more than just a "vent check," although that is the most common name for this procedure. The monitoring must always begin with a complete assessment of the patient before proceeding to the machine. This includes auscultation, vital signs, airway care, and evaluation for the presence of barotrauma or volutrauma.

Once the patient's response to ventilatory support has been evaluated, proper functioning of the equipment should be verified. This part of the check minimally should include the correlation of the settings with current physician orders or protocol, setting and functioning of alarms, temperature of inspired gas, and analysis of the F_IO_2. As always, if the work is not documented, the work was not done. Proper charting, therefore, is our only legal documentation that the patient-ventilator system check was done in a timely and proper manner.

The goals of mechanical ventilation must be clearly established and continually refined so that monitoring of the patient-ventilator system leads to the desired outcomes.

OBJECTIVES

Upon completion of this chapter, the student will be able to:

1. Apply infection control guidelines and standards associated with equipment and procedures, according to OSHA regulations and CDC guidelines.

2. Perform patient assessment techniques.

3. Properly verify and document the function of the ventilator.

4. Perform calculations to verify and document the patient's response to mechanical ventilation. These calculations specifically include effective **dynamic** compliance (EDC), effective **static** compliance (C_{ST}), resistance, and auto-PEEP or intrinsic PEEP.

5. Analyze and interpret waveforms and data generated by the patient-ventilator system.

6. Practice the documentation skills required for a patient-ventilator system check on a ventilator flow sheet and the skills necessary to generate a narrative or shift note.

7. Practice communication skills needed for the reporting of clinically significant data to the members of the health care team.

KEY TERMS
dynamic

extrinsic
intrinsic

static

weaning

EQUIPMENT REQUIRED

- Adult breathing circuits for ventilators available (needed for critical care and home care ventilators)
- HEPA bacteria filters
- Manufacturer's operation and maintenance manuals
- Water traps
- Humidifiers (HME, cascade, and wick)
- Sterile water
- Volume ventilators
- Home care ventilators
- 50 psi oxygen source
- 50 psig regulator
- Blender
- Bourdon gauge and Thorpe tube flowmeters
- High-pressure hoses
- Air compressor
- Wrench
- T-adaptor with small-bore tubing connection and cap
- Test lungs and lung simulator (if available)
- Watch with second hand
- Respirometer
- Oxygen analyzer and in-line adaptor
- Spring-loaded PEEP valve

- Stethoscope
- Intubated or tracheostomized airway management trainer
- Hospital bed

 E X E R C I S E S

EXERCISE 29.1 Basic Ventilator Monitoring

These exercises require the initiation of mechanical ventilation for various patient scenarios, as in Chapter 28, followed by the simulation of a complete patient-ventilator system check and documentation as on a legal medical document. The ventilator system must be assembled completely (including gas and electrical sources), and its function must be verified before initiation. Components needed for each setup must be selected and obtained by each student. It is recommended that each scenario be repeated for each available ventilator, and students should completely disassemble the ventilator setup after completion of each scenario.

Scenario 1

1. Set up a volume ventilator with an adult setup and HME.
2. Initiate ventilation. Mr. Lisanti is a 21-year-old, 150-lb man who has just come from the operating room (OR) after a craniotomy and evacuation of a subdural hematoma. He is orally intubated, has no documented lung pathology, and is not a smoker. Initiate ventilation with the following settings: mode = A/C, V_T = 800 ml, f = 12/min, and F_IO_2 = 0.35. All other settings and alarms are to be selected by you.
3. Perform a patient-ventilator system check, including "patient" assessment. Include oxygen analysis, cuff pressures, and airway care. *Record all pertinent data on the ventilator flow sheet provided in your laboratory report.*
4. Write a narrative note documenting your patient's status and any other data required to write a comprehensive shift note. *Record it on your laboratory report.* This will require you to use your imagination to create clinically relevant assessment data.

Scenario 2

1. Set up the ventilator with an adult setup and humidifier.
2. Initiate ventilation. Mrs. Kay is a 30-year-old, 110-lb woman who is in status asthmaticus. She is in severe acute respiratory acidosis with moderate hypoxemia and has just been nasally intubated. Initiate ventilation with the following settings: mode = A/C, V_T = 600 ml, f = 10/min, and F_IO_2 = 0.50.
3. Perform a patient-ventilator system check, including "patient" assessment. Include oxygen analysis, cuff pressures, and airway care. *Record all pertinent data on the ventilator flow sheet provided in your laboratory report.*
4. Write a narrative note documenting your patient's status and any other data required to write a comprehensive shift note. *Record it on your laboratory report.* This will require you to use your imagination to create clinically relevant assessment data.

Scenario 3

1. Set up the ventilator with an adult setup and humidifier.
2. Initiate ventilation. Miss Aswama is a 38-year-old, 100-lb woman who has myasthenia gravis. She has been on the ventilator for several weeks with a tracheostomy. Adjust her settings as follows: mode = SIMV, V_T = 500 ml, f = 12/min, F_IO_2 = 0.30, pressure support = 5 cm H_2O, and PEEP = 5 cm H_2O.
3. Perform a patient-ventilator system check, including "patient" assessment. Include oxygen analysis, cuff pressures, and airway care. *Record all pertinent data on the ventilator flow sheet provided in your laboratory report.*
4. Write a narrative note documenting your patient's status and any other data required to write a comprehensive shift note. *Record it on your laboratory report.* This will require you to use your imagination to create clinically relevant assessment data.

Scenario 4

1. Set up the ventilator with an adult setup. The mode of humidification should be selected by you.
2. Initiate ventilation. Mr. Lagoudakis is a 60-year-old, 160-lb man who is a known COPD patient with a superimposed respiratory infection, possibly pneumonia. His ABGs are pH = 7.16, $PaCO_2$ = 77 mm Hg, and PaO_2 = 49 torr on a 0.40 Venturi mask. The attending physician requests your recommendations for ventilator mode and settings. Initiate ventilation as you see fit. Orally justify to your laboratory partner the rationale for your choices, and *document the rationale on your laboratory report.*
3. Perform a patient-ventilator system check, including "patient" assessment. Include oxygen analysis, cuff pressures, and airway care. *Record all pertinent data on the ventilator flow sheet provided in your laboratory report.*
4. Write a narrative note documenting your patient's status and any other data required to write a comprehensive shift note. *Record it on your laboratory report.* This will require you to use your imagination to create clinically relevant assessment data.

EXERCISE 29.2 Data Generation for Evaluation of Patient Status

EXERCISE 29.2.1 Effective Dynamic and Static Compliance and Resistance Calculations

1. Using the equipment and settings in the preceding four scenarios, calculate the effective dynamic compliance (EDC) using the following formula. *Record the results on the ventilator flow sheet provided in your laboratory report.*

$$\frac{V_T}{\text{Peak pressure} - \text{PEEP}}$$

2. Using the same four scenarios, calculate the effective static compliance (C_{ST}) using the following formula. *Record the results on your laboratory report.*

$$\frac{V_T}{\text{Plateau pressure} - \text{PEEP}}$$

Remember that you have to obtain a plateau pressure by instituting an inspiratory pause or hold. This value is obtained in different ways depending on the brand of ventilator. Ventilators with external exhalation valves, such as home care ventilators or earlier models, may require that the exhalation valve tubing be kinked or pinched closed at peak inspiration to obtain an inspiratory hold until the plateau pressure is achieved. The tubing should then be released so exhalation can be completed.

3. From the preceding data, calculate resistance by using the following formula. *Record the results on your laboratory report.*

$$\frac{Peak\ pressure - Plateau\ pressure}{Flow\ rate}$$

EXERCISE 29.2.2 Determination of Auto-PEEP

To measure auto-PEEP, an expiratory hold must be implemented. How this is done depends on the type of ventilator used.

1. Consult the manufacturer's manual to determine the method of measuring auto-PEEP or implementing an expiratory hold.

2. Set up an adult ventilator on the following settings: mode = A/C, $V_T = 700$ ml, $f = 24/\text{min}$, $F_IO_2 = 0.21$, PEEP = 3 cm H_2O, and peak flow = 40 lpm (or percent inspiratory time = 20 percent).

3. Attach a test lung to the patient wye.

4. Initiate the expiratory hold or auto-PEEP measurement procedure.

5. Observe the pressure manometer or digital display for the final pressure reading once the pressure has equilibrated. If auto-PEEP is present the reading will be above the baseline PEEP value set. *Record the end-expiratory pressure observed on your laboratory report.*

6. Calculate auto-PEEP as follows, and *record on your laboratory report:* Auto-PEEP = End expiratory pressure – Baseline PEEP pressure.

7. Determine which ventilator parameters must be adjusted to eliminate the auto-PEEP. *Record on your laboratory report any recommendations you would make to a physician to change the ventilator orders.*

EXERCISE 29.3 Waveform Identification and Interpretation

EXERCISE 29.3.1 Identification of Pressure-Time Curves

Figure 29.1 shows a typical pressure-time curve. The horizontal *(x)* axis represents time; the vertical *(y)* axis represents pressure. Positive pressure inspiration is shown as a rise in pressure. The peak inspiratory pressure appears as the highest point of the curve. Exhalation is shown immediately after PIP and continues until the next inspiration. The beginning pressure is referred to as the baseline, which appears above zero

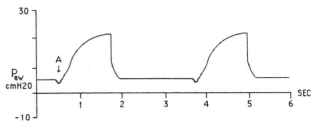

FIGURE 29.2 Patient-initiated mandatory (PIM) Nellcor Puritan Bennett Inc., Carlsbad, CA: Waveforms: The graphical presentation of ventilatory data. Form AA-1594, February 1991, p. 5, with permission.)

when PEEP/CPAP modes are in use. The average mean airway pressure is calculated from the shaded area under the curve.[1] A negative deflection immediately before a rise in pressure indicates the patient's effort in patient-initiated mandatory breaths (Fig. 29.2).[2]

Small fluctuations in pressure represent a patient's spontaneous breathing efforts (Fig. 29.3).[2] Breaths that rise to a plateau and display varying inspiratory times indicate pressure-supported breaths (Fig. 29.4).[3]

Breaths that rise to a plateau and display constant inspiratory time indicate pressure-controlled breaths (Fig. 29.5).[3]

In some cases, a ventilator may not be able to meet the required patient inspiratory demand, or the inspiratory flow may be set too low (Fig. 29.6).[4]

A stable static plateau pressure measurement is needed to accurately calculate resistance and compliance (Fig. 29.7).[5]

EXERCISE 29.3.2 Identification of Flow-Time Curves

Instead of using pressure measurements on the *y* axis, flow can also be plotted. One major difference in this type of graphical representation is that expiration is plotted below the baseline.

Figure 29.8 represents a typical flow-time curve in which inspiration is shown from *A* to *B* and expiration is shown from *B* to *C*. The peak inspiratory flow is the highest flow rate achieved during inspiration *(D)*. The peak expiratory flow rate is shown as *E*.[6]

Figure 29.9 illustrates various breath types.

Figure 29.10 shows a flow-time curve indicating auto-PEEP. Note that the expiratory flow does not return to baseline before the next breath is initiated.

Figure 29.11 shows inspiratory flow patterns that can be selected for mandatory, volume-based breaths on most ventilators.

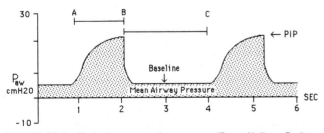

FIGURE 29.1 Typical pressure-time curve. (From Nellcor Puritan Bennett Inc., Carlsbad, CA: Waveforms: The graphical presentation of ventilatory data. Form AA-1594, February 1991, p. 3, with permission.)

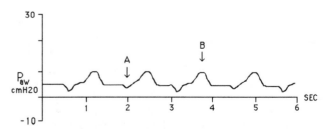

FIGURE 29.3 Spontaneous breathing. (From Nellcor Puritan Bennett Inc., Carlsbad, CA: Waveforms: The graphical presentation of ventilatory data. Form AA-1594, February 1991, p. 5, with permission.)

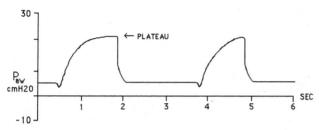

FIGURE 29.4 Pressure-supported breaths. (From Nellcor Puritan Bennett Inc., Carlsbad, CA: Waveforms: The graphical presentation of ventilatory data. Form AA-1594, February 1991, p. 6, with permission.)

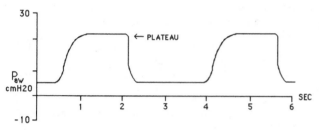

FIGURE 29.5 Pressure control ventilation. (From Nellcor Puritan Bennett Inc., Carlsbad, CA: Waveforms: The graphical presentation of ventilatory data. Form AA-1594, February 1991, p. 6, with permission.)

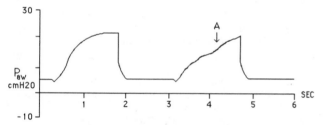

FIGURE 29.6 Inadequate flow rate. (From Nellcor Puritan Bennett Inc., Carlsbad, CA: Waveforms: The graphical presentation of ventilatory data. Form AA-1594, February 1991, p. 7, with permission.)

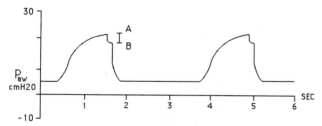

FIGURE 29.7 Static pressure measurements. (From Nellcor Puritan Bennett Inc., Carlsbad, CA: Waveforms: The graphical presentation of ventilatory data. Form AA-1594, February 1991, p. 9, with permission.)

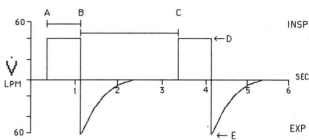

FIGURE 29.8 Typical flow-time curve. (From Nellcor Puritan Bennett Inc., Carlsbad, CA: Waveforms: The graphical presentation of ventilatory data. Form AA-1594, February 1991, p. 11, with permission.)

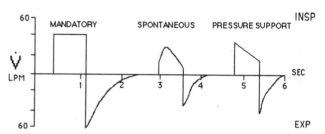

FIGURE 29.9 Flow-time curves indicating breath types. (From Nellcor Puritan Bennett Inc., Carlsbad, CA: Waveforms: The graphical presentation of ventilatory data. Form AA-1594, February 1991, p. 12, with permission.)

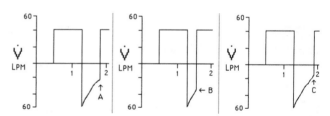

FIGURE 29.10 Flow-time curves indicating Auto-PEEP. (From Nellcor Puritan Bennett Inc., Carlsbad, CA: Waveforms: The graphical presentation of ventilatory data. Form AA-1594, February 1991, p. 13, with permission.)

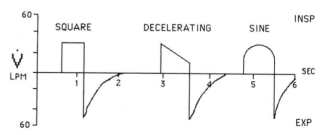

FIGURE 29.11 Flow patterns. (From Nellcor Puritan Bennett Inc., Carlsbad, CA: Waveforms: The graphical presentation of ventilatory data. Form AA-1594, February 1991, p. 15, with permission.)

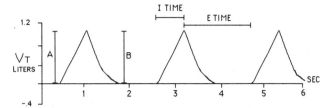

FIGURE 29.12 Typical volume-time curve. (From Nellcor Puritan Bennett Inc., Carlsbad, CA: Waveforms: The graphical presentation of ventilatory data. Form AA-1594, February 1991, p. 17, with permission.)

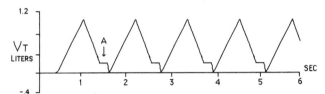

FIGURE 29.13 Detecting air trapping or leaks. (From Nellcor Puritan Bennett Inc., Carlsbad, CA: Waveforms: The graphical presentation of ventilatory data. Form AA-1594, February 1991, p. 18, with permission.)

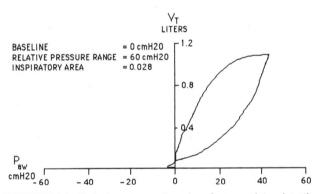

FIGURE 29.14 Typical pressure-volume loop for a mandatory breath. (From Nellcor Puritan Bennett Inc., Carlsbad, CA: Waveforms: The graphical presentation of ventilatory data. Form AA-1594, February 1991, p. 33, with permission.)

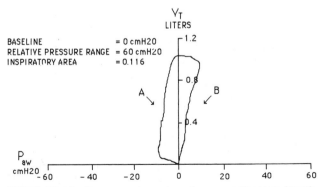

FIGURE 29.15 Pressure-volume loop for a spontaneous breath. (From Nellcor Puritan Bennett Inc., Carlsbad, CA: Waveforms: The graphical presentation of ventilatory data. Form AA-1594, February 1991, p. 34, with permission.)

EXERCISE 29.3.3 Identification of Volume-Time Curves

Figure 29.12 shows a typical volume-time curve in which the upslope indicates inspiratory volume and the downslope indicates expiratory volume. Inspiratory time is measured from the beginning of inspiration to the beginning of expiration. Expiratory time is measured from the beginning of exhalation to the beginning of the subsequent inspiration. In this figure, the patient has exhaled fully before the next breath. An increase in respiratory rate would be acceptable and would not cause air trapping.[7]

Figure 29.13 indicates an exhalation that does not return to zero. Volume in and volume out are not always equal.

EXERCISE 29.3.4 Pressure-Volume Loop

Figure 29.14 shows a typical pressure-volume loop for a mandatory breath. Pressure is plotted on the horizontal axis, volume on the vertical axis. The lower segment of the curve represents inspiration, the upper portion expiration. Inspiration is plotted first, and the loop moves counterclockwise.[8]

Figure 29.15 shows a pressure-triggered spontaneous breath with inspiration indicated by *A* and exhalation indicated by *B*. The entire inspiratory area appears to the left of the *y* axis and is plotted first so that the entire loop moves clockwise.[9]

Figure 29.16 shows a pressure-volume loop for an assisted breath. The patient initiates the breath and inspiration begins plotting clockwise to the left of the *y* axis, but when the ventilator takes over, the plot direction shifts to counterclockwise to the right of the *y* axis.[10]

EXERCISE 29.3.5 Interpretation of Waveforms

For Figures 29.17 through 29.23, identify the data indicated, and *record your interpretations on the laboratory report.*

1. Figure 29.17:
  a. Mode of ventilation.
  b. Inspiratory time for the first curve.
  c. Line *B–C.*
  d. What is occurring at point *D?*
  e. Suggested correction for point *D.*

2. Figure 29.18:
  a. Mode of ventilation.
  b. Explain the difference between curves *A* and *B*. What adjustment was made to correct curve *A?*

3. Figure 29.19:
  a. Explain the difference in *B* for curves 1 and 2.
  b. What possible treatment interventions would have caused this change?

4. Figure 29.20:
  a. Mode of ventilation.
  b. Respiratory rate.
  c. Events at points *A* and *B.*

5. Figure 29.21:
  a. Mode of ventilation.
  b. Respiratory rate.
  c. Events at points *A* and *B.*

6. Figures 29.22 and 29.23:
  a. Which curve illustrates the greater work of breathing?
  b. What modalities could be implemented to result in the change from curve VI to curve VII?

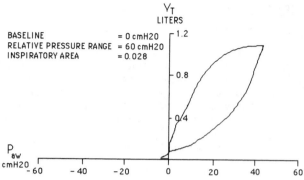

FIGURE 29.16   Pressure-volume loop for an assisted breath. (From Nellcor Puritan Bennett Inc., Carlsbad, CA: Waveforms: The graphical presentation of ventilatory data. Form AA-1594, February 1991, p. 35, with permission.)

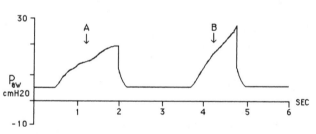

FIGURE 29.17   Evaluating respiratory events I. (From Nellcor Puritan Bennett Inc., Carlsbad, CA: Waveforms: The graphical presentation of ventilatory data. Form AA-1594, February 1991, p. 8, with permission.)

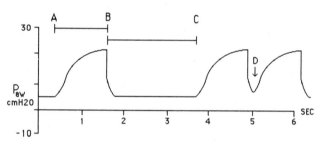

FIGURE 29.18   Evaluating respiratory events II. (From Nellcor Puritan Bennett Inc., Carlsbad, CA: Waveforms: The graphical presentation of ventilatory data. Form AA-1594, February 1991, p. 8, with permission.)

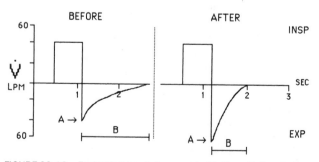

FIGURE 29.19   Evaluating respiratory events III. (From Nellcor Puritan Bennett Inc., Carlsbad, CA: Waveforms: The graphical presentation of ventilatory data. Form AA-1594, February 1991, p. 14, with permission.)

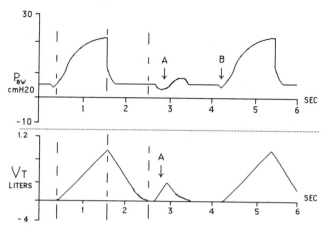

FIGURE 29.20   Evaluating respiratory events IV. (From Nellcor Puritan Bennett Inc., Carlsbad, CA: Waveforms: The graphical presentation of ventilatory data. Form AA-1594, February 1991, p. 18, with permission.)

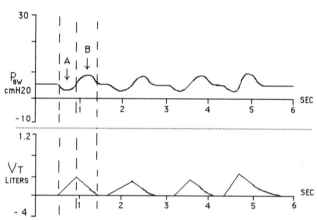

FIGURE 29.21   Evaluating respiratory events V. (From Nellcor Puritan Bennett Inc., Carlsbad, CA: Waveforms: The graphical presentation of ventilatory data. Form AA-1594, February 1991, p. 18, with permission.)

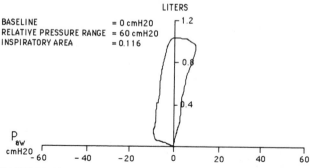

FIGURE 29.22   Evaluating respiratory events VI. (From Nellcor Puritan Bennett Inc., Carlsbad, CA: Waveforms: The graphical presentation of ventilatory data. Form AA-1594, February 1991, p. 37, with permission.)

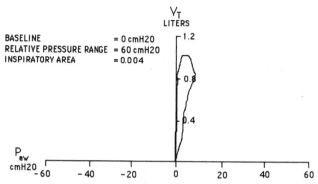

BASELINE = 0 cmH2O
RELATIVE PRESSURE RANGE = 60 cmH2O
INSPIRATORY AREA = 0.004

FIGURE 29.23 Evaluating respiratory events VII. (From Nellcor Puritan Bennett Inc., Carlsbad, CA: Waveforms: The graphical presentation of ventilatory data. Form AA-1594, February 1991, p. 38, with permission.)

EXERCISE 29.4 Setting Modification and Documentation

The following scenarios are continuations from the scenarios introduced in Exercise 29.1.

Scenario 1

Mr. Lisanti is a 21-year-old, 150-lb man who has just come from the OR after a craniotomy and evacuation of a subdural hematoma. He is orally intubated, has no documented lung pathology, and is not a smoker. Ventilation was initiated with the following settings: mode = A/C, V_T = 800 ml, f = 12/min, and F_IO_2 = 0.35. An arterial blood gas was drawn 30 min later with the following results: pH = 7.29, $PaCO_2$ = 45 mm Hg, HCO_3 = 21, and PaO_2 = 110. The physician has requested that you adjust the ventilator to hyperventilate the patient for the first 24 hours and maintain the PaO_2 at 80 to 90 mm Hg.

1. Formulate the clinical data required to make recommendations for changes in the ventilator settings, and *record them on your laboratory report.* Use any formulas or rules of thumb (see the Appendix) that are applicable to the situation.

2. With your lab partner acting as the physician, present your rationale orally.

3. The physician agrees with your recommendations. Implement the changes, and *record them on your laboratory report.*

The next day, the patient has regained consciousness. You have measured bedside **weaning** parameters and have decided that the patient is ready to be weaned.

1. Identify what the minimal acceptable values would be for VC, MIP, MVV, and V_T in this patient, and *record them on your laboratory report.*

2. State what method of weaning you would recommend, and *justify your answer on your laboratory report.*

Scenario 2

Mrs. Kay is a 30-year-old, 110-lb woman who is in status asthmaticus. She is in severe acute respiratory acidosis with moderate hypoxemia and has just been nasally intubated. Ventilation was initiated with the following settings: mode = A/C, V_T = 600 ml, f = 10/min, and F_IO_2 = 0.50. Before taking the initial blood gas on the ventilator, you observe that the high-pressure alarm is continually sounding with each breath and only 480 ml of exhaled volume is measured. Auscultation reveals markedly diminished breath sounds bilaterally.

Identify the two most likely causes of this situation, and make recommendations to correct these problems. *Record your answers on the laboratory report.*

Two days later, Mrs. Kay is stable and ready to be weaned. She is currently on SIMV 8/min, V_T 600 ml, and F_IO_2 = 40 percent. Total breath rate is 28/min, and spontaneous V_T = 200 to 250 ml. Blood gases reveal pH = 7.48, $PaCO_2$ = 32 mm Hg, HCO_3 = 25, and PaO_2 = 135 mm Hg.

What changes would you recommend to commence weaning at this time? *Record your suggestions and rationale on the laboratory report.*

Scenario 3

Miss Aswama is a 38-year-old, 100-lb woman who has myasthenia gravis. She has been on the ventilator for several weeks with a tracheostomy: mode = SIMV, V_T = 500 ml, f = 12/min, F_IO_2 = 0.30, pressure support = 5 cm H_2O, and PEEP = 5 cm H_2O. The capnometry reading has been stable at 38 mm Hg and SpO_2 = 94 percent, VC = 800 ml, and MIP = −30 cm H_2O. Weaning has begun on pressure support of 10 cm H_2O, CPAP = 3, and F_IO_2 = 0.30. One hour later, the capnometry reading is 45 mm Hg and SpO_2 = 88 percent.

What changes in vital signs and symptoms would you expect based on these values? What recommended changes would you make at this time? *Record your answers and rationale on the laboratory report.*

References

1. Nellcor, Puritan-Bennett: Waveforms: The graphical presentation of ventilatory data. Form AA-1594, February 1991, p 3.
2. Nellcor, Puritan-Bennett: Waveforms: The graphical presentation of ventilatory data. Form AA-1594, February 1991, p 5.
3. Nellcor, Puritan-Bennett: Waveforms: The graphical presentation of ventilatory data. Form AA-1594, February 1991, p 6.
4. Nellcor, Puritan-Bennett: Waveforms: The graphical presentation of ventilatory data. Form AA-1594, February 1991, p 7.
5. Nellcor, Puritan-Bennett: Waveforms: The graphical presentation of ventilatory data. Form AA-1594, February 1991, p 9.
6. Nellcor, Puritan-Bennett: Waveforms: The graphical presentation of ventilatory data. Form AA-1594, February 1991, p 11.
7. Nellcor, Puritan-Bennett: Waveforms: The graphical presentation of ventilatory data. Form AA-1594, February 1991, p 17.
8. Nellcor, Puritan-Bennett: Waveforms: The graphical presentation of ventilatory data. Form AA-1594, February 1991, p 33.
9. Nellcor, Puritan-Bennett: Waveforms: The graphical presentation of ventilatory data. Form AA-1594, February 1991, p 34.
10. Nellcor, Puritan-Bennett: Waveforms: The graphical presentation of ventilatory data. Form AA-1594, February 1991, p 35.

Related Readings

Eubanks, DH and Bone, RC: Principles and Applications of Cardiorespiratory Care Equipment. Mosby, St Louis, 1994.
McPherson, SP: Respiratory Care Equipment, ed 5. Mosby, St Louis, 1995.
Pilbeam, S: Mechanical Ventilation: Physiological and Clinical Applications. Mosby, St Louis, 1992.
Scanlan, C et al (eds): Egan's Fundamentals of Respiratory Care, ed 6. Mosby, St Louis, 1995.

Selected Journal Articles

American Association for Respiratory Care: The AARC clinical practice guideline: Patient-ventilator system checks. Respir Care 37:882–886, 1992.
Boysen, PG and Kacmarek, RM (eds): Special issue: Mechanical ventilation part II. Respir Care 32:497–640, 1987.
Brochard, L et al: Comparison of three methods of gradual withdrawal from ventilatory support during weaning from mechanical ventilation. Am J Respir Crit Care Med 150:896–903, 1994.

Kacmarek, R and Pierson, D (eds): Special issue: Positive end-expiratory pressure (PEEP) part I. Respir Care 33:397–501, 1988.

Kacmarek, R and Pierson, D (eds): Special issue: Positive end-expiratory pressure (PEEP) part II. Respir Care 33:523–637, 1988.

Lain, D et al: Pressure control versus inverse ratio ventilation as a method to reduce peak inspiratory pressure and provide adequate ventilation and oxygenation. Chest 95:1081–1088, 1989.

MacIntyre, N and Branson, RD (eds): Special issue: Consensus conference on the essentials of mechanical ventilators. Respir Care 37:965–1130, 1992.

Muir, J et al: Survival and follow up of tracheostomized patients with COPD treated by home mechanical ventilation. Chest 106:201–209, 1994.

Scheinhorn, DJ, Artinian, BM and Catlin, JL: Weaning from prolonged mechanical ventilation: The experience at a regional weaning center. Chest 105:534–539, 1994.

LABORATORY REPORT

CHAPTER 29: PATIENT-VENTILATOR SYSTEM CARE

Name _____   Date _____

Course/Section _____   Instructor _____

Data Collection

EXERCISE 29.1   Basic Ventilator Monitoring

Scenario 1

Mode = A/C, V_T = 800 ml, f = 12/min, F_1O_2 = 0.35.
Use the patient-ventilator system check flow sheet and progress note forms to document your settings.

Scenario 2

Mode = A/C, V_T = 600 ml, f = 10 min, F_1O_2 = 0.50.
Use the patient-ventilator system check flow sheet and progress note forms to document your settings.

Scenario 3

Mode = SIMV, V_T = 500 ml, f = 12 min, F_1O_2 = 0.30, pressure support = 5 cm H_2O, PEEP = 5 cm H_2O.
Use the patient-ventilator system check flow sheet and progress note forms to document your settings.

Scenario 4

Use the patient-ventilator system check flow sheet and progress note forms to document your settings.

Rationale: _____

_____

EXERCISE 29.2   Data Generation for Evaluation of Patient Status

EXERCISE 29.2.1   Effective Dynamic and Static Compliance and Resistance Calculations

Show your work!

Scenario 1

EDC = _____

C_{ST} = _____

R_{AW} = _____

Scenario 2

EDC = _____

C_{ST} = _____

R_{AW} = _____

Scenario 3

EDC = _____

C_{ST} = _____

R_{AW} = _____

Scenario 4

EDC = _____

C_{ST} = _____

R_{AW} = _____

EXERCISE 29.2.2   Determination of Auto-PEEP

End-expiratory pressure = _____

Calculated auto-PEEP (show your work!) = _____

Recommendations and adjustments: _____

_____

_____

_____

EXERCISE 29.3   Waveform Identification and Interpretation
EXERCISE 29.3.5   Interpretation of Waveforms
Figure 29.17

Mode of ventilation = _____

Inspiratory time for the first curve = _____

Line *B–C* = _____

What is occurring at point D? _____

_____

Suggested correction for point D: _____

_____

Figure 29.18

Mode of ventilation = _____

Explain the difference between curves *A* and *B*. What adjustment was made to correct curve *A*? _____

_____

_____

_____

Figure 29.19

Explain the difference in *B* for curves 1 and 2: _____

_____

_____

What possible treatment interventions would have caused this change? _____

_____

_____

Figure 29.20

Mode of ventilation = _____

Respiratory rate = _____

Event at point *A* = _____

Event at point *B* = _____

Figure 29.21

Mode of ventilation = _____

Respiratory rate = _____

Events at points *A* and *B* = _____

Figures 29.22 and 29.23

Which curve illustrates the greater work of breathing? What modalities could be implemented to result in a change

from curve VI to curve VII? _____

_____

_____

_____

_____

EXERCISE 29.4 Setting Modification and Documentation
Scenario 1

Clinical data required: _____

_____

_____

_____

_____

Formulas, rules of thumb used: _____

_____

_____

_____

_____

Changes implemented: _____

_____

_____

_____

Minimal acceptable values:

VC _____

MIP _____

MVV _____

V_T _____

Method of weaning recommended and rationale: _____

_____

_____

_____

_____

_____

_____

Scenario 2

Identify the two most likely causes: _____

_____

_____

Recommendation to correct these problems: _____

_____

_____

_____

What changes would you recommend 2 days later? _____

_____

_____

_____

Scenario 3

What changes in vital signs and symptoms would you expect based on these values? What recommended changes would you make at this time? _____

_____

_____

_____

_____

_____

_____

PATIENT-VENTILATOR SYSTEM CHECK										PT ID:	
DATE											
TIME											
MODE											
SET RATE											
TOTAL RATE											
SET VT/VE											
EXH. VT/VE											
SPONT. VT											
SET F_IO_2											
ANALYZED F_IO_2											
PSV											
PEEP/CPAP											
FLOW/%I-TIME											
FLOW PATTERN											
I : E RATIO											
SENSITIVITY											
PIP											
PLATEAU											
MAP											
HME/GAS TEMP											
HIGH P											
LOW P											
LOW VT/VE											
HI/LOW O_2											
LOW PEEP/CPAP											
TEMP ALARM											
AUTO-PEEP											
EDC											
CST											
RAW											
TUBE SIZE/TYPE											
TUBE PLACEMENT											
CUFF PRESS											
SpO_2											
$PECO_2$											
BP											
HR											
ECG											
TEMP											
pH											
$PaCO_2$											
PaO_2											
COHB/METHB											
C.O.											
PAP											
PWP											
PvO_2											
SvO_2											
$CavO_2$											
SIGNATURE											

DATE	TIME	RESPIRATORY CARE PROGRESS NOTES
		NOTES

PROCEDURAL COMPETENCY EVALUATION

Name _____ Date _____

Patient-Ventilator System Care

Setting: ☐ Lab ☐ Clinical   Evaluator: ☐ Peer ☐ Instructor

Conditions (describe): _____

_____

Equipment Used

_____

_____

	SATISFACTORY	UNSATISFACTORY	NOT OBSERVED	NOT APPLICABLE
Equipment and Patient Preparation				
1. Verifies, interprets, and evaluates physician's orders or protocol	☐	☐	☐	☐
2. Reviews any pertinent information (history and interview, lab data, x-rays) in the patient's chart as the acuity of the circumstances permits	☐	☐	☐	☐
3. Selects, gathers, and assembles the necessary equipment	☐	☐	☐	☐
4. Washes hands and applies standard precautions and transmission-based isolation procedures as appropriate	☐	☐	☐	☐
5. Identifies patient, introduces self and department	☐	☐	☐	☐
6. Explains purpose of the procedure and confirms patient understanding	☐	☐	☐	☐
Assessment and Implementation				
7. Evaluates the patient by performing	☐	☐	☐	☐
a. Vital signs	☐	☐	☐	☐
b. Physical assessment of the chest	☐	☐	☐	☐
c. Auscultation	☐	☐	☐	☐
d. Suctioning	☐	☐	☐	☐
e. Airway placement	☐	☐	☐	☐
f. Pulse oximetry	☐	☐	☐	☐
g. End-tidal CO_2	☐	☐	☐	☐
h. ECG monitoring	☐	☐	☐	☐
i. Subjective; comfort level, sensorium	☐	☐	☐	☐
8. Verifies airway size and placement	☐	☐	☐	☐
9. Performs cuff pressure measurement	☐	☐	☐	☐
10. Performs maintenance on humidifier	☐	☐	☐	☐
11. Analyzes the F_IO_2	☐	☐	☐	☐
12. Verifies all ventilator settings and makes any ordered adjustments	☐	☐	☐	☐
13. Verifies all alarm settings and adjusts if necessary	☐	☐	☐	☐
14. Measures mandatory and spontaneous rates and volumes	☐	☐	☐	☐
15. Measures bedside spirometry if applicable	☐	☐	☐	☐
16. Performs EDC, C_{ST}, R_{AW} measurement	☐	☐	☐	☐

	S A T I S F A C T O R Y	U N S A T I S F A C T O R Y	N O T O B S E R V E D	N O T A P P L I C A B L E
17. Measures auto-PEEP and adjusts any applicable parameters	☐	☐	☐	☐
18. Analyzes and interprets any displayed waveforms and adjusts any applicable parameters	☐	☐	☐	☐

Follow-up

19. Maintains/processes equipment	☐	☐	☐	☐
20. Disposes of infectious waste and washes hands	☐	☐	☐	☐
21. Records pertinent data in chart and departmental records	☐	☐	☐	☐
22. Notifies appropriate personnel and makes any necessary recommendations or modifications to the patient care plan	☐	☐	☐	☐

_____
Signature of Evaluator

_____
Signature of Student

PERFORMANCE RATING SCALE

5 EXCELLENT—FAR EXCEEDS EXPECTED LEVEL, FLAWLESS PERFORMANCE
4 ABOVE AVERAGE—NO PROMPTING REQUIRED, ABLE TO SELF-CORRECT
3 AVERAGE—THE MINIMUM COMPETENCY LEVEL, NO CRITICAL ERRORS
2 IMPROVEMENT NEEDED—PROBLEM AREAS EXIST; CRITICAL ERRORS, CORRECTIONS NEEDED
1 POOR AND UNACCEPTABLE PERFORMANCE—GROSS INACCURACIES, POTENTIALLY HARMFUL

PERFORMANCE CRITERIA	SCALE				
1. DISPLAYS KNOWLEDGE OF ESSENTIAL CONCEPTS	5	4	3	2	1
2. DEMONSTRATES THE RELATIONSHIP BETWEEN THEORY AND CLINICAL PRACTICE	5	4	3	2	1
3. FOLLOWS DIRECTIONS, EXHIBITS SOUND JUDGMENT, AND DEMONSTRATES ATTENTION TO SAFETY AND DETAIL	5	4	3	2	1
4. EXHIBITS THE REQUIRED MANUAL DEXTERITY	5	4	3	2	1
5. PERFORMS PROCEDURE IN A REASONABLE TIME FRAME	5	4	3	2	1
6. MAINTAINS STERILE OR ASEPTIC TECHNIQUE	5	4	3	2	1
7. INITIATES UNAMBIGUOUS GOAL-DIRECTED COMMUNICATION	5	4	3	2	1
8. PROVIDES FOR ADEQUATE CARE AND MAINTENANCE OF EQUIPMENT AND SUPPLIES	5	4	3	2	1
9. EXHIBITS COURTEOUS AND PLEASANT DEMEANOR	5	4	3	2	1
10. MAINTAINS CONCISE AND ACCURATE RECORDS	5	4	3	2	1

ADDITIONAL COMMENTS: INCLUDE ERRORS OF OMISSION OR COMMISSION, COMMUNICATIVE SKILLS, AND EFFECTIVENESS OF PATIENT INTERACTION:

SUMMARY PERFORMANCE EVALUATION AND RECOMMENDATIONS

SATISFACTORY PERFORMANCE—Performed without error or prompting, or able to self-correct, no critical errors.

_____ LABORATORY EVALUATION. SKILLS MAY BE APPLIED/OBSERVED IN THE CLINICAL SETTING.

_____ CLINICAL EVALUATION. STUDENT READY FOR MINIMALLY SUPERVISED APPLICATION AND REFINEMENT.

UNSATISFACTORY PERFORMANCE—Prompting required; performed with critical errors, potentially harmful.

_____ STUDENT REQUIRES ADDITIONAL LABORATORY PRACTICE.

_____ STUDENT REQUIRES ADDITIONAL SUPERVISED CLINICAL PRACTICE.

SIGNATURES

STUDENT: _____   EVALUATOR: _____

DATE: _____   DATE: _____

CHAPTER 30

Neonatal/Pediatric Respiratory Care

INTRODUCTION

Respiratory distress is most frequently the primary problem in many infant and pediatric disorders. Advances in medical technology and pharmacology have greatly increased the survival of newborns. The increasing incidence of pediatric asthma and long-term survival of children with genetic disorders such as cystic fibrosis have contributed to the significant increase in the need for perinatal/pediatric respiratory care specialists.

A family-centered approach to patient care is essential to cope with the additional psychological and emotional stress encountered when a child is sick.[1]

Although basic concepts of quality patient care are similar in adults and children, the indications, goals, and hazards associated with respiratory care must be modified to meet the special needs of this patient population. Techniques, procedures, equipment, and expected outcomes are frequently significantly altered from the adult population.

OBJECTIVES
Upon completion of this chapter, the student will be able to:

1. Practice communication skills needed for the instruction of patients and family members in respiratory care of neonatal and pediatric patients.

2. Apply patient assessment techniques to a neonatal or pediatric patient.

3. Modify respiratory care procedures to meet the special needs of the neonatal or pediatric patient.

4. Apply infection control guidelines and standards associated with equipment and procedures, according to OSHA regulations and CDC guidelines.

5. Select, assemble, verify, and document the function of a time-cycled, pressure-controlled ventilator.

6. Practice the documentation skills required for a neonatal or pediatric patient-ventilator system check on a ventilator flow sheet and the skills necessary to generate a narrative or shift note.

7. Practice communication skills needed for the reporting of clinically significant data to the members of the health care team.

KEY TERMS

abruptio placentae
acrocyanosis
amniotic fluid
anomaly
Apgar score
breech
cesarean
choanal atresia
chorionic villi
diaphragmatic hernia
ductus arteriosus
ductus venosus
dystocia
eclampsia
fetal asphyxia
foramen ovale
gestation
gravida
hyperbilirubinemia
lanugo
lecithin/sphingomyelin
  (L/S) ratio
meconium
Moro reflex
neonate
oligohydramnios
para
periodic breathing
placenta
placenta previa
polyhydramnios
postterm
preeclampsia
preterm
tocolytic
umbilical artery
umbilical vein
vernix

EQUIPMENT REQUIRED

- Infant airway management trainer
- Infant mannequin
- Pediatric care doll or mannequin
- Small volume nebulizers
- Large volume nebulizers
- Infant/pediatric ventilators
- High-frequency ventilator (optional)
- Endotracheal tube connector
- HEPA bacteria filters
- Manufacturer's operation and maintenance manuals
  (videos if available)
- 50 psi oxygen source

- Infant ventilator circuits
- 50 psig regulator
- Bourdon gauge and Thorpe tube flowmeters
- High-pressure hoses
- Air compressor
- Blender
- Wrenches
- T-adaptor with small-bore tubing connection and cap
- Watch with second hand
- Respirometer
- Respiratory transfer set (continuous feed system)
- Sterile water
- Wick humidifiers
- Water traps
- Infant test lungs
- Infant lung simulator (optional)
- Temperature probes
- Oxygen analyzers
- Cloth tape
- Neonatal and pediatric sizes of the following:
  Nasal cannula
  Oxygen masks
  Aerosol masks
  Spacers with masks
- Bulb syringe
- Suction catheters
- Infant nasal CPAP setup
- Percussion cups
- Ventilator circuits (heated-wire circuits if available)
- Stethoscopes
- Blood pressure cuffs
- Endotracheal and tracheostomy tubes
- Miller laryngoscope blades and handles
- Infant manual resuscitators with masks

● EXERCISES

EXERCISE 30.1 Patient Assessment in the Newborn

EXERCISE 30.1.1 Maternal Assessment

For this exercise, students either independently or as a group will need to get permission from a pregnant woman or any woman who has given birth to perform a "prenatal" history and interview.

1. Introduce yourself and your department to the mother.

2. Explain the purpose of the interview.

3. Interview the mother and take a history with special emphasis on the following:
   Date of birth
   Date of last menses
   Number of pregnancies (**gravida**) and number carried to term (**para**)
   Multiple **gestations**
   Any medications taken during pregnancy
   History of diabetes, hypertension, toxemia, **preeclampsia,** maternal hypertension, **eclampsia,** previous fetal loss, smoking, pulmonary disease, previous **breech** births, rH factors, **oligohydramnios, polyhydramnios,** previous **meconium** stains, previous placental problems, maternal sepsis, in utero infections, cardiac disease, drug use, alcohol use, sexually transmitted diseases

TABLE 30.1 **Neonatal Resuscitation Equipment**

Radiant warmer
Suction equipment
  Bulb syringe
  Vacuum
  Suction catheter
  DeLee trap
Ventilation equipment
  Resuscitation bag
  Masks
  Pressure manometer
  Oxygen tubing
Oxygen source
Laryngoscope
  Handles
  Batteries
  Blades
Endotracheal tubes (sizes 2.5–4 mm)
Nasogastric tubes
Umbilical vessel catheter equipment
Syringes
Blood gas analysis equipment

From Barnhart, SL and Czervinske, MP: Clinical Handbook of Perinatal and Pediatric Respiratory Care. WB Saunders, Philadelphia, 1995, p. 363, with permission.

EXERCISE 30.1.2 Preparation for Resuscitation of the Newborn

Table 30.1 shows the equipment and supplies needed for resuscitation of the **neonate.** Prepare a cart or table with all the equipment and supplies needed before performing the following exercises.

EXERCISE 30.1.3 Resuscitation of the Newborn

In the following scenarios the initiation of basic life support will be required. It is expected that the student will have already had instruction in basic life support for health providers before this laboratory. Refer to current American Heart Association (AHA) or American Red Cross (ARC) cardiopulmonary resuscitation (CPR) guidelines for specific details.

Table 30.2 shows the Apgar scoring system.

Using the algorithm shown in Figure 30.1, simulate on an infant mannequin what would need to be done in the following scenarios.

TABLE 30.2 **Apgar Scoring System**

	0	1	2
Heart rate	None	<100	>100
Respiratory rate	None	Weak, irregular	Strong cry
Color	Pale blue	Acrocyanosis	Pink
Reflex irritability	No response	Grimace	Cry, cough, or sneeze
Muscle tone	Limp	Some flexion	Well flexed

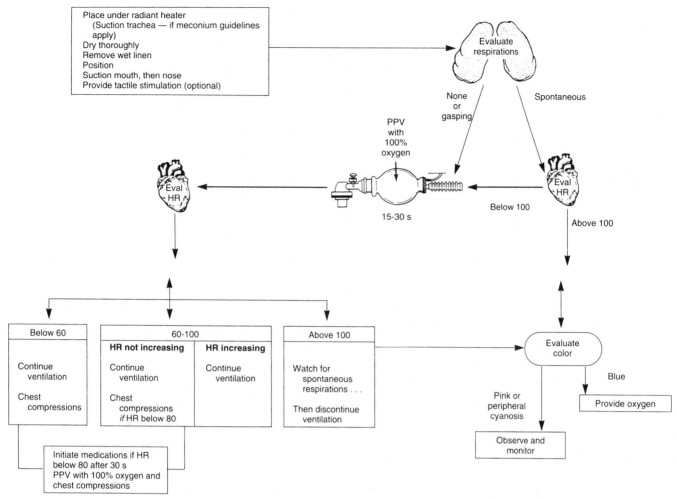

FIGURE 30.1   Overview of resuscitation in the delivery room. (Reproduced with permission. © *Textbook of Neonatal Resuscitation*, 1987, 1990, 1994. Copyright American Heart Association.)

Scenario 1: Baby Boy Marcos

You are present for the delivery of a 42-week-gestation neonate. The mother has been in labor for 30 hours and has evidence of meconium staining in the **amniotic fluid.**

The following is noted in the initial assessment of Baby Boy Marcos:

Weight 8.0 pounds
Central cyanosis
Grimaces noted when bulb suction of nares performed
Heart rate 90
Respiratory rate 40 with periods of apnea, retractions noted
Extremities some flexion

1. Perform an **Apgar score** for this scenario, and *record the score on your laboratory report.*

2. Referring to the resuscitation algorithm, perform the required resuscitation procedures. *"Chart" the event on your laboratory report.*

Scenario 2: Baby Girl A and Baby Girl B Williams

You have been called to the delivery room in anticipation of the delivery of 30-week-gestation twins.

The following is noted in the initial assessment of Baby Girl A:

Weight 3.5 pounds
Complete cyanosis
No grimaces noted when bulb suction of nares performed

Heart rate 60
Respiratory rate none
Limp

The following is noted in the initial assessment of Baby Girl B:

Weight 4.0 pounds
Acrocyanosis
Crying and sneeze stimulated with bulb suction of nares
Heart rate 130
Respiratory rate 60 and irregular
Well flexed

1. Perform an Apgar score for each twin, and *record the scores on your laboratory report.*

2. Referring to the resuscitation algorithm, perform the required resuscitation procedures for each twin. *"Chart"* the events on your laboratory report.

EXERCISE 30.2 Nasal Continuous Positive Airway Pressure for the Infant

1. For Baby Boy Marcos in Scenario 1, Exercise 30.1.3: After a successful resuscitation, the baby is placed on nasal CPAP of 5 cm H_2O and an F_IO_2 of 0.80. Set up the equipment needed as shown in Figure 30.2. (Also, see Fig. 24.2*B*.)

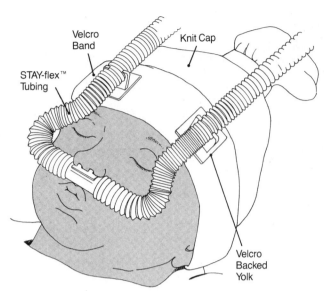

FIGURE 30.2 Infant nasal continuous positive airway pressure (CPAP) setup. (Courtesy of Ackrad Laboratories Inc., Cranford, NJ.)

2. Initiate CPAP using a mannequin. "Chart" the procedure, documenting your patient assessment and any other data required to write a comprehensive note, and *record it on your laboratory report*. This will require you to use your imagination to create clinically relevant assessment data. Include expected capillary blood gases and noninvasive monitoring results.

EXERCISE 30.3 Time-Cycled/Pressure-Limited Ventilators

EXERCISE 30.3.1 Ventilator Assembly

1. Select an infant ventilator, water traps, bacteria filters, humidifier, and infant test lung or mannequin.

Record the ventilator make and model on your laboratory report.

2. Obtain the maintenance manual for the ventilator selected. In the manual, find the manufacturer's recommendations for the following:
   Changing and cleaning of bacteria filters
   Fan filters
   Sterilization or disinfection instructions for internal and external parts and surfaces
   Requirements for routine maintenance
   Record this information on your laboratory report.

3. Locate the chronometer, and *record the number of hours of use on your laboratory report.*

4. Assemble the ventilator as shown in Figure 30.3.

5. Repeat this exercise for each ventilator provided.

EXERCISE 30.3.2 Identification of Controls

1. On the same infant ventilator used in Exercise 30.3.1, identify the following controls. It is important to note that not all ventilators have the same controls, but they have several controls in common (Fig. 30.4).
   High-pressure limit
   Rate
   F_IO_2
   Flow
   Inspiratory time
   Expiratory time
   Mode selection
   Low inspiratory pressure
   Low PEEP/CPAP
   Low oxygen pressure
   Low air pressure
   Prolonged inspiratory pressure
   Ventilator inoperative
   Overpressure relief valve

2. *Record the controls identified on your laboratory report.*

3. Repeat this exercise for each ventilator provided.

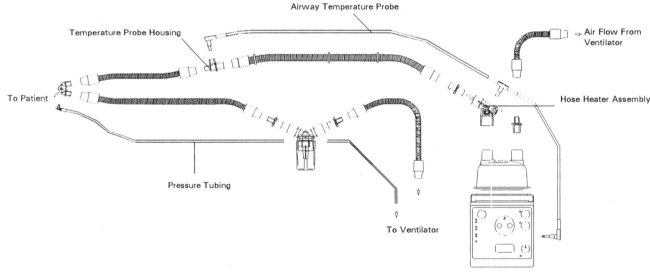

FIGURE 30.3   Infant ventilator assembly with heated wire circuit. (Courtesy of Fisher & Paykel Healthcare, Auckland, New Zealand.)

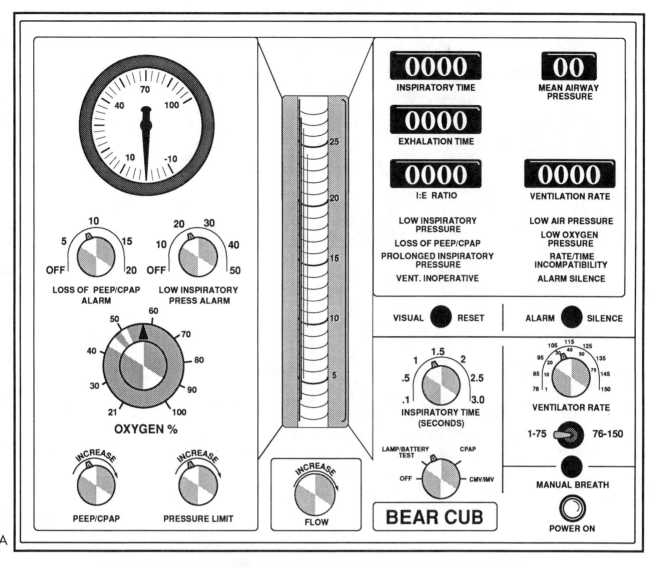

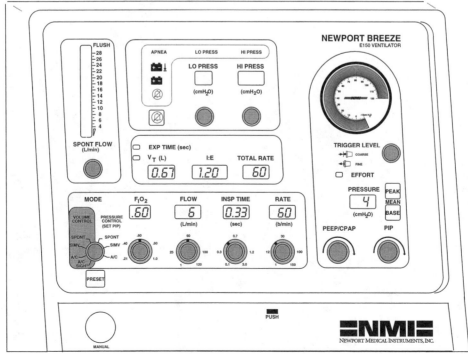

FIGURE 30.4   Infant ventilator panels: *(A)* Bear Cub. (From Branson, RD, Hess, DR and Chatburn, RL: Respiratory Care Equipment. JB Lippincott, Philadelphia, 1995, p. 319, with permission.) *(B)* Newport Breeze. (Courtesy of Newport Medical Instruments, Inc., Newport Beach, CA.)

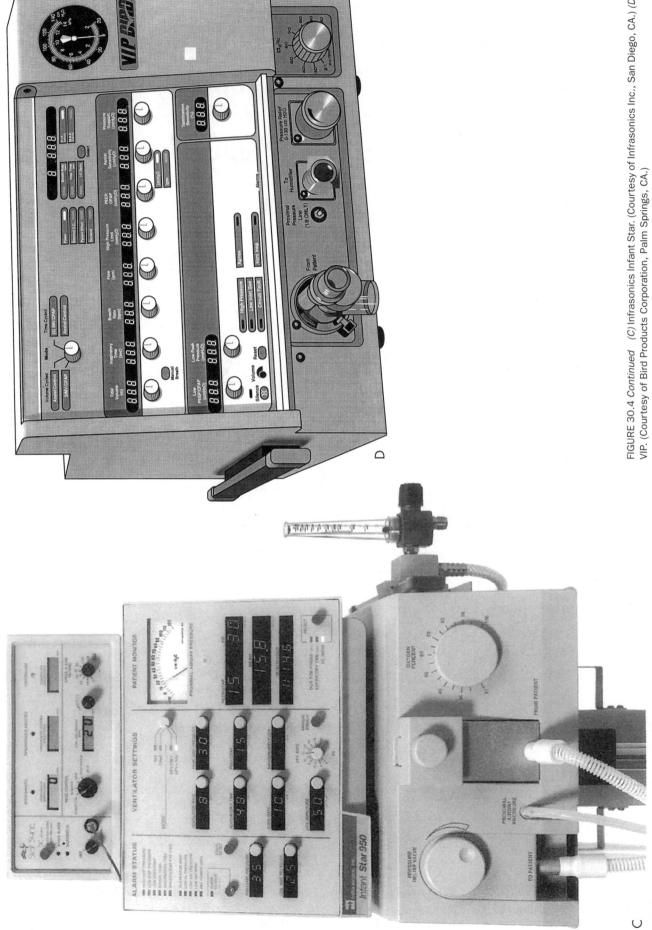

FIGURE 30.4 Continued (C) Infrasonics Infant Star. (Courtesy of Infrasonics Inc., San Diego, CA.) (D) Bird VIP. (Courtesy of Bird Products Corporation, Palm Springs, CA.)

C

D

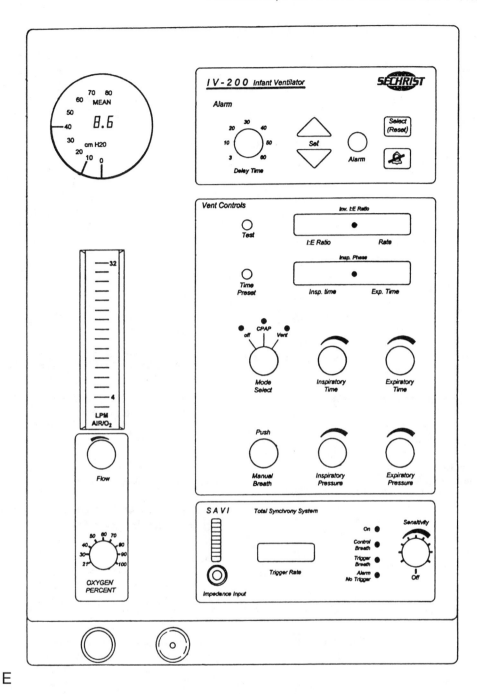

E

FIGURE 30.4 *Continued* (E) Sechrist Infant Ventilator. (Courtesy of Sechrist Industries Inc., Anaheim, CA.)

EXERCISE 30.3.3 Manipulation of Controls

1. Adjust the settings to the following:

Mode = IMV or SIMV
PIP = 20 cm H_2O
f = 20/min
Flow rate = 9 lpm
Inspiratory time = 0.4 sec
PEEP = 5 cm H_2O
F_1O_2 = 1.0

Make sure that all the alarms are set to the appropriate settings. *Record the alarm settings selected on your laboratory report.*

2. Attach the infant test lung to the patient wye connection.

3. Observe the inflation of the test lung, and *record your observations on your laboratory report.*

4. Squeeze the test lung several times to simulate an inspiratory effort and rate of 40/min. Observe the manometer. Count the rate at which you are squeezing the test lung, and compare it with the displayed rate on the machine. *Record the results on your laboratory report.*

5. Observe the test lung expansion, and compare it with step 3. *Record your observations on your laboratory report.*

6. Adjust the inspiratory time to 1 sec. Squeeze the test lung at a minimum rate of 40/min. Listen to the sound of the machine. Observe the manometer and alarms.

Record the results and observations on your laboratory report.

7. Observe the test lung expansion, and compare it with step 5. *Record the result on your laboratory report.*

8. Return the inspiratory time to 0.4 sec. Decrease the rate to 5/min.

9. Stop squeezing the test lung. Wait 1 min, and observe the ventilator response. Count the ventilator rate. *Record your results and observations on your laboratory report.*

10. Change the flow rate to 2 lpm. Continue simulating spontaneous respirations at a rate of 40/min. Observe the test lung expansion, manometer, and alarms. *Record your observations on your laboratory report.*

11. Change the flow rate to 12 lpm. Continue simulating spontaneous respirations at a rate of 40/min. Observe the test lung expansion, manometer, and alarms. *Record your observations on your laboratory report.*

12. Return the flow to 9 lpm. Adjust the PIP to 10 cm H_2O. Continue simulating spontaneous respirations at a rate of 40/min. Observe the test lung expansion, manometer, and alarms. *Record your observations on your laboratory report.*

13. Adjust the PIP to 30 cm H_2O. Continue simulating spontaneous respirations at a rate of 40/min. Observe the test lung expansion, manometer, and alarms. *Record your observations on your laboratory report.*

EXERCISE 30.4 High-Frequency Ventilators

Audiovisual training videotapes are available from several high-frequency ventilator manufacturers. Your instructor may have these available in the laboratory.

Because of the complexity of this technology and the lack of availability of the equipment for many respiratory care schools, it is recommended that arrangements be made for a manufacturer's demonstration of the equipment. An observational experience in the clinical setting would also be useful.

1. Obtain a high-frequency ventilator, if available. Set up the ventilator as shown in Figure 30.5.

2. Attach a test lung to the circuit.

3. Initiate high-frequency ventilation (HFV) using Table 30.3 as a guide.

4. Indicators for adequate inflation during HFV include the following[1]:
   Chest x-ray findings
   Stomach wiggle
   TCPO$_2$ and TCPCO$_2$ values
   SpO$_2$
   C$_{ST}$
   Hemodynamic status
   a/A ratio
   Alveolar ventilation is directly proportional to the amplitude setting.[2]

5. *"Chart" the initiation of high-frequency ventilation on Baby Girl A Williams on your laboratory report.*

6. Adjust the amplitude to 11. Observe the test lung, and *record your observations on your laboratory report.*

7. Adjust the amplitude to 51. Observe the test lung, and *record your observations on your laboratory report.*

8. Return the amplitude to 24. Adjust the settings to 10 Hz (600 beats or cycles/min). Determine the I:E ratio, and

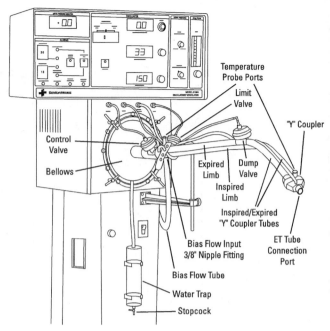

FIGURE 30.5 High-frequency oscillator ventilator. (Courtesy of SensorMedics Critical Care, Yorba Linda, CA.)

record your answer on your laboratory report. Observe the test lung, and *record your observations on your laboratory report.*

9. Adjust the settings to 22 Hz (1320 beats or cycles/min). Observe the test lung, and *record your observations on your laboratory report.*

EXERCISE 30.5 Initiating Mechanical Ventilation in an Infant

Scenario 1
Baby Boy Marcos is currently on CPAP of 5 cm H_2O and an F_IO_2 0.80. The following data are obtained:
   SpO$_2$ = 85 percent
   TcPCO$_2$ = 75 mm Hg
   Capillary stick pH = 7.20

1. The physician has asked you to initiate mechanical ventilation. Using Table 30.4 as a guide, adjust the ventilator and initiate mechanical ventilation.

TABLE 30.3 **Initial HFV Settings[2] (Premature Infants <2.5 kg)**

Frequency	15 Hz (900 bmp); range 6–15 Hz
	6–12 Hz with air leaks
Inspiratory time	Fixed at 18 ms (0.018 sec)
I:E Ratio	Dependent on rate
Amplitude	24 (11–51)
	Adjust until vigorous chest wall vibrations seen
	Titrate based on PaCO$_2$
	To change PaCO$_2$ ± 2–4 mm Hg ad change amplitude 3 units
	To change PaCO$_2$ ± 5–9 mm Hg ad change amplitude 6 units
PEEP	Equal to MAP on CMV

*BPM = beats per minute.

TABLE 30.4   **Initial Ventilator Parameters**

Suggested Initial Ventilator Settings for Newborn Infants*

	With Normal Lungs	With Noncompliant (Stiff) Lungs or RDS
PIP	12–18 cm H_2O	20–25 cm H_2O
Respiratory rate	10–20 breaths/min	20–40 breaths/min
PEEP	2–3 cm H_2O	4–5 cm H_2O
Flow rate	4–10 L/min	4–10 L/min
Inspiratory time	0.4–0.8 sec	0.3–0.5 sec
I/E ratio	1:2–1:10	1:1–1:3
F_{IO_2}	To maintain $Pa_{O_2} > 50$ mm Hg	To maintain $Pa_{O_2} > 50$ mm Hg

*RDS = respiratory distress syndrome; PIP = peak inspiratory pressure; PEEP = positive end-expiratory pressure; I/E ratio = inspiratory-expiratory ratio; F_{IO_2} = fractional concentration of oxygen in inspired gas; Pa_{O_2} = partial pressure of arterial oxygen.

From Whitaker, K: Comprehensive Perinatal and Pediatric Respiratory Care. Delmar, Albany, 1992, p. 508, with permission.

2. Perform a patient-ventilator system check, including "patient" assessment. Include oxygen analysis and airway care. *Record all pertinent data on the ventilator flow sheet provided in your laboratory report.*

3. A blood gas is obtained after your initial settings:
   pH = 7.32
   PaO_2 = 120 mm Hg
   $PaCO_2$ = 60 mm Hg

   Adjust the ventilator settings according to Table 30.6. Perform a patient-ventilator system check, including "patient" assessment. Include oxygen analysis and airway care. *Record all pertinent data on the ventilator flow sheet provided in your laboratory report.*

4. Write a narrative note documenting your patient's status and any other data required to write a comprehensive shift note. *Record it on your laboratory report.* This will require you to use your imagination to create clinically relevant assessment data.

Scenario 2

Baby Girl B Williams is presently in the NICU receiving an F_IO_2 of 0.40 via oxyhood. You have noticed increasing expiratory grunting, retractions, and periods of apnea and bradycardia over the last hour. As you are suctioning the patient, she has a complete respiratory arrest. The nurse is manually ventilating while you set up and initiate mechanical ventilation.

1. Select the appropriate size endotracheal tube, and *record your selection on your laboratory report.*

2. Baby Girl B Williams is now intubated. Determine the appropriate ventilatory parameters, and initiate ventilation. Perform a patient-ventilator system check, including "patient" assessment. Include oxygen analysis and airway care. *Record all pertinent data on the ventilator flow sheet provided in your laboratory report.*

3. A blood gas is obtained after your initial settings:
   pH = 7.45
   $PaCO_2$ = 35 mm Hg
   PaO_2 = 45 mm Hg

   Adjust the ventilator settings according to Table 30.6. Perform a patient-ventilator system check, including "patient" assessment. Include oxygen analysis and airway care. *Record all pertinent data on the ventilator flow sheet provided in your laboratory report.*

TABLE 30.5   **Guidelines for Pediatric Tracheal Tube Size**

CHILD'S AGE	INTERNAL DIAMETER (mm)
Premature	
1000 g	2.5
1000–1500 g	3.0
1500–2500 g	3.5
Normal newborns	3.5–4.0
6–12 months	4.0–4.5
1–2 years	4.5
4 years	5.0
6 years	5.5
8 years	6.0
10 years	6.5
Greater than 12 years	
Female	7.0–8.5
Male	8.0–10.0

From Barnhart, SL and Czervinske, MP: Clinical Handbook of Perinatal and Pediatric Respiratory Care. WB Saunders, Philadelphia, 1995, p. 387, with permission.

TABLE 30.6   **Suggested Neonatal Ventilator Adjustments**

SETTING	ADJUSTMENT INCREMENT	ANTICIPATED RESULTS
F_{IO_2}	2–5 (%)	Change in Pa_{O_2}
PIP	+1–2 (cm H_2O)	Increased Pa_{O_2} Decreased Pa_{CO_2}
PEEP	+1–2 (cm H_2O)	Increased Pa_{O_2} Decreased Pa_{CO_2}
T_i	+0.1–0.2 (sec) −0.1–0.2 (sec)	Increased Pa_{O_2} Better synchronization
Rate	2–5 (breaths per minute)	Change in Pa_{CO_2}

From Barnhart, SL and Czervinske, MP: Clinical Handbook of Perinatal and Pediatric Respiratory Care. WB Saunders, Philadelphia, 1995, p. 81 with permission.

4. Write a narrative note documenting your patient's status and any other data required to write a comprehensive shift note. *Record it on your laboratory report.* This will require you to use your imagination to create clinically relevant assessment data.

EXERCISE 30.6 Pediatric Ventilation

Obtain an appropriate ventilator for pediatric patients, set it up, and verify the function. *Record the make and model on your laboratory report.*

For each of the following scenarios, initiate mechanical ventilation according to the guidelines outlined in Table 28.1.

Scenario 1
Amanda Chung is an 8-month-old infant admitted with RSV pneumonia. She weighs 16 lb. Initial blood gases reveal the following:

pH = 7.15
$PaCO_2$ = 65 mm Hg
PaO_2 = 40 mm Hg

1. Select the appropriate size and type of airway, and *record your selection on your laboratory report.*

2. The physician asks you to determine the appropriate ventilatory mode and parameters and initiate ventilation. Perform a patient-ventilator system check, including "patient" assessment. Include oxygen analysis and airway care. *Record all pertinent data on the ventilator flow sheet provided in your laboratory report.*

3. Write a narrative note documenting your patient's status and any other data required to write a comprehensive shift note. *Record it on your laboratory report.* This will require you to use your imagination to create clinically relevant assessment data.

Scenario 2
Chiam Goldfarb is a 3-year-old child brought to the emergency room unconscious after ingestion of an unknown quantity of paint thinner. Initial assessment reveals a 35-lb, well-nourished child with the following findings:

Pulse 140/min
f = 45/min with sternal retractions
Stridor
Nasal flaring
Breath sounds diminished with diffuse bilateral wheezes
Color pale with circumoral cyanosis

An attempt to intubate the child is unsuccessful due to severe glottic edema.

1. Select the appropriate size and type of airway, and *record your selection on your laboratory report.*

2. The physician asks you to determine the appropriate ventilatory mode and parameters and initiate ventilation. Perform a patient-ventilator system check, including "patient" assessment. Include oxygen analysis and airway care. *Record all pertinent data on the ventilator flow sheet provided in your laboratory report.*

3. Write a narrative note documenting your patient's status and any other data required to write a comprehensive shift note. *Record it on your laboratory report.* This will require you to use your imagination to create clinically relevant assessment data.

References

1. Barnhart, SL and Czervinske, MP: Clinical Handbook of Perinatal and Pediatric Respiratory Care. WB Saunders, Philadelphia, 1995, p 79.
2. Klein, JM: Management Strategies with High Frequency Ventilation in Neonates: Infant Star Ventilator. Presented at 41st Annual AARC Convention, Orlando, FL, 1995.

Related Readings

Aloan, CA: Respiratory Care of the Newborn. JB Lippincott, Philadelphia, 1987.
American Red Cross: Standard First Aid. American National Red Cross, New York, 1991.
Barnhart, SL and Czervinske, MP: Perinatal and Pediatric Respiratory Care. WB Saunders, Philadelphia, 1995.
Barnhart, SL and Czervinske, MP: Clinical Handbook of Perinatal and Pediatric Respiratory Care. WB Saunders, Philadelphia, 1995.
Eubanks, DH and Bone, RC: Principles and Applications of Cardiorespiratory Care Equipment. Mosby, St Louis, 1994.
Koff, PB, Eitzman, D and Neu, J: Neonatal and Pediatric Respiratory Care, ed 2. Mosby, St Louis, 1993.
McPherson, S: Respiratory Care Equipment, ed 5. Mosby, St Louis, 1995.
Merenstein, G and Gardner, S: Handbook of Neonatal Intensive Care, ed 2. Mosby, St Louis, 1989.
Scanlan, C et al (eds): Egan's Fundamentals of Respiratory Care, ed 6. Mosby, St Louis, 1995.
Whitaker, K: Comprehensive Perinatal and Pediatric Respiratory Care. Delmar, Albany, 1992.
Wilkins, R and Dexter, J: Respiratory Diseases: Principles of Patient Care, ed 2. FA Davis, Philadelphia, 1997.

Selected Journal Articles

American Association for Respiratory Care: AARC clinical practice guideline: Selection of an oxygen delivery device for neonatal and pediatric patients. Respir Care 41:637–646, 1996.
American Association for Respiratory Care: AARC clinical practice guideline: Neonatal time-triggered, pressure-limited, time-cycled, mechanical ventilation. Respir Care 39:808–816, 1994.
American Association for Respiratory Care: AARC clinical practice guideline: Application of continuous positive pressure to neonates via nasal prongs or pharyngeal tube. Respir Care 39:817–823, 1994. (Errata: Respir Care 39:1050, 1994.)
American Association for Respiratory Care: AARC clinical practice guideline: Surfactant replacement therapy. Respir Care 39:824–829, 1994.
American Heart Association: Guidelines for cardiopulmonary resuscitation and emergency cardiac care: Recommendations of the 1992 national conference. JAMA 268:16, 1992.
Bernstein, G et al: Prospective randomized multicenter trial comparing synchronized and conventional intermittent mandatory ventilation (SIMV vs IMV) in neonates (abstract). Pediatr Res 31:4A, 1992.
Bernstein, G et al: Response time and reliability of three neonatal patient-triggered ventilators. Am Rev Respir Dis 148:358–364, 1993.
Derleth, DP: Clinical experience with low rate mechanical ventilation via nasal prongs for intractable apnea of prematurity (abstract). Pediatr Res 31:200A, 1992.
Kopotic, RJ: Concerns with HFV in neonatal transport (abstract). Respir Care 39:1061, 1994.
Patel, CA and Klein, J: Outcome of infants with birth weights less than 1000 g with respiratory distress syndrome treated with high-frequency ventilation and surfactant replacement therapy. Arch Pediatr Adolesc 140:317–321, 1995.
Plesko, L: Interview: Ventilation. An interview with Graham Bernstein, MD. Neonatal Intensive Care 36–39, 1994.

LABORATORY REPORT

CHAPTER 30: NEONATAL/PEDIATRIC RESPIRATORY CARE

Name _____   Date _____

Course/Section _____   Instructor _____

Data Collection

EXERCISE 30.1   Patient Assessment in the Newborn

EXERCISE 30.1.1   Maternal Assessment

_____

_____

_____

_____

_____

_____

_____

_____

_____

_____

EXERCISE 30.1.3   Resuscitation of the Newborn

Scenario 1: Baby Boy Marcos

Apgar score: _____

Charting: _____

_____

_____

_____

_____

_____

_____

_____

_____

_____

_____

Scenario 2: Baby Girl A and Baby Girl B Williams

BABY GIRL A

Apgar score: _____

Charting: _____

_____

_____

_____

_____

_____

_____

_____

_____

_____

BABY GIRL B

Apgar score: _____

Charting: _____

_____

_____

_____

_____

_____

_____

_____

_____

_____

_____

EXERCISE 30.2   Nasal Continuous Positive Airway Pressure for the Infant
Baby Boy Marcos

Charting: _____

_____

_____

_____

_____

_____

_____

_____

_____

_____

_____

EXERCISE 30.3   Time-Cycled/Pressure-Limited Ventilators
EXERCISE 30.3.1   Ventilator Assembly

Ventilator make and model: _____

Manufacturer's recommendations:

1. Changing and cleaning of bacteria filters: _____

2. Fan filters: _____

3. Sterilization or disinfection instructions for internal and external parts and surfaces: _____

4. Requirements for routine maintenance: _____

Number of hours of use: _____

EXERCISE 30.3.2   Identification of Controls

_____
_____
_____
_____
_____
_____
_____
_____
_____
_____

EXERCISE 30.3.3   Manipulation of Controls

Mode = IMV or SIMV
PIP = 20 cm H_2O
f = 20/min
Flow rate = 9 lpm
Inspiratory time = 0.4 sec
PEEP = 5 cm H_2O
F_IO_2 = 1.0

Alarm settings: _____

_____
_____
_____
_____
_____

Observation of the inflation of the test lung: _____

_____
_____

Spontaneous rate of 40/min: _____

Observation of the manometer: _____

Rate comparison: _____

Comparison of test lung expansion with step 3: _____

Inspiratory time 1 sec, spontaneous rate 40/min:

Observation of the manometer and alarms: _____

Comparison of the test lung expansion with step 5: _____

Inspiratory time 0.4 sec, rate 5/min, spontaneous rate 0:

Observation of ventilator response: _____

Flow rate 2 lpm, spontaneous rate 40/min:

Observation of the test lung expansion, manometer, and alarms:

_____

_____

_____

_____

_____

Flow rate 12 lpm: _____
Observation of the test lung expansion, manometer, and alarms:

_____

_____

_____

_____

_____

Flow rate 9 lpm, PIP 10 cm H_2O: _____
Observation of the test lung expansion, manometer, and alarms:

_____

_____

_____

_____

_____

PIP 30 cm H_2O: _____
Observation of the test lung expansion, manometer, and alarms:

_____

_____

_____

_____

_____

EXERCISE 30.4   High-Frequency Ventilators

"Charting" of HFV on baby girl A Williams: _____

_____

_____

_____

_____

_____

_____

_____

_____

Amplitude = 11:

Observations: _____

_____

_____

_____

Amplitude = 51: Observations: _____

_____

_____

Amplitude = 24: Frequency = 10 Hz (600 BPM):

Observations: _____

_____

_____

_____

I:E ratio (show your work!): _____

Observations: _____

_____

_____

_____

Frequency = 22 Hz (1320 BPM): Observations: _____

_____

_____

_____

_____

EXERCISE 30.5   Initiating Mechanical Ventilation in an Infant

Scenario 1

Baby Boy Marcos is currently on CPAP of 5 cm H_2O and an F_IO_2 0.80. The following data are obtained: SpO_2 = 85 percent, $TcPCO_2$ = 75 mm Hg, capillary stick pH = 7.20.
(Insert ventilator flow sheet at end of laboratory report.)

"Charting": _____

_____

_____

_____

_____

_____

_____

_____

Scenario 2: Baby Girl B Williams

Size endotracheal tube: _____
(Insert ventilator flow sheet at end of laboratory report.)

"Charting": _____

_____

_____

_____

_____

_____

_____

_____

_____

EXERCISE 30.6   Pediatric Ventilation

Make and model of ventilator: _____

Scenario 1: Amanda Chung

Size and type of airway: _____
(Insert ventilator flow sheet at end of laboratory report.)

"Charting": _____

_____

_____

_____

_____

_____

_____

_____

_____

_____

_____

_____

_____

Scenario 2: Chiam Goldfarb

Size and type of airway: _____
(Insert ventilator flow sheet at end of laboratory report.)

"Charting": _____

_____

_____

_____

_____

CRITICAL THINKING QUESTIONS

1. For the following respiratory care procedures, identify the major differences between adult and pediatric care and explain the rationale for the differences:
   a. Oxygen therapy
   b. Aerosol delivery
   c. Suctioning
   d. Airway care
   e. Chest physiotherapy
   f. Noninvasive monitoring
   g. Blood gas analysis

2. Baby Girl A Williams, as presented in Scenario 2 of Exercise 30.1.3, is going to receive surfactant replacement therapy with Exosurf. Calculate the dosage needed and show your work.

3. Explain how an incorrect flow rate setting (too high and too low) on a pressure-limited time-cycled ventilator affects the volume delivered.

4. Compare the procedures for basic life support in infants, children, and adults for the following:
   a. Age criteria
   b. Head position
   c. Location for pulse check
   d. Rate of compression for single rescuer
   e. Rate of compression for double rescuer
   f. Ratio of compression to ventilations for single rescuer
   g. Ratio of compression to ventilations for double rescuer
   h. Depth of compression
   i. Rate of rescue breathing
   j. Hand position
   k. Obstructed airway maneuvers
   l. Timing for activation of EMS

	PATIENT-VENTILATOR SYSTEM CHECK NEONATAL									PT ID:	
DATE											
TIME											
MODE											
SET RATE											
TOTAL RATE											
SET F_IO_2											
ANALYZED F_IO_2											
PEEP/CPAP											
FLOW/%I-TIME											
I:E RATIO											
SENSITIVITY											
PIP											
PLATEAU											
MAP											
GAS TEMP											
HIGH P											
LOW P											
HI/LOW O_2											
LOW PEEP/CPAP											
TEMP ALARM											
TUBE SIZE/TYPE											
TUBE PLACEMENT											
SpO_2											
$TcPO_2$											
$TcPCO_2$											
$PECO_2$											
BP											
HR											
ECG											
TEMP											
pH											
$PaCO_2$											
PaO_2											
COHB/METHB											
C.O.											
PAP											
PWP											
PvO_2											
SvO_2											
$CavO_2$											
SIGNATURE											

DATE	TIME	RESPIRATORY CARE PROGRESS NOTES
		NOTES

Name _____ Date _____

Neonatal Patient-Ventilator System Care

Setting: ☐ Lab ☐ Clinical

Evaluator: ☐ Peer ☐ Instructor

Conditions (describe): _____
_____

Equipment Used

_____
_____

	SATISFACTORY	UNSATISFACTORY	NOT OBSERVED	NOT APPLICABLE
Equipment and Patient Preparation				
1. Verifies, interprets, and evaluates physician's orders or protocol	☐	☐	☐	☐
2. Reviews any pertinent information (history and interview, lab data, x-rays) in the patient's chart as the acuity of the circumstances permits	☐	☐	☐	☐
3. Selects, gathers, and assembles the necessary equipment	☐	☐	☐	☐
4. Washes hands and applies standard precautions and transmission-based isolation procedures as appropriate	☐	☐	☐	☐
5. Identifies patient, introduces self and department to patient's family	☐	☐	☐	☐
6. Explains purpose of the procedure and confirms family's understanding	☐	☐	☐	☐
Assessment and Implementation				
7. Evaluates the patient by performing	☐	☐	☐	☐
a. Vital signs	☐	☐	☐	☐
b. Physical assessment of the chest	☐	☐	☐	☐
c. Auscultation	☐	☐	☐	☐
d. Suctioning if needed	☐	☐	☐	☐
e. Airway placement	☐	☐	☐	☐
f. Pulse oximetry or transcutaneous monitoring	☐	☐	☐	☐
g. ECG monitoring	☐	☐	☐	☐
8. Verifies airway size and placement	☐	☐	☐	☐
9. Performs maintenance on humidifier	☐	☐	☐	☐
10. Measures and records gas temperature	☐	☐	☐	☐
11. Analyzes the F_IO_2	☐	☐	☐	☐
12. Verifies all ventilator settings and makes any ordered adjustments	☐	☐	☐	☐
13. Verifies all alarm settings and adjusts if necessary	☐	☐	☐	☐
14. Measures mandatory and spontaneous rates and I:E ratio	☐	☐	☐	☐
Follow-up				
15. Maintains/processes equipment	☐	☐	☐	☐
16. Disposes of infectious waste and washes hands	☐	☐	☐	☐
17. Records pertinent data in chart and departmental records	☐	☐	☐	☐
18. Notifies appropriate personnel and makes any necessary recommendations or modifications to the patient care plan	☐	☐	☐	☐

_____
Signature of Evaluator

_____
Signature of Student

PERFORMANCE RATING SCALE

5 EXCELLENT—FAR EXCEEDS EXPECTED LEVEL, FLAWLESS PERFORMANCE
4 ABOVE AVERAGE—NO PROMPTING REQUIRED, ABLE TO SELF-CORRECT
3 AVERAGE—THE MINIMUM COMPETENCY LEVEL, NO CRITICAL ERRORS
2 IMPROVEMENT NEEDED—PROBLEM AREAS EXIST; CRITICAL ERRORS, CORRECTIONS NEEDED
1 POOR AND UNACCEPTABLE PERFORMANCE—GROSS INACCURACIES, POTENTIALLY HARMFUL

PERFORMANCE CRITERIA		SCALE			
1. DISPLAYS KNOWLEDGE OF ESSENTIAL CONCEPTS	5	4	3	2	1
2. DEMONSTRATES THE RELATIONSHIP BETWEEN THEORY AND CLINICAL PRACTICE	5	4	3	2	1
3. FOLLOWS DIRECTIONS, EXHIBITS SOUND JUDGMENT, AND DEMONSTRATES ATTENTION TO SAFETY AND DETAIL	5	4	3	2	1
4. EXHIBITS THE REQUIRED MANUAL DEXTERITY	5	4	3	2	1
5. PERFORMS PROCEDURE IN A REASONABLE TIME FRAME	5	4	3	2	1
6. MAINTAINS STERILE OR ASEPTIC TECHNIQUE	5	4	3	2	1
7. INITIATES UNAMBIGUOUS GOAL-DIRECTED COMMUNICATION	5	4	3	2	1
8. PROVIDES FOR ADEQUATE CARE AND MAINTENANCE OF EQUIPMENT AND SUPPLIES	5	4	3	2	1
9. EXHIBITS COURTEOUS AND PLEASANT DEMEANOR	5	4	3	2	1
10. MAINTAINS CONCISE AND ACCURATE RECORDS	5	4	3	2	1

ADDITIONAL COMMENTS: INCLUDE ERRORS OF OMISSION OR COMMISSION, COMMUNICATIVE SKILLS, AND EFFECTIVENESS OF PATIENT INTERACTION:

SUMMARY PERFORMANCE EVALUATION AND RECOMMENDATIONS

SATISFACTORY PERFORMANCE—Performed without error or prompting, or able to self-correct, no critical errors.

_____ LABORATORY EVALUATION. SKILLS MAY BE APPLIED/OBSERVED IN THE CLINICAL SETTING.

_____ CLINICAL EVALUATION. STUDENT READY FOR MINIMALLY SUPERVISED APPLICATION AND REFINEMENT.

UNSATISFACTORY PERFORMANCE—Prompting required; performed with critical errors, potentially harmful.

_____ STUDENT REQUIRES ADDITIONAL LABORATORY PRACTICE.

_____ STUDENT REQUIRES ADDITIONAL SUPERVISED CLINICAL PRACTICE.

SIGNATURES

STUDENT: _____   EVALUATOR: _____

DATE: _____   DATE: _____

Hemodynamic Monitoring

INTRODUCTION

The role of the respiratory therapist has evolved from the transporter of oxygen cylinders to the expert in sophisticated invasive monitoring. Diagnostic capabilities have progressed from obtaining basic vital signs to the performance of technologically advanced hemodynamic and laboratory techniques. Intensive care has radically improved patient diagnosis and the evaluation of therapeutic interventions.[1] The evaluation of the cardiovascular system and the efficiency of oxygen delivery are key factors in the care of the critically ill. Mastering the use of this equipment, including setup and troubleshooting, makes the respiratory therapist an indispensable member of the health care team. Application of physiologic principles and the interpretation of the data obtained from hemodynamic monitoring aid in the care of the critically ill and enhance ventilator management. Although the involvement of the respiratory therapist with hemodynamic monitoring varies from facility to facility, the National Board for Respiratory Care recognizes that advanced level practitioners must demonstrate a basic competency in this area.

OBJECTIVES
Upon completion of this chapter, the student will be able to:

1. Practice communication skills needed for the instruction of patients during hemodynamic monitoring.
2. Identify the components of a pulmonary artery catheter.
3. Identify the proper port for mixed venous blood sampling on a pulmonary artery catheter.
4. Select, assemble, and calibrate the equipment required for a fluid-filled monitoring system.
5. Calibrate a pressure transducer.
6. Simulate the procedure for obtaining a **cardiac output** using the thermodilution method.
7. Identify central venous, right ventricle, pulmonary artery, and pulmonary capillary wedge waveforms.
8. Identify and correct problems with a fluid-filled monitoring system.
9. Practice the calculations to obtain derived hemodynamic data: **body surface area,** Fick equation, mean arterial pressure, **cardiac index,** various shunt equations, **systemic vascular resistance,** and **pulmonary vascular resistance.**
10. Practice documentation and reporting of hemodynamic data collected.
11. Apply infection control guidelines and standards associated with equipment and procedures, according to OSHA regulations and CDC guidelines.

KEY TERMS
body surface area
cardiac index
cardiac output

central venous pressure
phlebostatic axis
pulmonary capillary wedge
  pressure

pulmonary vascular
  resistance

systemic vascular
  resistance

EQUIPMENT REQUIRED

- Quadruple-lumen or triple-lumen pulmonary artery catheter
- IV pole
- IV tubing (high pressure)
- Microdrip chamber
- IV saline solution (1-L bag)
- Heparin
- Medication label

- Alcohol prep pads
- Ice
- Basin
- Sterile normal saline
- Pressure and cardiac output monitor
- Equipment manual
- Pressure transducer
- Inflatable pressure bag or pressure infuser
- Female caps
- Intraflow or flush device

- Three-way stopcocks
- T-connectors
- Tuberculin syringe
- 10-ml syringes (five)
- Mercury manometer with inflation bulb
- Hemodynamic simulator (if available)
- DuBois body surface area chart
- Medical scale

⬤ E X E R C I S E S

EXERCISE 31.1 Identification of the Components of a Flow-Directed Pulmonary Artery Catheter

1. Select a pulmonary artery catheter as shown in Figure 31.1. *Identify the components on your laboratory report.*
   Thermistor connection
   Balloon inflation port
   Proximal port
   Distal port
   Thermistor opening
   Balloon
   Distal opening
   Centimeter markings
   Proximal opening
   Extra injection port

2. Using a tuberculin syringe, inflate the balloon with 0.5 ml of air. *Overinflation of the balloon will cause it to rupture. This is expensive in the laboratory setting and dangerous in the clinical setting.*

3. Feel the balloon.

4. Deflate the balloon.

5. Identify the port used for mixed venous blood sampling, and *record it on your laboratory report.*

EXERCISE 31.2 Assembly and Calibration of a Fluid-Filled Monitoring System[2]

1. Gather the necessary equipment and assemble it as shown in Figure 31.2. Make sure your handling of the equipment maintains the sterility of all ports. All ports should be capped with female caps to avoid inadvertent contamination.

2. Simulate heparinizing the IV solution, and label the bag. Use 10 mg of a 1-percent solution of heparin per 500 ml. *Record how much heparin is needed for the size IV solution bag used in your setup on your laboratory report.*

3. Insert the microdrip chamber spike and IV tubing into the bag.

4. Squeeze all the air out of the IV bag.

5. Gravity fill the tubing and transducer assembly.

6. Inspect for the presence of air bubbles. Remove any air bubbles found.

7. Place the IV bag into the inflatable pressure bag or pressure infuser.

8. Inflate the pressure bag or infuser to 300 mm Hg.

9. Turn on the pressure monitor and allow 5 to 10 min for warm-up.

10. Zero the monitor and transducer according to the manufacturer's instructions as shown in Figure 31.3.

11. Close the system by closing the stopcock to all ports.

12. Connect the proximal port of the catheter to the IV tubing.

13. The completed setup is shown in Figure 31.4.

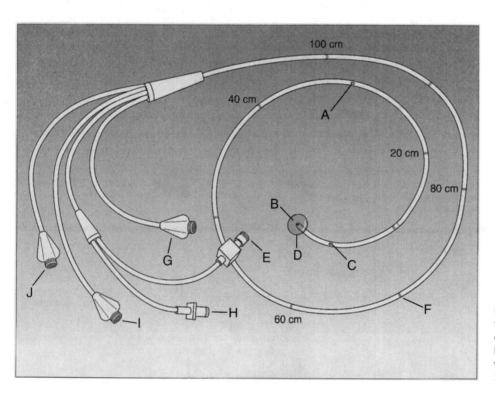

FIGURE 31.1 The components of a flow-directed pulmonary artery catheter. (From Persing, G: Advanced Practitioner Respiratory Care Review. WB Saunders, Philadelphia, 1994, p. 109, with permission.)

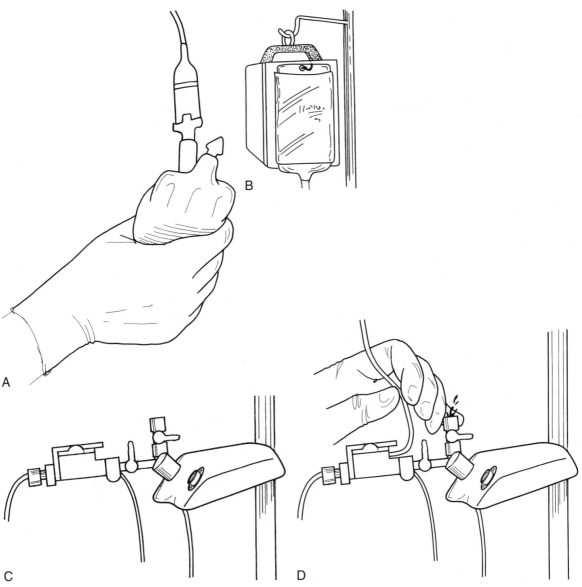

FIGURE 31.2 Components of a fluid-filled monitoring system.

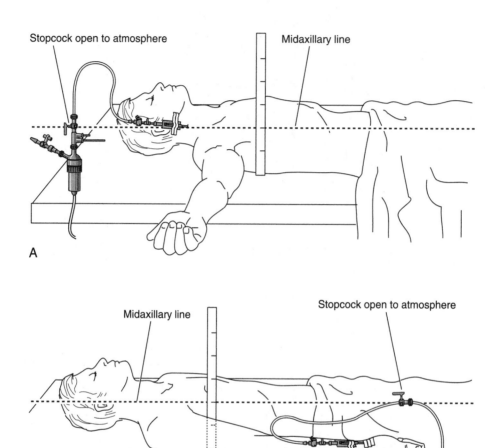

FIGURE 31.3 Zeroing the pressure transducer. (From Gardner, RM and Hollingsworth, KW: Optimizing the electrocardiogram and pressure monitoring. Crit Care Med 14:651, 1986, with permission.)

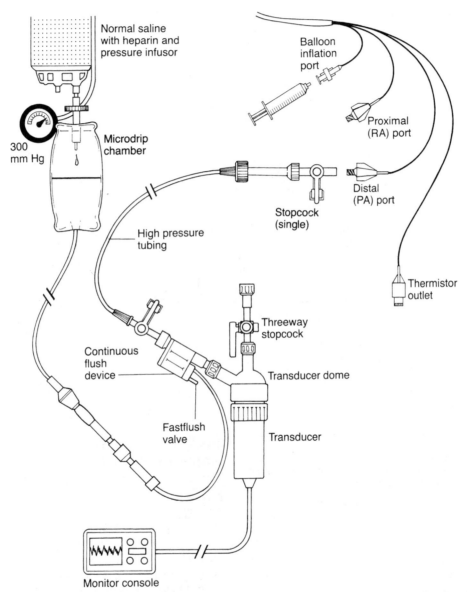

FIGURE 31.4   Completed assembly of a fluid-filled monitoring system. (From Darovic, GO: Hemodynamic Monitoring: Invasive and Noninvasive Clinical Application, ed 2. WB Saunders, Philadelphia, 1995, p. 266, with permission.)

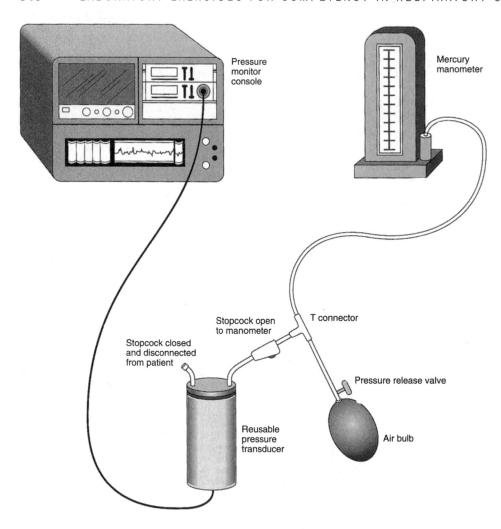

Pressure monitor console

Mercury manometer

Stopcock open to manometer

T connector

Stopcock closed and disconnected from patient

Pressure release valve

Reusable pressure transducer

Air bulb

FIGURE 31.5 Assembly of a pressure transducer and manometer for transducer calibration. (From Darovic, GO: Hemodynamic Monitoring: Invasive and Noninvasive Clinical Application, ed 2. WB Saunders, Philadelphia, 1995, p. 171, with permission.)

EXERCISE 31.3 Transducer Calibration[3]

1. Select and assemble the equipment as shown in Figure 31.5.
2. Open the stopcock to ensure communication between the manometer and the pressure monitor.
3. Inflate the manometer to 90 mm Hg by squeezing the bulb.
4. Observe the pressure monitor, and *record the pressure reading on your laboratory report.*
5. Disassemble the equipment.

EXERCISE 31.4 Identification of Pressure Waveforms

1. *Identify the pressure waveforms in Figures 31.6, 31.7, 31.8, and 31.9 on your laboratory report.*
2. Using a simulator (if available), generate and identify the following problem waveforms. *Print out (if possible) the waveforms associated with these problems and attach them to your laboratory report, or draw them on a separate sheet.* Common problems associated with a fluid-filled monitoring system are shown in Figure 31.10.
    Overdamped system
    Underdamped system

Flush
Catheter whip

EXERCISE 31.5 Thermodilution Cardiac Output Determination[4]

This exercise simulates the preparation of materials necessary to obtain a cardiac output.

1. Wash your hands and apply standard precautions and transmission-based isolation procedures as appropriate.
2. Explain the purpose of the procedure to the patient.
3. Prepare an ice/slush solution on the basin. Be sure to maintain the sterility of all solutions, ports, and connectors.
4. Make sure that the cardiac output pressure monitor is turned on and properly calibrated and zeroed according to the instructions in the manual.
5. Connect the temperature probe to the monitor.
6. Fill four 10-ml syringes with sterile normal saline. Be sure to maintain sterility. Inspect the syringes and ensure that they are free from any air bubbles.
7. Insert the probe into one of the syringes to verify injectate temperature.
8. Place the syringes in the ice/slush bath.

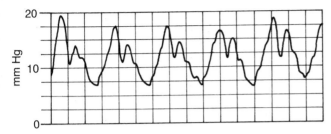

FIGURE 31.6 Waveform A. (From Darovic, GO: Hemodynamic Monitoring: Invasive and Noninvasive Clinical Application, ed 2. WB Saunders, Philadelphia, 1995, p. 272, with permission.)

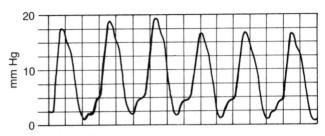

FIGURE 31.8 Waveform C. (From Darovic, GO: Hemodynamic Monitoring: Invasive and Noninvasive Clinical Application, ed 2. WB Saunders, Philadelphia, 1995, p. 272, with permission.)

9. Ensure that the thermistor port of the catheter is connected to the monitor. The system should be similar to Figure 31.11.

10. Position the patient in the supine position (not elevated more than 30°).

11. Verify catheter position by identification of the proper pressure waveform for the pulmonary artery.

12. Record the temperature of the injectate solution by pressing the appropriate key on the face of the monitor. The temperature should be between 0° and 4°C.

13. Take one of the injectate syringes and connect it to the proximal port of the catheter. A three-way stopcock may be used.

14. Press the start key on the monitor.

15. Steadily and rapidly inject the 10-ml solution. The injection should take no longer than 4 sec. Observe the waveform produced.

16. Observe the cardiac output reading.

17. Repeat the procedure at intervals of 90 sec until three readings have been obtained. The readings should be within 10 percent. If they are not, a technical error may have occurred. Using the fourth syringe, obtain another cardiac output. *Record all readings on your laboratory report.*

18. Average the three readings to report the cardiac output, and *record the results on your laboratory report.*

19. Ensure the patient's comfort after the procedure.

20. Clean the area and discard any medical waste in the appropriate containers.

21. Remove and properly dispose of any PPE. Wash your hands.

22. *Record any data and your observations on your laboratory report.*

EXERCISE 31.6 Hemodynamic Calculations

Normal hemodynamic data are shown in Table 31.1.

EXERCISE 31.6.1 Mean Arterial Pressure

Calculate the mean arterial pressure (MAP) using the following formula:

$$MAP = \frac{Systolic + 2(Diastolic)}{3}$$

1. Systolic = 120 mm Hg, diastolic = 80 mm Hg
2. Systolic = 170 mm Hg, diastolic = 100 mm Hg
3. Systolic = 90 mm Hg, diastolic = 40 mm Hg

EXERCISE 31.6.2 Cardiac Output Using the Fick Equation

Calculate the cardiac output using the Fick equation for the following data.

$$Cardiac\ output = \frac{Oxygen\ consumption}{C(a-v)O_2}$$

Record the cardiac output on your laboratory report.
PaO_2 = 85 mm Hg
$PaCO_2$ = 40 mm Hg
SaO_2 = 93 percent
Hb = 14 g/dl
PvO_2 = 38 mm Hg
$PvCO_2$ = 44 mm Hg
SvO_2 = 68 percent
F_IO_2 = 0.50
Oxygen consumption = 260 ml/min

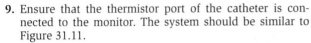

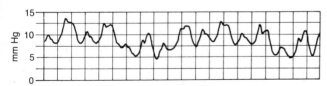

FIGURE 31.7 Waveform B. (From Darovic, GO: Hemodynamic Monitoring: Invasive and Noninvasive Clinical Application, ed 2. WB Saunders, Philadelphia, 1995, p. 273, with permission.)

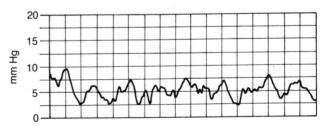

FIGURE 31.9 Waveform D. (From Darovic, GO: Hemodynamic Monitoring: Invasive and Noninvasive Clinical Application, ed 2. WB Saunders, Philadelphia, 1995, p. 271, with permission.)

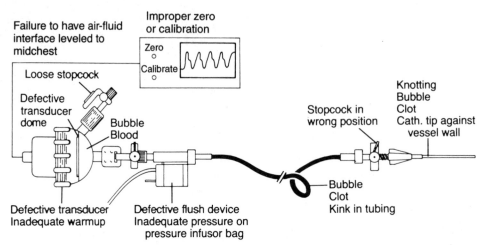

FIGURE 31.10   Step-by-step approach to problem identification. (From Darovic, GO: Hemodynamic Monitoring: Invasive and Noninvasive Clinical Application, ed 2. WB Saunders, Philadelphia, 1995, p. 312, with permission.)

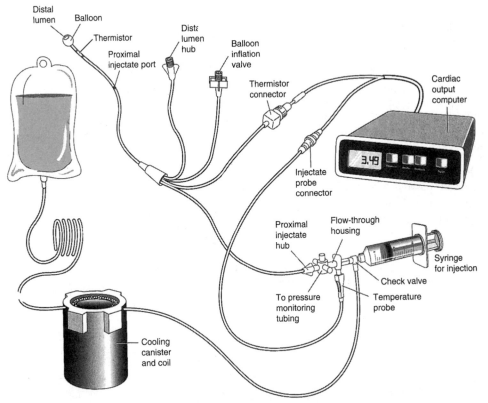

FIGURE 31.11   System for obtaining a thermodilution cardiac output. (From Baxter Healthcare Corporation, Edwards Critical Care Division, Santa Ana, CA, with permission.)

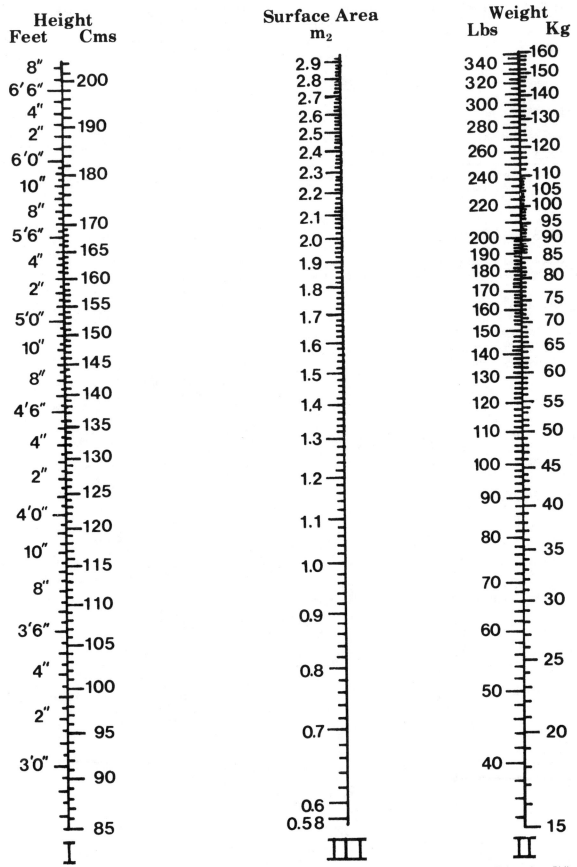

FIGURE 31.12   DuBois body surface area chart. (From Meschan, I and Ott, DJ: Introduction to Diagnostic Imaging. WB Saunders, Philadelphia, 1984, with permission.)

TABLE 31.1 **Normal Hemodynamic Data***

Cardiac output	4–8 lpm
Cardiac index	2.5–4.2 lpm/m²
Arterial blood pressure	100–140/60–90 mm Hg
Central venous pressure	0–8 mm Hg
Right ventricular pressure	15–25/0–8 mm Hg
Pulmonary artery pressure	15–25/6–12 mm Hg
Pulmonary wedge pressure	4–12 mm Hg
Percent shunt	3%–5%
Systemic vascular resistance	770–1500 dynes/sec^{-5}
Pulmonary vascular resistance	150–250 dynes/sec^{-5}

*It should be noted that normal values may vary from text to text, or even from institution to institution.

EXERCISE 31.6.3 Cardiac Index

1. Using your laboratory partner as the patient, obtain your partner's height and weight. *Record them on your laboratory report.*
2. Using the DuBois body surface area (BSA) chart in Figure 31.12, obtain your partner's body surface area. *Record it on your laboratory report.*
3. Calculate BSA using the following formula. *Record the BSA on your laboratory report.*

$$BSA = \frac{(4 \times \text{Weight in kg}) + 7}{\text{Weight in kg} + 90}$$

4. Assuming a cardiac output of 5.0 L, calculate the cardiac index using the following formula. *Record it on your laboratory report.*

$$\text{Cardiac index} = \frac{\text{Cardiac output}}{\text{Body surface area}}$$

EXERCISE 31.6.4 Systemic and Pulmonary Vascular Resistance

Using the data and formulas given, calculate systemic vascular resistance (SVR) and pulmonary vascular resistance (PVR):

$$\text{SVR dyne sec/cm}^{-5} = \frac{\text{Mean arterial pressure} - \text{CVP}}{\text{Cardiac output}} \times 80$$

$$\text{PVR dyne sec/cm}^{-5} = \frac{\text{Mean PAP} - \text{PWP}}{\text{Cardiac output}} \times 80$$

Blood pressure = 108/60 mm Hg
PAP = 24/12 mm Hg
PWP = 8 mm Hg
CVP = 0 mm Hg
C. O. Use answer from Exercise 31.6.2

EXERCISE 31.6.5 Shunt Calculation

Using the following data, calculate the percent shunt using all three formulas. *Record and compare the results on your laboratory report.*

Classic Shunt Formula

$$\text{Percent shunt} = \frac{CcO_2 - CaO_2}{CcO_2 - CvO_2} \times 100$$

$$CcO_2 = 1.0 (1.39 \times Hb) + (0.003 \times P_AO_2)$$

Modified Estimated Shunt Equation: Q_S/Q_T

$$\frac{(P_AO_2 - PaO_2) \times 0.003}{(CaO_2 - CvO_2) + [(P_AO_2 - PaO_2) \times 0.003]}$$

Can use 5 for $CavO_2$ in stable individuals or 3.5 in critically ill.

Estimated Shunt

$AaDO_2/5$ on room air

$PaO_2 = 485$ mm Hg	$PvO_2 = 380$ mm Hg
$PaCO_2 = 35$ mm Hg	$Pv = 47$ mm Hg
$SaO_2 = 99$ percent	$SvO_2 = 99$ percent
$Hb = 12$ g/dl	$F_IO_2 = 1.0$

References

1. Darovic, GO: Hemodynamic Monitoring: Invasive and Noninvasive Clinical Application, ed 2. WB Saunders, Philadelphia, 1995, p 3.
2. Darovic, GO: Hemodynamic Monitoring: Invasive and Noninvasive Clinical Application, ed 2. WB Saunders, Philadelphia, 1995, p 163.
3. Darovic, GO: Hemodynamic Monitoring: Invasive and Noninvasive Clinical Application, ed 2. WB Saunders, Philadelphia, 1995, p 170.
4. Darovic, GO: Hemodynamic Monitoring: Invasive and Noninvasive Clinical Application, ed 2. WB Saunders, Philadelphia, 1995, pp 335–336.

Related Readings

Daily, EK and Schroeder, JP: Techniques in Bedside Hemodynamic Monitoring, ed 5. Mosby, St Louis, 1994.
Darovic, GO: Hemodynamic Monitoring: Invasive and Noninvasive Clinical Application, ed 2. WB Saunders, Philadelphia, 1995.
Eubanks, DH and Bone, RC: Principles and Applications of Cardiorespiratory Care Equipment. Mosby, St Louis, 1994.
McPherson, S: Respiratory Care Equipment, ed 5. Mosby, St Louis, 1995.
Scanlan, C et al (eds): Egan's Fundamentals of Respiratory Care, ed 6. Mosby, St Louis, 1995.

Selected Journal Articles

Connors, AF et al: Hemodynamic status in critically ill patients with and without acute heart disease. Chest 98:1200–1206, 1990.
Fahey, PJ, Harris, K and Vanderwarf, C: Clinical experience with continuous monitoring of mixed venous oxygen saturation in respiratory failure via a pulmonary artery catheter. Chest 86:748–752, 1984.
Safcsak, K and Nelson, L: Detecting distal migration of pulmonary artery (PA) catheter with a right ventricular (RA) port 10 cm from the catheter tip. Heart Lung 20:302, 1991.

LABORATORY REPORT

CHAPTER 31: HEMODYNAMIC MONITORING

Name _____   Date _____

Course/Section _____   Instructor _____

Data Collection

EXERCISE 31.1   Identification of the Components of a Flow-Directed Pulmonary Artery Catheter

A: _____

B: _____

C: _____

D: _____

E: _____

F: _____

G: _____

H: _____

I: _____

J: _____

Blood sampling port: _____

EXERCISE 31.2   Assembly and Calibration of a Fluid-Filled Monitoring System

Amount of heparin used (show your work): _____

_____

EXERCISE 31.3   Transducer Calibration

Pressure reading: _____

EXERCISE 31.4   Identification of Pressure Waveforms

Figure 31.6 _____

Figure 31.7 _____

Figure 31.8 _____

Figure 31.9 _____

Overdamped system: _____

Underdamped system: _____

Flush: _____

Catheter whip: _____

EXERCISE 31.5   Thermodilution Cardiac Output Determination

CO 1: _____

CO 2: _____

CO 3: _____

CO 4: _____

Average CO (show your work!): _____

Observations: _____

_____

_____

_____

EXERCISE 31.6   Hemodynamic Calculations

Show all your work!

EXERCISE 31.6.1   Mean Arterial Pressure

1. MAP = _____

2. MAP = _____

3. MAP = _____

EXERCISE 31.6.2   Cardiac Output Using the Fick Equation

Cardiac output: _____

EXERCISE 31.6.3   Cardiac Index

Partner's height: _____

Partner's weight: _____

DuBois BSA: _____

Calculated BSA: _____

Cardiac index: _____

EXERCISE 31.6.4   Systemic and Pulmonary Vascular Resistance

Mean arterial pressure: _____

SVR dyne sec/cm^{-5}: _____

PVR dyne sec/cm^{-5}: _____

EXERCISE 31.6.5   Shunt Calculation

CcO_2: _____

CaO_2: _____

CvO_2: _____

Percent shunt (classic): _____

Percent shunt (modified): _____

Percent shunt (estimated): _____

CRITICAL THINKING QUESTIONS

For each of the pressure tracings shown in Figures 31.13 through 31.16, identify and interpret the waveforms for channels 1 (ECG tracing) and 2 (hemodynamic tracing). Identify what is being monitored in channel 3. If the tracing indicates a malfunction, state what corrective action(s) would be needed. Correlate the tracings with possible clinical findings, and recommend any necessary therapeutic interventions, if possible.

1. Figure 31.13, unknown *A*

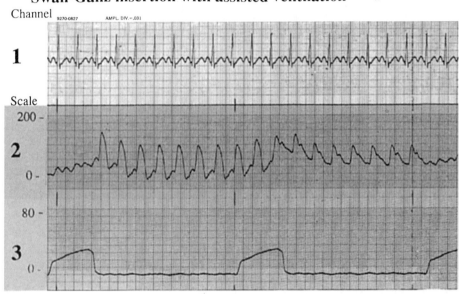

Swan-Ganz insertion with assisted ventilation

FIGURE 31.13 **Unknown A.** (From Laerdal Heartsim 2000 User's Manual, p. 46, with permission.)

2. Figure 31.14, unknown *B*

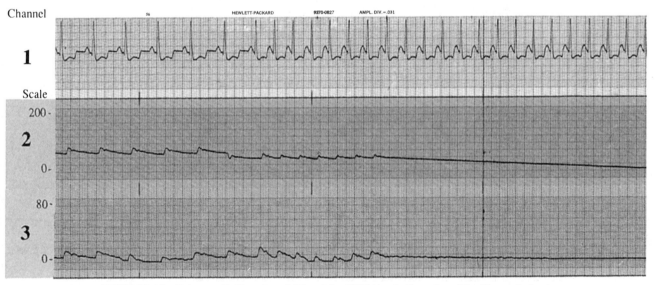

FIGURE 31.14 **Unknown B.** (From Laerdal Heartsim 2000 User's Manual, p. 47, with permission.)

Note that channel 2 is arterial pressure and channel 3 is the pulmonary catheter tracing.

3. Figure 31.15, unknown *C*

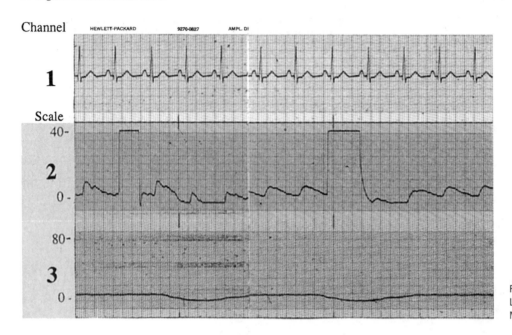

FIGURE 31.15   **Unknown C.** (From Laerdal Heartsim 2000 User's Manual, p. 50, with permission.)

4. Figure 31.16, unknown *D*

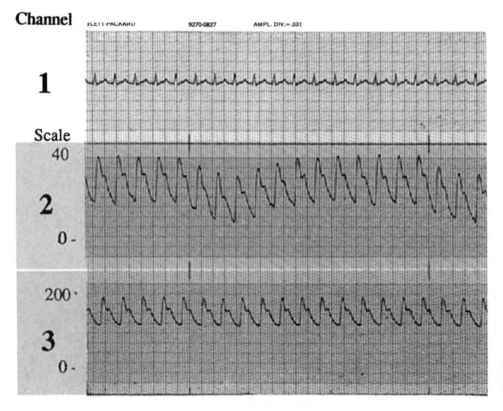

FIGURE 31.16   **Unknown D.** (From Laerdal Heartsim 2000 User's Manual, p. 49, with permission.)

PROCEDURAL COMPETENCY EVALUATION

Name _____   Date _____

Hemodynamic Monitoring

Setting: ☐ Lab ☐ Clinical   Evaluator: ☐ Peer ☐ Instructor

Conditions (describe): _____

_____

Equipment Used

_____

_____

	SATISFACTORY	UNSATISFACTORY	NOT OBSERVED	NOT APPLICABLE
Equipment and Patient Preparation				
1. Verifies, interprets, and evaluates physician's order or protocol	☐	☐	☐	☐
2. Scans chart for diagnosis and any other pertinent data and notes	☐	☐	☐	☐
3. Selects, gathers, and assembles the necessary equipment	☐	☐	☐	☐
4. Washes hands and applies standard precautions and transmission-based isolation procedures as appropriate	☐	☐	☐	☐
5. Identifies patient, introduces self and department	☐	☐	☐	☐
6. Explains purpose of the procedure and confirms patient understanding	☐	☐	☐	☐
Assessment and Implementation				
7. Assesses the patient before performance of testing	☐	☐	☐	☐
8. Identifies components of Swan-Ganz catheter	☐	☐	☐	☐
a. Inflation lumen port	☐	☐	☐	☐
b. Distal lumen port	☐	☐	☐	☐
c. Proximal lumen port	☐	☐	☐	☐
d. Thermistor connection	☐	☐	☐	☐
e. Proximal lumen orifice	☐	☐	☐	☐
f. Thermistor balloon	☐	☐	☐	☐
g. Distal orifice	☐	☐	☐	☐
9. Identifies pressure waves; states normal for each	☐	☐	☐	☐
a. CVP	☐	☐	☐	☐
b. RA	☐	☐	☐	☐
c. RV systolic	☐	☐	☐	☐
d. RV diastolic	☐	☐	☐	☐
e. PA systolic	☐	☐	☐	☐
f. PA diastolic	☐	☐	☐	☐
g. PAP mean	☐	☐	☐	☐
h. PWP	☐	☐	☐	☐
10. Corrects any malfunctions of pressure measuring system	☐	☐	☐	☐
11. Prepares five 10-ml syringes of dextrose or saline solution at 0 to 4°C or room temperature	☐	☐	☐	☐

	S A T I S F A C T O R Y	U N S A T I S F A C T O R Y	N O T O B S E R V E D	N O T A P P L I C A B L E
12. Identifies proper injectate site (proximal port)	☐	☐	☐	☐
13. Records cardiac output from monitor for a minimum of three injections within 10 percent	☐	☐	☐	☐
14. Averages three measurements	☐	☐	☐	☐
15. Interprets all data obtained	☐	☐	☐	☐

Follow-up

16. Maintains/processes equipment	☐	☐	☐	☐
17. Disposes of infectious waste and washes hands	☐	☐	☐	☐
18. Records pertinent data in chart and departmental records	☐	☐	☐	☐
19. Notifies appropriate personnel and makes any necessary recommendations or modifications to the patient care plan	☐	☐	☐	☐

_____   _____
Signature of Evaluator   Signature of Student

PERFORMANCE RATING SCALE

5 EXCELLENT—FAR EXCEEDS EXPECTED LEVEL, FLAWLESS PERFORMANCE
4 ABOVE AVERAGE—NO PROMPTING REQUIRED, ABLE TO SELF-CORRECT
3 AVERAGE—THE MINIMUM COMPETENCY LEVEL, NO CRITICAL ERRORS
2 IMPROVEMENT NEEDED—PROBLEM AREAS EXIST; CRITICAL ERRORS, CORRECTIONS NEEDED
1 POOR AND UNACCEPTABLE PERFORMANCE—GROSS INACCURACIES, POTENTIALLY HARMFUL

PERFORMANCE CRITERIA	SCALE				
1. DISPLAYS KNOWLEDGE OF ESSENTIAL CONCEPTS	5	4	3	2	1
2. DEMONSTRATES THE RELATIONSHIP BETWEEN THEORY AND CLINICAL PRACTICE	5	4	3	2	1
3. FOLLOWS DIRECTIONS, EXHIBITS SOUND JUDGMENT, AND DEMONSTRATES ATTENTION TO SAFETY AND DETAIL	5	4	3	2	1
4. EXHIBITS THE REQUIRED MANUAL DEXTERITY	5	4	3	2	1
5. PERFORMS PROCEDURE IN A REASONABLE TIME FRAME	5	4	3	2	1
6. MAINTAINS STERILE OR ASEPTIC TECHNIQUE	5	4	3	2	1
7. INITIATES UNAMBIGUOUS GOAL-DIRECTED COMMUNICATION	5	4	3	2	1
8. PROVIDES FOR ADEQUATE CARE AND MAINTENANCE OF EQUIPMENT AND SUPPLIES	5	4	3	2	1
9. EXHIBITS COURTEOUS AND PLEASANT DEMEANOR	5	4	3	2	1
10. MAINTAINS CONCISE AND ACCURATE RECORDS	5	4	3	2	1

ADDITIONAL COMMENTS: INCLUDE ERRORS OF OMISSION OR COMMISSION, COMMUNICATIVE SKILLS, AND EFFECTIVENESS OF PATIENT INTERACTION:

SUMMARY PERFORMANCE EVALUATION AND RECOMMENDATIONS

SATISFACTORY PERFORMANCE—Performed without error or prompting, or able to self-correct, no critical errors.

_____ LABORATORY EVALUATION. SKILLS MAY BE APPLIED/OBSERVED IN THE CLINICAL SETTING.

_____ CLINICAL EVALUATION. STUDENT READY FOR MINIMALLY SUPERVISED APPLICATION AND REFINEMENT.

UNSATISFACTORY PERFORMANCE—Prompting required; performed with critical errors, potentially harmful.

_____ STUDENT REQUIRES ADDITIONAL LABORATORY PRACTICE.

_____ STUDENT REQUIRES ADDITIONAL SUPERVISED CLINICAL PRACTICE.

SIGNATURES

STUDENT: _____   EVALUATOR: _____

DATE: _____   DATE: _____

Name _____ Date _____

Shunt Studies

Setting: ☐ Lab ☐ Clinical   Evaluator: ☐ Peer ☐ Instructor

Conditions (describe): _____

_____

Equipment Used

_____

_____

	SATISFACTORY	UNSATISFACTORY	NOT OBSERVED	NOT APPLICABLE
Equipment and Patient Preparation				
1. Verifies, interprets, and evaluates physician's order or protocol	☐	☐	☐	☐
2. Selects, gathers, and assembles the necessary equipment	☐	☐	☐	☐
3. Washes hands and applies standard precautions and transmission-based isolation procedures as appropriate	☐	☐	☐	☐
4. Identifies patient, introduces self and department	☐	☐	☐	☐
5. Explains purpose of the procedure and confirms patient understanding	☐	☐	☐	☐
Assessment and Implementation				
6. Assesses patient before performance of testing	☐	☐	☐	☐
7. Draws a mixed venous blood sample from the distal port of the pulmonary artery catheter	☐	☐	☐	☐
8. Draws an arterial blood gas	☐	☐	☐	☐
9. Analyzes and records results of both samples	☐	☐	☐	☐
10. Calculates	☐	☐	☐	☐
a. PAO_2	☐	☐	☐	☐
b. $PA\text{-}aDO_2$	☐	☐	☐	☐
c. a/A ratio	☐	☐	☐	☐
d. Oxygenation ratio	☐	☐	☐	☐
e. CaO_2	☐	☐	☐	☐
f. CvO_2	☐	☐	☐	☐
g. $CavO_2$	☐	☐	☐	☐
h. Percent shunt	☐	☐	☐	☐
i. MAP	☐	☐	☐	☐
j. SVR	☐	☐	☐	☐
11. Records data and interprets results	☐	☐	☐	☐
Follow-up				
12. Maintains/processes equipment	☐	☐	☐	☐
13. Disposes of infectious waste and washes hands	☐	☐	☐	☐
14. Records pertinent data in chart and departmental records	☐	☐	☐	☐
15. Notifies appropriate personnel and makes any necessary recommendations or modifications to the patient care plan	☐	☐	☐	☐

_____   _____
Signature of Evaluator   Signature of Student

PERFORMANCE RATING SCALE

5 EXCELLENT—FAR EXCEEDS EXPECTED LEVEL, FLAWLESS PERFORMANCE
4 ABOVE AVERAGE—NO PROMPTING REQUIRED, ABLE TO SELF-CORRECT
3 AVERAGE—THE MINIMUM COMPETENCY LEVEL, NO CRITICAL ERRORS
2 IMPROVEMENT NEEDED—PROBLEM AREAS EXIST; CRITICAL ERRORS, CORRECTIONS NEEDED
1 POOR AND UNACCEPTABLE PERFORMANCE—GROSS INACCURACIES, POTENTIALLY HARMFUL

PERFORMANCE CRITERIA		SCALE			
1. DISPLAYS KNOWLEDGE OF ESSENTIAL CONCEPTS	5	4	3	2	1
2. DEMONSTRATES THE RELATIONSHIP BETWEEN THEORY AND CLINICAL PRACTICE	5	4	3	2	1
3. FOLLOWS DIRECTIONS, EXHIBITS SOUND JUDGMENT, AND DEMONSTRATES ATTENTION TO SAFETY AND DETAIL	5	4	3	2	1
4. EXHIBITS THE REQUIRED MANUAL DEXTERITY	5	4	3	2	1
5. PERFORMS PROCEDURE IN A REASONABLE TIME FRAME	5	4	3	2	1
6. MAINTAINS STERILE OR ASEPTIC TECHNIQUE	5	4	3	2	1
7. INITIATES UNAMBIGUOUS GOAL-DIRECTED COMMUNICATION	5	4	3	2	1
8. PROVIDES FOR ADEQUATE CARE AND MAINTENANCE OF EQUIPMENT AND SUPPLIES	5	4	3	2	1
9. EXHIBITS COURTEOUS AND PLEASANT DEMEANOR	5	4	3	2	1
10. MAINTAINS CONCISE AND ACCURATE RECORDS	5	4	3	2	1

ADDITIONAL COMMENTS: INCLUDE ERRORS OF OMISSION OR COMMISSION, COMMUNICATIVE SKILLS, AND EFFECTIVENESS OF PATIENT INTERACTION:

SUMMARY PERFORMANCE EVALUATION AND RECOMMENDATIONS

SATISFACTORY PERFORMANCE—Performed without error or prompting, or able to self-correct, no critical errors.

_____ LABORATORY EVALUATION. SKILLS MAY BE APPLIED/OBSERVED IN THE CLINICAL SETTING.

_____ CLINICAL EVALUATION. STUDENT READY FOR MINIMALLY SUPERVISED APPLICATION AND REFINEMENT.

UNSATISFACTORY PERFORMANCE—Prompting required; performed with critical errors, potentially harmful.

_____ STUDENT REQUIRES ADDITIONAL LABORATORY PRACTICE.

_____ STUDENT REQUIRES ADDITIONAL SUPERVISED CLINICAL PRACTICE.

SIGNATURES

STUDENT: _____   EVALUATOR: _____

DATE: _____   DATE: _____

Normal and Critical Values, Formulas, and Rules of Thumb

CONTENTS

METRIC CONVERSIONS

1 L = 1000 ml
1 in = 2.54 cm
1 kg = 2.2 lb
Weight kg × 2.2 = lb
mm Hg × 1.36 = cm H_2O
cm H_2O/1.36 = mm Hg

Body Weight

Body Surface Area (BSA)

$$BSA = \frac{(4 \times weight\ kg)}{kg + 90} + 7$$

Normal adult average BSA = 2.5–4.2 m^2

Calculation of Ideal Body Weight (IBW)

Men IBW (lb) = 106 + [6 × (height in inches – 60)]

Women IBW (lb) = 105 + [5 × (height in inches – 60)]

Temperature Conversions

$$°C = \frac{(°F - 32)5}{9} \qquad °F = \left(°C\frac{9}{5}\right) + 32 \qquad °K = °C + 273$$

PATIENT ASSESSMENT

Vital Signs

Normal Respiratory Rate (f)

Adult = 12–20/min
Child = 20–40/min
Infant = 40–60/min

Normal Heart Rate

Adult = 60–100/min
<60 is bradycardia
>100 is tachycardia
Child = 100–120/min
Infant = 120–160/min

Blood Pressure (BP)

$$BP = \frac{120}{80} \qquad \frac{>140}{90} = hypertension \qquad \frac{<100}{60} = hypotension$$

Normal Temperature

98.6°F = 37°C

Lab Values

CBC

Hemoglobin (Hb) = 12–16 g/dl (15)
Hematocrit (Hct) = 35%–50%
White blood cells (WBC) = 5,000–10,000 mm^3
Red blood cells (RBC) = 5,000,000 mm^3
Platelets = 150,000–350,000 per mm^3

Electrolytes

Potassium (K^+) = 3.5–5.0 mEq/L
Sodium (Na^+) = 135–145 mEq/L
Chloride (Cl^-) = 95–105 mEq/L
Calcium (Ca^{++}) = 5–10 mEq/L
Magnesium (Mg) = 1.5–2.5 mEq/L
Phosphorus (PO_4) = 1.7–2.6 mEq/L

Chemistry

Blood urea nitrogen (BUN) = 8–25 mg/dl
Creatinine = 0.5–1.5 mg/dl
Glucose = 70–110 mg/dl
Albumin = 3.5–5.0 mg/dl
Triglycerides = 10–190 blood lipid
Cholesterol <200 g/dl
Creatine phosphokinase (CPK) 5–35 µ/ml
   >120 indicates myocardial infarction (MI)
   Myocardial bands (MB) > 5% total
   Rise within 4–6 hr of MI
   Ratio of CPK/MB > 2.2 males, 2.9 females → MI
Lactic dehydrogenase (LDH) 95–200 µ/L
Serum glutamic oxaloacetic acid (SGOT)
   Normal 5–40 µ/ml

Miscellaneous

Alcohol (ethyl)
   Normal 0%
   <0.05 no significant influence
   0.05–0.01 present
   0.10–0.15 influence reaction time
   >0.15 intoxication
   >0.25 severe
Urine output 100 ml/hr, <30 ml/hr renal failure
Theophylline: therapeutic range 10–20 µ/ml
   >20 nausea, vomiting, diarrhea, anorexia (may occur at
     lower levels also)
   >30 cardiac arrhythmias
   >40 seizures
Digitalis: therapeutic range 0.5–2.2
   >2.5 indicates dig toxicity
Chloride—sweat electrolyte
   <50 mEq/L normal
   >60 C/F: induced with pilocarpine (direct parasym-
     pathomimetic); must repeat twice for positive
     result

Pulmonary Mechanics

Compliance: $\Delta V/\Delta P$
Compliance C_L = 0.2 L/cm H_2O
Compliance C_T = 0.2 L/cm H_2O
Compliance C_{LT} = 0.1 L/cm H_2O
Resistance = 0.5–1.5 cm H_2O/L/sec

Respiration

Respiratory Quotient (RQ)

Normal = 0.8

$$\frac{VCO_2}{VO_2} = \frac{200\ ml/min}{250\ ml/min}$$

Respiratory exchange ratio or ventilation/perfusion
(V/Q) = 0.8 (0.7–1.0)

$$\frac{V_A}{Q_C} = \frac{4L}{5L}$$

Anatomic V_D = 1 ml/lb or 2 ml/kg (average adult 150 ml)
Anatomic shunt = 3%–5% of CO (from azygous, bronchial, thebesian cardiac veins)
Low V/Q < 0.7 = shunt
High V/Q > 1.0 = deadspace

Lung Volumes and Capacities

Four Volumes

Tidal volume (V_T): normal amount of air moved during inspiration or expiration, usually at rest
Inspiratory reserve volume (IRV): volume that can be inhaled after a normal inhalation
Expiratory reserve volume (ERV): volume that can be exhaled after a normal exhalation
Residual volume (RV): volume left in lungs after a maximal exhalation

Four Capacities

Inspiratory capacity (IC): maximal amount of air inhaled after a normal exhalation
Vital capacity (VC): Maximal amount of air exhaled after a maximal inhalation
Functional reserve capacity (FRC): amount of air left in lungs after a normal exhalation
Total lung capacity (TLC): amount of air in lungs after a maximal inhalation

IC = IRV + VT
TLC = IRV + VT + ERV + RV
TLC = IC + FRC
TLC = VC + RV
TLC = IC + ERV + RV
TLC = IRV + VT + FRC
VC = IRV + VT + ERV
VC = IC + ERV
VC = TLC − RV
FRC = ERV + RV
FRC = TLC − IC

"Normal" Values for Lung Volumes and Capacities

VT = 500 ml
IC = 3500 ml
IRV = 3000 ml
FRC = 2500 ml
ERV = 1000 ml
VC = 4500 ml (4.0–5.0 L)
RV = 1500 ml
TLC = 6000 ml (5–6 L)

Actual values depend on age, sex, height, and race.

Bedside Spirometry

Tidal volume (V_T) = 5–7 ml/kg (average adult = 500 ml or 400–700 ml)
Minute ventilation ($\dot{V}_E$) = 6–10 L/min; $V_T \times f$
Alveolar ventilation ($\dot{V}_A$) = 4.2 L/min; $(V_T - V_D) \times f$
Vital capacity (VC) = 50–70 ml/kg

Inspiratory:Expiratory Ratio

I:E ratio—normal 1:2 or 1:3
Inspiratory flow rate (Vi) = 20–30 lpm
$\dot{V}_E \times 3$ = estimated inspiratory flow
Peak flow = 300 – 600 lpm
Negative inspiratory force (NIF) or maximum inspiratory pressure (MIP) = −60 to −100 cm H_2O
Maximum voluntary ventilation (MVV) = 100 to 200 lpm; should approximate 35 × FEV_1

Critical Values

Minimal values needed to sustain spontaneous breathing (numbers less than these indicate impending respiratory failure):

VC = 10–15 ml/kg for adequate cough, sigh
= 2–3 × V_T

MIP (NIF) = 20 to −25 cm H_2O
Peak flow (asthmatics) < 80–100 lpm ominous sign
MVV < 2–3 × $\dot{V}_E$

MEDICAL GAS THERAPY: OTHER EQUIPMENT

Concentration of Gases in Atmosphere

Normal atmospheric barometric pressure (P_B) at sea level:

P_B = 760 mm Hg
P_B = 14.7 psi
P_B = 29.92 in Hg

Major gases:

N_2 = 78.3%
O_2 = 20.9%

Trace gas:

CO_2 = 0.04%

Partial pressure of gases in alveoli: P_B = 760 mm Hg

N_2	= 573 mm Hg
O_2	= 100 mm Hg
CO_2	= 40 mm Hg
H_2O	= 47 mm Hg
Total	= 760 mm Hg

Dalton's law: sum of partial pressure of a gas (Pp) = Total P_B
Saturated: $(P_B - P\ H_2O)F_I = Pp$
Dry: $P_B \times F_I = Pp$

Duration of Flow: Compressed Gas Cylinders

Factors: H tank = 3.14   Full tank = 2200 psi
E = 0.28

$$\frac{psi \times Factor}{Liter\ flow \times 60} = Duration\ of\ flow\ in\ hours$$

NOTE: Change *before* empty! (This may be at 500, 200, or 100 psi depending on use of cylinder and institutional policy.)

Duration of Liquid Cylinder

$$\frac{344 \times Liquid\ wt}{Flow}$$ Liquid wt = Total wt − Empty wt

Total Flow of Gas Mixtures

Oxygen	Air/O$_2$ Entrainment
24%	25:1
28%	10:1
30%	7:1
35%	5:1
40%	3:1
50%	1.7:1
60%	1:1
70%	0.6:1

Total flow = liter flow × (air + O$_2$ ratio)

$$\text{Total flow} = \frac{O_2 \times 0.79}{F_1O_2 - 0.21}$$

$$F_1O_2 = \frac{O_2\text{flow} + (0.21 \times \text{Air flow})}{\text{Total flow}}$$

Oxygen Delivery Percentages

O$_2$ Flow Rate	Oxygen
Cannula	
1 lpm	24%
2 lpm	28%
3 lpm	32%
4 lpm	36%
5 lpm	40%
6 lpm	44%

Low-flow system dependent on patient V_T
If patient hyperventilates, F_1O_2 decreases.
If patient hypoventilates, F_1O_2 increases.

Helium Mixtures: Conversion Factors

80%/20% use 1.8 × lpm
70%/30% use 1.6 × lpm

Humidity Deficits

Gas at body temperature and pressure, saturated
(BTPS) 37°C
Contains 44 mg/L H$_2$O, 47 mm Hg

$$\frac{\text{Absolute mg/L} \times 100}{\text{Capacity}} = \text{Relative humidity }\%$$

44 mg/L – mg/L inspired = Humidity deficit
Minimum 30 mg/L needed for adequate humidity with bypassed upper airway

Gas Laws

Boyle's law: $V_1 \times P_1 = V_2 \times P_2$ — Volume and pressure inversely related, temperature constant

Charles' law: $\dfrac{V_1}{T_1} = \dfrac{V_2}{T_2}$ — Volume and temperature directly related, pressure constant

Gay-Lussac's law: $\dfrac{P_1}{T_1} = \dfrac{P_2}{T_2}$ — Pressure and temperature directly related, volume constant

Combined gas law: $\dfrac{V_1P_1}{T_1} = \dfrac{V_2P_2}{T_2}$

Poiseuille's law: fluid flow through tubes

$$\dot{V} = \frac{P\Pi r^4}{8ln}$$

$\dot{V}$ = flow
P = pressure
r = radius
t = time
l = length
n = viscosity constant

Reynold's number: >2000 turbulent flow
　　　　　　　　　<2000 laminar flow
LaPlace's law: surface tension

$$P = \frac{2T}{r}$$

P = distending pressure
T = surface tension
r = radius of sphere
OHM's law
Voltage = Current × Resistance (V = IR)

AIRWAY CARE

Suctioning

ID = inner diameter
Fr = French size
(0.5 ID mm × 3) + 2 = Fr
Suction catheter size not to exceed ½ ID of tracheal tube

Suction Pressures

Adult: 100–120 (150 max) mm Hg
Child: 80–100 mm Hg
Infant: 60–80 mm Hg

Pediatric ET Tube Size

$$\frac{\text{Age} + 16}{4} = \text{mm}$$

Length of ET Tube Insertion

Oral Pediatric

$$12 + \frac{\text{Age}}{2} = \text{cm}$$

Nasal Pediatric

$$15 + \frac{\text{Age}}{3} = \text{cm}$$

Endotracheal Tube Placement

Tip of tube: adult 3–7 cm above carina, at the level of the aortic knob. Typical tube position: oral 21–23 cm mark; nasal 24–26 cm mark.

Tracheostomy decreases anatomical deadspace by up to 50%.

Endotracheal tubes decrease anatomical deadspace by up to 30%.

BLOOD GASES

Arterial	Venous
pH: 7.35–7.45	pH: 7.34–7.36
PaO_2: 80–100 mm Hg (100)	$P\bar{v}O_2$: 37–43 (40) mm Hg
$PaCO_2$: 35–45 mm Hg (40)	$P\bar{v}CO_2$: 46–48 mm Hg
HCO_3^-: 22–26 mEq/L	Same
SaO_2: 97%	$S\bar{v}O_2$: 70%–75%

Predicting PaO₂ on Room Air Based on Age (14–84)

Supine: $103.5 - (0.42 \times Age) \pm 4$
Seated: $104.2 - (0.27 \times Age) \pm 6$
PaO_2 decreases approximately 1 mm Hg/yr from 80 mm Hg for ages 60–90 yr.

Alveolar Air Equation

$$PAO_2 = [F_1O_2 (P_B - PH_2O)] - (PaCO_2 \times 1.25)$$

Alveolar-Arterial Oxygen Gradient (A-a Gradient)

$$AaDO_2 = PAO_2 - PaO_2$$

$AaDO_2$ increases 4 mm Hg for every 10 yr of age.
Normal A-a gradient: < 20 mm Hg on room air, < 50 mm Hg on 100% O_2.

Oxygen Content

Total O_2 content = Dissolved + Combined

Arterial

$$CaO_2 = [PaO_2 \times 0.003 \text{ (dissolved)}] + [Hb \times 1.39 \times SaO_2 \text{ (combined)}]$$

Venous

$$CvO_2 = [PvO_2 \times 0.003 \text{ (dissolved)}] + [Hb \times 1.39 \times SvO_2 \text{ (combined)}]$$

A-V Difference

Amount of oxygen used from each 100 ml of blood per minute:
$C(a - v)O_2 = CaO_2 - CvO_2$
Normal 4–6 vol%, < 4 vol% indicates decreased O_2 consumption (e.g., hypothermia), > 6 vol% indicates increased O_2 consumption or decreased tissue perfusion (e.g., hypotension, sepsis)

Estimation of F₁O₂ Needed for Desired PaO₂

Step 1: Calculate a/A.
$$a/A \text{ ratio} = PaO_2/PAO_2$$
Step 2: Determine desired PaO_2.

Step 3 Determine PAO_2 to achieve desired PaO_2.
$$PAO_2 \text{ needed} = \frac{PaO_2 \text{ desired}}{a/A \text{ ratio}}$$

$$F_1O_2 \text{ needed} = \frac{P_AO_2 + (PaCO_2 \times 1.25)}{P_B - 47}$$

Oxygenation Ratio (P/F)

$$\frac{PaO_2}{\%O_2}$$

$$\text{Estimated } F_1O_2 \text{ needed} = \frac{\text{Desired } PaO_2}{\text{Oxygenation ratio}}$$

Classic Shunt Formula

$$\text{Percent shunt} = \frac{C_{CO_2} - CaO_2}{C_{CO_2} - CvO_2} \times 100$$

Modified Estimated Shunt

$AaDO_2/5$ on room air
On 100% for every 50 mm Hg approximately 2% shunt
$$\frac{AaDO_2}{50} \times 2$$

Henderson-Hasselbach (H-H) Equation

$$pH = 6.1 + \log\left[\frac{\text{Base}}{\text{Acid}}\right] \qquad \text{normal ratio } 20:1$$

$$= 6.1 + \log\left[\frac{HCO_3}{PCO_2 \times 0.03}\right] \qquad \log 20 = 1.3$$

$HCO_3^- = [\text{inv log } (pH - 6.1)] \times (PCO_2 \times 0.03)$
Total $CO_2 = HCO_3^- + (PCO_2 \times 0.03)$
pH at or below 7.40: for every increase $PaCO_2$ 20 mm Hg = pH 0.1 decrease
pH at or above 7.40: for every decrease $PaCO_2$ 10 mm Hg = pH 0.1 increase

Minute Ventilation/CO₂ Disparity

For every doubling of $\dot{V}_E$, the CO_2 should decrease by 10 mm Hg. If the CO_2 has changed less than this, it most likely indicates increased deadspace.

For every decrease of $\dot{V}_E$ by ½ the CO_2 should increase by 20 mm Hg. If the CO_2 has changed more than this, it most likely indicates increased deadspace.

Base Excess (BE)

$$\text{bicarb} - 24 = BE$$

Determination of Bicarbonate Need in Patients with Metabolic Acidosis

$$HCO_3 \text{ needed} = \frac{\text{Body weight (kg)} \times BD}{4}$$

where BD = deficit in buffer (base), same number as BE
4 = factor that represents the extracellular space bicarbonate distribution

Infuse $\frac{1}{2}$ amount IV. Recheck ABGs 5 min. Repeat as necessary only if pH < 7.20, BD > −10, metabolic acidosis, with associated hyperkalemia.

HEMODYNAMICS

Cardiac output (CO) = Stroke volume × Heart rate
   Normal 4–8 lpm
Central venous pressure (CVP) 0–8 mm Hg
Ejection fraction = 65%–75%
Right ventricular pressure (RVP) = 15–25/0–8 mm Hg
Stroke volume = 40–80 ml
Pulmonary artery pressure (PAP) = 25/10 mm Hg
Mean PAP = 10–20 mm Hg
   >30/15 is pulmonary hypertension
Pulmonary capillary wedge pressure (PCWP) =
   4–12 mm Hg

Estimated Shunt Equation: $\dot{Q}_S/\dot{Q}_T$

$$\frac{(P_AO_2 - PaO_2) \times 0.003}{(CaO_2 - CvO_2) + [(P_AO_2 - PaO_2) \times 0.003]}$$

Can use 5 for $CaO_2 - CvO_2$ in normal individuals or 3.5 in critically ill

Fick Equation

$$\dot{V}O_2 \text{ ml/min} = (CO\ L \times 10)\ (C(av)O_2\ vol\%)$$

Cardiac Index (CI)

$$CI = \frac{CO}{BSA}$$

Normal = 2.5–3.5 lpm/m^2

Stroke Index (SI)

CI/HR or SV/BSA
Normal 30–65 ml/m^2

Mean Arterial Pressure (MAP)

Normal 60–100 mm Hg

$$\frac{BP\ systolic + 2\ (BP\ diastolic)}{3}$$

Mean Pulmonary Artery Pressure

$$\frac{PAP\ systolic + 2\ (PAP\ diastolic)}{3}$$

Systemic Vascular Resistance (SVR)

Right atrial pressure (RAP) = 2–6 mm Hg

$$SVR = \frac{(MAP - RAP)}{CO} \times 80$$

Normal: 900–1400 dynes × cm × sec^{-5}

Pulmonary Vascular Resistance (PVR)

$$PVR = \frac{(Mean\ PAP - PCWP)}{CO} \times 80$$

Normal: 150–250 dynes × cm × sec^{-5}

PHARMACOLOGY

0.05% = 1:2000
0.5% solution contains 5 mg/ml = 1:200 solution
1% solution contains 10 mg/ml = 1:100 solution
2% solution contains 20 mg/ml
3% solution contains 30 mg/ml
mg/ml × ml solution = mg

$$\frac{Actual\ mg}{ml} = \frac{Desired\ mg}{ml}$$

Cross multiply and solve for x.

Drug Dilution

$$Volume_1 \times Concentration_1 = Volume_2 \times Concentration_2$$
$$V_1C_1 = V_2C_2$$

Standard Adult Dosages for Aerosolized Medications

Racemic epinephrine (Vaponephrin, Micronephrin): 0.25–0.5 ml 2.25% solution
Isuprel (isoproterenol): 0.5% 1:200 solution, 0.25–0.5 ml
Bronkosol (isoetharine): 1:100 1% solution, 0.25–0.5 ml
Alupent (metaproterenol): 5% solution, 0.3 ml
Maxair (Pirbuterol) MDI, 0.2 mg/puff, 2 puffs q4–6h
Brethine (Terbutaline) MDI, PO, SC 1–2 mg of 0.1% solution
Proventil, Ventolin (albuterol): 2.5 mg (0.5 ml) of 0.5% solution
Tornalate (Bitolterol) MDI liquid 2.25%
Severent (Salmeterol xinafoate) MDI 2 puffs 42 µ OD or bid
Atropine: 1–2 mg 0.2% or 2% solution; side effects: 0.5 mg, dry mouth and skin; 2.0 mg, tachycardia, blurred vision, pupillary dilation; 5.0 mg, difficulty with speech, swallowing, urination, mental confusion
Atrovent (ipratropium bromide): 40–80 µ MDI, 500 µ of 0.02% solution 2.5 ml unit dose
Mucomyst (acetylcysteine)
   Two strengths
   20% solution 3–5 ml tid or qid
   10% solution 6–10 ml tid or qid
   Pulmozyme rhDNase or Dornase alpha
   2.5 ml of 1 mg/ml dose tid
   Has no effect on uninfected sputum
   Side effects: voice alteration, pharyngitis, laryngitis, rash, chest pain, conjunctivitis
Exosurf: 5 kg/ml via ET instillation—half dose given at a time, infant turned to side, then other half given, turned to other side; may need to be repeated once or twice in 12-hour intervals
Survanta, beractant (modified natural): 4 ml/kg comes in 8-ml vial already mixed; 25 mg/ml in 0.9% NSS; Given $\frac{1}{4}$ dose at a time, repeat at least 6 hours apart
Intal (Cromolyn Na) 20-mg dose qid 20 mg/2 ml = 1% solution

Pentam (pentamidine): DO NOT mix with bronchodilator, NSS; recommend 300 mg (1 vial)/6 ml (50 mg/ml) @ 6/pm with Respirgard nebulizer

Virazole (ribavirin): 6 g/100 ml vial + 300 ml H_2O (20 mg/ml = 2%); using SPAG 12–18 hr/day 3–7 days

Pediatric Dosages

Young's rule (age 1–12 yr.):

$$\text{Child's dose} = \frac{Age}{Age + 12} \times \text{Adult dose}$$

Clark's rule (infant or child):

$$\frac{\text{Weight in lb}}{150} \times \text{Adult dose}$$

Fried's rule (infant or child up to 2 years):

$$\frac{\text{Age in months}}{150} \times \text{Adult dose}$$

PATIENT ASSESSMENT (CRITICAL CARE)

Airway Resistance Estimated

PIP = peak inspiratory pressure

$$R_{AW} = \frac{\text{PIP-Pl}}{\text{Flow}} \text{ cm } H_2O/L/sec \qquad Pl = \text{plateau pressure}$$

Effective dynamic compliance (EDC):

$$EDC = \frac{V_T}{PIP - PEEP} \qquad L/cmH_2O$$

Static compliance (C_{ST}):

$$C_{ST} = \frac{V_T}{P1 - PEEP}$$

Time constant (represents alveolar filling time):

$$R_{AW} \times C_{ST}$$

Measured TI and TE should be at least 3 time constants for complete inspiration and expiration to occur.

Deadspace to tidal volume ratio:

$$V_D/V_T = \frac{PaCO_2\text{-}P_ECO_2}{PaCO_2}$$

Normal = 0.25 to 0.35, >0.60 ventilatory failure

Deadspace volume:

$$\frac{PaCO_2\text{-}P_ECO_2}{PaCO_2} \times V_T = V_D \text{ ml}$$

I:E ratio:
  T = Total time
  f = Frequency
  I = Inspiratory time
  E = Expiratory time

$$T = 60/f$$

If I known: $T - I = E$
If E known: $T - E = I$
If I and f known:

$$T = 60/f$$
$$T - I = E$$
$$I:E = \frac{I}{I}:\frac{E}{I}$$
$$I = \frac{T}{I + E}$$

If $\dot{V}_E$ and flow known:

$$\frac{I}{E} = \frac{\dot{V}_E}{\dot{V}_E} : \frac{\text{Flow rate} - \dot{V}_E}{\dot{V}_E}$$

Flow rate needed:

$$V_T = \frac{\dot{V}_E \times (I + E)}{\text{Flow} \times I}$$

Mean airway pressure:

$$\left[\frac{F \times I}{60} \times (\text{PIP} - \text{PEEP}) \right] + \text{PEEP}$$

$\dot{V}_E$ required for desired $PaCO_2$ (can substitute for V_T also):

$$\text{New } \dot{V}_E = \frac{\text{Current } \dot{V}_E \times PaCO_2}{\text{Desired } PaCO_2}$$

AUTO-PEEP

End-expiratory pressure with expiratory hold – baseline PEEP

ECG TRACINGS

Paper speed = 25 mm/sec
Each small box = 0.04 sec
5 small boxes = 1 large box
30 large boxes/min
1500 small boxes/min
Each 1 mm height = 1 mV
PR interval 0.12 to 0.20 sec (3 to 5 little boxes)
PR > 0.20 indicates heart block
QRS width < 0.10 sec
If lead I or II have completely negative deflections, check for limb lead placement reversal:

Lead Placement

  I = R arm neg/L arm pos/R leg ground
  II = R arm neg/L leg pos/L arm ground
  III = L arm neg/L leg pos/R arm ground
  Augmented—all three into common ground
  AVR: right arm ground
  AVL: left arm ground
  AVF: left foot ground

Standard Bipolar Hookup

RA: White
LA: Black
RL: Green
LL: Red
C: Brown

Precordial Lead Placement

V_1—4th intercostal space R sternal border
V_2—4th intercostal space L sternal border
V_3—between V_2 and V_4
V_4—midclavicular line 5th intercostal space
V_5—anterior axillary line (5th intercostal space)
V_6—midaxillary line (6th intercostal space)

Artifact (Interference with Normal Tracing)

1. Muscle tremor: multiple irregular spikes; causes: movement, tremor; most common type

2. 60-cycle interference; causes: AC electrical equipment, bad ground, broken or damaged wires, wires pulled too tight
3. Wandering baseline; causes: poor contact, poor skin prep, dried or lost gel, connections not secured, breathing
4. Isoelectric line; causes: intermittent loss of signal

Heart Rate Calculation

1. Approximation: Number of QRS/6 sec strip $\times$ 10
2. Dubin's method (approximation): Count from R wave on line to next R wave (300, 150, 100, 75, 60, 50, 43)
3. 1500 divided by number of small boxes between R-R or P-P; number of small boxes per minute (30 large boxes in 6 sec $\times$ 5 small boxes in each large box $\times$ 10 = 1500 per 1 minute)—*most accurate method*

PULMONARY FUNCTION

All volumes, flows recorded to 2 decimal places
All percentages to 1 decimal place
Labeled with appropriate units
ATPS to BTPS
For V_T, $\dot{V}_A$, SVC, FVC, FEV_1, $FEF_{25\%-75\%}$
ATPS value $\times$ Correction factor = BTPS value

$$FEV_1\% = \frac{FEV_1}{FVC} \times 100\%$$

ACCURACY OF SPIROMETERS

Calibrated at least daily
3 L $\pm$ 3% or 50 ml, whichever is greater

Validity of Spirometry

Three valid tracings, all of which are free from:
    Cough
    Glottic closure
    Baseline error
    Leaks
    Early termination
    Variable effort
    Excessive variability for FVC, FEV_1
    Early termination

Plateau is achieved when test is at least 6 sec duration with 0 volume change in last second of test.
Minimum paper speed: 20 mm/sec
Excessive variability: $\leq$5% or 200 ml, whichever is greater for FVC, FEV_1:

$$\frac{\text{Largest value} - \text{Next largest value}}{\text{Largest value}} \times 100 = \text{Percent}$$

Extrapolated volume: $\leq$5% or 150 ml, whichever is greater of FVC for that curve
Percent predicted for FVC, FEV_1, $FEF_{25\%-75\%}$:

$$\frac{\text{Actual BTPS value}}{\text{Predicted (race corrected)}} \times 100 = \text{Percent}$$

Race Correction for Nonwhites

Predicted value $\times$ 0.85 = Corrected predicted value

Changes in Surveillance Spirometry

For FVC, FEV_1, $FEF_{25\%-75\%}$:
Absolute = Largest value − Current value ml

$$\text{Percent change} = \frac{\text{Largest value} - \text{Current value}}{\text{Largest value}} \times 100$$

Expected Change Due to Aging Alone

Men

30 ml in FVC
25 ml in FEV_1

Women

25 ml in both FVC, FEV_1

Preshift to Postshift Surveillance

No greater than 200 ml change or 5% in FEV_1, FVC

Annual Surveillance

No greater than 10% change for FVC, FEV_1
No greater change than 5% at any time for $FEV_1\%$

Related Reading

Chang, DW. Respiratory Care Calculations. Delmar, Albany, 1994.

Glossary

abduction: movement away from axis of body

abruptio placentae: sudden separation of the placenta from the uterine wall

absolute refractory: period of complete resistance where there is no response to a stimulus

accuracy: the correct value; errorless

acid: substance that yields hydrogen ions or protons to another substance

acidosis: abnormal state of increased hydrogen ion in the blood

acrocyanosis: symmetric mottled cyanosis of hands and feet

actuator: device to initiate an action or process

acute: sudden onset, short course, severe

additive: two drugs in combination; effects equal the algebraic sum of each contribution

adduction: movement toward the midline of the body

adenopathy: any enlargement of a gland, especially lymphatic tissue

adhesion: molecular force exerted between two surfaces in contact

adjunctive: assisting or aiding; auxiliary

adrenergic: stimulating epinephrine receptors (sympathomimetic)

adventitious: foreign, acquired; occurring in unusual or abnormal places

adverse: unfavorable or bringing harm

aerobe: organisms requiring oxygen for metabolism

aerosol: liquid or dry particles suspended in gas

affinity: having attraction to

agonist: having affinity and efficacy; producing desired affect

alkalosis: abnormal state characterized by a decrease in blood hydrogen levels

ambient: atmospheric; surrounding

ambulatory: able to walk; not confined to bed rest

American Standard Safety System (ASSS): the connection between the outlet of a large medical gas cylinder and the pressure-reducing valve

amniotic fluid: the fluid in the sac surrounding the developing embryo

amplitude: fullness, breadth, or range or extent

anaerobe: organism that does not use oxygen for metabolism

analgesia: absence of sensibility to pain; relief of pain without loss of consciousness

anaphylaxis: severe allergic hypersensitivity; may result in shock, airway obstruction

anastomosis: intercommunication (natural or surgical) of blood vessels or other hollow organs or parts

anatomic deadspace: part of the tracheobronchial tree where there is ventilation without perfusion; the entire conducting airway

anemia: deficiency or decrease in amount of red blood cells or hemoglobin

aneroid: mechanical gauge, working without a fluid

anesthesia: loss of feeling or sensation

anhydrous: without water; dry

anion: negatively charged atom

anomaly: any deviation from what is regarded as normal

anoxia: without oxygen; antiquated term for hypoxia

antagonist: a drug having affinity but no efficacy; blocks, inhibits, or reverses effect

antecubital (fossae): triangular area in the bend of the elbow

anterior: the front of a structure

anticholinergic: synonym for parasympatholytic

anticholinesterase: blocks the action of the enzyme cholinesterase, which catalyzes breakdown of acetylcholine

anticoagulation: agent that prevents clotting

antihistamine: agent that counteracts the effect of histamine, a chemical agent believed to cause hypersensitive or allergic symptoms

antiseptic: chemical agent that interferes with infectious potential; usually applied to human body

antitussive: cough suppressant

Apgar score: evaluation of infant's physical condition; usually performed 1 min and again 5 min after birth

apical: pertaining to the pointed part of an organ (apex)

apnea: cessation of breathing

apneustic center: localized collection of neurons in the pons; moderates rhythmic breathing activity

arrhythmia: abnormal heartbeat pattern on ECG

arteriosclerosis: hardening of the arteries; loss of elasticity of artery walls

artifact: artificial or extraneous characteristic introduced by accident

asepsis: exclusion of pathogenic microorganisms

aseptic: free from infection or infectious matter

aspiration: act of sucking up or sucking in, such as inhaling a foreign body, vomitus; withdrawing fluids from a body cavity (e.g., suctioning)

asymmetrical: lack of similarity or correspondence of parts on each side of an organism

ataxia: incoordination of voluntary muscular action, particularly related to walking or reaching

atelectasis: collapse of the alveoli (air sacs in the lungs)

atherosclerosis: buildup of fatty deposits or plaque within a vessel

atmospheric temperature and pressure, saturated (ATPS): condition of exhaled air once breathed into a measuring device

atomizer: hand-bulb device to produce large particle spray

atopic: hereditary allergic state

atrium: upper chamber; connected to several other chambers or passageways

atrophy: the wasting away of an organ (e.g., muscle)

augment: to exacerbate or increase; supplement

auscultation: listening for sounds produced in the body

auxiliary: functioning as secondary, supplemental

bacteremia: presence of bacteria in the blood

bactericidal: agent that kills or destroys bacteria

bacteriostatic: agent that prevents growth and development of bacteria

baffle: surface in a nebulizer designed to impact large aerosol particles and reduce their size

barotrauma: physical injury sustained as a result of exposure to ambient pressures above normal

base: alkaline, yields hydroxyl ions; combines with acid to form salt

basilar: pertaining to the bases or widest part of pyramid-shaped organ

beta-agonist: drug that activates the beta-sympathetic receptors (lungs, cardiac)

bevel: angled tip

bifurcation: division into two branches

bilateral: on two sides

binaural: relating to both ears

Biot's respiration: an irregular, chaotic breathing pattern with periods of apnea associated with certain diseases

blanching: loss of color; becoming pale

bland: gentle, not irritating or stimulating; mild or soothing

bleb: blister; air cyst adjacent to the pleura

body surface area (BSA): mathematical calculation of the total physical volume the body takes up in space

body temperature and pressure, saturated (BTPS): condition of air in the lungs

boiling point: temperature at which a liquid turns to gaseous form

bradycardia: slow heart rate less than 60/min in an adult

breech: fetus positioned feet down

bronchoactive: any drug affecting the tracheobronchial tree

bronchoconstriction: narrowing or spasm of the smooth bronchial muscle lining the airways

bronchodilation: widening or relaxation of bronchial smooth muscle

bronchorrhea: excess mucus production from the lung

bronchospasm: same as bronchoconstriction

buffer: substance that prevents extreme swings in pH

bulla: thin-walled, air-filled area surrounded by normal tissue more than 1 cm in diameter

cachectic: characterized by severe generalized weakness, malnutrition, emaciation; wasted appearance with poor skin turgor

cachexia: condition of general ill health and malnutrition characterized by weakness and emaciation

calibration: determining the accuracy of an instrument

calorie: heat energy unit; quantity of heat required to raise one gram of water one degree Centigrade

capnography: measuring and recording a graphic display of exhaled carbon dioxide as a waveform

capnometry: numerical measurement of exhaled carbon dioxide pressure

cardiac index: standardized measure of cardiac performance; volume per minute of cardiac output per square meter of body surface area; normal resting average is 2.2 L

cardiac output: total amount of blood pumped per minute; heart rate multiplied by stroke volume

cardiomegaly: enlarged heart

cardioversion: application of (lower wattage than defibrillation) direct current to reverse abnormal rhythm (usually PAT) and resume normal sinus rhythm

caseation (caseous): collection of cheeselike material from coagulation necrosis of tissue, especially in tuberculosis

catecholamine: natural or synthetic chemicals similar in structure to epinephrine and norepinephrine

catheter: hollow tubular instrument for the passage of fluid from or into a body cavity

cation: positive ion

caudad: toward the tail

cell-mediated: physiologic mechanisms occurring by way of specific cells (as opposed to neurological or humoral)

central venous pressure: measurement of the blood pressure representing the filling pressure of the right atrium

cephalad: toward the head

cesarean: surgical procedure through an abdominal wall incision for delivery of a fetus

Cheyne-Stokes respiration: a regularly irregular increase and decrease in depth of breathing with periods of apnea

choanal atresia: abnormal closure of the normal opening of the posterior nares; failure to develop in utero

cholinergic: produces effect of acetylcholine (parasympathomimetic)

chorionic villi: numerous branching projections from the surface of the outermost layer of the fetal membranes

chronic: persisting for a long time; slow progression

chronometer: device to measure time

chronotropic: affecting time or rate

chylothorax: presence of milky lymph fluid in pleural space

clubbing: painless enlargement of the distal phalanges associated with chronic hypoxia

coagulation: blood clotting

coalescence: growing or blending together

cold stress: phenomenon of increased oxygen consumption when exposing the face of a newborn to cold air

collateral: accessory or secondary

colloid: homogeneous material of gluelike consistency; aggregate of molecules evenly dispersed in solution resisting sedimentation; cannot pass through a semipermeable membrane

colonization: organisms growing in a host where they are not normally found without invasion of tissue or toxic effects; contamination

colorimetric: relating to a procedure for quantitative chemical analysis based on a comparison of color to a standard

combustible: rapid oxidation of substance accompanied by production of heat and light; burning

commensalism: relationship in which an organism uses the host without harm or benefit; always capable of being potential pathogens

compensation: counterbalancing

compensatory: counterbalancing a lack or defect in body physiologic function

compliance: volume/unit pressure; ability to expand

compressibility factor: numeric constant for any given ventilator and circuit representing the amount of gas that will be lost in the circuit due to pressure increasing the density of the gas

compressible volume: amount of gas that will be lost in the circuit due to pressure increasing the density of the gas

condensate: changing of gas to liquid

consolidation: becoming solid; airless lung tissue

contraindication: any treatment that is inadvisable or improper; treatment that should not be done

contralateral: on the opposite side

copious: large amount

costophrenic: angle between rib cage and diaphragm

couplant: lower chamber of an ultrasonic nebulizer; upper chamber contains the medication solution separated from the couplant by a diaphram; couplant contains fluid to transmit the piezoelectric vibrations to the diaphram

crepitation: crackling noise or sensation

critical pressure: the pressure exerted by a gas in an evacuated container at its critical temperature

critical temperature: highest temperature at which a substance can exist as a liquid regardless of pressure

crystalloid: a substance that, when in solution, can pass through a semipermeable membrane

cuirass: breastplate or chestpiece of a negative pressure ventilator

cumulation: increasing amount in body when rate of removal or inactivation is slower than rate of administration

cyanosis: bluish color of the skin and mucous membranes associated with hypoxia; requires 5 grams of deoxygenated hemoglobin

deadspace: ventilation without or in excess of perfusion; high ventilation/perfusion (V/Q) relationship; rebreathed air

debilitated: weakened condition

decannulation: removal of a tracheostomy tube

decongestant: agent that reduces swelling or edema of mucous membranes

decontamination: initial cleaning of an object or person to make it safe to handle by unprotected personnel

decubitus (position): horizontal posture; ulcer caused by prolonged unrelieved pressure on bony prominence

defibrillation: electric shock applied to heart to reverse fibrillation and resume normal rhythm

dehydration: removal or deprivation of water

demographics: statistical study of groups of people

density: number per unit volume; closeness or compactness

denudation: the act of stripping or laying bare; remove covering

depolarization: the reduction of ion distribution differentials across a polarized semipermeable membrane usually resulting in nerve conduction or muscle contraction

deposition: collection of matter in any part

desiccation: depriving substance of moisture; to dry out

diagnosis: art of determining the nature of patient's disease; a conclusion reached

Diameter Index Safety System (DISS): safety system connection between a small high-pressure cylinder and the reducing valve

diapedesis: the passage of blood cells through unruptured wall of blood vessels into the tissue

diaphoresis: profuse sweating; cold and clammy

diaphragmatic hernia: protrusion of the intestines through the diaphragm and into the lung space

diastole: relation of the heart between contractions when filling occurs

diastolic pressure: pressure in the heart and blood vessels during relaxation of the heart

diffusion: movement of molecules from an area of higher concentration or pressure to an area of lower concentration or pressure

diluent: making more watery; substance used to dilute

discrimination: to distinguish; responding differently

disinfectant: chemical that kills vegetative cells; usually applied to equipment

disinfection: act of destroying pathogenic microorganisms (but does not sterilize), usually by chemical means

displacement: removal from the normal position or location

dissociation: act of separating

dissolved: a substance passed into solution

distal: farthest point away from point of origin

diuretic: drug or chemical that increases formation and release of urine

drugs: chemical substances that when taken into a living organism alters its function or processes

ductus arteriosus: fetal vessel connecting the left pulmonary artery to the descending aorta, creating a shunt

ductus venosus: fetal connection of the left umbilical vein through the liver to the vena cava

dynamic: characterized by energy or force, moving and changing

dyskinesia: abnormal or difficult movement

dysphagia: difficulty swallowing

dysphasia: difficulty in speaking or in understanding language

dysphonia: impairment of the voice

dyspnea: subjective feeling of shortness of breath; difficulty breathing

dysrhythmia: abnormal heart rhythm; arrhythmia

dystocia: difficult childbirth

ecchymosis: "black and blue," bruising or purplish patch caused by extravasation of blood into the subcutaneous tissues

eclampsia: sudden development of convulsions associated with late-stage pregnancy associated with hypertension, proteinuria, and edema

edema: abnormal increase of fluid in the intercellular spaces of the body; swelling

efficacy: usefulness, having the desired effect

egophony: modification of the transmission of the voice heard through the stethoscope over areas of lung consolidation; a bleating quality

elastance: tendency to recoil or collapse after stretching; opposite of compliance

electrolyte: substance that in solution can conduct electrical charge

embolism: obstruction of blood vessel by foreign matter (blood clot, fat, air) that travels from another area

emesis: the act of vomiting

empyema: accumulation of pus or infected fluid in the pleural space

endemic: present among particular people in specific locality

endocytosis: process by which a cell takes in material from its environment; bulk transport by enclosing in a membrane

endotoxin: substance found in bacterial cell walls, especially gram-negative bacteria associated with various physiologic effects, including fever and shock

enteric: pertaining to the gastrointestinal tract

entrainment: to carry along, as when air is pulled into the flow of a gas due to shearing forces

enzyme: complex proteins that act as catalysts in chemical reactions

epidemic: extensive outbreak or unusually high incidence at certain times or places

epidemiology: the study of the distribution and spread of disease

epistaxis: nosebleed

epithelium: covering of internal or external organs or vessels

equilibrium: state of balance

erosion: wearing away of a surface

erythema: redness of the skin, from blushing or inflammation

etiology: the study of the causes and sources of disease

eukaryotic: pertaining to cells with true nucleus, nuclear membrane, and capable of mitosis

eupnea: normal breathing

evaporation: change from liquid to gaseous form occurring below its boiling point

excretion: process of elimination as in waste matter or normal discharge

exocrine: secreting externally; glandular secretion to a duct or surface

exotoxin: excreted into environment by living organisms

expectoration: coughing up and spitting out of sputum

exsanguination: extensive loss of blood due to hemorrhage

extrapolation: to infer unknown data from known data

extrathoracic: outside of the chest cavity

extubation: removal of a tube

exudate: fluid with high protein content, resulting from abnormal capillary leakage or inflammation

facilitate: enhance or make easy

facultative: not obligatory; having the ability to adapt to changing conditions

fasciculation: small localized muscle tremors visible under the skin

fastidious: having very specific requirements; "picky"

febrile: body temperature greater than 100.4°F

fenestrated: having an opening, similar to a window

fetal asphyxia: suffocation of the fetus in the uterus caused by interruption of its blood supply

fetid: foul smelling; putrid

fibrillation: noncoordinated muscular twitching; abnormal, chaotic, irregular impulses from multiple foci

fissure: deep furrow or slit

fistula: any tubelike passage between two organs

flaccid: weak or soft muscles, limp

flammable: tending to ignite or burn easily

flange: projecting edge or rim

flaring: to open or spread outward

flip-flop phenomenon: paradoxical decrease in blood oxygen level when returning to a higher F_IO_2 after an initial decrease in F_IO_2

flow rate: volume per unit time; the speed of movement of a fluid through a tube

flush: to wash out

fomite: nonliving materials that may transmit infectious agents (e.g., bed linens, equipment)

foramen ovale: perforation or opening through the septum between the right and left atria as part of fetal circulation

fowler's position: sitting upright, head elevated

fractional distillation: process of successively separating the components of air to manufacture oxygen

frangible: breakable or fragile

fremitus: palpable vibrations

fusible: capable of being melted

gain: a control to increase a value of an electronic device

galvanic: creating steady direct current

gestation: duration of pregnancy

goal: measurable desired outcome

granuloma: tumorlike pathological structure composed of macrophage, lymphocytes resulting from inflammation; disordered repair

gravida: a pregnant woman

hematocrit: percentage of blood that is cells compared with liquid plasma

hematoma: localized collection of extravascular blood

hemoglobin: protein in red blood cells that transports oxygen

hemolysis: rupture of red blood cells

hemolytic: capable of rupturing red blood cells

hemoptysis: coughing up blood

hemorrhage: excessive bleeding

hemothorax: collection of blood in the pleural cavity

homeostasis: to remain relatively constant even when the environment is changing

homogeneous: uniform character and consistency

hormone: substance originating in an organ or gland and transported by bloodsteam to other areas where it has a regulatory effect

humoral: pertaining to physiologic mechanisms in body fluids by way of chemical or biological mediators (as opposed to neurological or cell-mediated)

hydration: absorption of water

hydrolysis: cleavage of a compound by addition of water

hygrometer: instrument for measuring atmospheric moisture

hygroscopic: absorbing moisture

hyperbilirubinemia: excess of bilirubin in the blood as a result of liver dysfunction or destruction of red blood cells

hypercapnia: excess carbon dioxide in the blood greater than 45 mm Hg

hypercarbia: excess carbon dioxide in the blood greater than 45 mm Hg

hyperextension: movement of stretching or straightening of limb or part beyond the normal limit

hyperinflation: overdistention with air

hyperlucent: excess radiolucency; dark or black on x-ray

hyperoxia: excess oxygen supply

hyperpnea: increase in depth of breathing

hyperresonant: increase in vibration sound created by percussion on a body cavity or part, usually indicating a more air-filled condition

hypersensitivity: increased threshold of response to irritating stimuli

hypertension: high blood pressure, greater than 150/90 in an adult

hyperthermia: elevated body temperature

hypertonic: having a greater osmotic pressure; concentration of solute is higher causing water to move across a semipermeable membrane toward the hypertonic solution in an attempt to dilute the solution

hypertrophy: enlargement of tissue or organ (e.g., muscle)

hyperventilation: alveolar air exchange in excess of that needed for metabolic needs; signified by a PCO_2 < 35 mm Hg in arterial blood

hypervolemia: increase in blood volume

hypocapnia: decreased carbon dioxide in the blood

hypoglycemia: low blood sugar

hypopnea: decreased depth of breathing

hypostasis: stagnant blood flow in a dependent part of the body

hypotension: low blood pressure; less than 100/60 in an adult

hypothermia: low body temperature

hypotonic: decreased concentration of solute with lower osmotic pressure than the solution with which it is compared

hypoventilation: alveolar air exchange less than required to meet metabolic needs, as signified by an arterial $PaCO_2$ greater than 45 mm Hg

hypovolemia: reduced blood volume

hypoxemia: insufficient oxygen in the blood; PO_2 less than 80 mm Hg

hypoxia: insufficient oxygenation to the tissues

hysteresis: phenomenon in which two related phenomena fail to keep pace with each other (e.g., compliance of the lung during inspiration and expiration)

iatrogenic: physician-induced; usually adverse effect

idiopathic: unknown cause or origin

immunology: study of the defense mechanisms by which the body wards off diseases (the immune system)

immunosuppressed: reducing the host's ability to defend against infection, such as from disease or medications

immunosuppression: reduced ability of the immune system to respond; may be purposefully induced by medication

impaction: condition of being tightly wedged or retained in a part; stuck

indication: a sign or circumstance that points to a particular diagnosis or treatment

induction: causing something to occur

infarction: formation of area of necrosis as a result of loss of blood supply

infection: introduction of pathogenic organisms into a host, where they may thrive to a point of disruption of homeostasis

inferior: below; bottom portion

infiltrate: to penetrate the interstices of a tissue

infiltration (infiltrates): radiodense accumulation in a tissue

infrared absorption: amount of electromagnetic radiation of a wavelength greater than that of the red end of the spectrum penetrating a substance; can be used to measure the amount of the substance present

inhibition: checking or restraining the action of organ, cell, or chemical

inotropic: affecting the force of muscle contraction

insidious: coming on gradually or almost imperceptibly

inspissated: thickened or dried by fluid evaporation as in secretions

instillation: direct administration of a liquid by drops

insufflation: blowing a gas into a body cavity

interaction: process of acting on each other

intersection: site at which one structure crosses another

interstitium: situated between parts of a tissue; extracellular space

intracranial pressure: pressure of the subarachnoid fluid in the sac between the skull and the brain

intradermal: injection into the skin

intraflow: device in the path of flow of a fluid system to control the flow

inverse: inside out or opposite

iodophor: iodine-based disinfectant

ionization: dissociation of a substance in solution into ions

irrigation: washing out of a wound or body cavity with fluid

ischemia: localized reduction of perfusion to part or organ

isoelectric: the baseline on an ECG rhythm strip

isotonic: containing equal concentration of solute to body fluids, 0.9%

jaundice: yellow coloration of tissues

jet: a narrowing in a tube creating a rapid stream of fluid

Kussmaul's respiration: extreme hyperventilation associated with diabetic acidosis

kymograph: rotating drum for recording variations or undulations

kyphosis: abnormal increase in curvature of spine with backward convexity

laceration: a tearing wound

laminar: consisting of layers

lancet: small, pointed, two-edged surgical puncturing device

lanugo: soft fluffy hair on a fetus

laryngospasm: constriction of the laryngeal muscles

latent: not manifest; dormant, potential

lateral: pertaining to the side or away from the midline

latex: sap produced in certain plants used to make rubber

lavage: washing out of an organ or cavity as in the lungs, stomach, intestines

lecithin/sphingomyelin (L/S) ratio: test compares the measurement of the two substances to determine fetal lung maturity

lesion: broad term indicating any injury or loss of function to body tissue

lethargic: sleepy

leukotriene: chemical mediator of immediate inflammation

lobe: distinct division or portion of an organ

lobule: smaller division of an organ or subdivision of a lobe

logarithm: the exponent value indicating the power to which a fixed number must be raised

lordosis: forward curvature of the spine

lordotic: positioned with the spine curved forward

Luer-Lok: locking mechanism to secure a syringe in place, usually by twisting

lumen: the channel within a tube

lymphadenopathy: disease and enlargement of lymph nodes

malacia: abnormal softening

malaise: generalized feeling of illness or discomfort

mandatory: required

mass: physical property of weight

meatus: opening or tunnel through a body part

mechanical deadspace: artificial adjunct or extension to the conducting airway where ventilation exists without perfusion and gas exchange

meconium: first fetal fecal matter

medial: pertaining to the midline

melting point: temperature at which a substance changes from a solid to a liquid

metabolism: sum of all physical and chemical changes that take place within an organism

metabolite: any product of metabolism

metastasis: process of tumor cells spreading to distant parts of the body

miliary: lesions resembling millet seeds as in tuberculosis

monitoring: continuous observation or collection of data

morbidity: state of being ill

moro reflex: normal reflex in an infant elicited by a sudden loud noise

morphology: study of the shape and structure of organisms

mortality: number of deaths per unit population in specific group

mucoid: resembling mucus; clear white secretions

mucokinetic: movement of mucus

mucolytic: breaking down of mucus

mucopurulent: containing mucus and pus

multifocal: originating from multiple points

muscarinic: stimulation of parasympathetic neuroeffector sites; includes increased mucous and salivary gland discharge, decreased heart rate, vasodilation, hypotension

mutualism: mutually beneficial relationship

mycology: study of fungi

myelitis: inflammation of the spinal cord with associated motor or sensory dysfunction

myocardial infarction: blockage of a coronary blood vessel leading to death of heart muscle; heart attack

myopathy: disease of muscle

nebulizer: device that produces aerosol (fine spray or mist) powered by external gas source (air or oxygen)

necrosis: death of cell or tissue

neonate: newborn infant

neoplasm: new growth of abnormal tissue

neutral thermal environment: environment created to maintain the normal body temperature of an infant to minimize oxygen consumption and caloric expenditure

nicotinic: stimulation of acetylcholine ganglionic (sympathetic and parasympathetic) sites and skeletal muscle receptors; increased blood pressure, vasoconstriction, heart rate

nodule: small round lesion

nomogram: graphic representation of normal values

nosocomial: hospital-acquired; an infection that develops in the hospital

obligate: able to live only in the way specified

obtunded: insensitive to pain or other stimuli due to decreased level of consciousness

obturator: removable device used to plug a tube during insertion

opacification: less able to transmit light; increased density on x-ray

opportunistic: commensal organisms that become pathogens when proper route of entry available

opsonin: antibody or complement product that enhances phagocytosis

optimum: most favorable; ideal or best

orthopnea: ability to breath easily only in the upright position

orthostatic: related to or caused by body position

osmosis: movement of fluid across a semipermeable membrane to a greater solute concentration

osteoporosis: decrease in mass-to-volume ratio of mineralized bone

oxidation: chemical reaction in which electrons are removed

palliative: relieves or soothes symptoms without a cure

pallor: paleness of the skin

palpation: examination by means of the hands

para: a woman who has given birth to infant; denoted by numerical prefix for each occurrence

paradoxical respiration: type of breathing in which part of lung deflates during inspiration and expands during expiration; opposite from expected

paralysis: loss of power of voluntary movement through injury or disease

paramagnetic: a substance that is in the same direction in an induced magnetic field as the magnetizing field

parasitism: organisms having harmful relationship to host

parasympatholytic: antagonist to parasympathetic system (anticholinergic)

parasympathomimetic: mimics effects of parasympathetic system

parenchyma: functional tissue of an organ (as opposed to supporting structures)

parenteral: denoting any route other than the gastrointestinal tract

paresis: partial or incomplete paralysis; muscle weakness

paresthesia: tingling sensation in extremities; "pins and needles"

parietal: pertaining to the walls of an organ or cavity

paroxysmal (cough): sudden attack, violent

particulate: in the form of fine particles, very small piece or portion of solid or liquid

patency: condition of being wide open and unblocked

pathogen: disease-producing organism

pathology: study of abnormal structure

pathophysiology: study of mechanisms of disordered function

pectoriloquy: increased transmission of vocal sound through consolidated lung tissue

pectus carinatum: condition of an abnormally protruding sternum; pigeon breast

pectus excavatum: condition of an abnormally concave sternum; funnel chest

penetration: process or capacity of entering within a part

percussion: diagnostic technique of manually striking on a body part, using short, sharp blows, to produce a sound in order to determine the size, position, or density of the underlying structures

perforation: to pierce through and make a hole

perfusion: passage of a fluid through the body (usually blood)

periodic breathing: irregular breathing pattern with recurring intervals of apnea common in premature infants

permeability: state of permitting passage of a substance

phagocytosis: process by which cell "eats" by engulfing particles; type of endocytosis

phalanges: (plural of phalanx) digits; any bone of the fingers or toes

pharmaceutical: study or phase of drugs including dosage, preparation, dispensation, and routes of administration

pharmacodynamics: study of drug mechanisms, actions, effects, and side effects

pharmacognosy: branch of pharmacology studying natural drugs and their constituents, sources

pharmacokinetics: study of absorption, distribution, metabolism, and elimination of drugs

pharmacology: study of drugs, their processes, origin, nature, properties, uses, and effects

phlebostatic axis: location of the right atrium, found by drawing an imaginary line from the fourth intercostal space at the right side of the sternum to an intersection with the midaxillary line

phlebotomy: opening of a vein to draw blood

phonation: utterance of vocal sounds; speech

phycology: study of algae

piezoelectric: the generation of a voltage in a solid when a mechanical stress is applied; conversion of one form of energy to another, such as electrical into mechanical

Pin Index Safety System (PISS): used to connect regulators to small, high-pressure cylinders

pinna: auricle or external ear

placenta: highly vascular organ to supply oxygen and nutrients to a developing fetus

placenta previa: malposition of the placenta in which it is blocking the opening to the cervix

plateau: a level or stable event or place

pleural effusion: abnormal accumulation of fluid in the pleural space

pleural friction rub: grating noise heard on auscultation associated with inflammation of the pleural linings

pleural space: potential space between visceral and parietal layers of the lining of the lungs

pleuritic (pain): pertaining to the pleura, a sharp stabbing localized pain

pneumatic: pertaining to gas or air

pneumatocele: large, thin-walled, air-filled cyst

pneumoconiosis: lung disease associated with the inhalation of dust, often occupation related

pneumotachometer: a device that measures the flow of respiratory gases

pneumotaxic center: specialized cells in the respiratory centers located in the pons, which controls the rhythmic output of breathing

pneumothorax: accumulation of air in the pleural space

polarograph: device that works by estimating the concentration of elements in an electrochemical cell that can be reduced or produce electrons during an oxidation-reduction reaction

polycythemia: increase in amount of red blood cells or hemoglobin

polyps: a growth or mass protruding from a mucous membrane

poncho: a blanketlike cloak with a hole for the head

positive pressure: force exerted greater than atmospheric pressure

posterior: toward the back

postterm: postmature; being born after a prolonged gestational period

potency: power or strength of a medicinal agent to produce desired effect

potentiation: enhancement of one agent by another to increase effect (e.g., 1 + 1 = 3)

pounds per square inch (psi): a unit of measure for pressure

pounds per square inch above gauge (psig): a unit of measure for pressure in which atmospheric pressure is the baseline and only the pressure above atmospheric is measured

preanalytical: occurring before analysis or laboratory examination of a specimen

precision: repeatability; statistical quality control of a measurement

preeclampsia: condition during late pregnancy characterized by edema, proteinuria, and hypertension; can lead to eclampsia or seizures if not treated

preterm: being born before completion of the normal gestational period; premature

proficiency: competency; performance with correctness and facility

prokaryotic: a cell without a true nucleus

proliferation: rapid growth and multiplication

prone: lying face down

prophylactic: preventive agent

prophylaxis: prevention of development or spread of disease

protein binding: bonding of drug with plasma albumen, decreasing biological availability

proximal: nearest point of reference

pulmonary capillary wedge pressure: intravascular pressure measured by the distal tip of a flow-directed pulmonary artery catheter (Swan Ganz) when the balloon is inflated; this lodges the catheter tip into the vessel and occludes all blood flow past that point, giving a pressure measurement equivalent to the left ventricular preload

pulmonary vascular resistance: force opposing flow through the pulmonary capillary bed, related to density, velocity, length, and radius of the vessels

purulent: consisting of pus

pus: collection of dead cells and debris associated with infection; product of liquefaction necrosis

quadriplegia: paralyzed in all four extremities, usually from the neck down

racemic: containing equal parts of both l and d stereoisomers

radiodense: resistant to penetration of x-rays; radiopaque or "white"

radiolucent: able to be penetrated by x-rays; "black"

rales: crackles heard on auscultation created by fluid-filled alveoli, or small airways, or atelectasis

reagent: substance used in a chemical reaction to detect, measure, or produce other substances

receptor: specialized area in a cell that recognizes and bonds with specific substances producing some effect on the cell

recoil: to return to original shape

reducing valve: a device used to decrease the high pressure in a gas cylinder to a lower working pressure

redundancy: duplication or repetition; excess above what is required

refractory: resisting stimulation or treatment

regression equation: formula for calculation of a variable approaching the mean value in a statistically significant relationship among several variables

regulator: a combination reducing valve and flowmeter; used to decrease the pressure of a gas cylinder and control the output flow

relative humidity: percent of the actual atmospheric moisture to the maximum capacity that could be present at a specific temperature

relative refractory period: period during which there is resistance to change, but a strong enough stimulus could initiate a response

reliability: the extent of reproducibility of a test or device with different investigators, or administration of a test over time

repolarization: return of ionic distribution to resting state

reproducibility: repeatability; duplication of a similar structure, situation, or phenomenon

reservoir: storage chamber or receptacle for fluids

resistance: opposition to force or flow

resolution: imaging process to distinguish adjacent structures; state of having made a firm decision

resonance: an echo or sound produced by percussion of an organ or cavity; related to the frequency of vibration

respiration: exchange of gases across a semipermeable membrane

resuscitation: process of sustaining the vital functions of a person in respiratory or cardiac failure while reviving him or her

retractions: drawing back of soft tissue between the ribs during labored breathing

rhonchi: rumbling sounds on auscultation from fluid in the larger airways; usually more pronounced on expiration and clearing with a cough

scoliosis: lateral curvature of the spine

sedation: administration of a drug to allay irritability or excitement; calming effect

segment: smaller distal portion of an organ or structure

sensitivity: capacity to feel, transmit, or react to a stimulus

sensor: device designed to respond to a physical stimulus and transmit the resulting impulses

sensorium: psychiatric consciousness; intelligent functional ability

sepsis: presence of disease-producing organisms in the blood causing a systemic infection, shock

septicemia: presence of bacteria in the blood to a point of disruption of homeostasis

serous: resembling serum; thin, watery, delicate

shunt: perfusion without ventilation (true shunt) or in excess of ventilation (shunt effect); low ventilation/perfusion ratio (V/Q)

slope: angle of incline upward or downward

solubility: ability to be dissolved

soluble: able to dissolve

solute: substance that dissolves in another substance

solution: a homogeneous mixture of two or more substances

solvent: the liquid portion of a solution capable of dissolving another substance

somnolent: sleepy, drowsy

spacer: auxiliary device used on a metered dose inhaler (MDI) to reduce the impaction of aerosol particles on the pharynx

specific gravity: weight of a substance compared with the weight of an equal amount of some other substance (usually water for liquids) taken as a standard

specificity: quality of reacting with only certain substances or having only certain actions or effects

spectrophotometry: technique of measurement using the absorption of visible light by a substance

sphygmomanometer: instrument for measuring arterial blood pressure

spirometer: instrument for measuring inhaled or exhaled lung volumes

splint: support; device to fix movable parts in order to lessen pain or promote healing

standard deviation (SD): statistical term measuring the dispersion of a random variable; the square root of the average squared deviation from the mean; for data with a normal distribution, 68% of data points will fall within 1 SD, and 95% will fall within 2 SD

static: at a constant level; stoppage of flow

stenosis: abnormal constriction or narrowing

sterilization: removal or destruction of *all* living organisms, including spores

stoma: hole or opening; similar to a mouth

stridor: high-pitched crowing sound on inspiration usually due to an upper airway obstruction

subcutaneous: beneath the layers of skin

subcutaneous emphysema: air in the tissue under the skin; creates crepitus

subglottic: below the glottis; cricoid area

sublimation: process of vaporizing a solid to a gas without passing through the liquid phase

superimposed: on top of; occurring at the same time

superior: above or top portion

supine: lying face upward on back

supraglottic: above the glottis or opening to the larynx

surfactant: surface-active, or detergent-like, agent; phospholipid substance secreted by type II alveolar cells to reduce surface tension

surrogate: substitute

symbiosis: mutualism; mutually beneficial relationship

symmetrical: correspondence in size, form, and arrangement of parts on opposite sides

sympatholytic: antagonist to sympathetic system (antiadrenergic)

sympathomimetic: mimics the sympathetic system

synchrony: occurs at the same time

syncope: fainting

synergism: joint action of agents or organisms; combined effect is greater than the sum of individual actions; enhances action (1 + 1 = 3)

systemic: pertaining to or affecting the body as a whole

systemic vascular resistance: forces opposing blood flow in the main circulation

systole: period of contraction of the heart

systolic pressure: peak force executed during contractor phase of heart

tachycardia: abnormally rapid heart rate, greater than 100/min in an adult

tachyphylaxis: sudden marked decrease in effect from repeated administration; rapid tolerance

tachypnea: rapid rate of breathing

tandem: an arrangement of two or more objects

tenacious: adhesive, thick

tetany: sustained muscle contraction or spasm, without twitching

thermophilic: heat loving

thoracic pump: phenomenon in which the subatmospheric pressure in the chest cavity aids in venous return

thrombus: blood clot, often obstructing a vessel

titrate: to analyze by incrementally adding a fluid of a known strength until a given endpoint is reached

tolerance: decreased response or sensitivity to subsequent repeated doses of same substance or need for increasing doses to maintain constant response

tomography: image technique producing single-image planes or slices

tonicity: the effective osmotic pressure

topical: applied to certain area, such as skin or mucous membrane, for localized effect

torr: a unit of pressure = 1 mm Hg

tourniquet: device for compression of a blood vessel

toxicology: study of harmful effects of drugs in an organism

tracheostomy: tube inserted into an opening in the windpipe to provide an airway, or the opening itself

tracheotomy: surgical procedure to create a tracheostomy

tragus: cartilaginous projection anterior to the meatus of the ear

transcutaneous: through the skin

transducer: device that converts one physical quantity to another (e.g., pressure to electrical)

transillumination: passage of strong light through a body structure to permit inspection of an observer on the opposite side

transpulmonary pressure: difference in pressure between the alveoli and pleural space

transudate: fluid low in protein; passed through membrane by altered hydrostatic or osmotic pressure

transverse: extending from side to side

Trendelenburg position: patient lying inclined with head lower than the feet

turbulent: flow with chaotic, irregular eddies

turgor: condition of fullness; extent of swelling or congestion

tympanitic: drumlike

umbilical artery: vessel in the cord that connects the fetus to the placenta; returns blood from the fetal heart to the placenta

umbilical vein: vessel in the cord that connects the fetus to the placenta; returns blood from the placenta to the fetus

unifocal: originating from one point

unilateral: affecting one side only

uvula: a pendentlike, fleshy mass; structure in back of the throat

vacuum: absence or decrease pressure, creating suction

validity: extent to which a measuring device measures what it intends or purports to measure; must be precise, accurate, reliable, and reproducible

vallecula: depression or furrow; groove behind the epiglottis

valve stem: projection used to turn a control device or stopcock

vane: a thin, flat or curved object that is rotated about an axis by a flow of fluid

variability: differences among items; quality of being changeable

vascular: pertaining to blood vessels

vasoconstriction: decrease in diameter of blood vessels

vasodilation: relaxation or widening of blood vessels

vector: agent such as insect that transmits disease from sick human to another person; directional force

ventilation: bulk movement of gases in and out of the lungs

ventricle: a cavity or chamber of a body part or organ; the lower heart chambers

venturi: a tube designed with a constricted point to increase the velocity of flow in order to entrain air or fluid into the main flow of gas

vernix: a cheesy coating on the skin of the fetus

virology: study of viruses

virulence: degree of pathogenicity; ability to invade, proliferate, and cause disease

virulent: agent that has an increase in the degree of pathogenicity

viscosity: resistance to flow; physical property dependent on friction; thickness

volatile: evaporating rapidly

volutrauma: physical injury to lung tissue caused by excessive volumes

vortex: a whorl or spiral pattern; a structure having the appearance of rotating around an axis

weaning: process of gradually withdrawing from life support

wheal: a raised, round, red lesion of the skin, usually edematous and itchy; welt

wheezing: making a polyphonic high-pitched noise, a whistling sound, usually due to narrowing of the airways

wye: a branching or bifurcated connection shaped like the letter "Y" (e.g., from a ventilator circuit to an artificial airway)

Index

"f" following a page number indicates a figure; "t" following a page number indicates a table.

PT 4-12
PTT = 24-32 sec.

1. Jet Nebulizer
2. Sterile H₂O
3. 1 sterile entrainment Neubizer
4. Corrugated tubing
5. T-tube
6. scissor
7. Measure
8. Calibrated tube

61

At last—a workbook that leads you step-by-step to **competent respiratory care!**

This comprehensive laboratory manual with a multitude of laboratory activities and 47 Procedural Competency Evaluations is designed to provide the hands-on technical and communication skills necessary to integrate theory and clinical practice. It can be used in both respiratory therapy and respiratory therapy technician programs and in conjunction with any textbook.

This workbook is up to date and, unlike other respiratory care laboratory manuals, maintains a clinical/laboratory orientation. It is structured to provide for hands-on investigation and practice with procedures and equipment, yet provides sufficient general instructions that can be modified to meet specific needs.
—Lawrence A. Dahl, EdD, RRT
Hawkeye Community College, Waterloo, Iowa

Key Features:
- Addresses equipment maintenance and trouble-shooting
- Exercises, many including case studies, are designed to promote your critical thinking
- Equipment discussed is generic, not brand specific
- Emphasizes documentation and communication skills
- Addresses home/alternative site care
- Covers newborn, infant, and pediatric patients
- Over 400 figures clearly illustrate step-by-step instructions
- Perforated and 3-hole-punched for easy removal/storage of laboratory reports and Procedural Competency Evaluation forms
- Each chapter includes:
  - ➤ Learning objectives
  - ➤ Key terms
  - ➤ Equipment required
  - ➤ Step-by-step instructions to perform the laboratory and trouble-shooting exercises
  - ➤ Related readings
  - ➤ A removable laboratory report with critical thinking questions
  - ➤ Procedural Competency Evaluation forms for preclinical and clinical application

Available at your local health science bookstore
or from F. A. Davis Company.
Call (800) 323-3555.
In Canada, call (800) 665-1148.
Visit us at www.fadavis.com

ISBN 0-8036-0248-0

90
9 780803 602489
EAN